T. C. WESTFALL

Cutting's Handbook of Pharmacology

Cutting's Handbook of Pharmacology

THE ACTIONS AND USES OF DRUGS

Sixth Edition

T. Z. Csáky, M.D.
Professor of Pharmacology
and Toxicology
University of Kentucky
College of Medicine
Lexington, Kentucky

Adjunct Professor of Pharmacology
and Toxicology
University of Louisville
School of Medicine
Louisville, Kentucky

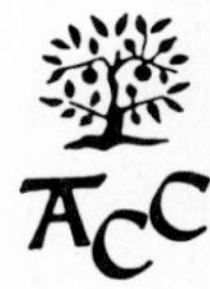

APPLETON-CENTURY-CROFTS/New York

79 80 81 82 83 / 10 9 8 7 6 5 4 3 2 1

Prentice-Hall International, Inc., London
Prentice-Hall of Australia, Pty. Ltd., Sydney
Prentice-Hall of India Private Limited, New Delhi
Prentice-Hall of Japan, Inc., Tokyo
Prentice-Hall of Southeast Asia (Pte.) Ltd., Singapore
Whitehall Books Ltd., Wellington, New Zealand

Library of Congress Cataloging in Publication Data
Csáky, T Z
Cutting's Handbook of pharmacology.

Prior editions by W. C. Cutting published under title: Handbook of pharmacology
Includes index.
1. Pharmacology. I. Cutting, Windsor Cooper, 1907– Handbook of pharmacology. II. Title.
RM300.C83 1978 615′.7 78-10784
ISBN 0-8385-1417-0

Cover design: **Susan F. Rich**

PRINTED IN THE UNITED STATES OF AMERICA

To Cathy and Karl and their Mother

and to the memory of the late Windsor Cutting,
an enthusiastic pharmacologist.

Contents

GANGLIONIC AND MYONEURAL AGENTS

ANESTHETICS

ANALGESICS

SEDATIVES AND RELATED AGENTS

STIMULANTS AND ADDICTING AGENTS

Preface

The unique feature of Cutting's Handbook is the presentation, in concise form, of the relationship between the chemical structure and the pharmacologic action of a large number of drugs. The wide acceptance of the previous editions by professionals and students fully justifies the need for such an approach.

In this new edition the basic structure of the book has remained unchanged. In the description of the drug-classes, those changes that were necessary because of alterations in basic concepts were made. An attempt was made to continue the custom of including new compounds even if these are still only experimental.

Thanks are due to several readers of the previous edition, especially Dr. Joseph Jerome, who, besides helping to update the previous edition was instrumental in securing the continuing cooperation of the U. S. Adopted Names Council. My wife rendered substantial assistance. The skillful technical contribution of Mrs. Virginia Crutcher is acknowledged.

Cutting's Handbook of Pharmacology

1. The Sulfonamides

Paul Ehrlich in 1906 crystallized the hope of every chemotherapist since that time in the words "therapia sterilisans magna," by which he meant complete eradification of an infecting organism by a drug. Ehrlich before this had been working in immunotherapy, but now he created the concept of chemotherapy, meaning the treatment of infections by small, often synthetic, molecules, instead of larger protein antibodies.

Before Ehrlich only a handful of specific chemotherapeutic agents were known: aspidium, mercury, ipecac, quinine. At present, with the partial exception of viral infections, all the groups of infectious agents are at least accessible to chemotherapy.

The Ehrlich influence lasted until the 1920's and added atoxyl, arsphenamine, suramin, and bismuth to the therapeutic list. With these agents most protozoal infections became reasonably susceptible to treatment. Most importantly, it had been demonstrated that man might make drugs without precedent in nature.

Until the early 1930's it seemed that chemotherapy against bacteria was impossible, or at least too toxic for clinical use. However, when the sulfonamides were appreciated and exploited, modern chemotherapy became perhaps the most important field of therapy.

The sulfonamides were responsible for two major innovations: the effective treatment of bacterial infections, and the antimetabolite explanation of drug action. Even though now replaced for most uses by other drugs, they are of profound historical and theoretical interest, and the excitement of their discovery has not been forgotten.

1. History. a. Gelmo (1908) synthesized *p*-aminobenzenesulfonamide.

b. Heidelberger and Jacobs (1919) showed the antibacterial property of an azosulfonamide, but unfortunately the lead was not followed up.

c. Domagk (1932) discovered the antibacterial property of Prontosil.

d. Trefuël, Trefuël, Nitti and Bovet (1935) showed that sulfanilamide was the active portion of Prontosil.

e. Colebrok and Kenny (1936) furnished clinical proof of the efficacy of Prontosil in puerperal fever.

f. Woods and Fildes (1940) showed that *p*-aminobenzoic acid (PABA) was an inhibitor of sulfanilamide.

2. Chemistry. Prontosil, the earliest of the sulfonamides, is a diazo compound, one half of which is *p*-aminobenzenesulfonamide (sulfanilamide), the active moiety. Derivative sulfonamides are made by substitutions in the amide of the sulfonamide group.

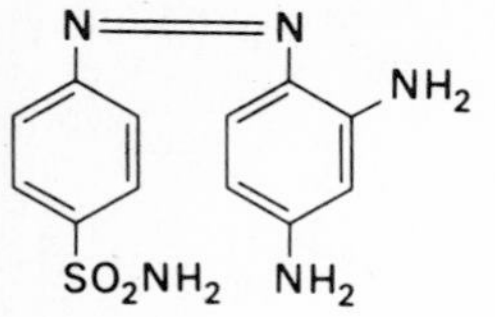

Prontosil 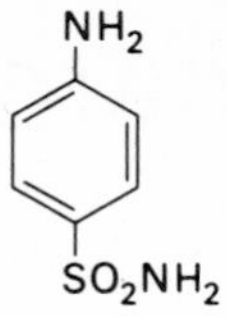 sulfanilamide 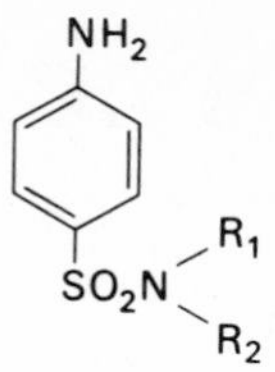 derivatives

3. Action. a. In ordinary dosage, the sulfonamides exert inhibitory effects, largely bacteriostatic, on many microorganisms; the host assists by phagocytosis and immune mechanisms.

b. General effectiveness:

a′. Gram-positive bacteria: Most are susceptible: e.g., streptococci, staphylococci, pneumococci.

b′. Gram-negative bacteria. Many are no longer susceptible because of the development of resistant strains.

c′. Other susceptible microorganisms: Actinomyces, "large viruses" of trachoma and lymphogranuloma venereum.

c. Different sulfonamides vary in effectiveness. Inside the bacterial cell, sulfanilamide is theoretically the most active member of the series as it resembles PABA most closely. However, sulfadiazine and others are more active in practice, possibly because of better penetration into the parasite.

A general comparison of in vivo effects at therapeutic dosage is shown in the following table (relative effectiveness varies to some extent with the infecting organism):

DRUG	RELATIVE EFFECTIVENESS
sulfapyridine	125
sulfathiazole	125
sulfadiazine	100
sulfamethazine	75
sulfamerazine	50
sulfisoxazole	50
sulfacetamide	25

4. Mechanism. a. Woods noted that sulfanilamide was inactive in the presence of pus or yeast; then that yeast contained PABA; and finally that sulfanilamide and PABA were competitive antagonists of each other. This led to the important thesis that substances with structural resemblances to each other might compete with each other, and that this could be a mechanism of action of drugs.

b. The competition between PABA and sulfanilamide is for incorporation into folic acid (or probably more accurately, for attachment to the enzyme which carries them into this incorporation). This mechanism is general for all the sulfonamides:

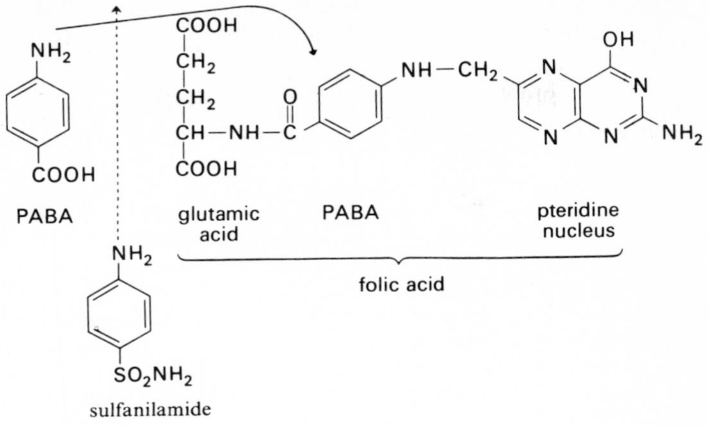

PABA

glutamic acid

PABA

pteridine nucleus

folic acid

sulfanilamide

c. The basis for the selective action upon bacteria and not on higher cells probably lies in the following hypothesis: susceptible bacteria need PABA, as they are impermeable to folic acid, or use some other derivative of PABA than folic acid; therefore a block in the utilization of PABA is lethal. Nonsusceptible bacteria are probably permeable to folic acid and so may use it directly from the medium. Humans require premade folic acid and therefore a lack of PABA is inconsequential.

d. Resistance to sulfonamides may involve increased production of PABA (gonococci).

5. Pharmacodynamics. a. Except for toxicity, sulfanilamide comes close to being an ideal drug as it is soluble, well absorbed, easily estimated, widely distributed in the body, and well excreted. Unfortunately, the more potent sulfonamides are less ideal.

b. The following are general characteristics for most members of the series: Absorption, alimentary or parenteral, rapid, in minutes; estimation, easy, by diazotization to colored compounds (Bratton, A. C., and Marshall, E. K. J. Biol. Chem., 128 : 537, 1939); distribution, widespread, with the water of the body, including penetration into the spinal fluid; metabolism, varying degrees of acetylation (of the para-NH_2), with some sulfonamides producing insoluble derivatives; excretion, moderately rapid, in 24 to 48 hours via the urine.

6. Toxicity. a. Most sulfonamides may produce mild toxic effects: nausea, dizziness.

b. Most also can produce severe sensitivity phenomena: dermatitis and rash, agranulocytosis, hepatitis.

c. Other manifestations are peculiar to certain sulfonamides. Thus, sulfanilamide may produce acidosis, cyanosis (met- or sulf-hemoglobinemia), and anemia; sulfapyridine and many others may produce renal damage and renal block by the insolubility of the parent compound or the acetyl derivative.

d. Long-acting sulfonamides may be potent and slowly excreted, allowing accumulation of the agent and severe toxicity of the erythema multiforme type.

7. Uses. a. Although effective in perhaps the majority of bacterial diseases, the sulfonamides have been replaced in large measure by more potent agents, primarily the antibiotics.

b. However, they still have application in patients sensitive to relevant antibiotics, and also are commonly used in urinary tract infections. Other instances in which they may be desirable include meningococcal meningitis and bacillary dysentery.

c. A number of therapeutic principles were developed more or less as part of the sulfonamide era. This was in part because of the heavy usage, but particularly because the ability to estimate the amount of drug in body tissues allowed a more satisfactory study than with most previous drugs.

a′. Effective plateau. The principle of continuous high blood and tissue level of drugs developed from experience with the sulfonamides more clearly than before.

b′. Initial and maintenance administration. The principle of a large initial dose to saturate to the desired therapeutic level, followed by maintenance doses at intervals which would maintain this level, although recognized before as with digitalis, became clearer because of the opportunity to follow blood levels.

c′. Certain therapeutic principles special to the sulfonamides were also developed. Alkalinization of the urine was found to increase the solubility of most of the sulfonamides and their acetyl derivatives, and so to help prevent renal damage. Mixtures of sulfonamides were found in most instances to exert additive therapeutic effect with mutual solubility, again furnishing a means of limiting renal damage. The intravenous administration of sodium salts was found to establish a rapid initial saturation of the tissues at the desired level.

8. Preparations

a. Systemic sulfonamides: Scores of sulfonamides have been synthesized and a considerable number have come into clinical use. In this section the more prominent members that have been used to treat systemic infections are considered.

a′. Early preparations, largely obsolete

SULFANILAMIDE (Prontylin *)

After Prontosil, the earliest of the series; obsolete.

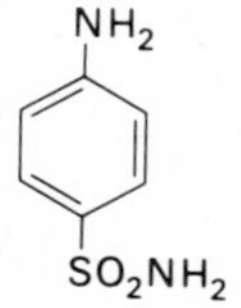

NH_2 / SO_2NH_2

SULFAPYRIDINE (Dagenan, M & B 693, and others)

Greatly increased potency over sulfanilamide but both sulfapyridine and the acetyl derivative insoluble, giving renal damage; obsolete for general use, but used in dermatitis herpetiformis and other dermatological conditions.

Dose: 1 gm 4 times a day by mouth, reduced to 1 or 2 times a day.

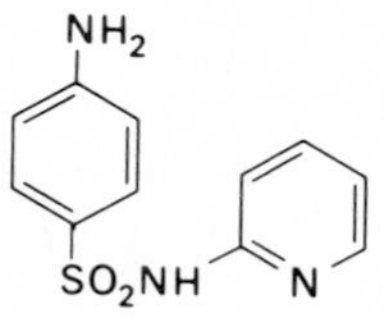

NH_2 / SO_2NH / N

* Trademark: throughout the book limited to one or two common examples.

SULFATHIAZOLE (Thiazamide, and others)

Also potent, but toxicity common, especially to skin and marrow; obsolete.

b′. Short-acting preparations

SULFADIAZINE (Pyrimal, and others)

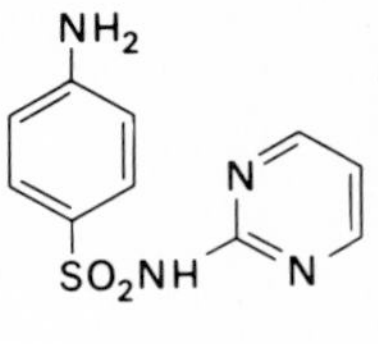

The standard general purpose sulfonamide, with which others are usually compared. Nearly as potent as sulfathiazole, but less toxic; serious reactions, i.e., blood dyscrasias and hepatitis, occur in about 0.1% of patients.

Dose: 4 gm initially by mouth, then 1 gm every 4 hours for maintenance.

NH_2 — SO_2NH — N — N

Sodium sulfadiazine, 0.5 to 4 gm intravenously in 5% solution.

SULFAMERAZINE (Methylpyrimal; etc.) and SULFAMETHAZINE (Diazil; etc.)

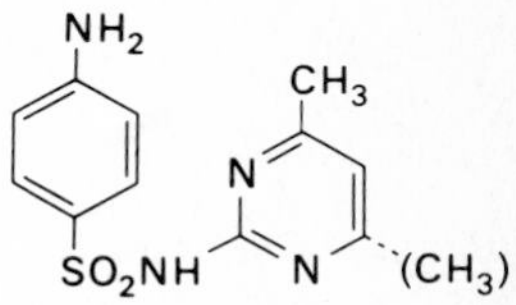

The methyl and dimethyl derivatives of sulfadiazine, somewhat more slowly excreted.

Dose: As for sulfadiazine.

NH_2 — CH_3 — N — SO_2NH — N — (CH_3)

Trisulfapyrimidines (triple sulfonamides)

Combinations of equal parts of sulfadiazine, sulfamerazine and sulfamethazine.

Dose: as for sulfadiazine.

c′. Long-acting preparations

SULFADIMETHOXINE (Madribon)

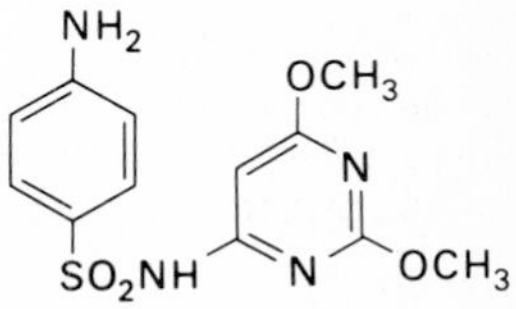

Similar to sulfamethoxypyridazine but slowly converted into the favorably soluble glucuronide instead of the usual acetyl derivative. Cumulation may lead to severe toxicity, as for sulfamethoxypyridazine.

Dose: 2 gm by mouth (initial), then 1 gm daily.

NH_2 — OCH_3 — N — SO_2NH — N — OCH_3

SULFADOXINE (Fanzil)

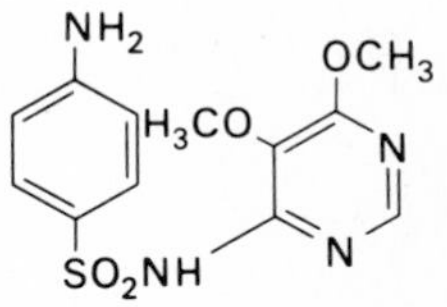

Dose: 1 gm by mouth (single administration).

NH_2 — OCH_3 — H_3CO — N — SO_2NH — N

SULFALENE (Kelfizina)

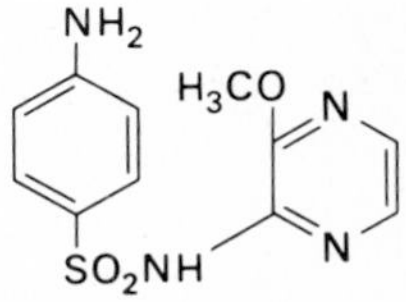

Extremely long acting. Used with pyrimethamine in resistant malaria.

Dose: 1 gm by mouth as a single dose under trial.

NH_2 — H_3CO — N — SO_2NH — N

SULFAMETER (Sulla)

Dose: 0.5 gm by mouth twice on first day, then 0.5 gm daily.

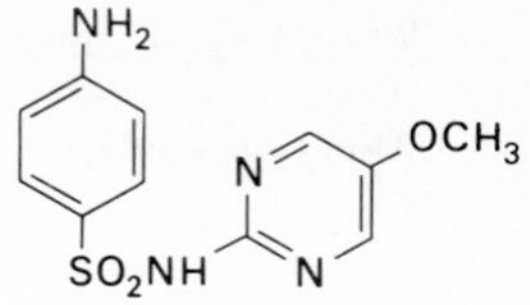

SULFAPHENAZOLE (Sulfabid)

Dose: 3 gm initially by mouth, then 1 gm twice daily.

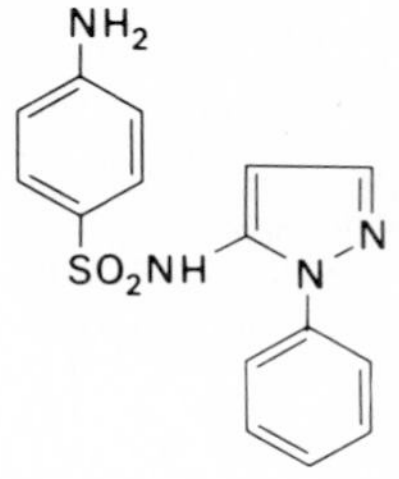

SULFAMETHOXYPYRIDAZINE (Kynex)

Potent, soluble, well absorbed, slowly excreted, allowing a small dose and infrequent administration. Used for general purposes and urinary tract infections; also in long term prophylaxis of rheumatic fever. Slow excretion may lead to cumulation and severe toxicity; Stevens-Johnson syndrome (erythema multiforme) reported.

Dose: 0.5 gm 2 times a day by mouth.

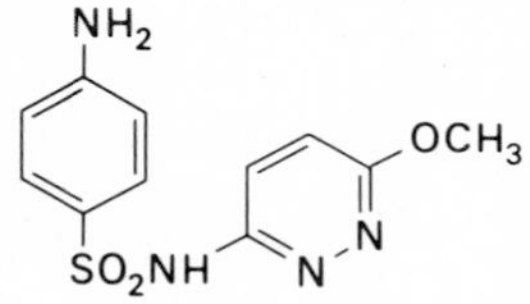

Acetyl sulfamethoxypyridazine (Kynex Acetyl)

Tasteless, for pediatric use; also adjunct to sulfones in leprosy.

Dose: Same as for sulfamethoxypyridazine.

b. Urinary sulfonamides: A number of sulfonamides are used particularly for urinary tract infections. They tend to be weaker than the systemic sulfonamides, to be excreted rapidly, and to produce blood levels too low for satisfactory systemic effects. Their generally high solubility reduces the chance of renal damage while allowing high concentration in the urinary tract.

SULFACETAMIDE (Sulamyd)

High solubility, low toxicity.

Dose: 1 gm 3 or 4 times a day by mouth.

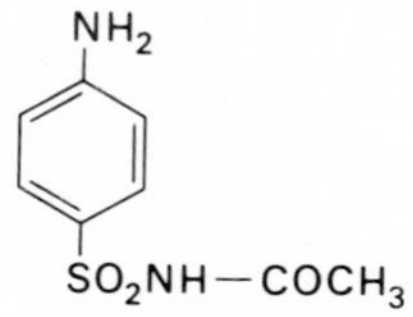

SULFACHLORPYRIDAZINE (Sonilyn)

High solubility; generally resembles sulfisoxazole.

Dose: 1 to 4 gm initially by mouth, then 1 gm 3 to 6 times a day.

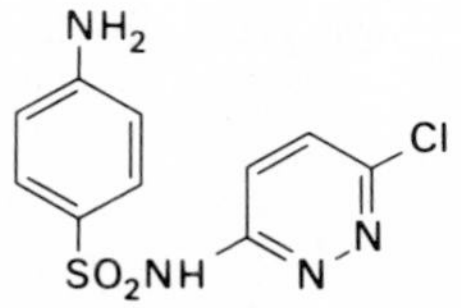

SULFACYTINE (Renoquid)
Short acting, rapidly excreted.
Dose: 250 mg 4 times a day by mouth.

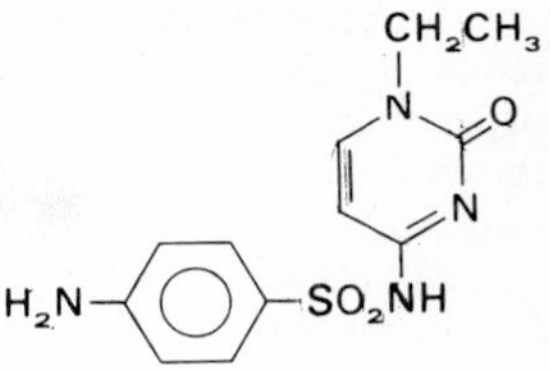

SULFAETHIDOLE (Sul-spansion)

Excreted rapidly and therefore given in sustained-release preparations.

Dose: 1 to 2 gm by mouth 2 times a day.

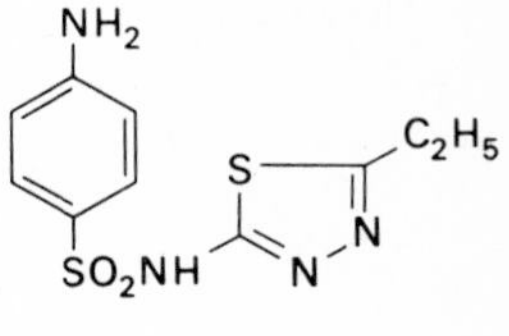

SULFAMETHIZOLE (Thiosulfil)

Good solubility, fair potency.
Dose: 0.25 to 0.5 gm 4 to 6 times a day by mouth.

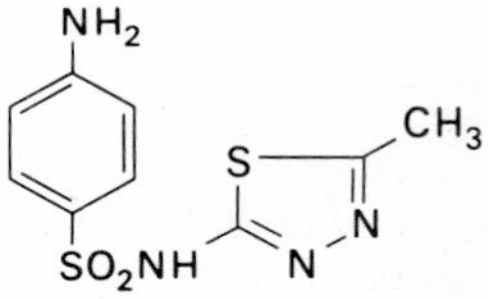

SULFAMETHOXAZOLE (Gantanol)

Less well absorbed and more slowly excreted than sulfisoxazole. Rare nausea and vomiting.

Dose: 2 gm initially by mouth, then 1 gm every 12 hours.

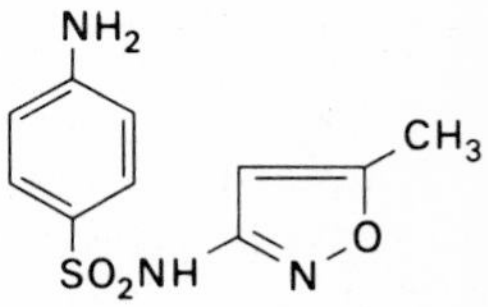

SULFISOMIDINE (Elkosin)

High solubility, low toxicity.
Dose: 1 gm 3 times a day by mouth.

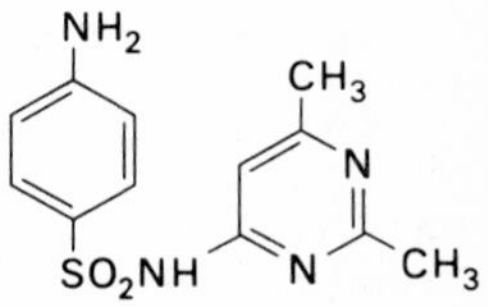

SULFISOXAZOLE (Gantrisin)

Popular urinary antiseptic; highly soluble and unlikely to produce crystalluria; occasional sensitivity manifestations, especially of skin.

Dose: 4 gm by mouth (initial), then 1 to 2 gm every 4 hours.

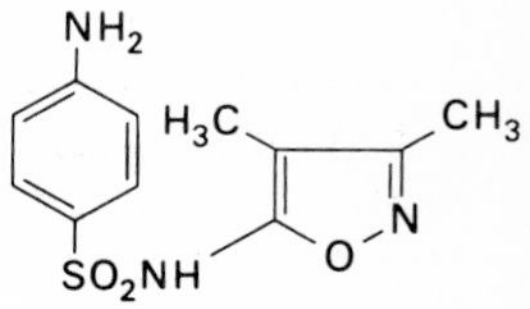

Sulfisoxazole diolamine

Acetylsulfisoxazole
Split to sulfisoxazole in the intestine; may be preferred for administration in emulsions to children.

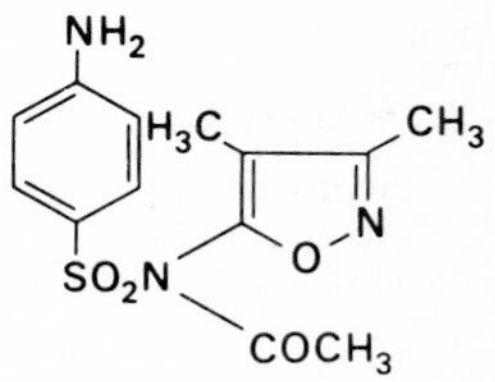

c. Alimentary sulfonamides: Poorly absorbed sulfonamides are used to reduce the bacterial flora in the bowel before abdominal surgical operations in order to lessen the danger of peritoneal contamination. Except for sulfaguanidine, the compounds act by slowly breaking down to sulfathiazole or sulfapyridine in the intestine.

Some antibiotics, especially neomycin, are used, alone or with the sulfonamides, for the same purpose.

PHTHALYLSULFATHIAZOLE (Sulfathalidine)

About 5% absorbed from the bowel; relatively effective and nontoxic.

Dose: 2 gm 4 times a day by mouth.

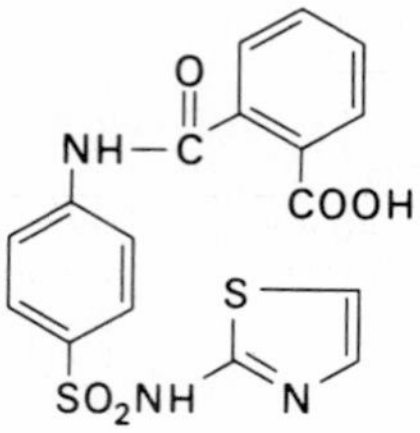

O
NH—C
COOH
S
SO_2NH
N

SULFASALAZINE (formerly Salicylazo-sulfapyridine) (Azulfidine and others)

Presumably breaks down slowly to sulfapyridine; used in ulcerative colitis.

Dose: 1 gm 4 to 6 times daily by mouth.

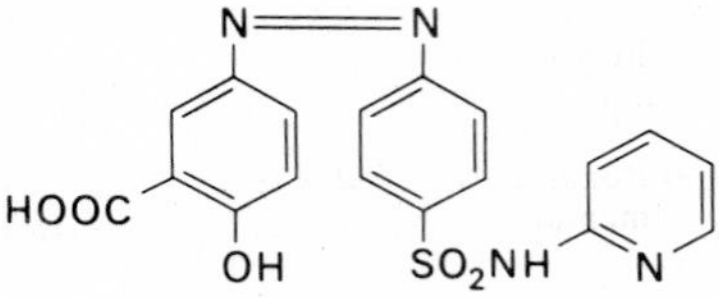

N═N
HOOC
OH
SO_2NH
N

SUCCINYLSULFATHIAZOLE (Sulfasuxidine)

More potent and more toxic than phthalylsulfathiazone; similarly used, and also in ulcerative colitis and in bacillary dysentery carriers.

Dose: 2 gm 4 to 6 times a day by mouth.

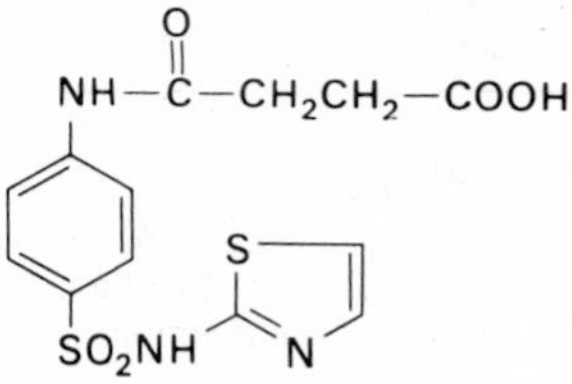

O
$NH—C—CH_2CH_2—COOH$
S
SO_2NH
N

SULFAGUANIDINE

The first of the series, obsolete.

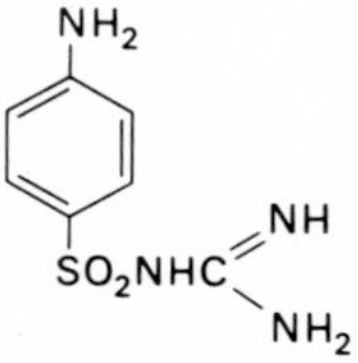

NH_2
NH
SO_2NHC
NH_2

d. Related sulfonamides: Para-amino group not present. Mechanism of action probably similar to sulfonamides.

MAFENIDE (Sulfamylon)

Analogue without the para-amino group; is not inactivated by PABA.

Dose: 10% suspension locally for burn and wound antisepsis.

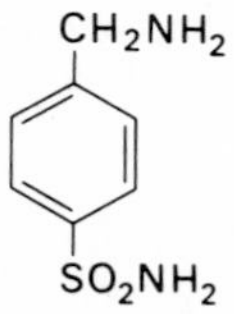

CH_2NH_2
SO_2NH_2

PARA-NITROSULFATHIAZOLE (Nisulfazole)

Used in ulcerative colitis.
Dose: 10 ml of a 10% suspension by rectum.

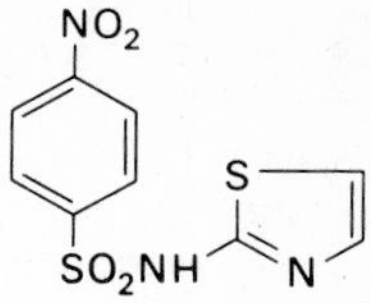

NO_2 … SO_2NH … S … N

SUMMARY: THE SULFONAMIDES

TYPE	*ACTION AND MECHANISM*	*TOXICITY*	*USE*	*EXAMPLES*
Sulfonamides, systemic	Bacteriostatic gram-pos. gram-neg. Block formation of folic acid by competition with PABA	Sensitization, crystalluria, erythema multiforme	Meningococcal meningitis bacillary dysentery	Sulfadiazine
Sulfonamides, urinary	Same	Sensitization	Urinary tract infection	Sulfisoxazole
Sulfonamides, alimentary	Same	Minor	Bacillary dysentery Surgical preparation	Succinyl-sulfathiazole
Sulfonamides, other	Probably similar	Minor	Local burns, wounds	Mafenide

Reviews

Burchall, J., Ferone, R., and Hitchings, G. Antibacterial chemotherapy. Ann. Rev. Pharmacol., 5:53, 1965.

Struller, T. Long-acting and short-acting sulfonamides. Antibiot. Chemother., 14:179, 1968.

2.
The Penicillin Group

A. The Antibiotics

Antibiotics are specific chemical compounds derived from or produced by living organisms that even in small amounts can inhibit the life processes of other organisms (Burkholder). They may thus be of use as chemotherapeutic agents.

Antibiotics are usually of microbial origin, but some have come from higher forms of life, and some are now made synthetically. Their selective toxicity is often of a high order; that is, in small doses they may greatly harm infecting organisms, while even large doses may not harm the host.

Many observations of antibiotic action were made in the early days of bacteriology. Some of the pioneers were as follows: Pasteur in 1878 noted the antagonistic effect of other bacteria on the anthrax organism. Vuillemin in 1889 coined the word antibiosis, which came to be used largely in reference to competition between microbes. Fleming in 1929 introduced the first highly potent antibiotic, penicillin, though mainly as a laboratory antibacterial. Dubos in 1939 isolated an antibiotic in crystalline form (gramicidin).

B. Natural Penicillins

In many ways penicillin is the most remarkable of drugs. It does its specific work with great effectiveness and, save in one particular, is nontoxic for man. However, this particular, allergic hypersensitivity, is a serious one and together with bacterial resistance has limited the once premier position of penicillin among drugs.

1. History. a. Fleming (1929) discovered that cultures of *Penicillium* had antibacterial powers.

b. Chain and Florey (1940) used penicillin in treating disease.

c. Du Vigneaud (1946) synthesized the molecule.

2. Chemistry. a. Penicillin is produced by *Penicillium notatum* and related species. Present strains and media are much more productive than the originals. The first commercial production was in fermentation bottles; later it was made on a large scale by submerged culture in fermentation vats. Extraction from the medium is with organic solvents and this process and subsequent concentration are in the cold.

b. The molecule contains the previously unknown penicillinic acid. Of the many derivatives which show antibacterial activity the benzyl is the most common.

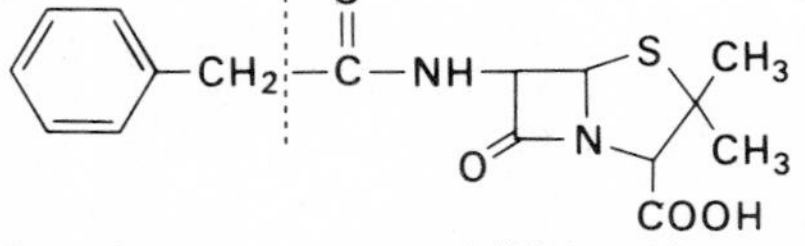

C_6H_5–CH_2 ⋮ –C(=O)–NH– [β-lactam ring (O=, N) fused to thiazolidine ring with S, CH_3, CH_3, COOH]

benzyl penicillinic acid

benzylpenicillin

Other natural penicillins are made by alterations in the strain or culture medium.

3. Action. a. Gram-positive bacteria are generally susceptible to penicillin, but many staphylococci are now resistant; gram-negatives are generally resistant, but some (gonococcus) are sensitive, and others are responsive to high concentrations.

b. Spirochetes (*Treponema pallidum*) are highly susceptible; actinomycetes (actinomycosis) and the large viruses (trachoma, lymphogranuloma venereum) are relatively susceptible.

c. Tubercle bacilli, protozoa, most fungi, and all true viruses are resistant.

4. Mechanism. a. Penicillin acts by blocking synthesis of the bacterial cell wall. This deceptively simple statement obscures the many steps which had to be taken in the development of this idea.

b. Fleming early noted that bactericidal effects were produced in growing organisms, and that bizarre giant forms were sometimes produced. Strominger and Smith (1957) finally found that penicillin caused the accumulation of a nucleotide which otherwise should have been utilized in the manufacture of the bacterial cell wall.

c. Normal cell wall synthesis.

a′. Cell wall (20% of dry weight of the bacterial cell) protects the osmotically sensitive, fragile protoplast from high osmotic pressure (20 atmospheres).

b′. Chemical linkages in the cell wall are continuously broken and new material introduced as the cell grows.

c′. Essential building materials vary (gram-negative more complex than gram-positive), but most bacteria have 4 constituents not found in animal tissues: diaminopimelic acid, D-glutamic acid, D-alanine, and muramic acid.

d′. One particular precursor of cell wall containing 3 of these building materials is uridine pyrophosphate-N-acetylmuramic acid peptide:

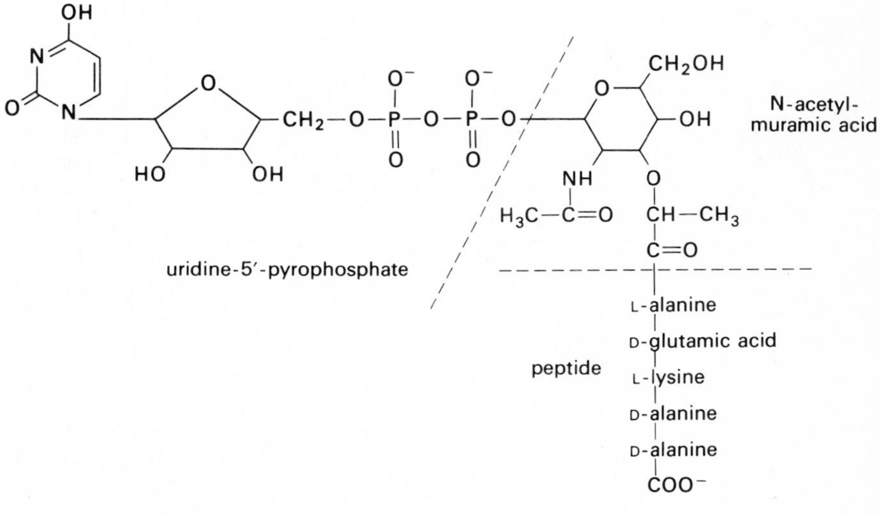

OH
N
O N
O
HO OH
$CH_2—O—P(O^-)(=O)—O—P(O^-)(=O)—O$
CH_2OH
O
OH
NH
$H_3C—C=O$
O
$CH—CH_3$
$C=O$
N-acetyl-muramic acid

uridine-5′-pyrophosphate

L-alanine
D-glutamic acid
peptide L-lysine
D-alanine
D-alanine
COO^-

d. Inhibition of cell wall synthesis.

a′. Low concentration of penicillin (or depletion of nutrients, or pH changes) cause filamentous or threadlike bacterial forms.

b′. High levels of penicillin (or severe shortage of nutrients, etc.) cause large bulbous or spherical forms with lysis; or protoplasts, or L forms.

e. Mechanism of penicillin action.

a′. Penicillin prevents the incorporation of uridine-muramic-peptides into the cell wall, and therefore in growing cells such compounds and fragments accumulate instead of being used.

b′. The basic mechanism appears to be an interference at the last step in cell wall manufacture. Normally transpeptidation provides cross linking of 2 linear glycopeptide strands by the elimination of a terminal alanine residue. Penicillin is an analogue of D-alanyl-D-alanine and reacts preferentially with the transpeptidase, thus making it (the peptidase) unavailable for cell wall synthesis (Strominger, Fed. Proc., 26:9, 1967).

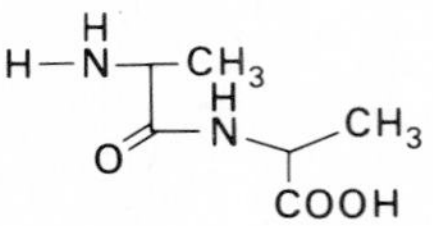

alanylalanine 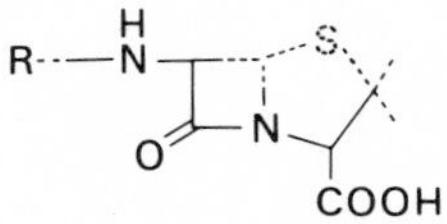 penicillin

5. Pharmacodynamics. a. Many forms of penicillin suffer destruction by gastric acid, but absorption from the intestine is excellent.

b. Estimation is by microbiological assay.

c. Distribution is widespread; moderately good into CNS.

d. Excretion is extremely rapid, via the renal tubules.

6. Toxicity. The only toxicity in man is allergic, but such sensitization is common and fatalities occur from anaphylactoid reactions; skin reactions are frequent. Sensitivity appears to be to the 6-aminopenicillanic acid moiety.

7. Uses. a. Penicillin is the most desirable drug for infections by susceptible microorganisms in nonsensitive persons. It is highly effective in infections with pyogenic cocci (except resistant staphylococci), gonococci, most gram-positives, and in syphilis. It should not be used unless the organisms are susceptible, because the patient may be sensitized and later therapy with penicillin precluded.

b. Therapeutic principles include:

a′. Intermittent vs. plateau blood levels. A continuous high (plateau) level, as is desirable with the sulfonamides, may be less necessary with penicillin because bacteria are killed only during the growing phase. However, a high, prolonged blood level is usually sought.

b′. Blood levels in the neighborhood of 0.1 units per ml of blood are effective against the most susceptible organisms; levels of 2.5 or more are required against the less susceptible.

c′. Excretion can be inhibited, and the blood level raised, by probenecid, but increased dosage of penicillin is usually preferable as it is less expensive and less toxic.

d′. Administration by injection is preferable for severe infections (endocarditis, meningitis, peritonitis) but may be oral for mild infections.

8. Preparations

a. Benzylpenicillin derivatives: Penicillin produced in modern corn steep liquor media (which contains β-phenylethylamine) is mainly benzylpenicillin, and this form has become the most widely used, and the standard by which others are compared. Prototype benzylpenicillin contains 1,667 units per mg.

a′. Soluble forms

BENZYLPENICILLIN (penicillin G), sodium or potassium salt

Preferred forms for immediate, intensive effects (by injection); oral absorption adequate, especially when combined with buffers.

Dose: 100,000 to 1,000,000 or more units intramuscularly every 3 hours (intensive); 500,000 units orally 3 times a day (less intensive).

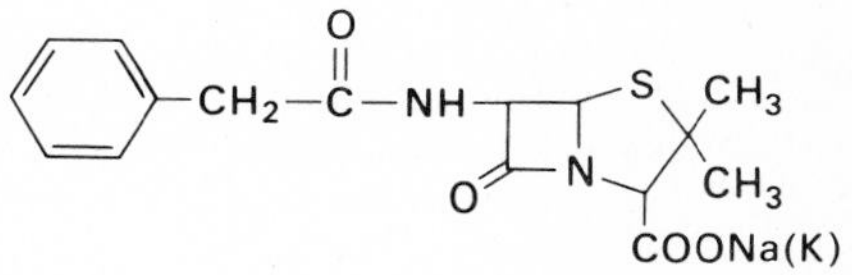

b′. Repository forms

PROCAINE PENICILLIN G (Crysticillin, and others)

The procaine salt delays absorption and so produces a sustained effect (12 to 24 hrs). Prepared in aqueous or oil suspensions.

Dose: 300,000 units or more 2 times a day intramuscularly.

BENZATHINE PENICILLIN G (Bicillin, Permapen)

This salt has still lower solubility than procaine penicillins and effective levels may be present 7 to 10 days after a single intramuscular injection. Little affected by acid and therefore also gives prolonged effects by mouth.

Dose: 200,000 units or more 4 times a day by mouth; 300,000 to 600,000 units intramuscularly in a single dose for susceptible infections (gonorrhea), or 1,200,000 units (syphilis); 600,000 units every 2 weeks, prophylactic for rheumatic fever.

b. Phenoxymethylpenicillin derivatives: Penicillin produced by *Penicillium chrysogenum* in media containing phenoxyacetic acid.

PHENOXYMETHYL PENICILLIN (Penicillin V, Pen Vee, V-Cillin)

Resistant to acid and gives rapid, high blood levels after oral administration, measurable for 4 hours.

Dose: 125 to 250 mg 3 times a day by mouth (gives peak blood levels of 0.5 to 1 mcg or more per ml of blood).

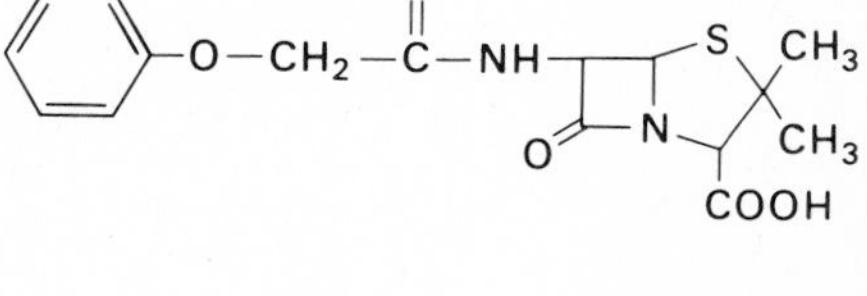

Potassium phenoxymethyl penicillin (Compocillin VK)
Absorbed more rapidly than the acid form; similarly used.

Hydrabamine phenoxymethyl penicillin (Compocillin V Hydrabamine)
Water insoluble, but releases phenoxymethyl penicillin rapidly in the gastrointestinal tract.

Benzathine phenoxymethyl penicillin (Pen-Vee Suspension)

C. Biosynthetic Penicillins

1. Chemistry. a. Batchelor (1959) showed that, by omission of the side-chain precursor, the production of penicillin could be interrupted at the 6-amino-penicillanic stage. From this latter building block many other penicillins have been made synthetically, including compounds resistant to acid or to penicillinase, or with activity against gram-negative as well as gram-positive bacteria.

b. Later work showed that natural penicillins could also be cleaved by penicillin acylase or amidase to 6-aminopenicillanic acid.

penicillinic acid
6-aminopenicillanic acid
penicillanic acid

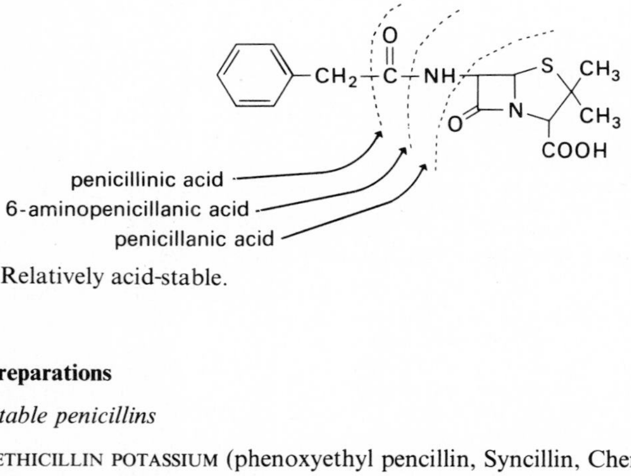

c. Relatively acid-stable.

2. Preparations

a. Acid-stable penicillins

PHENETHICILLIN POTASSIUM (phenoxyethyl pencillin, Syncillin, Chemiphen)

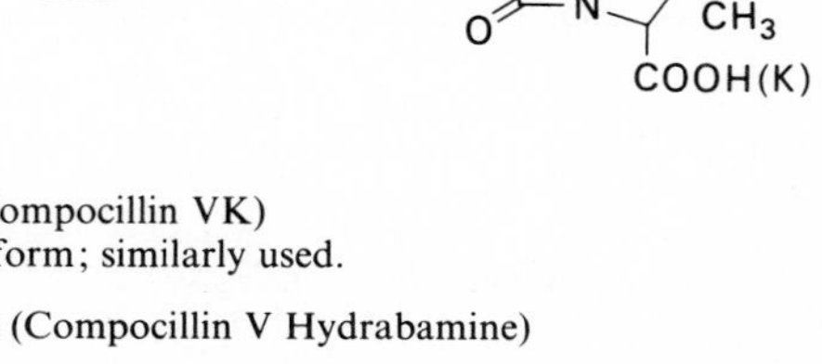

Similar to phenoxymethyl penicillin but produces brief, higher blood levels; probably no therapeutic advantage.

Dose: 125 to 250 mg 3 times a day by mouth (gives peak blood levels of 1 to 2 mcg or more per ml of blood).

Potassium phenoxymethyl penicillin (Compocillin VK)
Absorbed more rapidly than the acid form; similarly used.

Hydrabamine phenoxymethyl penicillin (Compocillin V Hydrabamine)

b. *Broad-spectrum penicillins*

AMPICILLIN (Polycillin)

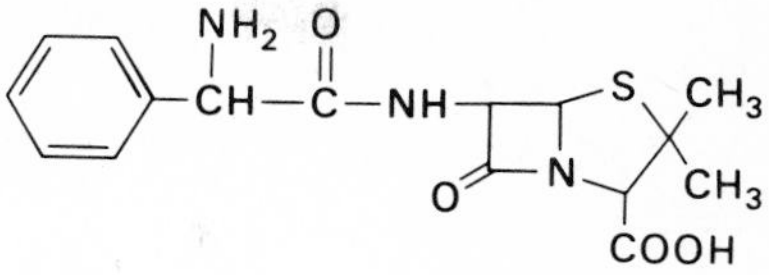

Active against both gram-positives and gram-negatives; comparable to tetracycline against the latter. Usually susceptible: *Haemophilus influenzae*, *Escherichia coli*, *Shigella*, *Salmonella*, *Klebsiella*, some *Proteus*. Usually resistant: *Pseudomonas*, *Aerobacter*, some *Proteus*, some *E. coli*. Not stable to penicillinase and ineffective against resistant staphylococci.

Absorbed by mouth (stable to acid); not metabolized in body; not highly bound to serum. Toxicity: transient rashes; allergic cross sensitivity; diarrhea.

Uses: Useful against most bacterial infections but especially against gram-negative organisms, where other penicillins have little effect.

Dose: 500 to 1,000 mg every 4 to 6 hours by mouth; up to 10 gm per day intramuscularly or intravenously.

Ampicillin sodium
Suncillin sodium (sulfoamino derivative)

CARBENICILLIN (calcium, disodium, or potassium)

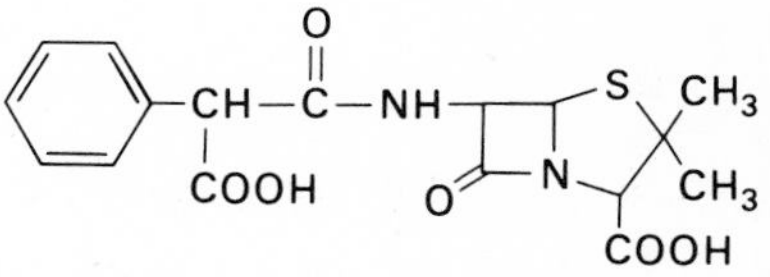

Active against *Pseudomonas*; variable activity against *Proteus*, *E. coli*, enterobacteria; not active against *Klebsiella*.

Poorly absorbed by mouth; resistance develops rapidly.

Carbenicillin calcium, *disodium*, or *potassium* (Geopen).

Dose: 1 gm every 6 hours intramuscularly (urinary tract); 10 to 30 gm per day for systemic infections.

Carbenicillin sodium indanyl

OTHERS

Largely relatives of ampicillin that break down in the body to ampicillin.

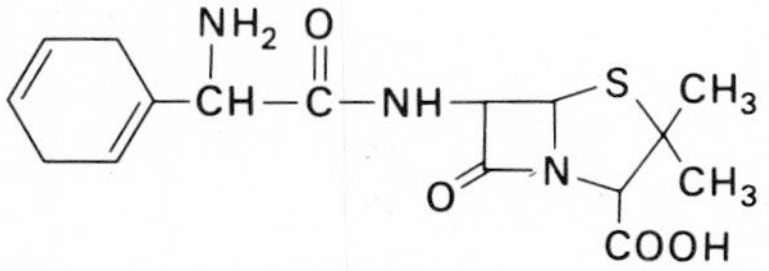

epicillin

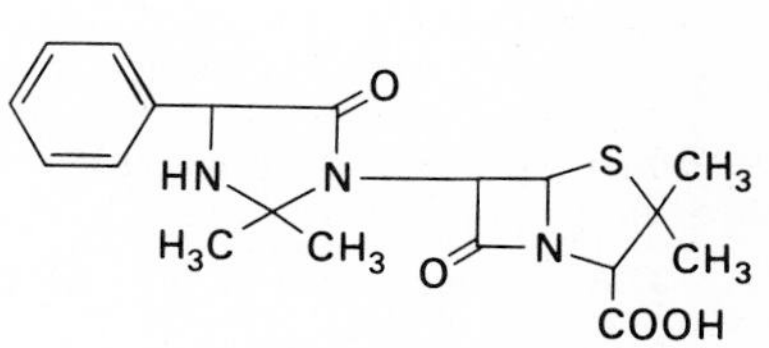

hetacillin
(Versapen)

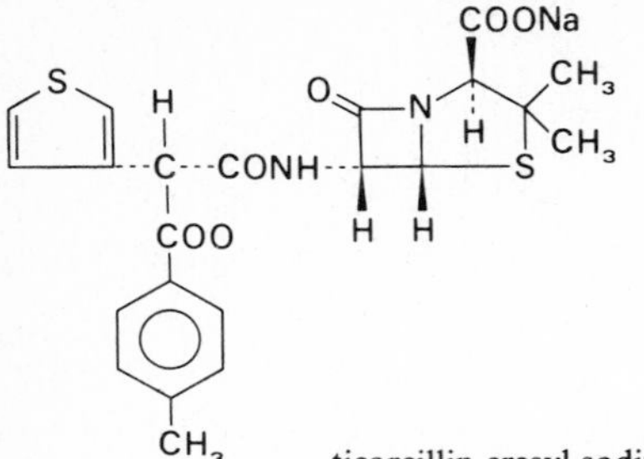

ticarcillin cresyl sodium

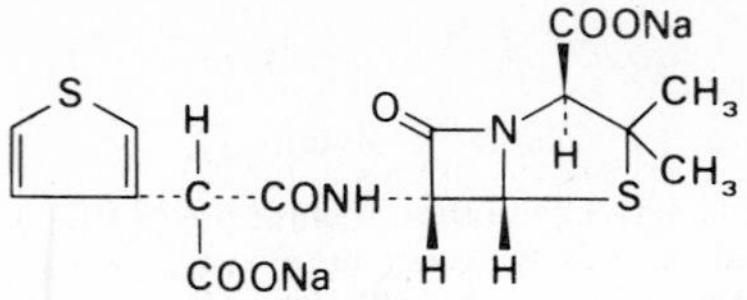

ticarcillin bisodium

c. *Penicillinase-stable penicillins*

CLOXACILLIN SODIUM (Orbenin)

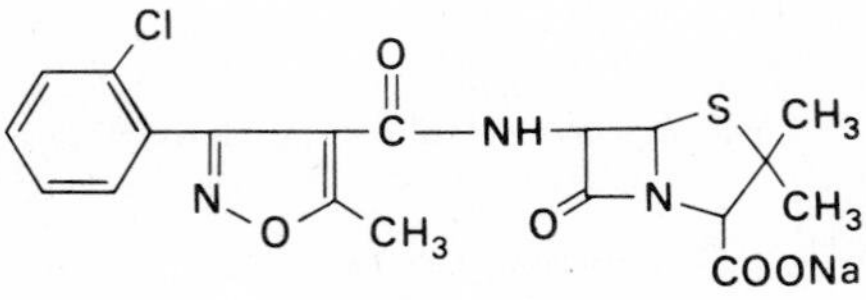

Similar to oxacillin against resistant staphylococci; both bound to protein, but serum level higher with cloxacillin; resistant to acid. Toxicity, minor; should be reserved primarily for use against resistant staphylococci. (Sidell, Clin. Pharmacol. Ther., 5:26, 1964.)

Dose: 0.5 to 1 gm every 4 to 6 hours by mouth. Parenteral forms also available.

DICLOXACILLIN (Veracillin, Orbenin)

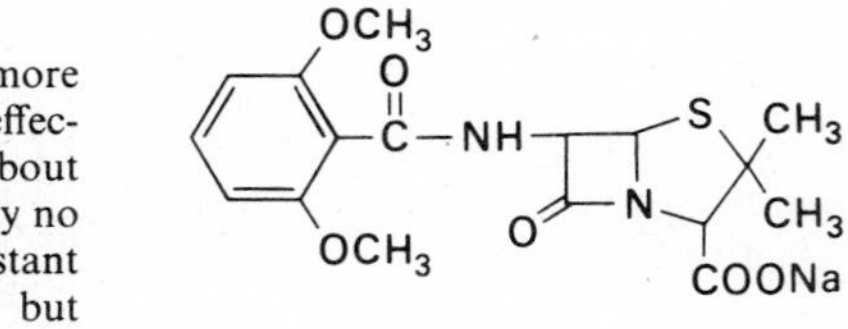

Resistant to acid and penicillinase.

Dose: 125 to 250 mg, or more, every 6 hours.

Sodium dicloxacillin monohydrate.

METHICILLIN SODIUM (Staphcillin, Dimocillin)

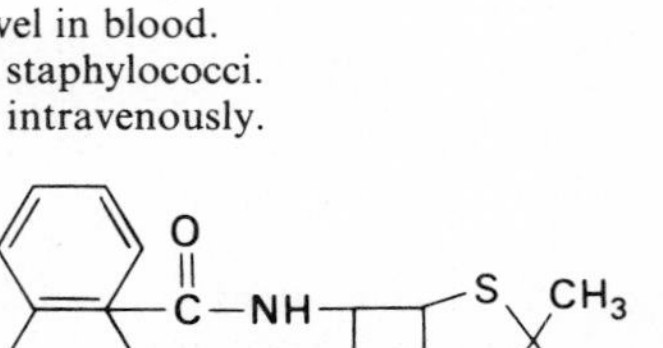

Inactivated by penicillinase 100 times more slowly than benzylpenicillin; hence may be effective against resistant staphylococci. Only about 1/20 as potent as benzylpenicillin. Apparently no cross-resistance with benzylpenicillin; resistant mutants may be produced experimentally but show low virulence.

Not absorbed orally; enters spinal fluid to 1/10 level in blood.

Should be limited to hospital use against resistant staphylococci.

Dose: 1 gm every 4 to 6 hours intramuscularly or intravenously.

NAFCILLIN SODIUM (Unipen)

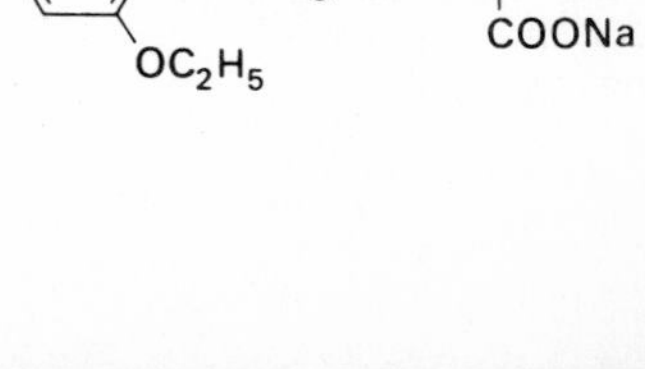

Highly resistant to penicillinase.

Dose: 500 mg every 6 hours by mouth, intramuscularly, or intravenously.

OXACILLIN SODIUM (Prostaphylin, Resistopen)

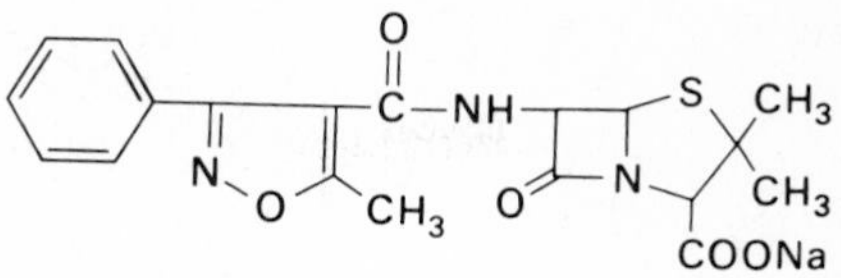

Resistant to penicillinase but also moderately stable toward acid and hence can be given by mouth. More active than methicillin (3 to 8 times), but this advantage partly offset by greater binding to plasma protein.

Rapidly excreted; effective blood levels last 2 to 3 hours.

Toxicity: rashes, gastrointestinal distress, fever, increased SGOT.

Used in oral therapy of penicillin-resistant staphylococcal infection.

Dose: 0.5 to 1 gm every 4 to 6 hours by mouth (1 to 2 hours before meals). Parenteral forms also available.

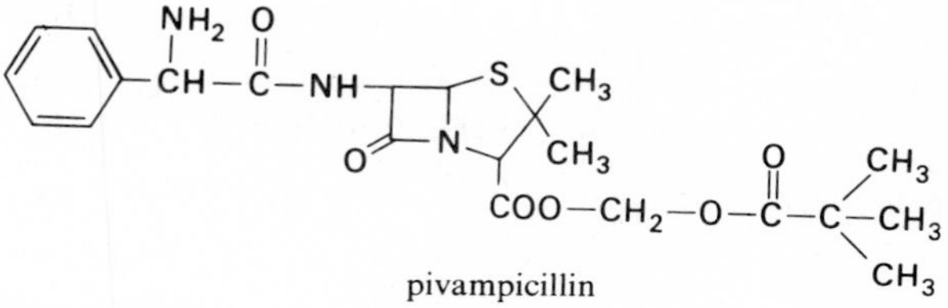

pivampicillin

D. Cephalosporins

1. Chemistry. A number of antibiotics closely related to penicillin derived from species of *Cephalosporium*.

2. Action and Mechanism. a. Active against gram-positives and some gram-negatives: staphylococci, enterococci, *Klebsiella*, sometimes *Aerobacter*, and *Proteus*.

b. Relatively resistant to penicillinase.

c. Infrequent microbial cross-sensitivity with penicillin.

d. Mechanism probably similar to that of penicillin.

3. Pharmacodynamics. Some are poorly absorbed and should be administered only parenterally. Excretion rapid in urine (Probenecid slows it).

4. Toxicity. Hypersensitivity reactions, frequent diarrhea, rash, malaise, fever, headache; doses of cephaloridine above 4 gm daily may cause renal tubular necrosis.

5. Uses. a. Used in urinary tract infections; against resistant staphylococci; in patients sensitive to penicillin.

b. Cephaloglycin used orally in urinary tract infections caused by some strains of colon and proteus bacilli and other sensitive organisms, but ampicillin ordinarily more satisfactory.

6. Preparations

CEFAZOLIN SODIUM (Ancef, Kefzol)

Dose: 250 to 500 mg 3 times a day intramuscularly or intravenously.

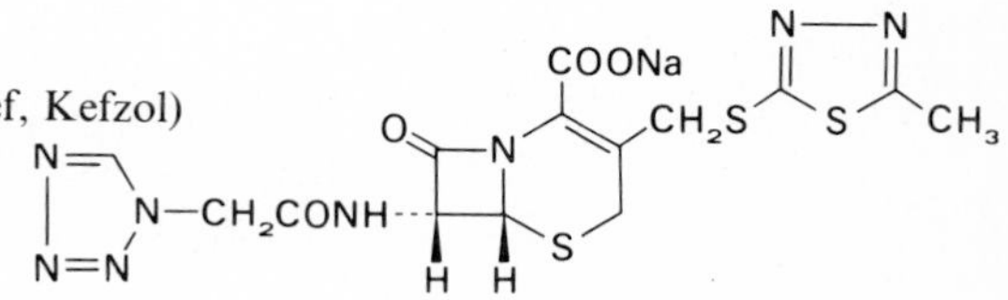

CEPHALEXIN (Keflex, Keforal)

Dose: 0.25–1.0 gm by mouth 4 times a day.

CEPHALOGLYCIN

Cephaloglycin dihydrate (Kafocin)

Dose: 250 to 500 mg by mouth 4 times a day.

CEPHALORIDINE (Keflordin, Loridine)

Dose: 0.5 to 1 gm 3 times a day intramuscularly or intravenously.

CEPHALOTHIN SODIUM (Keflin)

Dose: 0.5 gm every 6 hours intramuscularly or intravenously.

CEPHAPIRIN SODIUM (Cefadyl)

Dose: 0.5 to 1 gm 4 times a day intramuscularly or intravenously.

CEPHRADINE (Velosef, Anspor)

Dose: 250 to 500 mg by mouth 4 times a day.

OTHERS

cefadroxil

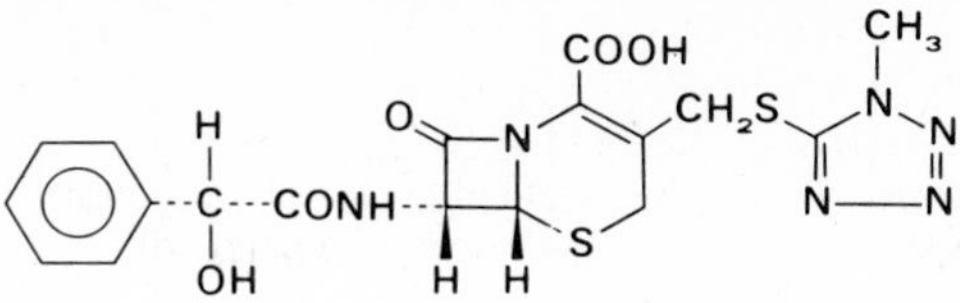

cefamandole

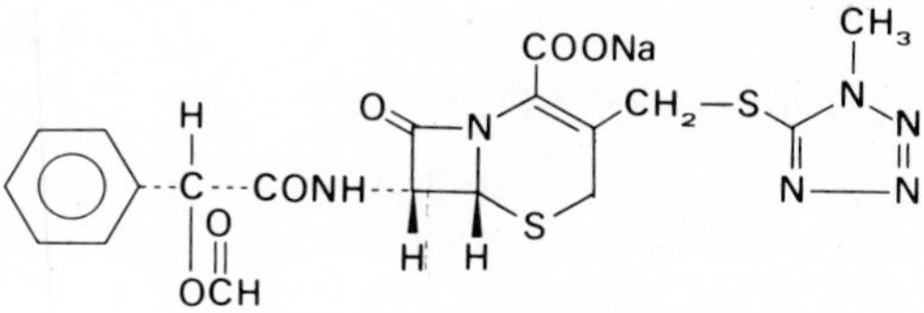

cefamandole nafate

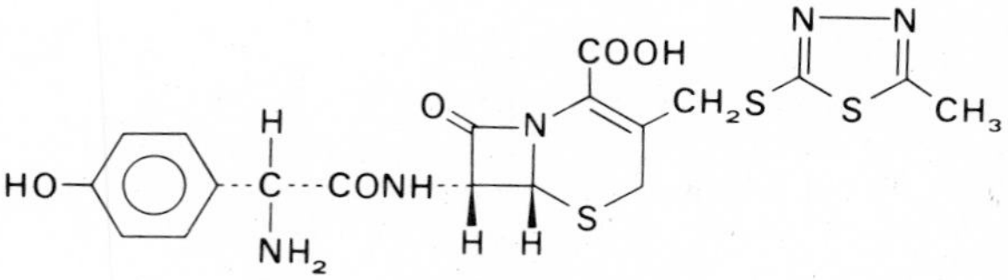

cefaparole

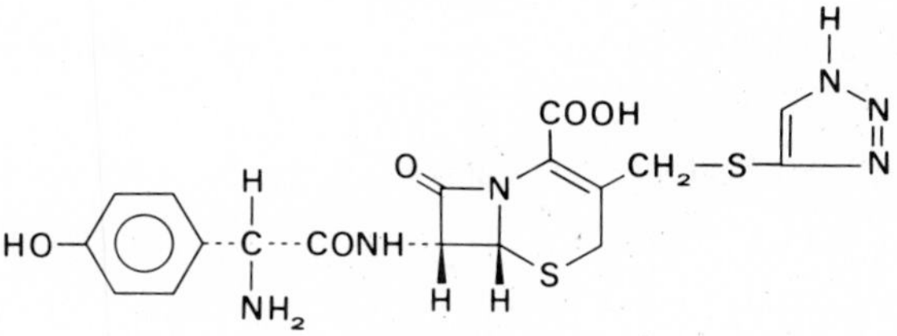

cefatrizine

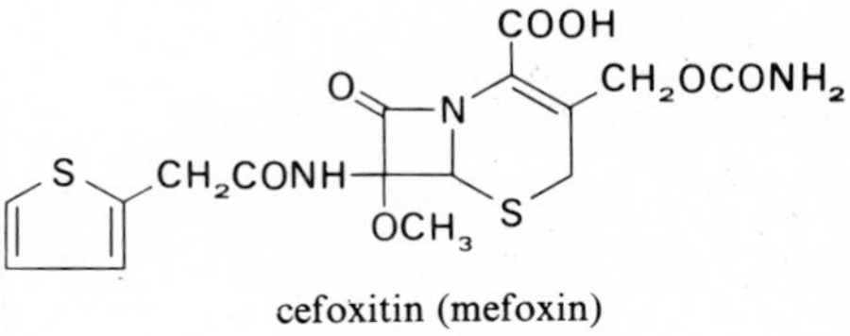

cefoxitin (mefoxin)

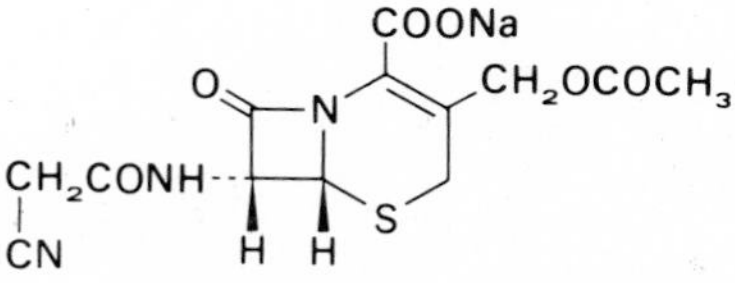

cephacetrile sodium (celospor)

E. Penicillinase

Some organisms appear to owe their resistance to penicillin, at least in part, to their ability to produce the enzyme penicillinase (β-lactamase), which destroys penicillin. Penicillinase has therefore been used therapeutically to destroy penicillin in patients undergoing penicillin reactions.

Other enzymes (acylase and amidase) hydrolyze penicillin to the inactive 6-aminopenicillanic acid, but this appears not to be the mechanism of resistance of gram-negative bacteria.

1. Chemistry. A purified enzyme prepared from *Bacillus cereus* (1958).

2. Action and Mechanism. a. Hydrolyzes the beta-lactam ring (β-lactamase) of penicillin to penicilloic acid, removing the antigenicity of penicillin.

b. Ineffective against methicillin and related penicillins.

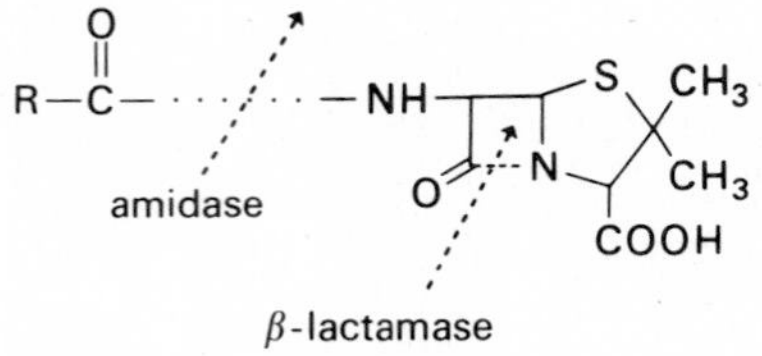

R—C(=O)—NH— S CH₃ N CH₃ COOH O

amidase

β-lactamase

3. Pharmacodynamics. Effective within an hour of injection; keeps penicillin level near zero for four to seven days.

4. Toxicity. May cause febrile reactions; may itself be antigenic; gives local pain and tenderness.

5. Uses. Penicillin reactions are of two types:

a. Immediate: Anaphylaxis, asthma, vascular collapse. Use epinephrine immediately; may follow with penicillinase.

b. Delayed. Urticaria, rashes, "serum sickness," exfoliative dermatitis. Penicillinase may be used if reaction severe.

6. Preparation

PENICILLINASE INJECTABLE (Neutrapen)

Dose: 800,000 units intramuscularly; 1 unit neutralizes 1 unit of penicillin.

SUMMARY: THE PENICILLIN GROUP

TYPE	*ACTION AND MECHANISM*	*TOXICITY*	*USE*	*EXAMPLES*
Penicillins, natural	Bactericidal vs. gram-pos., gram-neg., treponema Block synthesis of bacterial cell wall by competition with alanine in glycopeptide	Sensitization	Generally preferred vs. susceptible organisms when patient not sensitive	Benzyl-penicillin
Penicillins biosynthetic	Same	Same	Same	
acid-stable				Phenethicillin
penicillinase-stable				Oxacillin
broad-spectrum				Ampicillin
Cephalosporins	Probably similar to penicillin Several active on gram-neg.	Same	Largely in urinary tract infections	Cephaloglycin
Penicillinase	Hydrolyzes penicillin	Fever, local pain	Delayed penicillin reactions	Penicillinase injectable

Reviews

Burchall, J., Ferone, R., and Hitchings, G. Antibacterial chemotherapy. Ann. Rev. Pharmacol., 5:53, 1965.

Childress, S. Chemical modifications of antibiotics. Topics Med. Chem., 1:109, 1967.

Hoeprich, P. The penicillins, old and new. Calif. Med., 109:301, 1968.

Jones, R. G. Antibiotics of the penicillin and cephalosporin family. Amer. Sci., 58:404, 1970.

3. Erythromycin and Penicillin Substitutes

Erythromycin and a number of other antibiotics, mostly produced by *Streptomyces*, resemble penicillin in showing a preferential action on gram-positive bacteria. Although their potency is in general less than that of penicillin they have become important therapeutically because of the high incidence of infections resistant to penicillin, and the inadvisability of using penicillin in patients sensitive to it. The availability of penicillins not affected by penicillinase, such as oxacillin, lessens the importance of this group.

A. Erythromycin and Related Agents

1. History. a. McGuire (1952) isolated erythromycin from *Streptomyces erythraeus*.

b. Tanner (1952) isolated carbomycin from *Streptomyces halstedii*.

c. Sobin (1954) isolated oleandomycin from *Streptomyces antibioticus*.

2. Chemistry. Structures that are known contain large rings (13 to 16 carbons and an oxygen) and attached sugars and amino sugars (macrolides).

3. Action. a. Active against gram-positives, slightly on gram-negatives, rickettsia, and protozoa; ineffective against tubercle bacilli.

b. Effective against penicillin-resistant staphylococci, but resistance may also develop to the erythromycin group. Cross resistance between the members of the erythromyces group is to be expected.

4. Mechanism. a. Inhibits bacterial protein synthesis.

b. Result of interaction with ribosomal RNA, preventing incorporation of phenylalanine into assembly of new protein (Wolfe, Science, 143:1445, 1964).

5. Pharmacodynamics. a. Absorption good by mouth; partly destroyed by gastric juice.

b. Estimation in body fluids by biological test as for penicillin.

c. Distribution adequate except poor into spinal fluid.

d. Excretion in urine minimal; primarily in bile and feces.

6. Toxicology. a. Erythromycin is relatively free of serious toxic effects, but doses over 0.5 gm frequently cause nausea, vomiting, and diarrhea.

b. Esterification of the OH of the desosamine (estolate; troleandomycin) may lead to hepatitis (intrahepatic cholestatic jaundice), presumably because the derivatives act as haptenes in allergic hypersensitivity (Gilbert, J.A.M.A., 182:1048, 1962).

7. Uses. Primary use is in infections with gram-positive, penicillin-resistant bacteria, or in patients sensitive to penicillin; also used against enterococci.

8. Preparations

ERYTHROMYCIN (Ilotycin, Erythrocin)

The first member of the group to be introduced.

Dose: 200 to 500 mg every 6 hours by mouth; topically 0.5% to 1%.

Erythromycin ethyl carbonate and *erythromycin stearate*

Resemble erythromycin base in actions and dosage.

Erythromycin estolate (Ilosone)

More stable in acid than preceding preparations and therefore need not be given fasting; suspensions palatable. May produce hepatitis.

Dose: 250 to 500 mg every 6 hours.

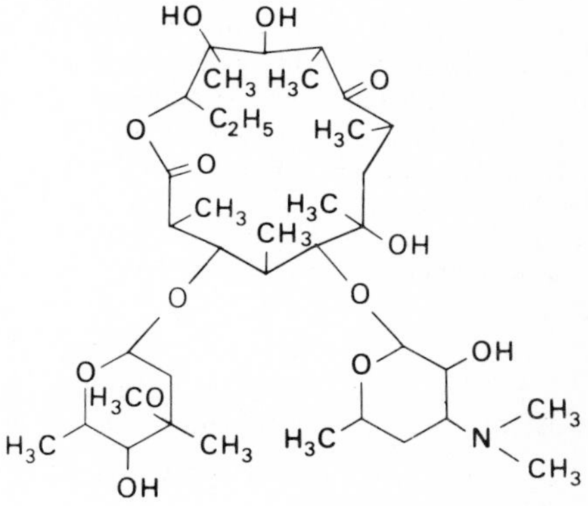

Erythromycin gluceptate, *ethylsuccinate*, and *lactobionate*

Parenteral forms for initial therapy in patients unable to take the drug orally.

Dose: 250 mg (as base) every 6 hours intramuscularly (ethylsuccinate) or intravenously (glucoheptonate or lactobionate); initial stock solution prepared only in water or dextrose solution.

OLEANDOMYCIN PHOSPHATE (Matromycin)

Similar to erythromycin in effect.

Dose: 250 to 500 mg 4 times a day by mouth or intravenously.

TROLEANDOMYCIN (triacetyloleandomycin; Cyclamycin; Tao)

Similar to oleandomycin but more stable in acid and absorption is more rapid and complete, giving higher blood levels. Liver damage may occur after 3 or 4 weeks. Esterification presumably favors sensitization by providing a haptene for combination with body protein.

Dose: Same as oleandomycin, but given orally.

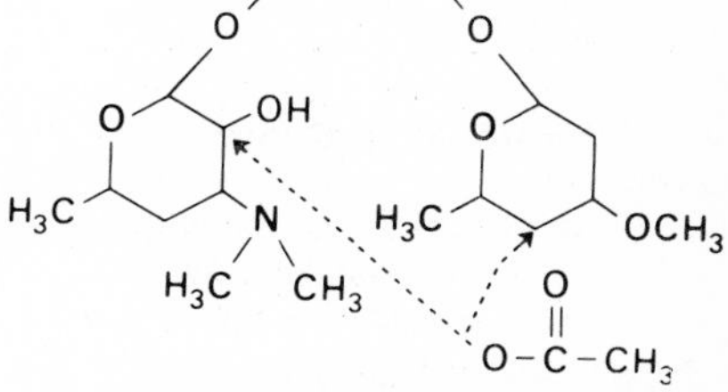

oleandomycin(troleandromycin has acetyl groups as indicated)

OTHER MACROLIDE ANTIBIOTICS

Berythromycin, kitasamycin, spiramicin.

B. Lincomycin Group

1. Chemistry. Pyrrolidine-carboxamido-pyranosides; from *Streptomyces lincolnensis*.

2. Action and Mechanism. a. Active gram-positive bacteria.

b. Mechanism similar to that for macrolides—i.e., interaction with ribosomal RNA, interfering with protein synthesis.

c. Bacteria may develop cross resistance with erythromycin.

3. Pharmacodynamics. Oral absorption rapid, but partial (30%); food in stomach retards it.

4. Toxicity. Nausea, cramps, diarrhea (sometimes severe), headache, local pain, allergic reactions.

5. Uses. Similar to erythromycin; primary use in infections with penicillin-resistant staphylococci (Holloway, Amer. J. Med. Sci., 249:691, 1965).

6. Preparations

LINCOMYCIN (Lincocin)

Dose: 500 mg every 6 to 8 hours by mouth.

Lincomycin hydrochloride
Dose: 600 mg once or twice daily intramuscularly, or 2 or 3 times intravenously.

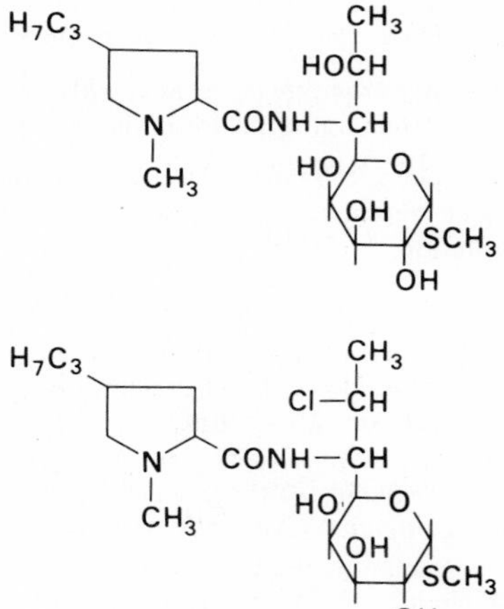

CLINDAMYCIN (Cleocin)

Shows antiparasitic as well as antibacterial action. May be effective against bacteroides. Less diarrhea than with lincomycin.

Dose: 150 to 450 mg 4 times a day by mouth.

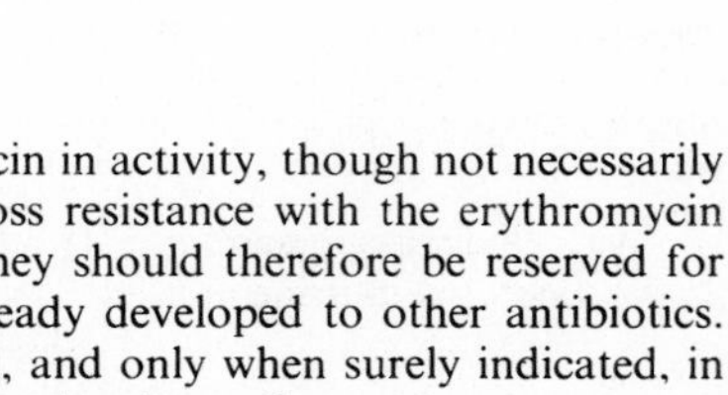

C. The Reserve Group

Certain antibiotics resembling erythromycin in activity, though not necessarily in structure, fortunately show little or no cross resistance with the erythromycin group, but are too toxic for ordinary use. They should therefore be reserved for serious infections in which resistance has already developed to other antibiotics. Also they should be used only in the hospital, and only when surely indicated, in order to prevent the development of a widespread resistant flora.

VANCOMYCIN

1. History. Isolated from *Streptomyces orientalis* (1958).

2. Chemistry. Structure not determined.

3. Action and Mechanism. a. Strongly active against gram-positive cocci including enterococci.

b. Resistance slow to develop and cross-resistance not reported.

c. Mechanism: presumed to inhibit cell wall synthesis.

4. Pharmacodynamics. Absorption minimal by mouth; distribution relatively good. Excretion via the urine.

5. Toxicity. Skin rashes, fever, ototoxicity, nephrotoxicity; thrombophlebitis of vein of injection.

6. Uses. Most important of the reserve antibiotics for use in resistant staphylococcal infections. Also used orally in micrococcal ileocolitis.

7. Preparation

VANCOMYCIN (Vancosin)

Dose: 0.5 gm intravenously 4 times a day.

NOVOBIOCIN

1. History. Welsh (1955) isolated from *Streptomyces spheroides*.

2. Chemistry

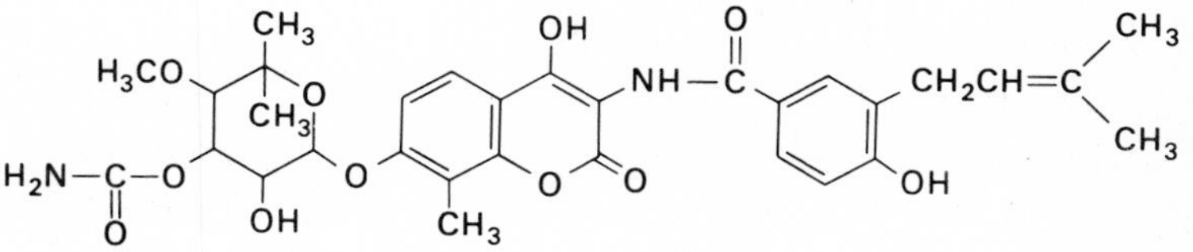

3. Action. a. Moderate effectiveness against penicillin-resistant staphylococci; also proteus. Resistance develops rapidly.

b. Mechanism: Inhibition of cell wall synthesis; induction of intracellular Mg deficiency (Brock, Science, 136:316, 1962).

4. Pharmacodynamics. Absorbed rapidly by mouth. Distributed widely in body. Excreted in urine and feces (bile).

5. Toxicity. Skin rashes, urticaria, fever, leukopenia, jaundice.

6. Uses. Formerly commonly used in resistant staphylococcal and other infections. Now almost entirely replaced by the newer penicillins, cephalosporins, and other compounds of low toxicity.

7. Preparation

NOVOBIOCIN (Albamycin; Cathomycin)

Dose: 0.25 gm 4 times a day by mouth; diluted solutions parenterally.

D. Other Antibiotics with Principal Effects on Gram-Positives

Alamecin, amphomycin, bluensomycin, chalcomycin, coumermycin, erizomycin, fosfomycin, fusidate sodium, monensin (Coban), nebramycin, neutramycin, rancomycin, ranimycin, relomycin, ristocetin (Spontin), spectinomycin (Trobicin), staphylomycin, steffimycin, thiostrepton, tobramycin, zorbamycin.

SUMMARY: ERYTHROMYCIN AND PENICILLIN SUBSTITUTES

TYPE	*ACTION AND MECHANISM*	*TOXICITY*	*USE*	*EXAMPLES*
Erythromycin group	Active vs. gram-pos. bacteria including penicillin-resistants	Minor except hepatitis from esters	Gram-pos. infections in which penicillin contraindicated	Erythromycin
Lincomycin group	Same	Minor except allergic reactions	Same	Lincomycin
Reserve group				
Vancomycin	Active vs. gram-pos. including staph resistant to penicillin	Rashes, ototoxicity and nephrotoxicity Thrombo-phlebitis	Same	Vancomycin
Novobiocin	Same	Rashes, leukopenia, jaundice	Same	Novobiocin

Reviews

Hammond, J. B., and Griffith, R. S. Factors affecting the absorption and excretion of erythromycin and two of its derivatives in humans. Clin. Pharmacol. Ther., 2:308, 1961.

Childress, S. Chemical modifications of antibiotics. Topics Med. Chem., 1:109, 1967.

4. The Tetracyclines and Other Broad-Spectrum Antibiotics

Penicillin and the erythromycin group are most useful against gram-positive microorganisms; the streptomycin group against the tubercle bacillus and serious systemic infections with gram-negatives. The tetracyclines and chloramphenicol are potent in both gram-positive and gram-negative infections, and also against the larger subbacterial parasites, such as the rickettsias. For this reason they are often called broad-spectrum or polyvalent antibiotics.

A. The Tetracyclines

1. History. a. Duggar (1948) isolated chlortetracycline from *Streptomyces aureofaciens*.

b. Finley (1950) isolated oxytetracycline from *Streptomyces rimosus*.

2. Chemistry. The tetracyclines are hydronaphthalene derivatives, with minor changes in substitutions on the characteristic 4-ring molecule differentiating the various members.

3. Action. a. Gram-positive bacteria are susceptible, but the effect is usually inferior to that of penicillin: pneumococci, streptococci, and staphylococci.

b. Gram-negatives are susceptible: *Haemophilus influenzae, Escherichia coli*, shigella, salmonella, proteus, pseudomonas; however, there are marked differences among different strains, some being highly resistant.

c. The rickettsias, large viruses (trachoma, lymphogranuloma venereum), and treponemas are generally susceptible.

d. Although relatively effective in amebiasis, the inhibition is largely on the bacterial flora that nourish the amebae.

e. Bacterial resistance may develop; cross resistance then present to entire group.

4. Mechanism. Primarily bacteriostatic, probably by interference with protein synthesis as a result of combination with ribosomes.

5. Pharmacodynamics. Absorption is fairly good by mouth. Distribution in the tissues is also good except into the spinal fluid and bile. Excretion is slow, about half and half in urine and stool (from bile).

6. Toxicity. a. Nausea, vomiting, diarrhea, lightheadedness, and Herxheimer reactions may occur.

b. More serious are alimentary and mucous membrane changes, related to alterations in resident bacterial flora with possible induction of vitamin deficiency, and to entry of monilia. Glossitis, and especially diarrhea, may be severe and prolonged. The antifungal agents, nystatin or amphotericin B, may be given simultaneously to suppress monilial growth.

c. Photosensitivity reactions, characterized by erythema and sometimes edema, may be seen.

d. Yellow discoloration and interference in development of teeth in utero and early childhood; result of chelation with calcium phosphate.

7. Uses. a. The tetracyclines are widely used as general, polyvalent antibiotics, particularly for gram-negative bacillary infections, gram-positive infections resistant to penicillin, rickettsial infections, and infections in patients sensitive to other agents.

b. There is little to choose between the various related members of the series.

8. Preparations

CHLORTETRACYCLINE HYDROCHLORIDE (Aureomycin)

Somewhat less well absorbed than tetracycline.

Dose: Orally and topically as for tetracycline hydrochloride.

Chlortetracycline calcium

For palatable oral suspensions.

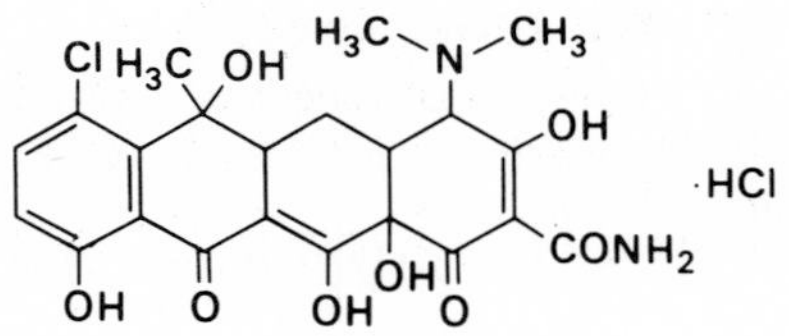

DEMECLOCYCLINE HYDROCHLORIDE (Declomycin)

More stable to acid and alkali than other forms, and excreted more slowly, giving higher, more protracted blood levels than others, but effect partly nullified by greater serum protein binding; penetration into spinal fluid poor. Photosensitivity reactions may be more common than with others.

Dose: 150 mg 4 times a day by mouth.

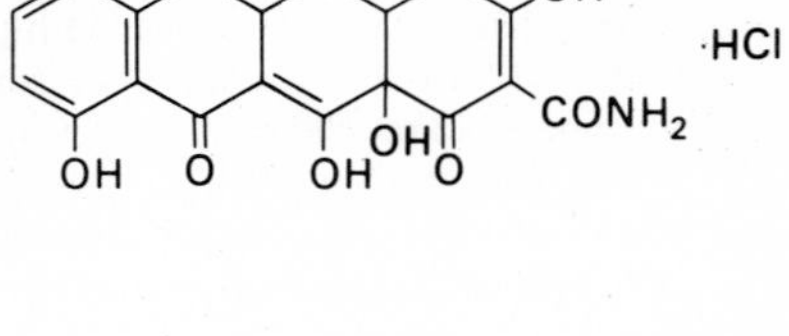

DOXYCYCLINE (Vibramycin)

Increased absorption allows once daily administration.

Dose: 100 mg twice on the first day, then once daily thereafter, by mouth.

Doxycycline hyclate; monohydrate

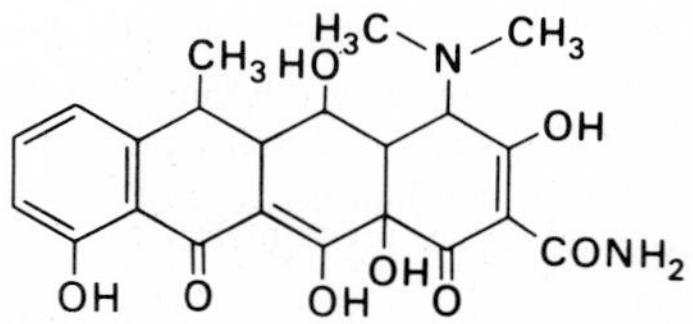

METHACYCLINE (Rondomycin)

Rapid absorption; brief action; effective in urinary infections.

Dose: 150 mg 4 times a day by mouth.

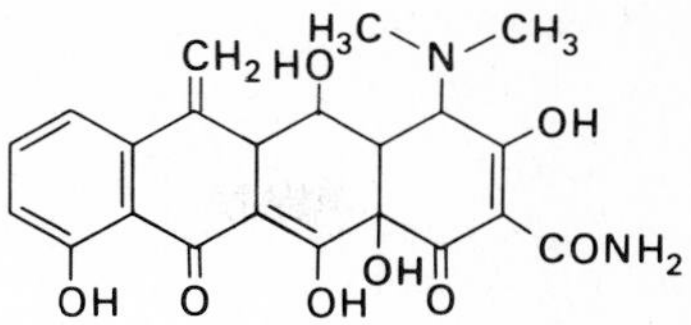

OXYTETRACYCLINE (Terramycin)

Similar to chlorotetracycline.

Dose: As for tetracycline.

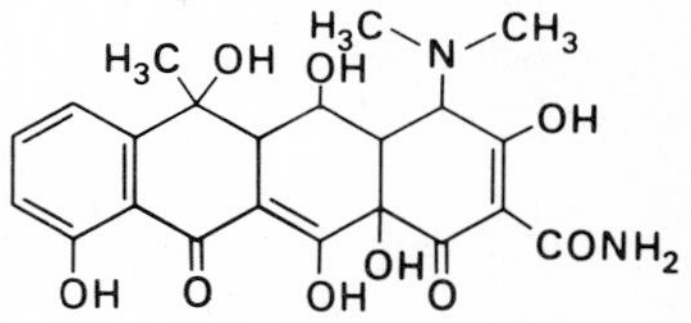

Oxytetracycline hydrochloride

Dose: Orally and topically as for tetracycline. Intravenous and intramuscular forms also available.

ROLITETRACYCLINE (Syntetrin)

Synthetic modification for intramuscular use. Increased water solubility.

Dose: 350 mg intramuscularly every 12 hours.

Rolitetracycline nitrate (Tetrim; Tetriv)

For intramuscular or intravenous use, respectively.

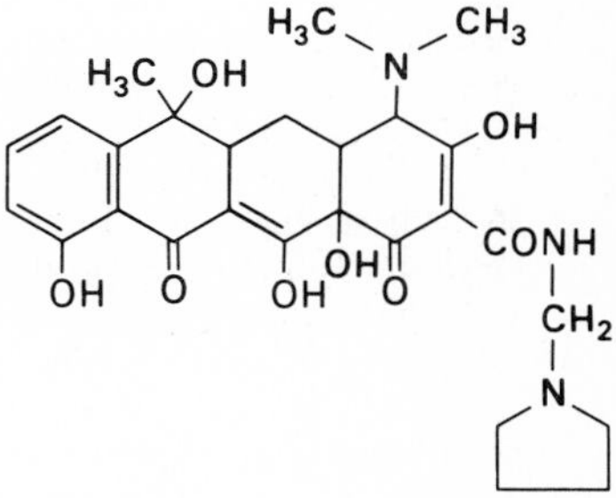

TETRACYCLINE

Natural or synthetic; usually considered as the fundamental member of the series. Absorption and passage through blood-brain barrier superior to others.

Dose: 0.25 gm 4 times a day by mouth.

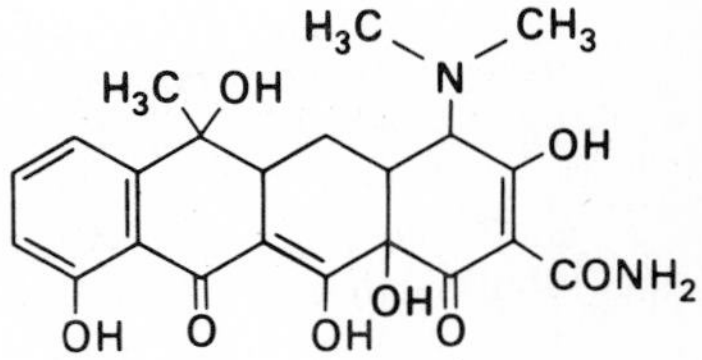

Tetracycline hydrochloride (Achromycin and others)

Effects similar to tetracycline.

Dose: Orally as for tetracycline; also topically 0.5 % to 3 %, intramuscularly or intravenously.

Tetracycline phosphate complex (Panmycin, Sumycin, and others)

Relatively insoluble complex, but more rapidly absorbed than tetracycline, producing higher blood levels.

Dose: As for tetracycline.

Tetracycline hyclate

OTHERS

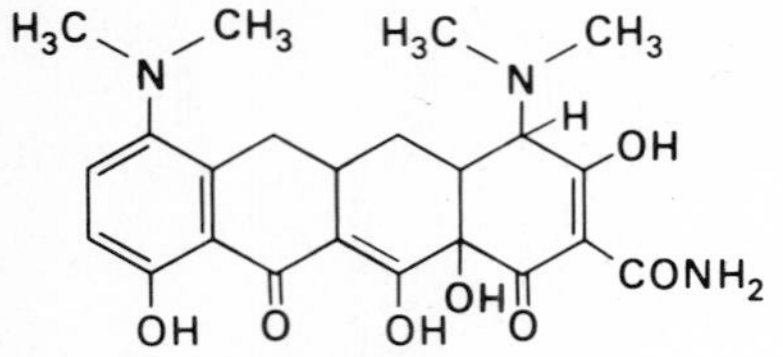

minocycline (Minocin)

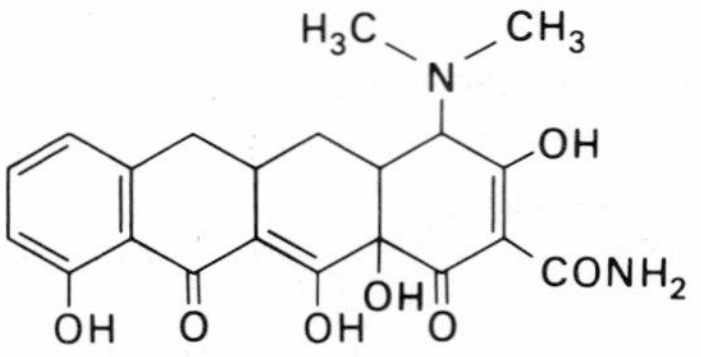

sancycline (Bonomycin)

B. Chloramphenicol

1. **History.** Burkholder (1948) isolated from *Streptomyces venezuelae.*

2. **Chemistry.** A relatively simple nitrobenzene derivative.

3. **Action.** a. Gram-positive and gram-negative bacteria, including typhoid and proteus, and rickettsias and large viruses (such as ornithosis and lymphopathia venereum viruses) are susceptible.

b. Resistant gram-negatives may also be resistant to the tetracyclines.

4. **Mechanism.** a. Inhibits protein synthesis by interfering with the incorporation of amino acids into the ribosomes.

b. The action is irreversible (except by removal of the drug) and noncompetitive; it is not clear why the effect is selectively on bacteria.

5. **Pharmacodynamics.** a. Absorption rapid, and high in the gastrointestinal tract, giving little effect on the flora lower in the intestine.

b. Estimation is by a modification of the sulfonamide method.

c. Distribution is widespread; blood level 5 to 10 mg % after an ordinary dose; spinal fluid level about one-half blood level; bile contains an inactive conjugate.

d. Excretion is rapid, in 24 to 48 hours; 90% as glucuronide.

6. **Toxicity.** a. Nausea and vomiting; in dogs, experimental glomerular and tubular damage.

b. Newborn infants are unable to carry out the glucuronide conjugation and so may be severely poisoned, developing abdominal distension, cyanosis, vascular collapse, and sometimes death.

c. Marrow damage with agranulocytosis or aplastic anemia; the latter, usually with fatal outcome, is a most serious hazard and should limit the use of chloramphenicol to serious infections in which no other agent would suffice. Temporary erythroid hypoplasia may also occur after large dosage (4 to 12 gm per day), possibly because of deficiency of an enzyme necessary for hemaglobin formation.

7. **Uses.** May be used justifiably in typhoid fever and influenzal meningitis, and in severe salmonella and resistant staphylococcal infections. Alternate choice in treatment of Rickettsial infections.

8. Preparations

CHLORAMPHENICOL (Chloromycetin)

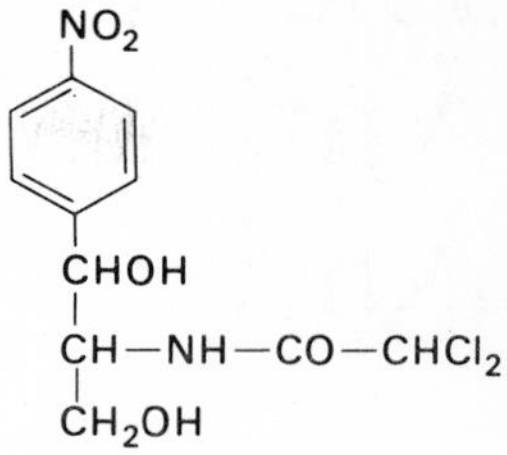

Usual oral preparation.
Dose: 12.5 to 25 mg per kg 4 times a day by mouth.

Chloramphenicol palmitate
Tasteless ester more palatable than bitter base.
Dose: As for chloramphenicol.

Chloramphenicol sodium succinate
Highly soluble derivative suitable for parenteral administration.

Dose: 1 gm every 6 to 8 hours (10% solution subcutaneously; 25% to 40% intramuscularly; 10% intravenously, slowly).

NO_2

CHOH

CH—NH—CO—$CHCl_2$

CH_2OH

C. Severe Antibiotic Reactions

With the accumulation of several years of experience it has become possible to generalize on the relative toxicities of different groups of antibiotics. It is apparent that, for the majority, penicillin is responsible for the allergic changes, the tetracyclines for the alimentary flora changes, and chloramphenicol for the blood dyscrasias.

SUMMARY: BROAD-SPECTRUM ANTIBIOTICS

TYPE	*ACTION AND MECHANISM*	*TOXICITY*	*USE*	*EXAMPLES*
Tetracycline group	Bacteriostatic vs. both gram-pos. and gram-neg. Probably acts by preventing protein synthesis by combining with ribosomes	Changes in alimentary flora may give diarrhea Photosensitivity	Infections with gram-neg. or penicillin resistant gram-pos. bacteria	Tetracycline
Chloramphenicol group	Same	Serious danger of aplastic anemia	Typhoid or other very severe gram-neg. infection	Chloramphenicol

Reviews

Ory, E., and Yow, E. Use and abuse of the broad-spectrum antibiotics. J.A.M.A., 185:273, 1963.

Burchall, J., Ferone, R., and Hitchings, G. Antibacterial chemotherapy. Ann. Rev. Pharmacol., 5:53, 1965.

5.
The Streptomycin Group: Antituberculosis and Antileprosy Drugs

A. Aminoglycoside Antibiotics

Streptomycin and a number of other antibiotics produced by species of *Streptomyces* show similarities in structure and action. They are organic bases containing unusual amino sugars, and most show chemotherapeutic effects on gram-negative bacteria and tubercle bacilli as well as on gram-positive organisms. Also, several of the members produce toxic effects on the ear or the kidney.

Historically the group is of great interest because streptomycin first extended the scope of practicable antibiotic treatment beyond penicillin, to include gram-negative infections and tuberculosis.

1. History. a. Waksman (1947) separated a number of antibiotics, including streptomycin, from *Streptomyces griseus*.

b. Waksman (1949) isolated neomycin from *Streptomyces fradiae* and showed a general resemblance in activity to streptomycin.

c. Umezawa (1957) isolated kanamycin from *Streptomyces kanamyceticus*.

d. Shafei (1959) isolated paromomycin from *Streptomyces* sp.

2. Chemistry. Aminoglycoside group; organic bases containing characteristic sugars, such as streptose, and bases, such as streptidine; oligoaminosaccharide group.

3. Action. a. Active against gram-positives and -negatives, often including organisms relatively unresponsive to most chemotherapy: *Streptococcus mitis* (viridans), *Streptococcus faecalis* (enterococcus), penicillin-resistant staphylococci, proteus, pseudomonas, coliforms, brucella.

b. Active against the tubercle bacillus and spirochetes.

c. Resistance (best documented with streptomycin) may develop with extreme rapidity, even to dependence (meningococci).

d. Cross-resistance exists, at least partially, between all the members of the group.

4. Mechanism. a. Inhibition of protein synthesis; streptomycin prevents proper attachment of messenger RNA to ribosomes. This "jams" the ribosome site and causes misreading of the code, resulting in decreased or abnormal protein.

b. Sites of antibacterial actions of antibiotics. Cell wall: impaired by penicillin, cephalosporin, novobiocin, vancomycin, bacitracin, cycloserine, ristocetin. Protoplast membrane: tyrothricin, polymyxin. Protein synthesis: chloramphenicol, tetracycline, erythromycin, puromycin, streptomycin, kanamycin, neomycin, paromomycin, gentamicin, viomycin. Nucleic acid synthesis: dactinomycin.

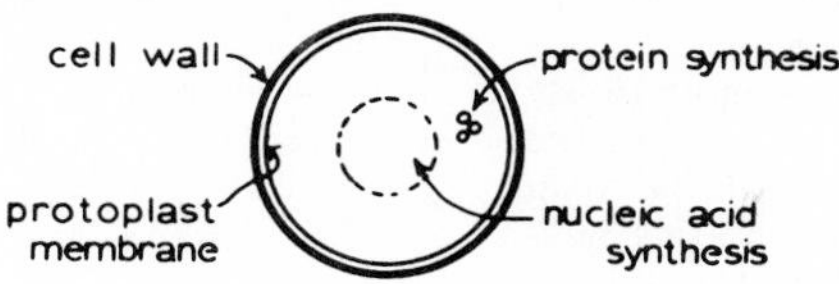

5. Pharmacodynamics. a. Absorption poor by mouth (4% for streptomycin), but complete after injection.

b. Distribution follows body water but poor into CNS.

c. Excretion glomerular, slow, majority in 24 hours.

6. Toxicity. a. Oral administration (neomycin, paromomycin) may produce nausea, vomiting, cramping, and loose stools; excessive dosage may allow overgrowth of *Candida albicans*.

b. Ototoxicity (parenteral administration): Streptomycin may produce severe vestibular damage, and dihydrostreptomycin, neomycin, and kanamycin severe auditory damage, which may appear after withdrawal and progress in spite of withdrawal of the drug.

c. Nephrotoxicity (parenteral administration): Neomycin, kanamycin may produce renal damage. Hepatotoxicity (parenteral): paromomycin.

d. Other: Fever, rash, allergic manifestations, loss of hair (gentamycin).

7. Uses. a. Systemic in tuberculosis (streptomycin), severe gram-negative infections, and in penicillin-resistant staphylococcal infections; in combination with penicillin in viridans or enterococcus endocarditis.

b. Locally (by mouth) in preparation of bowel for surgery (neomycin, kanamycin, paromomycin); may be given in combination with a poorly absorbed sulfonamide.

c. Amebiasis (paromomycin); not clear whether effects direct or secondary to antibacterial action.

8. Preparations

GENTAMICIN (Garamycin)

Derived from *Micromonospora purpurea*. A mixture of C_1, C_2, C_3 forms. Use especially in skin and urinary tract (alkaline urine) infections.

Dose: 0.4 mg per kg body wt 2 to 4 times per day intramuscularly.

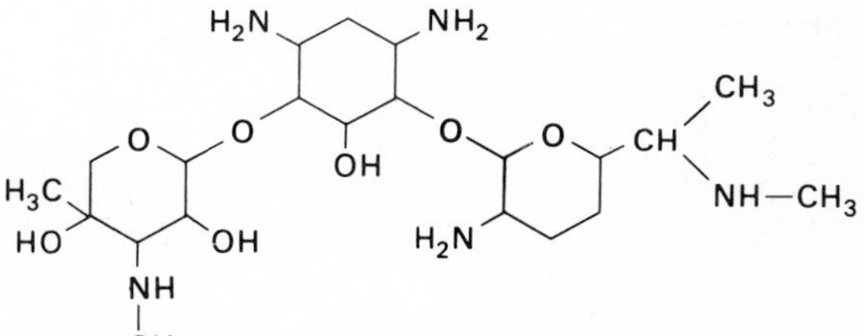

gentamicin C_1

KANAMYCIN (Kantrex)

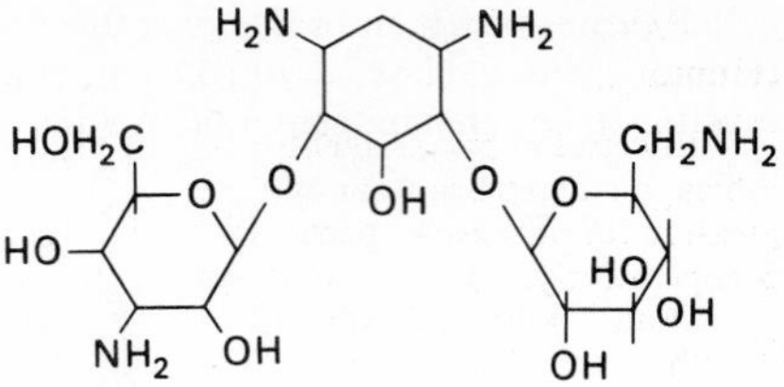

Limited use in severe, resistant proteus and coliform infections; most pyocyaneus resistant; not a drug of choice in tuberculosis or resistant staphylococcal infections.

Resistance develops more slowly than to streptomycin, with incomplete cross-resistance. More likely than streptomycin to produce hearing damage; most dangerous when renal function impaired.

Dose: 0.5 gm intramuscularly 4 times a day, but for not more than a total of 40 gm, or period of 8 days; 1 gm daily by mouth (preoperative).

AMIKACIN SULFATE
Dose: Same as Kanamycin.

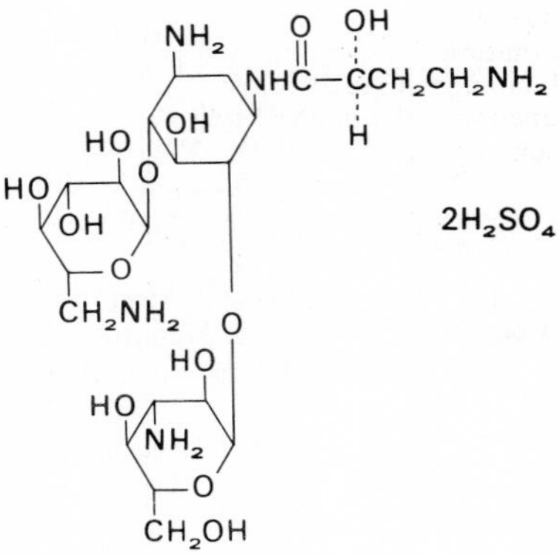

$2H_2SO_4$

NEOMYCIN SULFATE
(Mycifradin)

Used topically in superficial infections, and orally for suppression of bacterial flora in intestine, especially in preoperative preparation of the bowel; parenterally with caution for severe gram-negative infections resistant to other agents or penicillin-resistant staphylococcal infections; obsolete in tuberculosis.

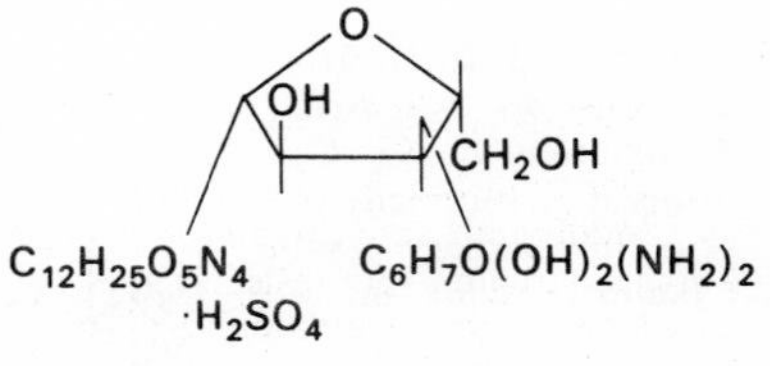

Dose: 1 gm every hour for 4 doses, then 1 gm every 4 hours up to 3 days, by mouth (preoperative); 0.5% topically.

$C_{12}H_{25}O_5N_4 \cdot H_2SO_4$ $C_6H_7O(OH)_2(NH_2)_2$

Neomycin palmitate
Neomycin undecylenate

Paromomycin (Humatin)

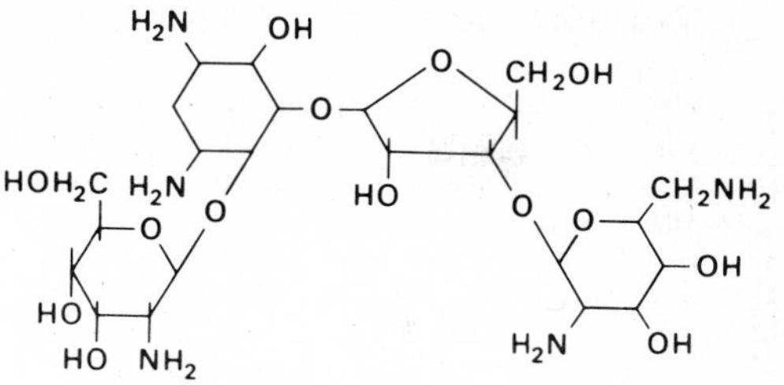

Effective in bacterial enteritidies; in amebiasis; for suppression of intestinal bacteria preoperatively.

Dose: 4 gm initially by mouth, then 2 gm daily, in divided doses.

Streptomycin sulfate

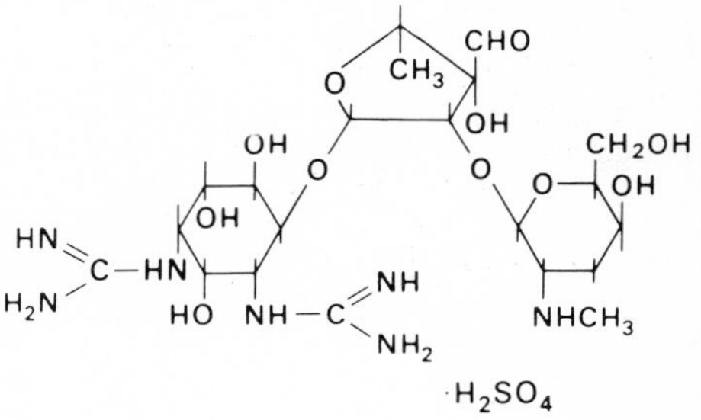

Used in tuberculosis and severe gram-negative infections.

Dose: 0.25 to 1 gm 2 to 4 times daily subcutaneously, intramuscularly, intravenously, or intrathecally in severe acute infections; 1 to 2 gm 2 times a week intramuscularly for 3 months in tuberculosis, in conjunction with aminosalicylic acid or isoniazid.

Tobramycin (Nebcin)

Produced by Streptomyces tenebrarius. Not absorbed orally.

Dose: 3 mg per kg per day by injection.

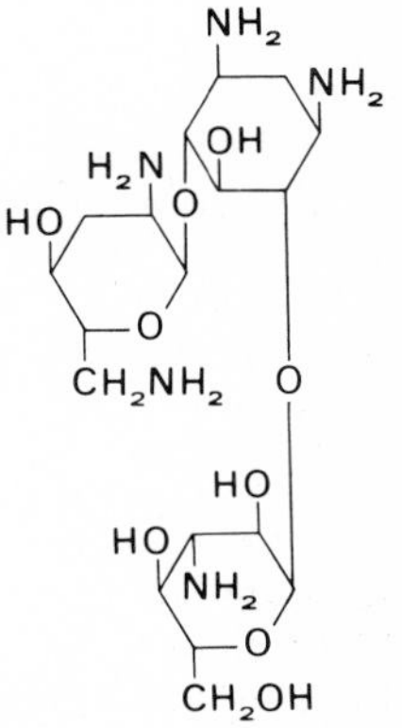

Viomycin (Vinactane; Viocin)

Derived from *Streptomyces puniceus.*

Moderately active against tubercle bacilli and used in combination with PAS or other agent in streptomycin resistance. May produce auditory and renal toxicity.

Dose: 1 gm intramuscularly given twice every third day for 4 to 6 months.

Others

Butirosin sulfate (mixture of A and B forms); sisomycin netilmicin.

B. The Sulfones

Effective chemotherapy of the acid-fast infections, tuberculosis and leprosy, began in 1940–41 when the sulfones were tried in tuberculosis and replaced chaulmoogra oil for leprosy. It was greatly stimulated when streptomycin proved to be valuable in tuberculosis and thus led to the search for other effective antibiotics (see The Streptomycin Group). Most of the synthetic compounds active against tuberculosis and leprosy bear a relationship to the sulfonamides.

1. History. a. Fromm and Wittman synthesized diaminodiphenylsulfone.

b. Buttle (1937) showed that it possessed strong antibacterial properties.

c. Feldman, Hinshaw, and Moses (1940) used glucosulfone in tuberculosis; Faget (1941) in leprosy.

2. Chemistry. Dapsone (diaminodiphenyl sulfone, DDS), the parent compound of the series, bears a rather close resemblance to the sulfonamides:

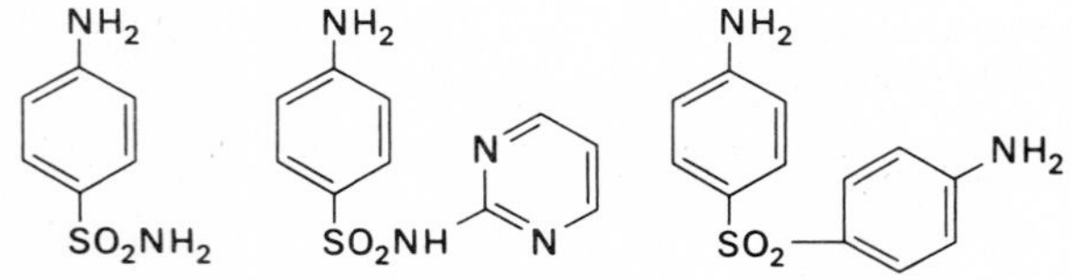

NH_2 — SO_2NH_2 — sulfanilamide

NH_2 — SO_2NH — N, N — sulfadiazine

NH_2 — SO_2 — NH_2 — dapsone

3. Action. a. DDS was early shown to be more effective than sulfanilamide on such microorganisms as streptococci and pneumococci, but it was not widely used because of toxicity.

b. Bacteriostatic on both tubercle and lepra bacilli.

4. Mechanism. a. DDS is presumably the active compound, the other members being converted into it in the body.

b. Although PABA is only a partial antagonist, the mechanism of action, i.e., competition with PABA, is probably similar to that of the sulfonamides.

5. Pharmacodynamics. a. The sulfones are difficult agents pharmacologically because of toxicity, but otherwise resemble the sulfonamides.

b. Absorption is complete after oral administration for DDS; variable for the others.

c. Distribution is satisfactory to all body tissues.

d. DDS is excreted slowly in the urine over a period of two weeks, partly because of recirculation from bile.

6. Toxicity. a. DDS is the most toxic of the sulfone series but appears to have as favorable a therapeutic margin as any of the others.

b. Excitement, dermatitis, and hemolytic anemia may be produced; there is no urinary tract damage.

7. Uses. a. The treatment of leprosy depends primarily upon the use of the sulfones, especially DDS. In the lepromatous type such drugs should be continued indefinitely; in the tuberculoid type their value is less certain, but they should be given if the disease is active.

b. The sulfones have no current use in tuberculosis.

c. Used to supplement other antimalarials in resistant falciparum malaria.

8. Preparations

DAPSONE (diaminodiphenylsulfone; DDS; Alvosulfon)

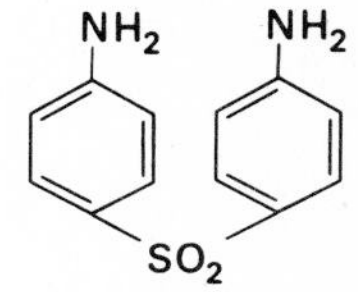

Formerly given intravenously; more recently the oral route has come to be preferred if the patient can be relied on to take the medication.

Dose: 0.5 mg per kg body weight daily by mouth, increased over several weeks to 2 to 3 mg; or, 1 mg per kg intravenously 2 times a week, increased to 8 mg.

ACEDAPSONE (DADDS)

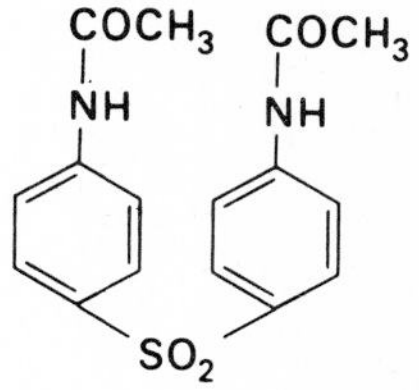

Longer-acting derivative.

In resistant malaria in combination with antimalarials

ACEDAPSONE DERIVATIVE (PSBA)

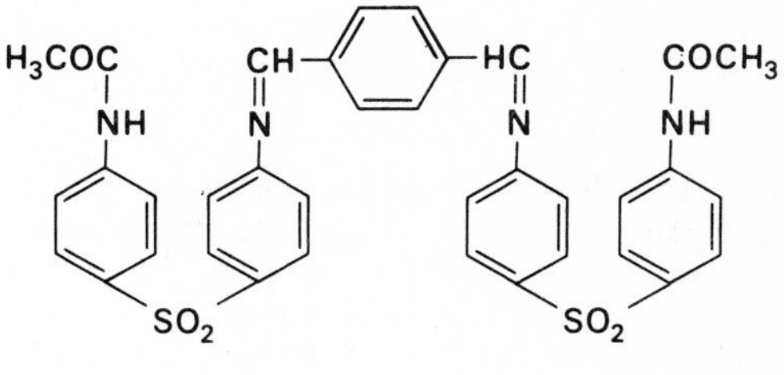

Produces a long, repository effect.

OBSOLETE SULFONES

Glucosulfone (Promin), hydroxyethylsulfone, acetosulfone sodium (Promacetin), sulfoxone (Diasone), thiazolsulfone (Promizole).

C. The Aminosalicylates

1. History. Lehmann (1946) introduced *p*-aminosalicyclic acid (PAS) for treatment of tuberculosis.

2. Chemistry. Analogues of *p*-aminobenzoic acid (PABA).

3. Action. a. Moderately antibacterial against the tubercle bacillus; not against other bacteria.

b. Exert an additive effect with streptomycin or isoniazid, presumably because different types of action involved; it has been suggested that one may make the bacterial wall penetrable to the other.

c. Resistance develops more slowly than with streptomycin; inhibition of growth by PAS lessens likelihood of mutation conferring streptomycin resistance; also bacterial line must make two mutations in order to become resistant to both drugs.

4. Mechanism. General assumption is that PAS competes with PABA, probably at the site of union of the pteridine nucleus with the rest of the molecule.

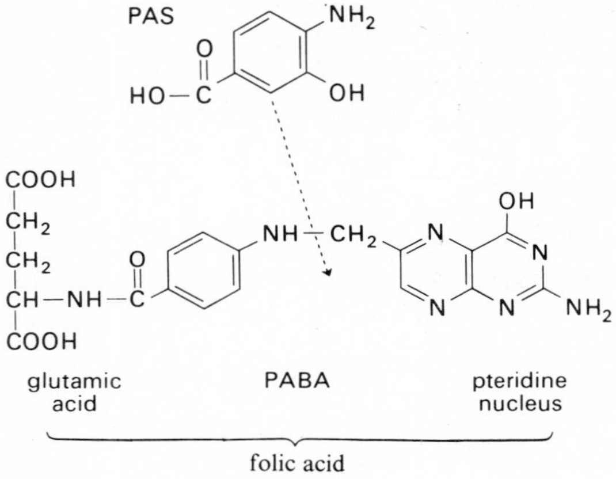

PAS

glutamic acid | PABA | pteridine nucleus

folic acid

5. Pharmacodynamics. Absorption is good by mouth; fair diffusion into spinal fluid. Excretion is satisfactory, via the renal tubules.

6. Toxicity. Highly unpleasant taste and gastric irritation make therapy difficult. Rare hypersensitivity; goiter; hepatitis.

7. Uses. PAS is widely used as a supplement to streptomycin, isoniazid, or other antituberculosis drugs. In addition to its antitubercle bacillus action, and its action to delay the emergence of resistant strains, it acetylates more readily than isoniazid, and thereby reduces the quantity of acetyl groups available to acetylate and inactivate isoniazid (Badger, New Eng. J. Med., 261:74, 1959).

8. Preparations

AMINOSALICYCLIC ACID (Pamisyl; Parasal; PAS)

Dose: 3 gm 4 times a day by mouth, commonly given as the Na, K, or Ca salt, to reduce gastric irritation.

Calcium aminosalicylate (Parasal calcium)
Potassium aminosalicylate (Parasal potassium)
Sodium aminosalicylate (Pamisyl sodium).

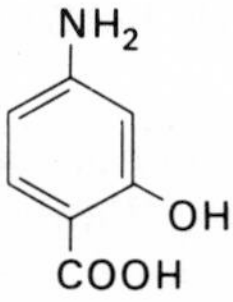

PHENYLAMINOSALICYLATE (Tebamin)

Absorbed intact from the intestine without gastric irritation; later split in the tissues to liberate PAS.

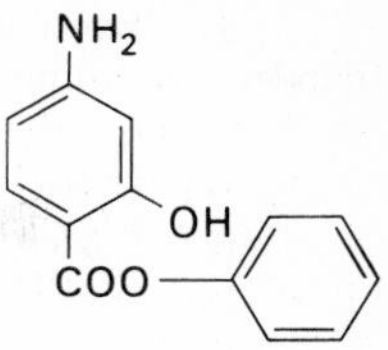

NH_2 … OH … COO

CALCIUM BENZOYLPAS (Benzapas)

Similar to phenyl-*p*-amino salicylate in action.

Dose: 3 gm 4 times a day by mouth.

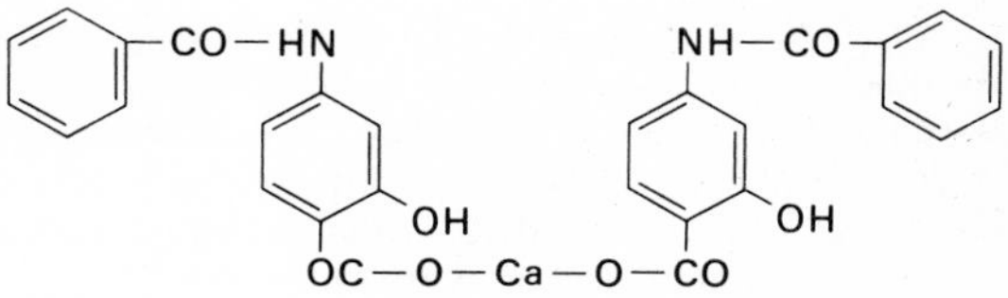

CO—HN … NH—CO … OH … OH … OC—O—Ca—O—CO

D. Pyridine Derivatives (Isoniazid)

1. History. a. Chorine (1945) tested pyridine and pyrimidine analogues of amithiozone and showed that nicotinamide had tuberculostatic activity.

b. Fox (1952) synthesized isoniazid.

2. Chemistry. Resemblance to other pyridines.

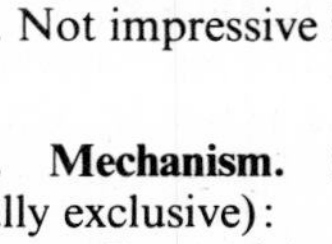

$CONH_2$ … N — nicotinamide

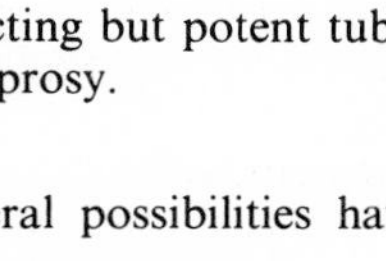

$CO—NH—NH_2$ … N — isoniazid

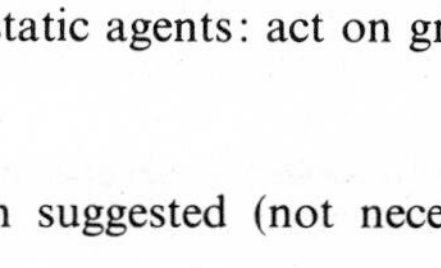

CHO … HO … CH_2OH … H_3C … N — pyridoxal

3. Action. Slowly acting but potent tuberculostatic agents: act on growing bacilli. Not impressive in leprosy.

4. Mechanism. Several possibilities have been suggested (not necessarily mutually exclusive):

a. Competition with pyridoxal.
b. Chelation of some metal essential to the tubercle bacillus.
c. Interference with nucleotide or porphyrin synthesis.
d. Inhibition in synthesis of a component (lipid?) in cell envelope.

5. Pharmacodynamics. a. Well absorbed by mouth.

b. Widely distributed, spinal fluid concentration about one-fourth that of blood.

c. Excretion adequate with ordinary doses.

d. Inactivated by acetylation in about one half of the patients; PAS may help by competing for the acetylation mechanism.

6. Toxicity. a. Mild euphoriant; vertigo, headache, dry mouth.

b. Toxicity is usually not severe, but large doses may produce excessive excitement or peripheral neuritis, which may be partially prevented by the simultaneous administration of pyridoxine, though this may possibly reduce effectiveness.

7. Uses. Current medicinal treatment of tuberculosis is almost always by combination of drugs, primarily because this delays the appearance of resistant bacteria. Any two of the three drugs, streptomycin, PAS, or isoniazid, may constitute such a combination, but many physicians believe that all plans should include isoniazid. Isoniazid and PAS, holding streptomycin in reserve, probably constitutes the most common basis of treatment.

8. Preparations

ISONIAZID (Nydrazid, INH, Rimifon, and others)

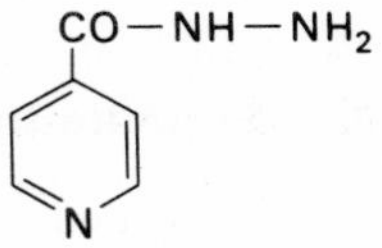

CO—NH—NH$_2$ (pyridine ring, N)

Dose: 1.5 to 2.5 mg per kg body weight by mouth or intramuscularly 2 times a day; usually accompanied by pyridoxine, 50 mg daily, to offset neurotoxicity.

ETHIONAMIDE (Trecator)

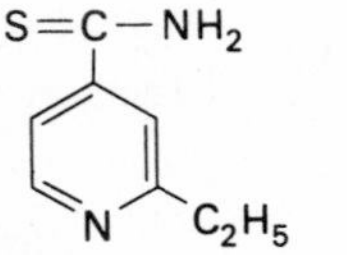

S=C—NH$_2$ (pyridine ring, N, C$_2$H$_5$)

Active against strains of the tubercle bacillus resistant to streptomycin, PAS, isoniazid, and kanamycin; but laboratory resistance can be developed to it.

Metabolized slowly. Toxicity may include stomatitis, severe abdominal discomfort, peripheral neuritis, mental disturbances, jaundice, gynecomastia, fetal abnormalities in pregnant women.

Used in tuberculosis when bacilli resistant or patient sensitive to other agents.

Dose: 0.5 to 1 gm by mouth daily.

E. Pyrazine Derivatives (Pyrazinamide)

1. History. Kushner (1952) introduced pyrazinamide.

2. Chemistry. Pyrazine analogue of nicotinamide.

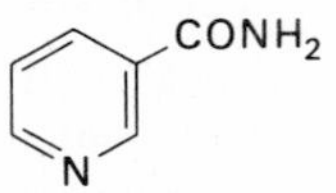

CONH$_2$ (ring, N) — nicotinamide

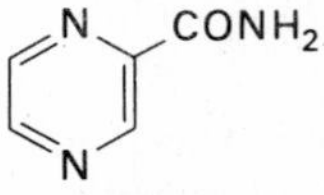

N, CONH$_2$ (ring, N) — pyrazinamide

3. Action on Bacteria. a. Moderately effective against the tubercle bacillus. b. Resistance develops rapidly, though delayed when given in combination with isoniazid only.

4. Mechanism. Probably by a mechanism similar to that of isoniazid.

5. Pharmacodynamics and Toxicity. Absorbed adequately. May produce hepatic damage and hyperuricemia.

6. Uses. A second line drug, but sometimes used for "surgical coverage" during and after an operation in a patient with streptomycin-isoniazid resistant disease.

7. Preparation

PYRAZINAMIDE (Aldinamide; PZA)

Dose: 3 gm by mouth daily for 2 weeks before and 2 weeks after the operation.

F. Other Compounds

ACETYL SULFAMETHOXYPYRIDAZINE (Kynex Acetyl)

Adjunct to sulfones in the treatment of leprosy (see Sulfonamides).

CAPREOMYCIN (Capastat)

From *Streptomyces capreolus*. Cyclic peptide.
Used to some extent in tuberculosis (with PAS) and leprosy.

CLOFAZIMINE

Under trial against both tuberculosis and leprosy. May cause skin pigmentation.

Dose: 100 to 300 mg per day by mouth.

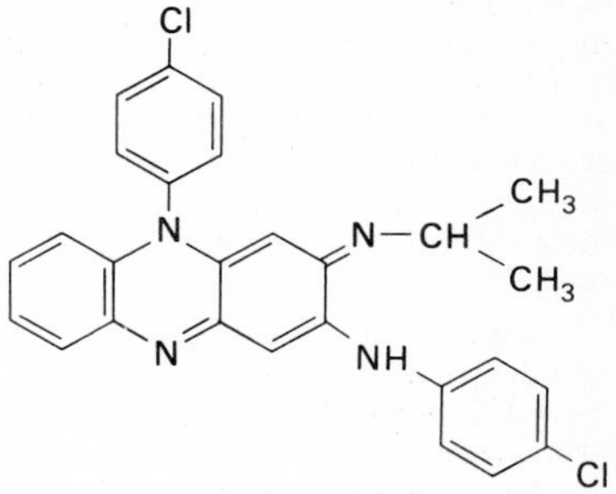

Cl

N

N

N—CH

CH_3

CH_3

NH

Cl

CYCLOSERINE (Oxamycin; Seromycin)

Derived from *Streptomyces orchidaceus*; competes with D-alanine as a cell wall precursor. Neurotoxicity, principally convulsions, in higher doses. In spite of low potency has had some use in tuberculosis, lepromatous leprosy, and urinary tract infections.

Dose: 250 mg daily by mouth.

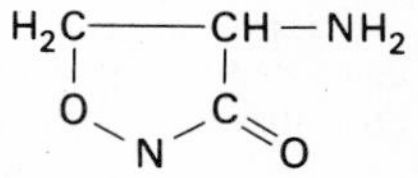

H_2C—CH—NH_2

O N C O

ETHAMBUTOL HYDROCHLORIDE (Myambutol)

Active against mycobacteria resistant to isoniazid and streptomycin. Orally comparable to isoniazid; parenterally to streptomycin. May cause reversible visual disturbances, including optic neuritis.

Dose 15 to 25 mg per kg body weight daily by mouth.

$$CH_3CH_2-\overset{H}{\underset{CH_2OH}{C}}-NHCH_2CH_2NH-\overset{CH_2OH}{\underset{H}{C}}-CH_2CH_3 \cdot 2HCl$$

ISOXYL (4,4′-diisoamyloxythiocarbanilide)

Promising in tuberculosis.
Dose: 0.5 gm daily by mouth.

RIFAMPIN (Rifadin)

Semisynthetic derived from rifamycin B, produced by *Streptomyces mediterranii.* Active against tubercle bacilli, leprosy, gram-negative and gram-positive bacteria, trachoma, vaccinia, and adenoviruses. Inhibits synthesis of RNA by binding directly to RNA polymerase; resistance may appear.

Absorption good by mouth. Toxicity includes increased SGOT, rash, leukopenia, thrombocytopenia, deafness. May diminish the effectiveness of glucocorticoids and estrogens (Buffington, G. A. et al, J.A.M.A., 236:1958, 1976).

Used in tuberculosis combined with isoniazid, ethambutol, or other agent.

Dose: 0.6 gm daily by mouth.

For parenteral use only.

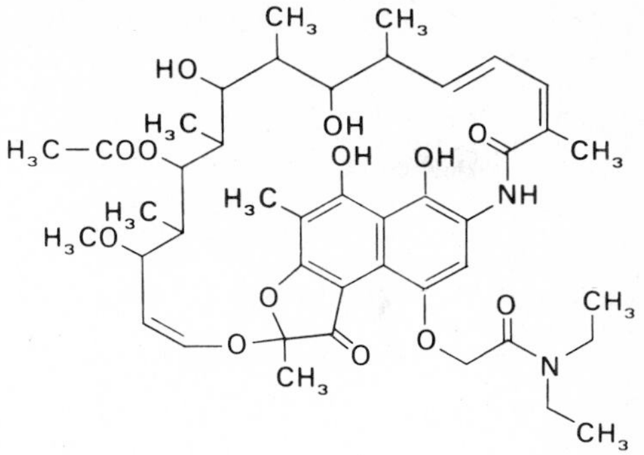

THALIDOMIDE

Effective against erythema nodosum in lepromatous leprosy; does not affect leprosy per se.

Dose: 100 mg 4 times a day by mouth (see Sedatives).

SUMMARY: THE STREPTOMYCIN GROUP: ANTITUBERCULOSIS AND ANTILEPROSY AGENTS

TYPE	*ACTION AND MECHANISM*	*TOXICITY*	*USE*	*EXAMPLES*
Streptomycin group	Active vs. gram-pos., gram-neg., tuberculosis Inhibit protein synthesis by interference with mRNA attachment to ribosome	Ototoxicity, nephrotoxicity, allergic sensitivity	Tuberculosis Severe gram-neg. infections Preparation for bowel surgery Amebiasis	Streptomycin
Sulfones	Bacteriostatic on tubercle and lepra bacilli Mechanism probably like that of sulfonamides	Dermatitis, hemolytic anemia	Leprosy	Dapsone
Aminosalicylates	Active vs. tbc Mechanism probably by competition with PABA	Bad taste	Tuberculosis	Aminosalicyclic acid
Pyridine derivatives	Tuberculostatic Mechanism uncertain	Excitement Neuritis	Tuberculosis	Isoniazid
Pyrazine derivatives	Probably similar	Hepatic damage Hyperuricemia	Tuberculosis	Pyrazinamide
Rifamycin group	Active vs. most bacteria	Rash, marrow damage	Tuberculosis	Rifampin

Reviews

D'Esopo, N. Present status of treatment of tuberculosis. Ann. N.Y. Acad. Sci., 106:85, 1963.

Robson, J. M., and Sullivan, F. M. Antituberculosis drugs. Pharmacol. Rev., 15:169, 1963.

Feingold, D. S. Antimicrobial chemotherapeutic agents: The nature of their action and selective toxicity. New Eng. J. Med., 269:900, 1963.

Burchall, J., Ferone, R., and Hitchings, G. Antibacterial chemotherapy. Ann. Rev. Pharmacol., 5:53, 1965.

Kunin, C. Effects of antibiotics on the gastrointestinal tract. Clin. Pharmacol. Ther., 8:495, 1967.

Shepard, C. Chemotherapy of leprosy. Ann. Rev. Pharmacol., 9:37, 1969.

6.
Polypeptide Antibiotics

The first modern antibiotic used clinically was tyrothricin, and it was probably in part this demonstration of the therapeutic possibilities of microbial substances that led to the reinvestigation of penicillin and its subsequent rapid introduction and use.

The polypeptide antibiotics differ from the groups previously considered both in their chemical nature and in their usual derivation from bacteria rather than molds. As a group they tend to be nonsensitizing, but to produce renal or other toxicity on systemic administration.

A. Agents Effective on Gram-Positive Bacteria

TYROTHRICIN

1. **History.** Dubos (1939) isolated the first preparations from *Bacillus brevis.*

2. **Chemistry.** Tyrothricin is a mixture of two cyclic decapeptides, gramicidin and tyrocidine. Gramicidin contains two unusual amino acids, L-ornithine and D-phenylalanine; tyrocidine also contains two D-phenylalanine groups.

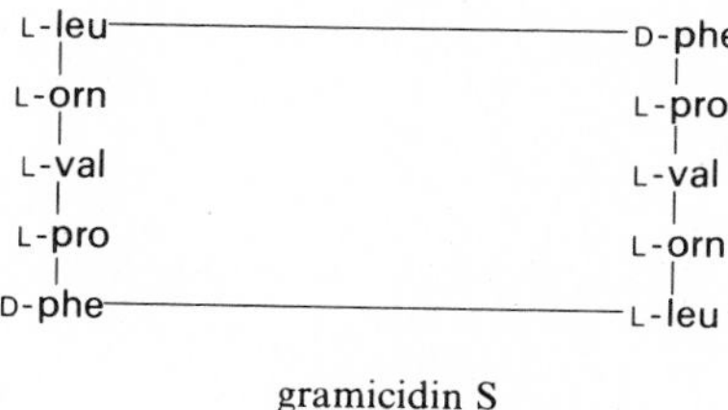

gramicidin S

3. **Action.** Bactericidal on gram-positive bacteria.

4. **Mechanism.** The basic polypeptides, positively charged, act as cationic detergents which damage cell membranes (see Antiseptics).

5. **Pharmacodynamics.** Not absorbed; ineffective orally.

6. **Toxicity.** Hemolytic on parenteral use. Allergically nonsensitizing.

7. Uses. Solutions and ointments used on body surfaces; solutions used to a limited extent in body cavities, especially the pleural cavity.

8. Preparation

TYROTHRICIN (Soluthricin)

Dose: Locally in solutions containing 500 mcg per ml.

BACITRACIN

1. History. Meleney (1945) isolated from *Bacillus subtilis.*

2. Chemistry. Complex polypeptide of suggested formula:

```
                        D-phe ———— L-his
                          |          |
                        L-ileu     L-asp — D-aspNH2
                          |          |
                        D-orn ———— L-lys
                                     |
H3C       NH2                      D-glu
   \       |         S ¬             |
    CH — CH ——— <    |             L-leu
   /                 N ————————————  C=O
H3C
```

bacitracin A

3. Action. Both gram-positive bacteria and amebae are susceptible.

4. Mechanism. Bacitracin inhibits the incorporation of amino acids into bacterial cell walls, with the accumulation of uridine nucleotides (resembling the action of penicillin).

5. Pharmacodynamics. Absorption poor by mouth.

6. Toxicity. Locally nonirritating and relatively nonsensitizing. Systemically may produce renal tubular necrosis.

7. Uses. a. Locally has had moderate use as a general antiinfective on the skin; it has been used by mouth in amebiasis.

b. It has also been used systemically in severe infections with penicillin-resistant organisms, but is ordinarily avoided because of its toxicity.

8. Preparation

BACITRACIN (Baciguent)

Dose: 500 units per ml locally; 25,000 units 4 times a day by mouth; 10,000 units or more 3 times daily intramuscularly; 10,000 to 20,000 units intrathecally.

B. Agents Active on Gram-Negative Bacteria

THE POLYMYXINS

1. History. a. Brownlee (1947) isolated from *Bacillus aerosporus* (also obtained from *Bacillus polymyxa*).

b. Koyama (1950) isolated colistin from *Aerobacillus colistinus.*

2. Chemistry. A number of polypeptides (A,B,C,D, and others), characteristically cyclic with a long fatty acid side chain.

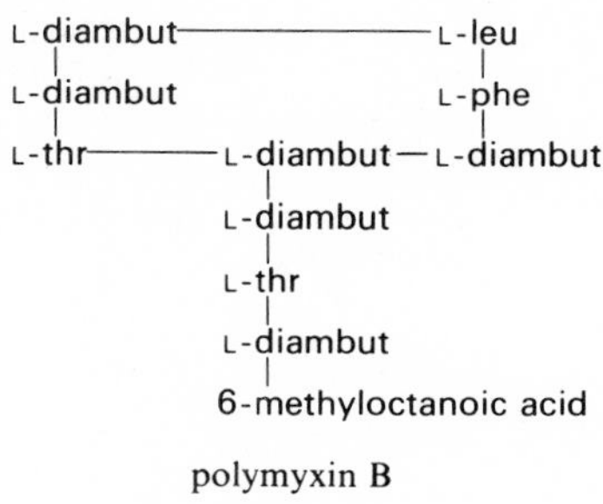

polymyxin B

3. Action. a. Potent bactericides against most gram-negative bacilli (except proteus); gram-positives and gram-negative cocci resistant.

b. Resistance slight and slow to develop; cross-resistance between polymyxins B and E.

4. Mechanism. a. Probably attach to anionic binding sites on cell membrane (Burchall, Ann. Rev. Pharmacol., 5:53, 1965).

b. Then damage cell membrane by surface effects, with disorganization of cell contents and final rupture.

5. Pharmacodynamics. a. Not absorbed by mouth; do not appear in spinal fluid after injection; blood levels low; urine levels high.

b. Partly inactivated in the presence of serum.

c. Rapidly excreted in the urine.

d. Colistin released from methanesulfonate complex slowly, with minor local irritation.

6. Toxicity. a. Polymyxins A and D may cause nausea, fever, and damage to renal tubules.

b. Polymyxins B and E are less toxic, but may cause bizarre neurological effects, including ataxia and paresthesias, and possibly renal damage with large doses.

c. All are relatively nonsensitizing.

7. Uses. a. Used effectively in pertussis, Friedländer's bacillus infection, tularemia, brucellosis, bacterial diarrheas, pseudomonas infections, and urinary tract infections, but customarily only in severe infections not responsive to less toxic agents; also locally.

b. The low blood levels limit systemic effect, but concentrations are adequate in urine or, after local injection, in spinal fluid.

8. Preparations

COLISTIMETHATE SODIUM (polymyxin E; Coly-Mycin M Intramuscular)

Dose: 2 to 5 mg per kg daily intramuscularly in 2 to 4 divided doses.

COLISTIN SULFATE (Coly-Mycin S oral suspension)

For the oral treatment of enteritis in infants and children.

Dose: 3 to 5 mg per kg body weight of a suspension by mouth daily, divided into 3 doses.

POLYMYXIN B SULFATE (Aerosporin)

Dose: 1.5 to 2.5 mg per kg body weight daily intramuscularly, divided into 3 doses; 0.1% to 0.25% locally; 5 mg intrathecally daily.

Polymyxin methane sulfonate

SULFOMYXIN (Dynamyxin)

Mixture of polymyxins.

SUMMARY: THE POLYPEPTIDE ANTIBIOTICS

TYPE	*ACTION AND MECHANISM*	*TOXICITY*	*USE*	*EXAMPLES*
Gram-positive	Cationic detergents Disrupt cell membranes Act on gram-pos. bacteria	Hemolytic, nephrotoxic	Local irrigations and ointments	Tyrothricin, bacitracin
The polymyxins	Active vs. gram-neg. bacteria Same as above	Nephrotoxic neurotoxic	Severe gram-neg. systemic infections	Polymyxin

Review

Barber, M., and Chain, E. B. Antibacterial Chemotherapy. Ann. Rev. Pharmacol., 4:115, 1964.

7. Other Antibacterials

A. Nitrofurans

1. History. Dodd and Stillman (1944) showed the bactericidal property of furan derivatives.

2. Chemistry. A series of stable derivatives of 5-nitro-2-furaldehyde. The 5-NO_2 group is essential for activity.

3. Action. a. Bacteriostatic or bactericidal against most gram-positive and gram-negative bacteria; most strains of pseudomonas are rather insensitive.
b. Bacterial resistance is negligible.

4. Mechanism. a. Crucial mechanism not defined; principal evidence is for inhibition of the formation of acetyl coenzyme A from pyruvic acid, impairing energy production, as indicated in the suggested sequence:

```
                                                 probable site of inhibition
                                                     ↓
glucose → hexose      → triose      → pyruvate → acetyl → Krebs
          phosphates    phosphates                S-CoA    cycle
```

b. Inhibition of dehydrogenase systems has also been suggested as a possible mechanism.
c. DNA synthesis depressed.

5. Pharmacodynamics. a. Nitrofurantoin is readily absorbed by mouth; excreted in the urine at antibacterial levels.
b. Furazolidone is poorly absorbed after oral administration.

6. Toxicity. Sensitization may occur from topical or systemic use.

7. Uses. a. Nitrofurazone is used locally as an ointment or solution in bacterial infections of skin, including wounds and burns, conjunctivae, bladder, and other cavities.
b. Nitrofurantoin is used as an antibacterial agent in the urinary tract.
c. Furazolidone has been used as an intestinal antibacterial agent.

8. Preparations

NITROFURAZONE (Furacin)

Dose: 0.02% to 0.2% in solutions; 0.2% to 1% in ointments.

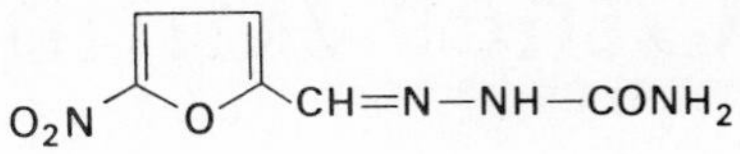

NITROFURANTOIN (Furadantin)

Dose: 50 to 100 mg 4 times a day by mouth.

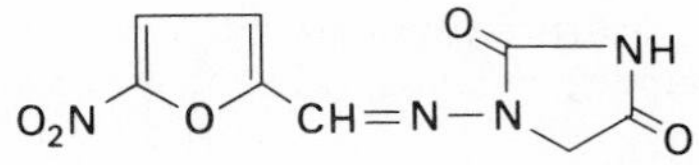

FURAZOLIDONE (Furoxone)

Dose: 100 mg 4 times a day by mouth. for intestinal infections.

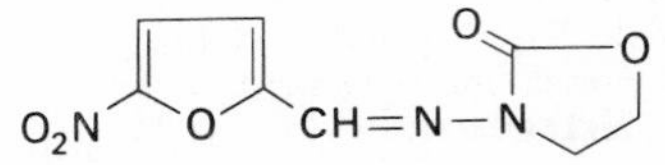

OTHERS

Furalazine, levolfuraltadone, nifuradene, nifuraldezone, nifuratel, nifuratrone, nifurdazil, nifurimide, nifurmerone, nifurpirinol, nifurquinazol, nifursemizone, nifursol, nifurthiazole.

B. Methenamine and Mandelic Acid

METHENAMINE MANDELATE

1. History. Methenamine has been known since 1860. Rosenheim (1935) introduced mandelic acid.

2. Chemistry. A combination of methenamine and mandelic acid.

3. Action. a. Moderately effective against most urinary pathogens when the urine can be brought to pH 5.5 or lower.

b. Ineffective in infections with ammonia-producing bacteria (*Proteus vulgaris*); usually ineffective in infections with *Pseudomonas aeruginosa* (pyocyaneus).

4. Mechanism. a. The methenamine and mandelic acid act separately but additively.

b. Methenamine, a condensation product of formaldehyde and ammonia, liberates formaldehyde in the presence of acid and thus is antibacterial.

c. Mandelic acid is excreted unchanged and is antibacterial in an acid urine. However, in ordinary dosage the action is primarily to contribute to the acidification of the urine.

5. Pharmacodynamics and Toxicity. a. Absorbed well, although part of the formaldehyde is liberated in the stomach.

b. Toxicity minor but there may be gastric irritation and nausea.

6. Uses. a. In urinary tract infections. Generally somewhat less active than the sulfonamides, but a useful alternative.

b. Should be given with ammonium chloride or other acidifiers to maintain urinary pH below 5.5.

7. Preparations

METHENAMINE MANDELATE (Mandelamine)

Dose: 1 gm 3 to 4 times a day. As the dose of mandelic acid when used alone is 12 gm daily, methenamine mandelate does not represent intensive therapy with mandelic acid.

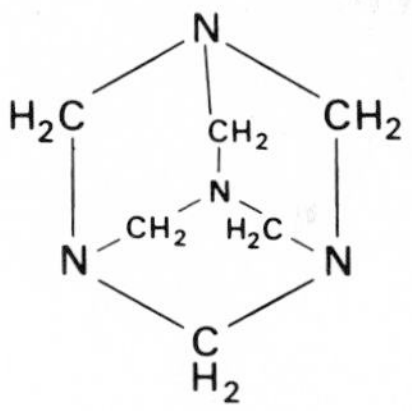

methenamine

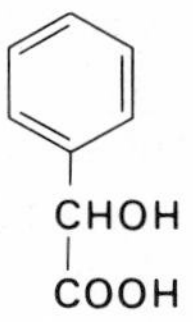

mandelic acid

METHENAMINE HIPPURATE (Hippramine)

Similar to methenamine mandelate.

C. Naphthyridine Derivatives

1. Chemistry. A naphthyridine derivative; described by Lesher (1962).

2. Action and Mechanism. a. Active against most gram-negatives: coliforms, proteus, aerobacter, klebsiella, typhoid, dysentery; pseudomonas resistant; others may develop resistance.

b. Inhibits synthesis of DNA, or cross links strands (Rosenkranz, Proc. Soc. Exp. Biol. Med., 120:549, 1965).

3. Pharmacodynamics and Toxicity. a. Effective orally or parenterally; excreted rapidly in urine (maximum at 6 hours).

b. May cause nausea, gastric distress, pruritis, chills.

4. Uses. Used against gram-negative infections, both systemic and urinary (Lishman, Brit. J. Urol., 35:116, 1963).

5. Preparation

NALIDIXIC ACID (NegGram; Wintomylon)

Dose: 0.5 gm every 4 hours by mouth.

Sodium nalidixate

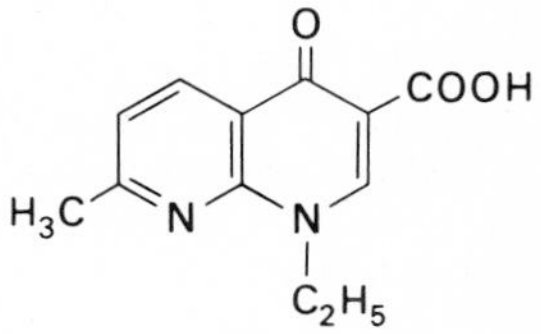

D. Others

OXOLINIC ACID (Utibid)

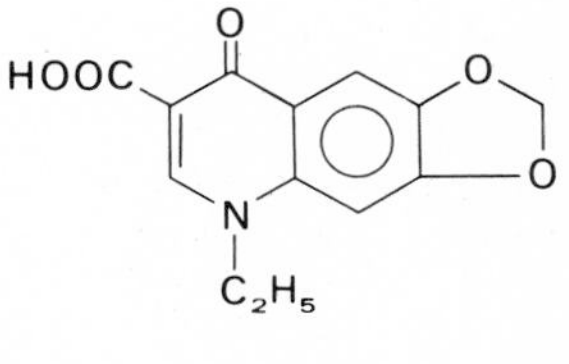

PHENAZOPYRIDINE HYDROCHLORIDE (Pyridium)

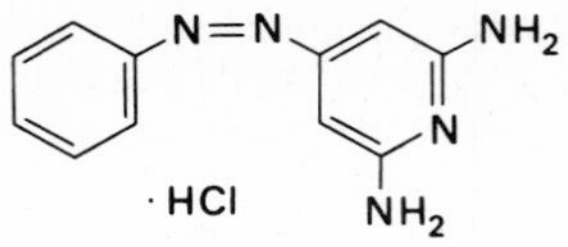

A diazo dye, ineffective chemotherapeutically, but possibly exerting an analgesic effect.

Dose: 200 mg daily by mouth.

ORMETOPRIM (in Rofenaid)

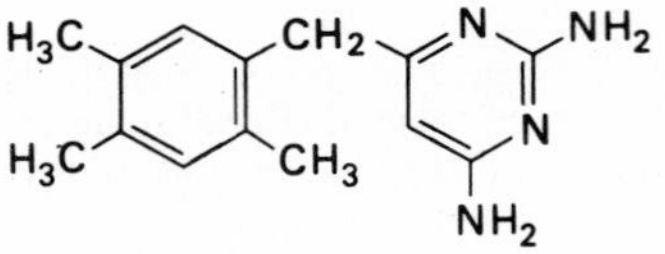

Antibacterial.

SUMMARY: OTHER ANTIBACTERIAL AGENTS

TYPE	*ACTION AND MECHANISM*	*TOXICITY*	*USE*	*EXAMPLES*
Nitrofurans	Active vs. most bacteria Mechanism uncertain	Sensitization	Antibacterial in urinary tract, skin, and other areas	Nitrofurantoin
Methenamine	Antibacterial Liberates formaldehyde in presence of acid	Minor	Urinary tract infections	Methenamine mandelate
Naphthyridines	Active vs. most gram-neg.	Nausea, pruritis convulsions	Against gram-neg. infections, especially of urinary tract	Nalidixic acid

8.
Antifungal Agents

Although iodides are still used for their nonspecific liquefying effects on granulomas, most systemic fungous infections remained resistant to chemotherapy for a considerable period after antibacterial therapy was well established. The principal exception was actinomycosis, which is quite responsive to sulfonamides, penicillin, and streptomycin. The situation is now changed, and potent therapy is possible in a number of systemic diseases caused by fungi.

A. The Polyene Group

1. History. a. Nystatin isolated by Hazen and Brown (1950) from *Streptomyces noursei.*

b. Amphotericin B (introduced 1958) isolated from *Streptomyces nodosus.*

c. Candicidin isolated from *Streptomyces griseus.*

2. Chemistry. a. The polyenes contain aliphatic rings or chains with unsaturation (—CH=CH—CH=CH—); vitamin A is a common example.

b. Empirical formula for nystatin $C_{46}H_{83}NO_{18}$; for amphotericin B (a heptaene) $C_{17}H_{73}NO_{20}$.

3. Action. a. Active against various fungi and yeast, including *Candida albicans*, *Coccidioides immitis*, and the organisms of blastomycosis and histoplasmosis; ineffective against bacteria and actinomycetes.

b. Laboratory resistance has been developed in several fungi, with cross resistance between nystatin and amphotericin B.

4. Mechanism. a. Fungistatic rather than fungicidal.

b. Inhibit selective permeability of cell membrane by specific affinity for sterols (50:1) in cells that do not have a rigid capsule or wall (fungal protoplasts; protozoa).

c. As a result of the changed permeability, protein leaks from the cell, and it may lyse (Ghosh, Antibiot. Chemother. (N.Y.), 12:204, 1962).

5. Pharmacodynamics. a. Most poorly soluble; oral absorption nil or minimal.

b. After injection excretion is slow; blood levels of amphotericin B may be measurable for 18 hours after a single intravenous dose.

6. Toxicity. a. Oral administration relatively nontoxic; occasional nausea, diarrhea.

b. Parenteral administration may be toxic, probably because of damage to cell walls similar to that upon fungi: fever, chills, anorexia, vomiting; cardiac depression, hypokalemia, hemolysis; renal damage, indicated by a rising blood urea, may be reversible.

7. Uses. a. Nystatin is used orally for intestinal moniliasis, and topically for stomatitis and vaginitis of monilial origin.

b. Amphotericin B is more stable than nystatin in aqueous preparations, and somewhat more active against monilia, and has the same local uses as nystatin.

c. Amphotericin B is probably the best agent to date for coccidioidomycosis, North and South American blastomycosis (hydroxystilbamidine an alternative), histoplasmosis, cryptococcosis, chromoblastosis, sporotrichosis, and systemic candidiasis.

d. Candicidin is used topically for vaginal moniliasis.

8. Preparations

AMPHOTERICIN B (Fungizone)

Dose: 1 mg per kg body weight daily intravenously for 1 to 2 months (given slowly in 5% dextrose solution stabilized with desoxycholate); 2 to 10 mg per day by mouth but relatively ineffective; 3% locally.

CANDICIDIN (Candeptin)

Dose: 3 mg in suppository or ointment locally in the vagina twice daily for 14 days.

FILIPIN

From *Streptomyces filipenenisis.*

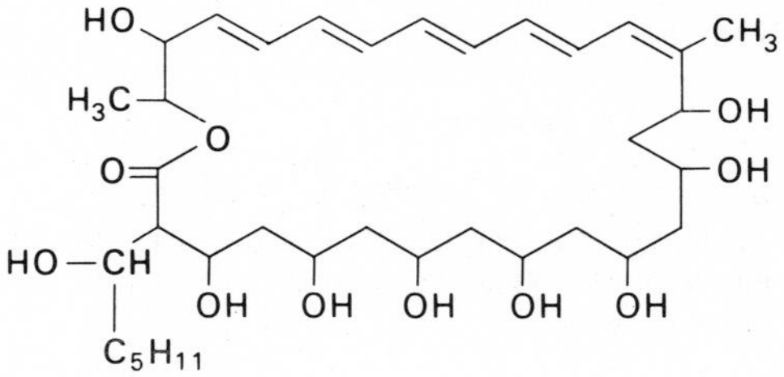

FUNGIMYCIN (Perimycin)

Antifungal antibiotic of heptaene type derived from *Streptomyces coelicolor* var. *aminophilus.*

NYSTATIN (Mycostatin)

Dose: 500,000 to 1,000,000 units 3 times a day by mouth; locally in suspensions containing 100,000 units per ml.

B. Griseofulvin

1. History. Formerly (1939) tried as an agricultural fungicide.

2. Chemistry. Derived from *Penicillium griseofulvin.*

3. Action. a. Effective against species of *Microsporon*, *Epidermophyton*, and *Trichophyton*.

b. Ineffective in blastomycosis, moniliasis, chromoblastosis, histoplasmosis, actinomycosis, coccidioidomycosis.

c. Resistance has not been demonstrated.

4. Mechanism. Deposited in the keratin precursor cells, rendering the keratin resistant to fungi in skin infections.

5. Pharmacodynamics. Absorbed satisfactorily by mouth. Excreted rapidly, in hours.

6. Toxicity. a. Relatively nontoxic, but headache, insomnia, nausea, and mild rashes have been observed.

b. Occasional severe reaction resembling serum sickness, with fever and joint pains.

c. Leukopenia has been reported, and large doses in experimental animals depress the hematopoietic system.

d. In animals, interference with mitosis (similar to colchicine) and spermatogenesis have been noted.

e. Carcinogenic in mice.

7. Uses. a. Unique agent; first means of oral treatment of mycotic infections of hair, nails, and skin (ringworm).

b. Effective in tinea capitis, corporis, unguium and pedis, favus, and other mycotic infections.

c. Adjunctive use of local keratolytic or desquamating preparations may be necessary.

8. Preparation

GRISEOFULVIN (Fulvicin; Grifulvin)

Dose: 1 to 2 mg daily by mouth for 1 to 3 months; micronized formulation, 125 to 150 mg four times a day.

H_3CO O OCH_3 =O H_3CO O Cl CH_3

C. Flucytosine

1. Chemistry. Structure similar to 5–fluorouracil (5–FU), an antimetabolite to uracil.

2. Action. Effective against candida and cryptococcus.

3. Mechanism. Assumed to be converted in the fungus to 5–FU and acts as an antimetabolite.

4. Pharmacodynamics. Absorbed by mouth. No significant metabolism; excreted by the kidneys.

5. Toxicity. Nausea, vomiting, diarrhea, rash, bone marrow depression (leucopenia, thrombopenia, anemia), liver and kidney damage.

6. Uses. In serious systemic infections.

7. Preparation

FLUCYTOSINE (Ancobon)

Dose: 50 to 150 mg per kg per day.

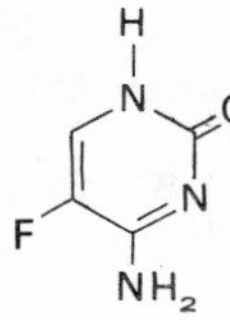

H N O N F NH$_2$

D. Other Systemic Antifungal Agents

Aromatic diamidines (hydroxystilbamidine), azaserine, cycloheximide (Actidione), denofungin, ethyl vanillate, flucytosine (Ancobon), hamycin, kalafungin, lomofungin, lydimycin, nifungin, scopafungin, viridofulvin.

E. Local Fungicides

1. Action. Exfoliating agents or superficial fungicides.

2. Uses. In various types of fungal infections, ringworm and dermatophytosis.

3. Preparations

CAPRYLIC COMPOUND (sod. and zinc caprylate); ZINC UNDECYLENATE: $CH_2=CH(CH_2)_8COOH \cdot \frac{1}{2}Zn$; ZINC UNDECATE (undecylenic acid and zinc salt; Desenex)

Bland powders of little use in epidermatophytosis.

CHLORDANTOIN (Sporostacin)

Used in vulvovaginal moniliasis; fungal infections of the skin; 1% in cream, lotions, solutions.

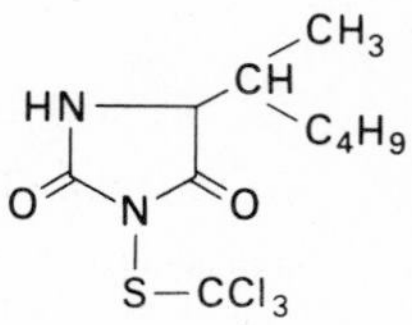

CH$_3$ CH HN C$_4$H$_9$ O N O S—CCl$_3$

CLOTRIMAZOLE

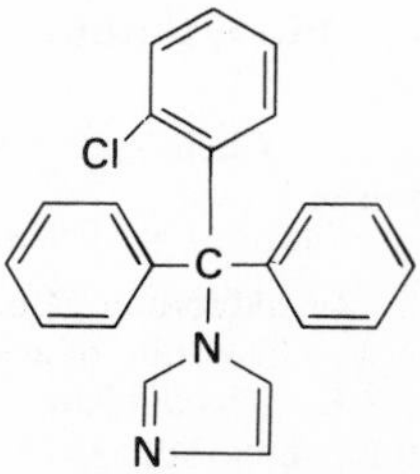

Cl C N N

ETHONAM NITRATE

Local fungicide against various dermatophytes.

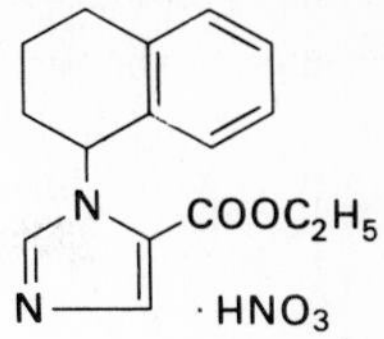

MICONAZOLE NITRATE

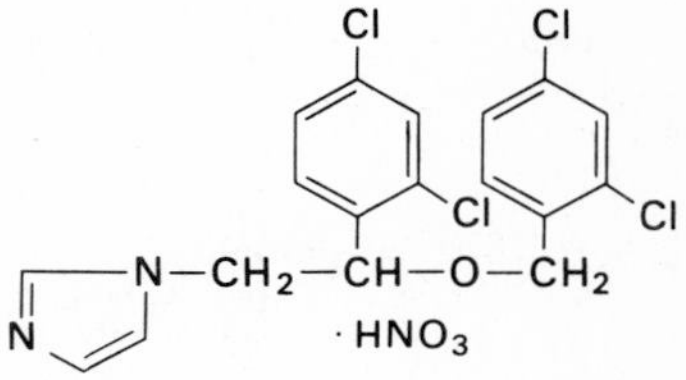

PYRROLNITRIN

From *Pseudomonas aureofaciens*

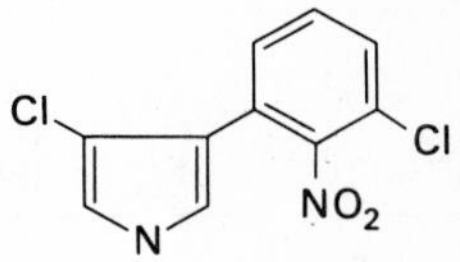

SALICYLIC ACID

Exfoliative and antiseptic fungicide.

Dose: 6% locally in ointment; with 12% benzoic acid in benzoic and salicylic ointment (Whitfield's ointment).

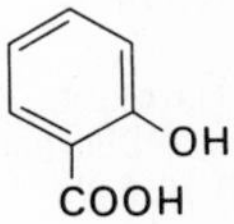

TICLATONE (Landromil)

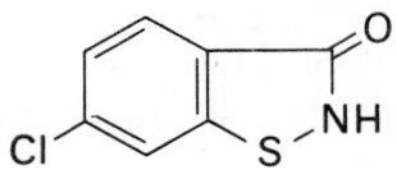

TOLNAFTATE (Tinactin)

Topical antifungal.

Dose: 0.1 to 0.2 ml of 1% solution locally.

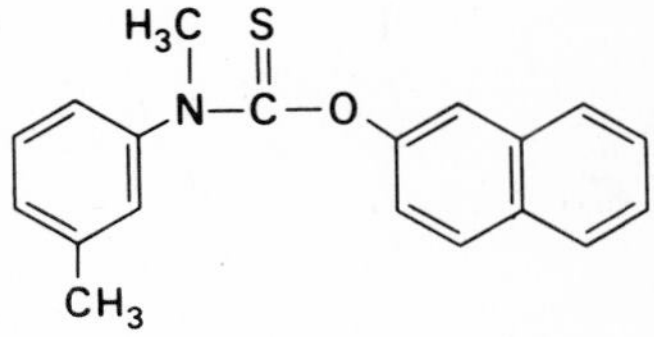

TRIACETIN (Enzactin)

Introduced in 1956 as a typical agent for dermatomycoses; acts by slow liberation of acetic acid; of dubious value.

$CH_2OOC{-}CH_3$
$CH{-}OOC{-}CH_3$
$CH_2OOC{-}CH_3$

ZINC PYRITHIONE (Zinc Omadine)

Fungicide and bactericide; used in shampoos.

$$\left[\text{pyridine } N\text{-oxide}\!-\!S- \right]_2 Zn$$

SUMMARY: ANTIFUNGAL AGENTS

TYPE	*ACTION AND MECHANISM*	*TOXICITY*	*USE*	*EXAMPLES*
The polyenes	Fungistatic vs. various fungi and yeasts Inhibit permeability of cell membranes by attachment to sterols	Systemic: fever, hypokalemia, hemolysis, renal damage	Moniliasis, systemic mycoses	Amphotericin B
Griseofulvin	Effective vs. local skin fungi Make keratin resistant to fungi	Fever, joint pains, leukopenia	Oral treatment of mycoses of hair, nails, skin	Griseofulvin

Reviews

Harrell, E. F., and Bocobo, F. C. Modern treatment of the systemic fungus diseases. Clin. Pharmacol. Ther., 1:104, 1960.

Utz, J. P. Current concepts in therapy: Chemotherapeutic agents for the systemic mycoses. New Eng. J. Med., 268:938, 1963.

Giorlando, S., Torres, J., and Muscillo, G. New antifungal antibiotic preparation. Amer. J. Obst. Gynec., 90:370, 1964.

Butler, W. T. Pharmacology, toxicity and therapeutic usefulness of amphotericin B. J.A.M.A., 195:127, 1966.

Kinsky, S. Antibiotic interaction with model membranes. Ann. Rev. Pharmacol., 10:119, 1970.

9.
Antimalarial Agents

Malaria continues to be a disease of great consequence despite several effective drugs. This is in part because of the development of resistance of parasites to drugs, and in part because of the complexity of the disease.

When a mosquito injects sporozoites into a victim they enter the tissues, especially the liver, and emerge as merozoites to parasitize red cells. The schizont cycle from red cell to red cell provokes the chills and ague of clinical disease. These schizont forms may be killed by the therapeutic drugs quinine, chloroquine, or chloroguanide, and the acute attack ended. Or these drugs may act as suppressives, preventing the schizonts from appearing. If continued for a time after exposure they may also be curative of falciparum malaria, but not of vivax malaria in which tissue forms are not extinguished and may reseed the blood. The cure of vivax malaria may require drugs of the primaquine group, which eradicate tissue forms.

A. Quinine Alkaloids

1. History. a. Cinchona bark was imported from South America into Europe as early as 1647, although doubt has been expressed of the truth of the legend of the cure of the Countess of Chinchon in 1638.

b. Quinine and other alkaloids were isolated from the bark by Pelletier and Caventou in 1820.

c. Quinine was synthesized by Woodward and Doering in 1944.

2. Chemistry. a. Two isomeric pairs of alkaloids exist in cinchona bark: quinine and quinidine, and cinchonine and cinchonidine.

b. All are quinoline derivatives.

3. Action. Antimalarial against asexual and erythrocytic forms; also neuromuscular inhibitor.

4. Mechanism. Underlying mechanism not clarified, but may involve interference in oxidation of glucose.

5. Pharmacodynamics. a. Absorption by mouth good.

b. Distributed widely in tissues, including the liver.

c. Most of the drug is destroyed in the body, but a portion is excreted in the urine.

6. Toxicity. a. Cinchonism, characterized by impaired hearing, tinnitus, vertigo, and nausea.

b. Massive overdosage may produce cardiac depression.

c. Hypersensitivity reactions not uncommon.

7. Uses. a. Quinine is the oldest effective suppressant and therapeutic agent in malaria, but has now been almost altogether replaced by chloroquine and other newer drugs. In emergency situations, as in cerebral malaria, the soluble hydrochloride allows rapid therapy, which may be lifesaving. Quinine may be used against malaria resistant to chloroquine, but unfortunately strains resistant to quinine are also appearing.

b. Quinine's action of neuromuscular inhibition is used to inhibit night cramps in elderly people, and also may have some usefulness in myotonia congenita.

c. It has been used as a bitter, and as a sclerosing agent.

d. Weak antiarrhythmic, only of historic interest.

8. Preparations

QUININE SULFATE

Dose: 0.4 gm by mouth daily (suppressive); 0.6 to 1 gm 3 times a day by mouth (therapeutic).

N

OCH_3

CHOH

$\cdot H_2SO_4$

$N \cdot CH_2CH_2$

$CH{=}CH_2$

Quinine hydrochloride

Dose: 0.6 gm intravenously.

B. Acridines and 4-Aminoquinolines (Chloroquine Group)

1. History. a. Ehrlich (1891) found that the thionine dye, methylene blue, had antimalarial action.

b. Mauss and Mietsch (1933) synthesized, and Kikuth (1938) introduced quinacrine.

c. Chloroquine was synthesized in Germany in 1934, but more fully developed under the incentive of World War II by the OSRD program in the United States (1944).

2. Chemistry. Quinacrine is an acridine derivative and chloroquine the analogous 4-aminoquinoline derivative.

3. Action. a. Active antimalarials against the asexual and erythrocytic forms of the parasites; thus similar to quinine in scope.

b. Ameliorate autoimmune diseases, possibly by suppression of antigen formation.

c. Cardiac depressants in arrhythmias.

4. Mechanism. a. Quinacrine inactivates DNA by combining with it 1:4 stoichiometrically. In the complex the absorption spectrum of quinacrine is altered, and the viscosity of the DNA increases and it becomes resistant to DNAase. Chloroquine is similar but requires more drug per unit DNA (Kurnick, J. Lab. Clin. Med., 60:669, 1962).

b. Mechanism of greater susceptibility of malaria parasites than host cells probably involves inhibition of parasite DNA replication, but there is also damage to digestive and pigment vesicles (lysosomes); vesicles coalesce and may be extruded; effect greatest in vesicles where hemoglobin is being digested (Warhurst, Nature, 214: 935, 1967; Macomber, Nature, 214: 937, 1967).

c. In autoimmune disease, suggested mechanism is removal of autogenous DNA to which patient is sensitive (Levin, New Eng. J. Med., 264: 535, 1961).

d. Another effect, possibly secondary to inactivation of DNA, is inhibition of polysaccharide synthesis (Whitehouse, Nature, 94: 984, 1962).

5. Pharmacodynamics. a. Well absorbed by oral or parenteral routes.

b. Distribution markedly localized to leucocytes, liver, spleen, heart, and lungs.

c. Excreted slowly in the urine over several days.

6. Toxicity. a. Not highly toxic, but may produce anorexia, nausea, diarrhea, headache, blurred vision, pruritis.

b. Quinacrine more toxic than the aminoquinoline derivatives and may produce temporary mental symptoms and yellowness of the skin.

c. Chloroquine has caused retinitis and blindness (Okun, Arch. Ophth., 65:59, 1963) in prolonged treatment (500 gm total), as in rheumatoid arthritis; also eighth nerve damage with deafness and imbalance.

7. Uses. a. Most useful drugs for suppression of malaria and termination of acute attacks; no action against exoerythrocytic forms in the liver or other tissues. However, the preeminent position is being threatened by the appearance of resistant strains.

b. Also useful against other protozoa, especially giardia and amebae (chloroquine).

c. Anthelmintic against tapeworms (quinacrine).

d. In autoimmune diseases. Rheumatoid arthritis, lupus erythematosus (local and possibly systemic), and other light sensitive dermatoses. Several weeks of therapy necessary before anti-inflammatory effects develop, but may allow replacement or reduction of dosage of corticosteroids, phenylbutazone, or gold salts.

8. Preparations

AMODIAQUIN HYDROCHLORIDE (Camoquin)

Infrequent nausea and vomiting; skin pigmentation (melanosis) reported. Used similarly to chloroquine as an antimalarial.

Dose: 0.6 gm by mouth daily (suppressive); 1.2 gm by mouth followed in 6 hours by 0.6 gm, then 0.6 gm daily for 2 days (therapeutic).

Cl N ·HCl NH CH_2N C_2H_5 C_2H_5 OH

CHLOROQUINE PHOSPHATE or DIPHOSPHATE (Aralen)

The most generally used antimalarial; also used in giardiasis and tissue amebiasis (see Amebicides), and in connective tissue disease.

Dose: 0.5 gm once weekly by mouth (suppressive); 1.0 gm by mouth followed in 6 hours by 0.5 gm, then 0.5 gm once daily for 2 days (therapeutic) in malaria; 0.2 to 0.3 gm intramuscularly. Prophylactic for resistant malaria: 500 mg plus 45 mg primaquine weekly, and 25 mg dapsone daily.

Cl, N, NH, $CHCH_2CH_2CH_2N(C_2H_5)_2$, CH_3, $\cdot 2H_3PO_4$

HYDROXYCHLOROQUINE SULFATE (Plaquenil)

May produce less gastrointestinal distress than chloroquine. Possibly weaker as an antimalarial than chloroquine but preferred in some reports for connective tissue diseases.

Dose: 0.5 gm, then 0.4 gm in 6 hours, and 0.4 gm on each of 2 successive days by mouth (antimalarial); 0.4 to 0.6 gm by mouth daily, initially, reduced gradually to maintenance dose of 0.2 to 0.4 gm daily or 1 or 2 times a week (connective tissue diseases).

Cl, N, NH, $CHCH_2CH_2CH_2N(C_2H_4OH)(C_2H_5)$, CH_3, $\cdot H_2SO_4$

QUINACRINE HYDROCHLORIDE (Atabrine, Mepacrine)

Largely replaced by chloroquine as an antimalarial, but used in tapeworm infestation (see Anthelmintics), in amebiasis (see Amebiasis), and in connective tissue disease.

Dose: 0.1 gm daily by mouth (suppressive); 0.2 gm 4 times on first day, then 0.1 gm 3 times a day for 6 days (therapeutic) in malaria.

Cl, N, OCH_3, NH, $CHCH_2CH_2CH_2N(C_2H_5)_2$, CH_3, $\cdot HCl$

OTHERS: Amquinate, Mefloquine

C. Biguanides and Phenylaminopyrimidines

1. History. a. Curd and Rose (1942) synthesized biguanide series.
b. Davey (1945) introduced to clinical use.

c. Hitchings (1949) developed pyrimethamine while studying drugs with anticancer effect.

2. Chemistry. Phenylaminopyrimidines in which the pyrimidine ring may be opened producing a biguanide.

3. Action. a. Act against asexual erythrocytic forms by inhibiting chromatin division in schizonts, thus preventing the appearance of merozoites.

b. Lesser action against tissue forms, but approach causal prophylaxis against *P. falciparum:* little action on gametocytes.

c. Plasmoidal resistance frequently develops early and easily; cross resistance between members.

4. Mechanism. a. Interference with reductases that convert folic acid into folinic acid, thus impairing the production of purine and pyrimidine bases needed for nucleic acid synthesis.

b. Reason for greater sensitivity of malarial parasites than of man not clear.

5. Pharmacodynamics. a. Absorbed slowly by mouth.

b. Distributed widely, but with localization in red and white blood cells, kidneys, and liver.

c. Excreted slowly by the kidneys, in part unchanged.

d. Cycloguanil is a metabolite of chloroguanide (and may be the active form).

6. Toxicity. a. Minimal, but may produce nausea, vomiting, diarrhea.

b. High doses of pyrimethamine may cause dermatitis, marrow depression, and convulsions.

7. Uses. a. Chloroguanide is almost an all-around antimalarial, but fails to prevent infection with vivax malaria, or to terminate it. Little used in the United States.

b. Pyrimethamine acts too slowly for therapy in acute episodes of malaria, but is a valuable suppressant. It also has been reported to be of value in toxoplasmosis, with side effects reduced by simultaneous use of folinic acid.

c. Development of resistance a drawback.

8. Preparations

CHLOROGUANIDE HYDROCHLORIDE
(proguanil; Paludrine)

Dose: 0.3 gm by mouth weekly (suppressive); 0.1 gm 3 times a day by mouth for 10 days (therapeutic).

$$Cl-C_6H_4-NH-C(=NH)-NH-C(=NH)-NH-CH(CH_3)_2 \cdot HCl$$

CHLORPROGUANIL (Lapudrine)

Similar to chloroguanide, but longer acting.

Dose: 20 mg by mouth once weekly.

$$Cl_2C_6H_3-NH-C(=NH)-NH-C(=NH)-NH-CH(CH_3)_2$$

CYCLOGUANIL

Insoluble salt; long acting (up to 6 months), but rapid excretion limits toxicity. May be a valuable suppressant. Also useful in leishmaniasis.

Cycloguanil pamoate (Camolar)

Dose: 2 to 5 mg per kg body weight intramuscularly.

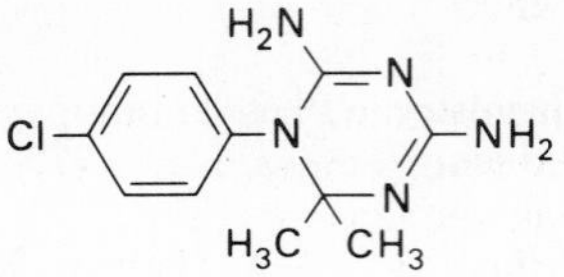

PYRIMETHAMINE (Daraprim)

Dose: 0.25 mg by mouth weekly (suppressive) in malaria. Has been used in combination with quinine in resistant malaria.

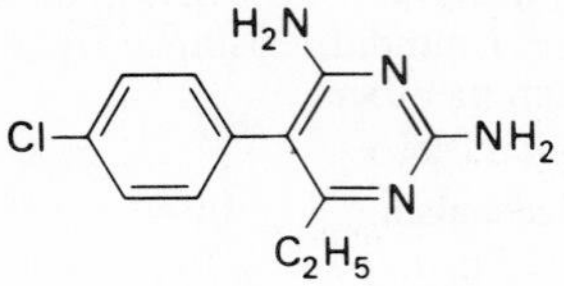

TRIMETHOPRIM (Syraprim)

In combination with long-acting sulfonamides in chronic urinary infections with E. coli, Kl. enterobacter, Proteus mirabilis, and Proteus vulgaris. Also tried in treatment of pneumocystis carini pneumonia.

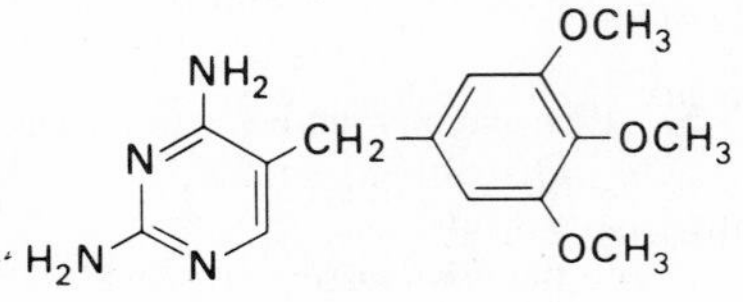

D. 8-Aminoquinolines (Primaquine Group)

The 8-aminoquinolines differ from the antimalarials previously considered in possessing activity against exoerythrocytic forms. This means, practically, that they have the potentiality of eradicating vivax malaria.

1. History. a. Schulemann and Memmi (1927) synthesized pamaquine, the first synthetic antimalarial.

b. The improved derivative, pentaquine, was developed under the OSRD program in 1946, and primaquine by Alving in 1948.

2. Chemistry. Related series of 8-aminoquinoline derivatives.

3. Action. Effective against exoerythrocytic (tissue) forms. Also effective on gametocytes (sexual forms).

4. Mechanism. May cause alteration in pentose phosphate pathway resulting in decrease of triphosphopyridine nucleotide (TPNH) in cells and in parasites; result may be more susceptible parasites and decrease in nutrients available to parasites.

5. Pharmacodynamics. a. Absorbed adequately by mouth.

b. Rapidly degraded in the body; slight localization in liver, lungs, and brain.

6. Toxicity. a. Nausea, vomiting, abdominal cramps.

b. Acute hemolytic anemia in patients with genetic deficiency of glucose-6-phosphate dehydrogenase, the enzyme that catalyzes the initial oxidative step of the pentose pathway of glucose metabolism. This deficiency predisposes to hemolysis by several drugs and foods; commonest in Mediterranean people and Negroes. Pamaquine is most toxic, pentaquine intermediate, and primaquine least.

7. Uses. a. Primaquine is used to terminate relapsing vivax malaria.

b. As it is active against gametocytes it is a potential agent to produce transmission blockade; however, the difficulties of such therapy have prevented its general use.

8. Preparations

PRIMAQUINE PHOSPHATE

Dose: 15 mg (base) by mouth daily. For gametocyte control: 45 mg by mouth once weekly.

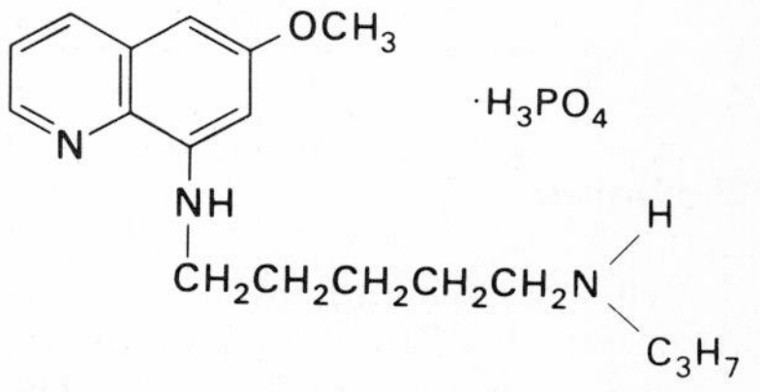

6-Methoxy-8-(5-propylaminoamylamino) quinoline phosphate

Comparable to primaquine in effect and toxicity, but also has schizonticidal activity almost equal to chloroquine.

OCH_3 · H_3PO_4 N NH H $CH_2CH_2CH_2CH_2CH_2N$ C_3H_7

E. Sulfones and Sulfonamides

Resistant strains of malaria, particularly of *P. falciparum*, have arisen in several parts of the world. Most commonly the resistance is to chloroquine and the other 4-aminoquinolines.

Combinations of an antimalarial (quinine, pyrimethamine, trimethoprim, chloroguanide, cycloguanil) with a sulfone (dapsone, acedapsone) or a sulfonamide (acetyl sulfamethoxypyridazine, sulfalene, sulfadoxine) have been variously used. Of perhaps greatest promise is the combination of trimethoprim and sulfalene.

SUMMARY: THE ANTIMALARIALS

TYPE	*ACTION AND MECHANISM*	*TOXICITY*	*USE*	*EXAMPLES*
Quinine	Active vs. red cell forms Mechanism not clear	Cinchonism, cardiac depression hypersensitivity	Suppressant and therapeutic in acute attack	Quinine sulfate
Chloroquine group	Active vs. red cell forms Combines with parasite DNA	Blurred vision pruritis, retinitis, deafness	Same	Chloroquine phosphate

(cont.)

SUMMARY: THE ANTIMALARIALS (cont.)

TYPE	*ACTION AND MECHANISM*	*TOXICITY*	*USE*	*EXAMPLES*
Biguanide group	active vs. red cell forms Interferes with conversion of folic to folinic acid	Dermatitis, marrow depression	Same	Chloroguanide hydrochloride
Primaquine group	Active vs. tissue forms and gametocytes May alter pentose phosphate pathway	Hemolytic anaemia	To terminate relapsing vivax malaria	Primaquine phosphate

Reviews

Powell, R. Chemotherapy of malaria. Clin. Pharmacol. Ther., 7:48, 1966.

Thompson, P. Parasite chemotherapy. Ann. Rev. Pharmacol., 7:77, 1967.

Neva, F. Malaria. Recent progress and problems. New Eng. J. Med., 277:1241, 1967.

Powell, R., and Tigertt, W. Drug-resistance of parasites causing human malaria. Ann. Rev. Med., 19:81, 1968.

10. Amebicides and Other Antiprotozoals

I. AGENTS ACTIVE ON AMEBAE, GIARDIA, TRICHOMONAS, AND THE LIKE

Although less complex than malaria, amebiasis also has a somewhat complicated natural history. Cystic forms of the parasite are ingested in food or drink and in the bowel grow out into motile, vegetative forms. Some of these later form cysts, and both vegetative and cystic forms appear in the stool, the vegetative forms more characteristically while there is acute diarrhea, and the cysts after the acute stage is over. At any time vegetative forms may penetrate the wall of the bowel, enter the tissues, and produce abscesses, particularly in the liver. Vegetative forms in the tissues are not transformed into cystic forms.

As there is not significant immune response, amebicides must be relied on to cure the disease. The therapeutic problem resolves itself into the use of drugs which will eliminate vegetative forms from the intestine and from the tissues. Cystic forms are probably resistant to attack, but cease to be formed when the vegetative forms are eliminated. Some drugs are direct amebicides; others are principally bactericides which reduce the bacteria that serve as food supply for the amebae in the intestine.

A. Alkaloids and Glycosides

EMETINE

1. History. a. Ipecacuanha brought from South America in 1658.
b. Pelletier (1816) isolated the alkaloid emetine.
c. Rogers (1912) used emetine in amebiasis.

2. Chemistry. Emetine is a hydroisoquinoline derivative.

3. Action. a. Highly effective amebicide against vegetative forms, either in bowel or in tissues (liver).
b. Also is an emetic, but slow in action.

4. Mechanism. Inhibition of protein synthesis; emetine blocks transfer of amino acids from sRNA to the ribosomes where the proteins are assembled.

5. Pharmacodynamics. a. By mouth it is a local irritant and produces vomiting, and therefore parenteral administration is necessary for systemic effect.

b. Distribution widespread. May cumulate in the body.

6. Toxicity. Local irritation, cardiac depression, cardiac damage, and muscle weakness.

7. Uses. May be used as initial therapy in amebiasis as it controls the intestinal symptoms, sometimes with amazing celerity, and at the same time sterilizes any systemic implants which may already have occurred. Course of emetine usually followed by alternating courses of an arsenical and a hydroxyquinoline.

8. Preparation

EMETINE HYDROCHLORIDE

Dose: 60 mg subcutaneously daily for 5 days (dysentery) to 10 days (hepatitis).

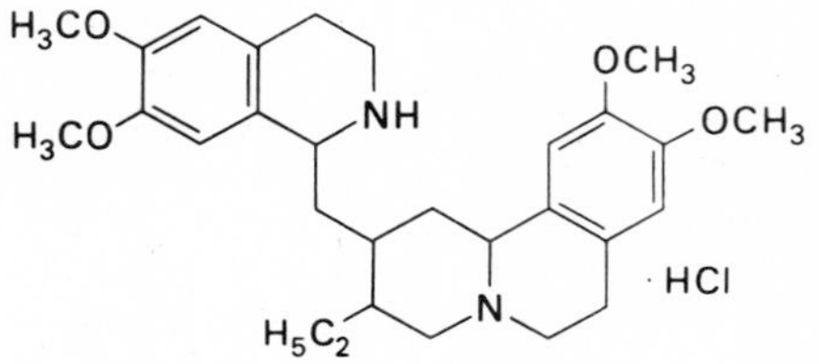

H_3CO H_3CO NH OCH_3 OCH_3 · HCl H_5C_2 N

OTHERS: Dehydroemetine; glaucarubin (Glarubin).

B. Halogenated Hydroxyquinolines (Chiniofon Group)

1. History. a. Mühlens and Merck (1920) first used chiniofon in amebiasis; synthesized (1892).

b. Leake (1931) introduced iodochlorhydroxyquin.

2. Chemistry. Halogenated hydroxyquinolines.

3. Action. Directly amebicidal, and also antitrichomonal and antibacterial.

4. Mechanism. May be based on chelation.

5. Pharmacodynamics. Absorption by mouth generally poor; moderate for iodochlorhydroxyquin.

6. Toxicity. May cause local irritation of the bowel. Rarely may produce iodism.

7. Uses. a. Useful in intestinal amebiasis, especially after the acute symptoms have been controlled with emetine or chloroquine.

b. Also useful locally in trichomonas vaginitis, infected wounds, dermatitis.

c. Widely advised in "turista" (diarrhea of travelers) but apparently ineffective.

8. Preparations

CHINIOFON (Yatren)

Dose: 0.5 gm by mouth twice daily for 10 days.

SO_3H I OH N

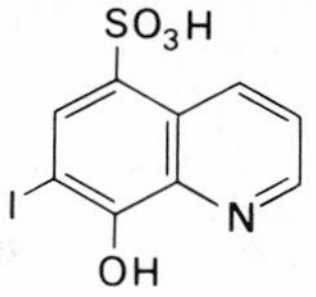

CLAMOXYQUIN HYDROCHLORIDE

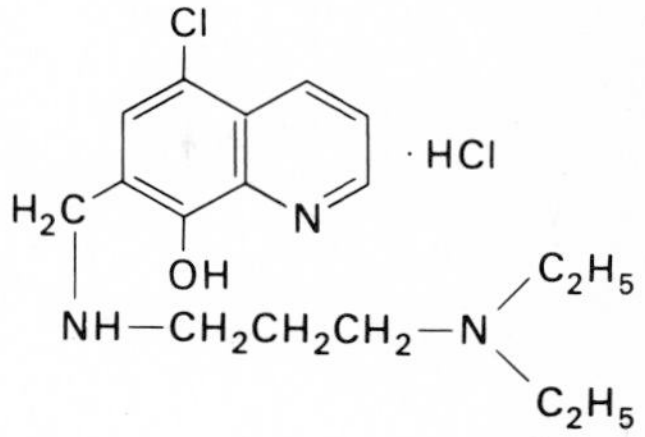

Cl H_2C OH N · HCl

$NH{-}CH_2CH_2CH_2{-}N(C_2H_5)_2$

DIIODOHYDROXYQUIN (Diodoquin)

Dose: 0.5 gm 4 times daily by mouth for 10 to 20 days; locally in powders or suppositories.

I I OH N

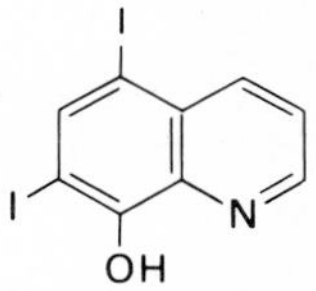

IODOCHLORHYDROXYQUIN (Vioform)

Dose: 0.5 gm by mouth twice daily for 10 days in amebiasis; locally in powders or suppositories.

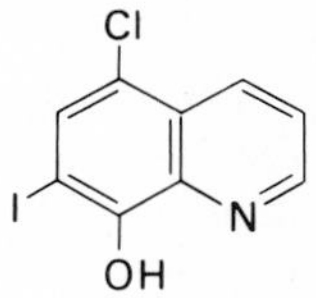

Cl I OH N

CLOXYQUIN

OH N Cl

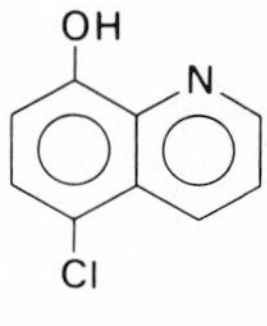

C. Other Antimalarial Quinolines (Chloroquine)

See Antimalarials and Topical Agents for further discussion of antiinfective quinolines.

1. Action and Mechanism. a. Directly amebicidal on tissue forms of amebae.

b. Not effective on intestinal forms, presumably because of prior absorption higher in the bowel.

2. Uses. a. Chloroquine is often preferred to emetine in the treatment of amebic hepatitis because of lesser toxicity.

b. Quinacrine is an alternative to chloroquine; preferred by some physicians in the treatment of giardiasis.

3. Preparations

CHLOROQUINE PHOSPHATE

Dose: 0.5 gm 2 times a day for 2 days, then 0.5 gm daily for 2 weeks in amebic hepatitis.

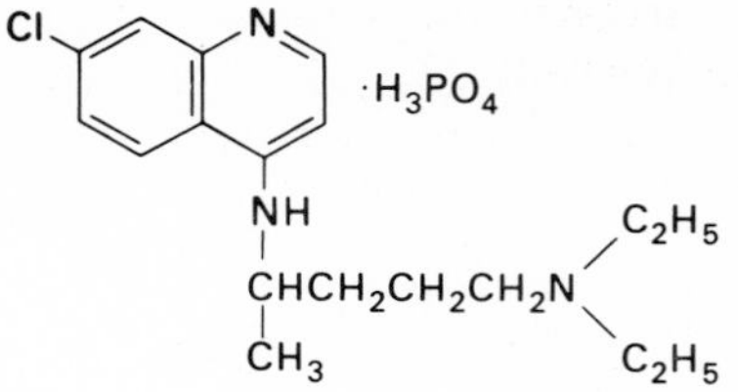

Cl N $\cdot H_3PO_4$

NH C_2H_5

$CHCH_2CH_2CH_2N$

CH_3 C_2H_5

OTHERS
Entobex; Quinacrine.

D. Pentavalent Arsenicals

See carbarsone and glycobiarsol under Pentavalent Organic Arsenicals in the second section of this chapter.

E. Antibiotics

The growth of amebae in culture is always associated with bacteria, and it is generally assumed that the principal effect of most antibacterials on amebae is an inhibition of the associated bacteria. In any case, the effect of a number of antibacterials in amebiasis has been beneficial, though usually with a lower percentage of final cure than with direct amebicides. The tetracyclines, erythromycin, paromomycin, bacitracin, and puromycin have all been rather extensively used.

Fumagillin (Fumadil), unlike most antibiotics, exerts a direct amebicidal effect, but is of questionable value because of toxicity and because the incidence of cure is not outstanding.

F. Benzylamine Group (Bialamicol)

1. Chemistry. Benzylamine derivatives.

2. Action and Mechanism. Apparently directly amebicidal.

3. Pharmacodynamics. Well absorbed and widely distributed. Slow excretion.

4. Toxicity. a. May produce headache, anorexia, nausea, cramps, diarrhea.

b. Skin reactions including exfoliative dermatitis; possibly agranulocytosis.

5. Uses. Bialamicol used for symptomatic relief of acute amebic dysentery; permanent cure only fair.

6. Preparations

BIALAMICOL HYDROCHLORIDE (Camoform)

Dose: 250 to 500 mg 3 times a day for 5 days by mouth.

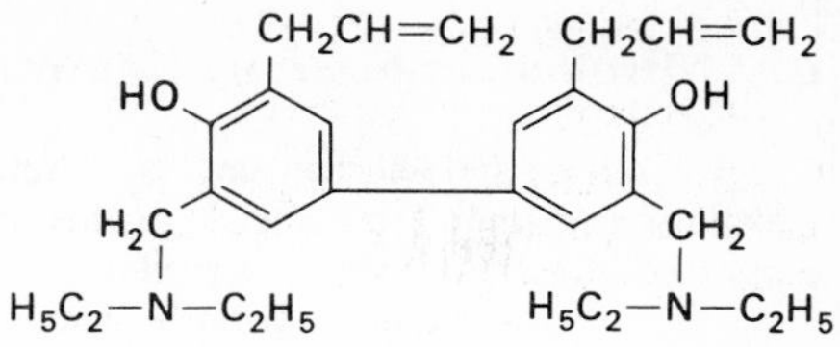

OTHERS

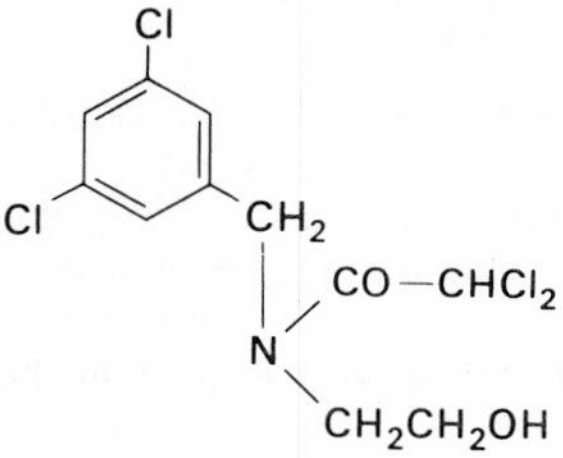

chlorbetamide (Mantomide)

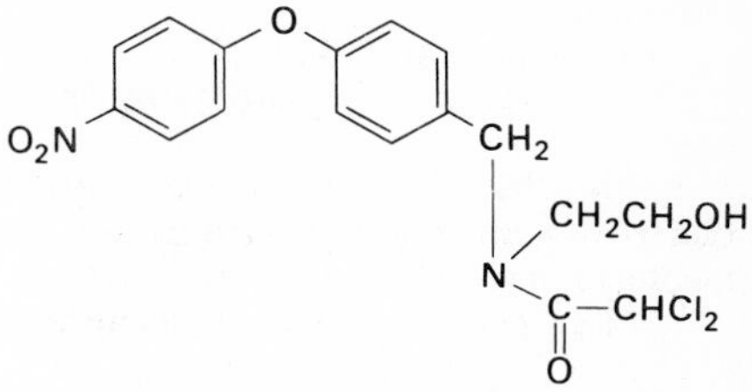

Clefamide (chlorphenoxamide)

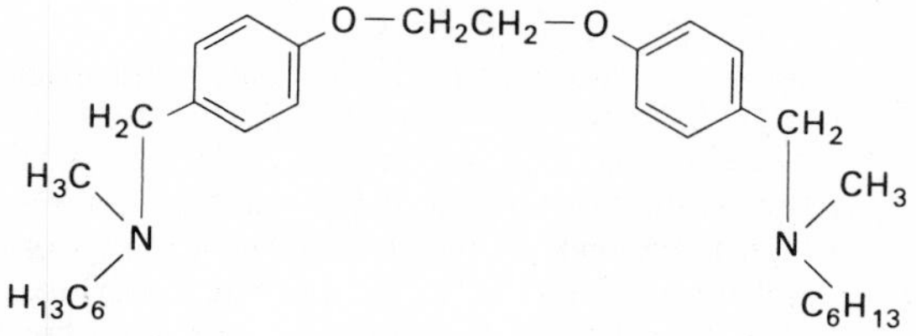

symetine HCl

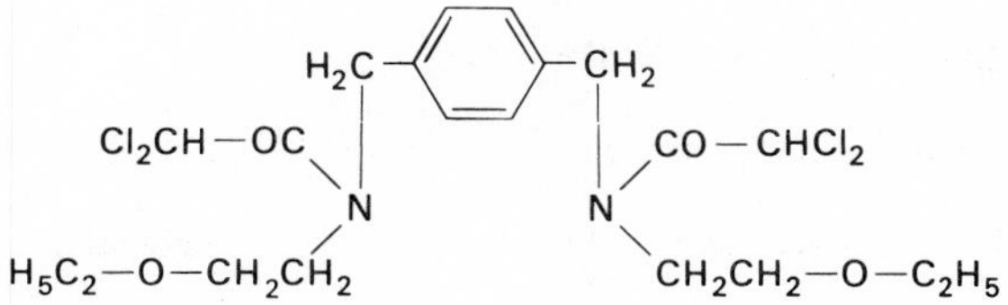

teclozan (Falmonox)

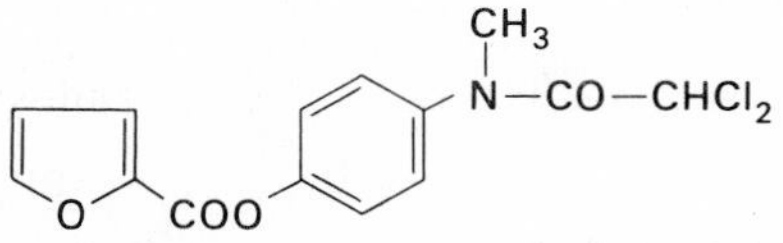

diloxanide furoate (Entamide)

G. Nitroimidazole Group (Metronidazole)

1. Action and Mechanism. a. Active against *Trichomonas vaginalis* and in giardiasis and amebiasis; inactive against monilia.

b. Resistance not observed.

c. May decrease adrenocorticosteroidism (Taylor, J.A.M.A., 181:776, 1962).

2. Pharmacodynamics. Well absorbed by mouth; excreted over 12 hours, largely in the urine.

3. Toxicity. a. Ordinarily only mild gastrointestinal symptoms and dizziness.

b. Rarely more severe: drowsiness, insomnia, bitter taste, backache, blurred vision, edema, vaginal itching, sore throat, transient leukopenia; in experimental animals, testicular damage, ataxia, tremor.

c. Secondary monilial or fungal infection may occur in mouth or vagina.

4. Uses. a. Curative in 80% of trichomonas vaginitis and useful in giardiasis, amebiasis, and trypanosomiasis.

b. Should not be used in pregnancy until possible effects on fetus have been determined.

5. Preparations

METRONIDAZOLE (Flagyl)

Dose: 250 mg 2 or 3 times a day by mouth for 10 days; may be supplemented by 500 mg suppositories, but advantage doubtful.

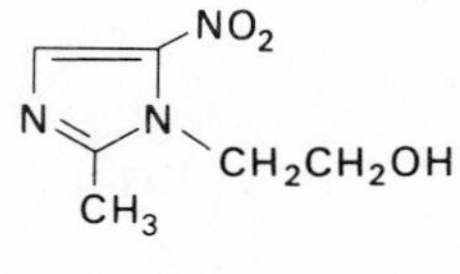

NO_2 N N CH_2CH_2OH CH_3

OTHERS

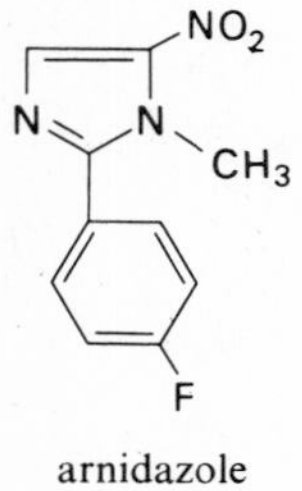

NO_2 N N CH_3 F

arnidazole

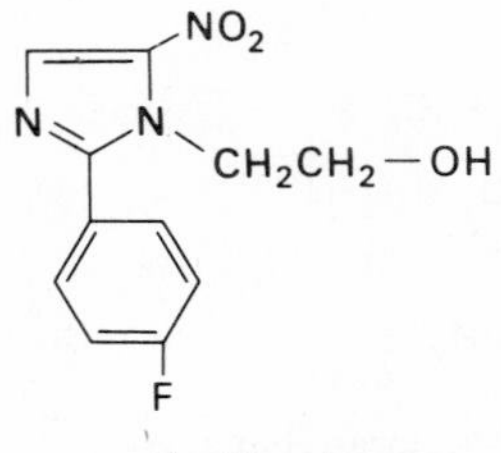

NO_2 N N CH_2CH_2-OH F

flunidazole

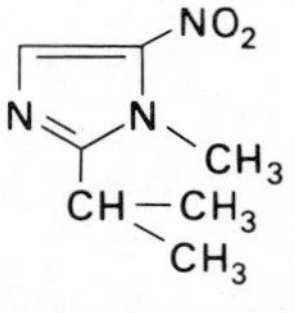

NO_2 N N CH_3 $CH-CH_3$ CH_3

ipronidazole (Ipropran)

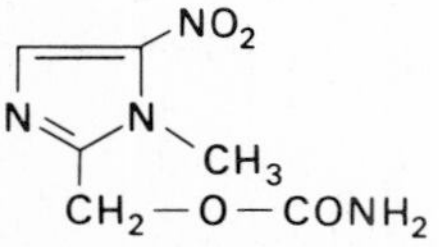

NO_2 N N CH_3 $CH_2-O-CONH_2$

ronidazole (Dugro)

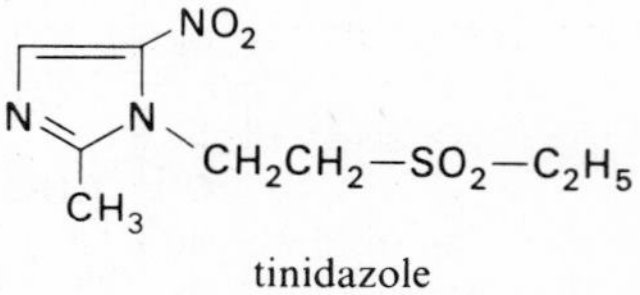

NO_2 N N $CH_2CH_2-SO_2-C_2H_5$ CH_3

tinidazole

II. AGENTS ACTING ON TRYPANOSOMES, LEISHMANIA, AND THE LIKE

A. Trivalent Organic Arsenicals

1. History. a. Ehrlich in 1907 synthesized arsphenamine (Salvarsan), one of the great drugs of all time, and with it introduced the concept of chemotherapy.

b. A series of related compounds followed arsphenamine, characterized by lesser toxicity or greater ease in handling.

2. Chemistry. a. Contain trivalent As, or break down to such compounds.

b. The principal members of the arsphenamine family are as follows:

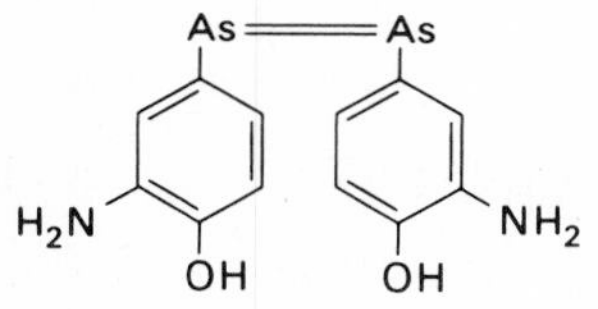

arsphenamine

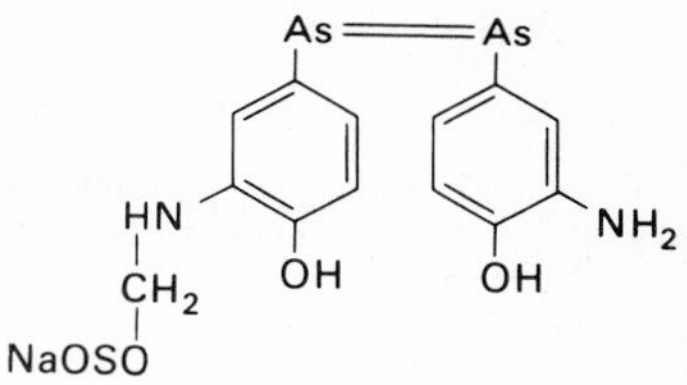

neoarsphenamine

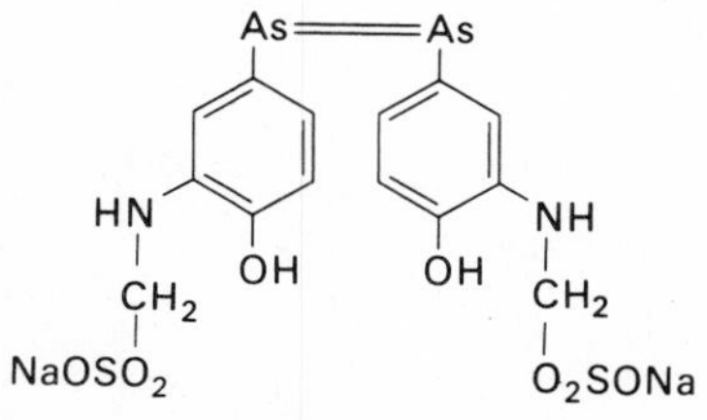

sulfarsphenamine

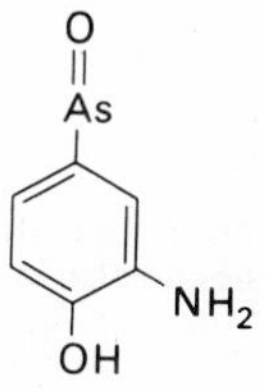

oxophenarsine

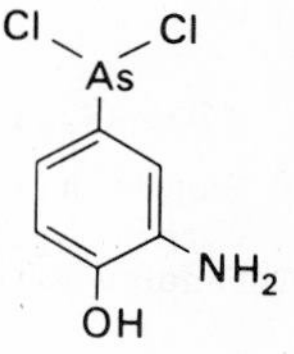

dichlorophenarsine

c. Melarsoprol is a combination of an arsenical with the antidote dimercaprol.

3. Action. General inhibitory action on spirochetes and protozoa.

4. Mechanism. All the compounds are presumably converted to "arsenoxide," perhaps identical with oxophenarsine, and in this form act as protoplasmic poisons through affinity for sulfhydryl groups, as in glutathione (Voegtlin, 1920).

5. Pharmacodynamics. a. Absorption poor, usually requiring parenteral use.

b. Distribution wide, but not into the CNS except for melarsoprol.

c. Excretion renal.

6. Toxicity. a. Local irritation, nitritoid reactions, acid arsphenamine reaction Herxheimer reaction, jaundice, neuritis, bone marrow depression, hemorrhagic encephalitis, purpura.

b. In many cases the initial recognition of important prototype toxic reactions later seen with other drugs came with the use of the arsphenamines.

c. Melarsoprol may produce a toxic encephalopathy.

d. For the arsphenamine group dimercaprol is an antidote, but it is less effective against melarsoprol.

7. Uses. The arsphenamines are no longer used, but formerly were used in syphilis as follows: vigorously for early stages, cautiously in later years; given in courses, over periods as long as two years, in alternation with mercury and later bismuth. All quickly replaced with the advent of penicillin.

b. Melarsoprol is a preferred agent in CNS trypanosomiasis, especially when the trypanosomes are resistant to tryparsamide.

8. Preparations

MELARSOPROL (Mel B)

Dose: 2 to 3.6 mg per kg, slowly, intravenously, for 3 daily doses; may repeat in 1 and 3 weeks.

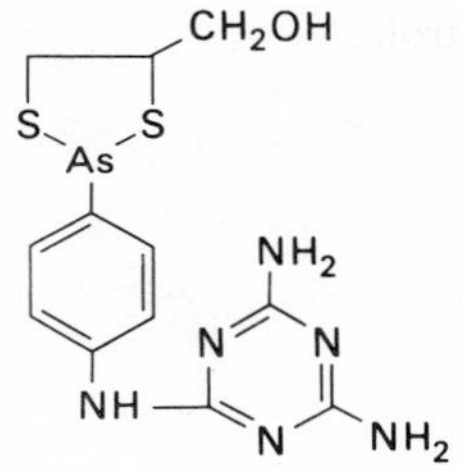

CH_2OH
S S
As
NH_2
N N
NH N NH_2

MELARSONYL (Mel W)

Water-soluble; given intramuscularly.

Used in trypanosomiasis and also in filariasis, where it may affect adult worms.

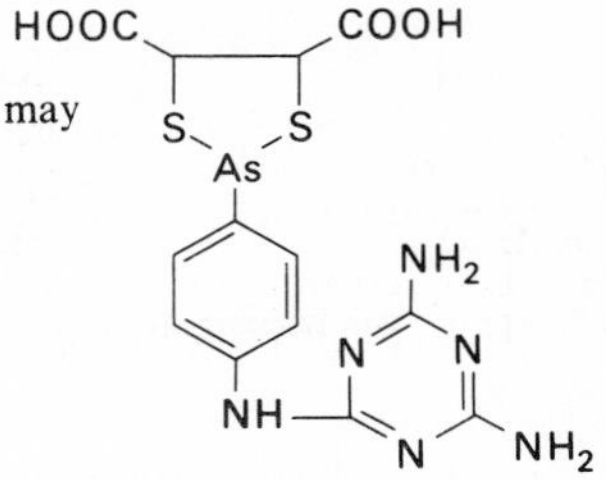

HOOC COOH
S S
As
NH_2
N N
NH N NH_2

B. Pentavalent Organic Arsenicals

1. History. a. Thomas and Breinl (1905) introduced atoxyl after much earlier synthesis by Becamp (1860).

b. Tryparsamide introduced by Brown and Pearce (1919) after synthesis by Jacobs and Heidelberger.

c. Ehrlich and Bertheim (1909) synthesized carbarsone; introduced by Leake (1930), replacing the earlier, more toxic acetarsone.

d. Hauer (1943) synthesized glycobiarsol; introduced by Dennis (1949).

2. Chemistry. Pentavalent arsenicals, derived from atoxyl.

3. Action and Mechanism. The pentavalent arsenicals are probably not active as such, but penetrate more widely than the trivalents, including the CNS, and then slowly liberate trivalent arsenic compounds of the arsenoxide type. They thus make the treatment of CNS disease possible.

4. Pharmacodynamics. Relatively poorly absorbed by mouth.

5. Toxicity. In general much less toxic than the trivalent arsenicals, but capable of producing optic atrophy.

6. Uses. a. Atoxyl was early replaced by the less toxic tryparsamide for use both against CNS trypanosomiasis and CNS syphilis. Penicillin has replaced tryparsamide in CNS syphilis, but the latter remains the only useful agent in the extremely refractory CNS stages of trypanosomiasis.

b. Carbarsone and glycobiarsol are used in courses, alternating with a hydroxyquinoline, in amebiasis after the acute stage of the disease has been controlled with a more rapidly effective drug.

7. Preparations

CARBARSONE

Dose: 0.25 gm 2 times daily by mouth for 10 days.

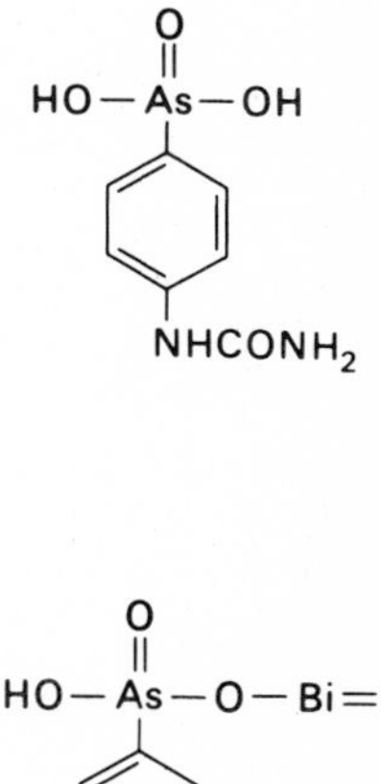

O
||
HO—As—OH
(benzene ring)
$NHCONH_2$

GLYCOBIARSOL (Milibis)

Less potent than carbarsone; useful in milder disease.
Dose: 0.5 gm 3 times a day for 7 days by mouth.

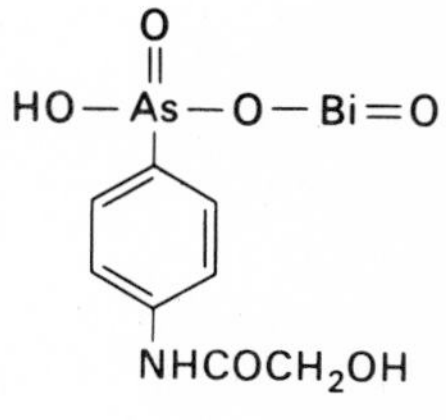

O
||
HO—As—O—Bi=O
(benzene ring)
$NHCOCH_2OH$

TRYPARSAMIDE

Dose: 1.0 gm intravenously.

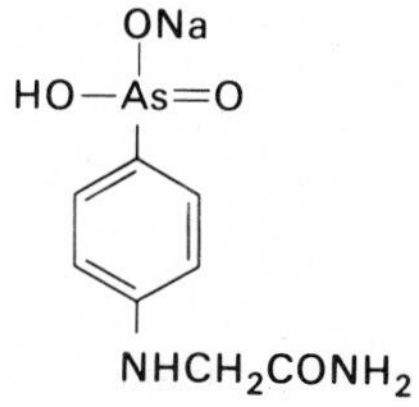

ONa
|
HO—As=O
(benzene ring)
$NHCH_2CONH_2$

C. Bismuth and Mercury

1. History. a. Levaditti (1929) introduced bismuth compounds as alternatives to mercurials in the treatment of syphilis. Hanzlik (1935) made orally absorbable compounds.

b. Mercury was the most effective agent in syphilis from the 1490's until the introduction of arsphenamine, but had been largely replaced by bismuth as the drug to alternate with arsenic even before penicillin made all metals obsolete.

2. Chemistry. A great variety of organic and inorganic preparations.

3. Action and Mechanism. Spirocheticidal effects probably on the basis of an affinity for —SH groups, as with arsenic.

4. Pharmacodynamics and Toxicity. a. Mostly poorly soluble and slowly absorbed; distribution good; excretion in urine (Bi), and urine and stool (Hg).

b. Bismuth may cause nephritis, jaundice; mercury damage to intestinal mucosa and kidney tubules.

5. Uses. a. No present use in syphilis, but formerly given in alternating series with arsenicals.

b. See bismuth compounds as constipating agents, and mercurial compounds as antiseptics and diuretics.

D. Suramin

1. History. Ehrlich in 1904 investigated the chemotherapeutic activity of benzopurpurin because it dyed cotton without a mordant. A series of trypanocidal dyes followed this beginning: trypan red, trypan blue, Afridol violet, and finally suramin, which was synthesized by Heyman et al. in the early 1920s and separately by Fourneau in 1924.

2. Chemistry. Suramin is a highly substituted urea.

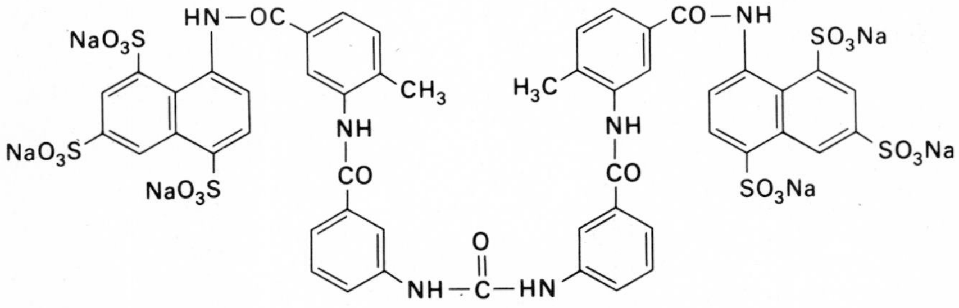

suramin sodium

3. Action. Active against African trypanosomes.

4. Mechanism. a. Combines first with a receptor on the trypanosome, then blocks cell division several generations later, producing a latent period of 24 hours (Hawking, Brit. J. Pharmacol., 15:567, 1960).

b. Crucial mechanism of inhibition not clear; but a number of enzymes have been demonstrated to be interfered with: hexokinase, urease, decarboxylase, succinic dehydrogenase, trypsin.

5. Pharmacodynamics. a. Not absorbed orally.

b. After injection does not enter the cells, but stays in extracellular transit for a prolonged period and is excreted slowly by the kidneys over several months.

6. Toxicity. Albuminuria, amblyopia, hemolysis, dermatitis, and agranulocytosis have been noted.

7. Uses. a. Used both for prophylaxis against trypanosomiasis and in the treatment of the early stages.

b. Ineffective in the late stages when there is CNS involvement because it does not enter the brain.

8. Preparation

SURAMIN SODIUM (Naphuride; Germanin; Bayer 205, and others)

Dose: 1 gm intravenously repeated once in a week, and then with repetition of the 2 doses at 3-monthly intervals (prophylactic); 1 gm weekly intravenously for 5 to 10 weeks (therapeutic).

E. Aromatic Diamidines (Stilbamidines)

1. History. a. Yorke (1944) introduced stilbamidine.

b. Development suggested by trypanocidal power of synthalin; trypanosomes need glucose, and synthalin produces hypoglycemia.

2. Chemistry. Series of aromatic diamidines related to synthalin.

3. Action. Inhibit trypanosomes; also organisms of babesia, leishmaniasis, North American blastomycosis.

4. Mechanism. May be related to enzyme inhibition, or to inhibition of nucleic acid synthesis; no latent period, as with suramin.

5. Pharmacodynamics. Effective by intravenous injection. Penetration into CNS poor.

6. Toxicity. a. Stilbamidine and pentamidine may provoke histamine release with faintness, sweating, dizziness, tachycardia, vomiting, and circulatory collapse; hypoglycemia; light sensitivity; late paresthesias, degenerative changes in the CNS, especially in the trigeminal nucleus.

b. Hydroxystilbamidine less toxic, especially as to trigeminal neuralgia.

7. Uses. a. Effective in early trypanosomiasis and in prophylaxis.

b. May also be tried in babesia, leishmaniasis, and North American blastomycosis (but amphotericin B preferred in the latter).

c. Formerly tried in multiple myeloma with doubtful results.

8. Preparations

2-AMINOSTILBAMIDINE

Under recent trial.

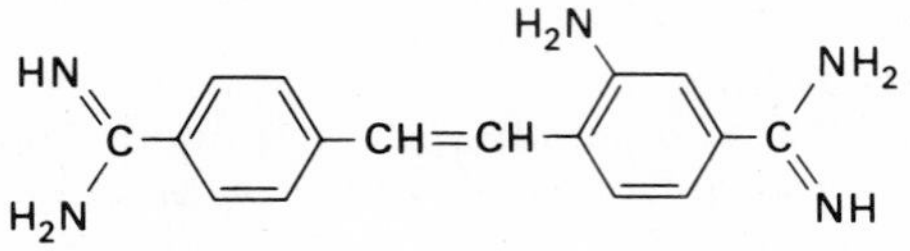

HYDROXYSTILBAMIDINE ISETHIONATE

Dose: 225 mg intramuscularly or intravenously, slowly.

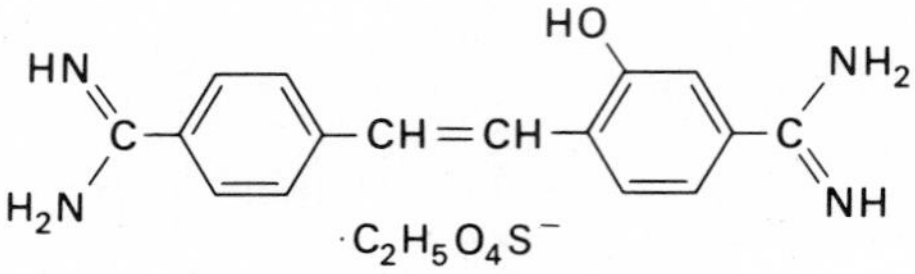

$\cdot C_2H_5O_4S^-$

PENTAMIDE ISETHIONATE (Lomidine)

Prophylactic for trypanosomiasis.

Dose: 5 mg per kilo body weight intramuscularly.

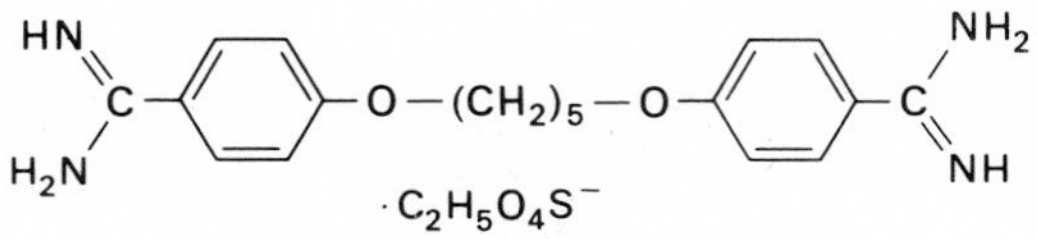

$\cdot C_2H_5O_4S^-$

STILBAMIDINE ISETHIONATE

Dose: 2 mg per kg body weight intravenously daily for 8 days.

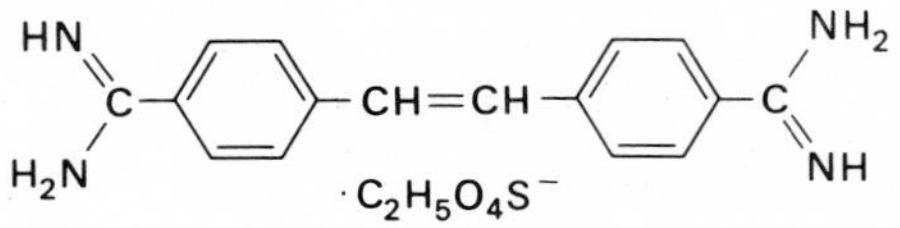

$\cdot C_2H_5O_4S^-$

F. Metamidium

1. History. Wragg (1958) introduced metamidium.

2. Chemistry. Derived from phenanthridinium compounds and the aromatic diamidines.

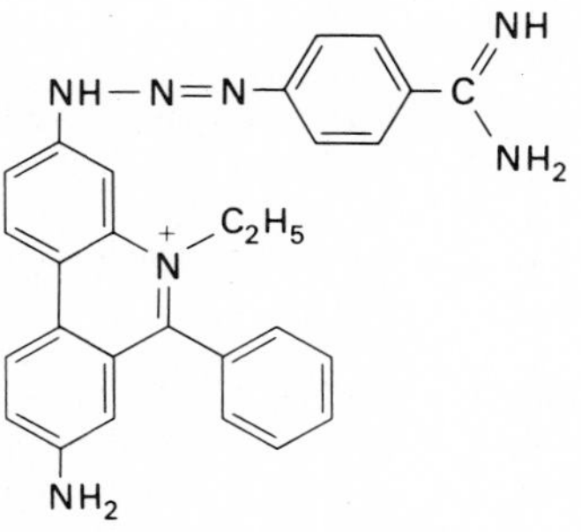

isometamidium (red compound)

3. Action and Mechanism. Antitrypanosomal. Mechanism unknown.

4. Uses. Gives promise in African trypanosomiasis, both as a prophylactic and as a curative (Wragg, Nature, 182:1005, 1958).

G. Antrycide

1. History. Introduced by Curd and Davey (1949).

2. Chemistry. A quinaldine derivative.

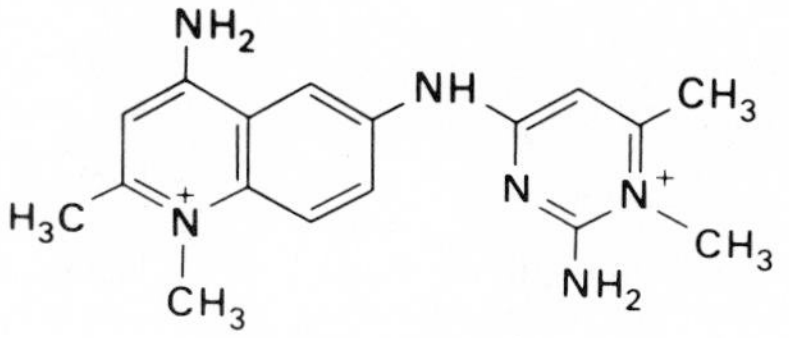

NH2 NH CH3 H3C N+ CH3 N N+ CH3 NH2

antrycide

3. Action and Mechanism. Trypanocidal. Mechanism not determined, possibly by pteridine competition. Resistance may develop.

4. Uses. a. Protective against trypanosomes for many weeks (two to three months for antrycide "prosalt").

b. May be curative in animals.

H. Veterinary Coccidiostats and Other Antiprotozoal Agents

Aclomide (in Novostat), clopindol (Coyden), dinsed (in Polystat), gloxazone, nitasone (in Histostat), nitromide (in Tristat), roxarsone (in Polystat 3).

SUMMARY: AMEBICIDES AND OTHER ANTIPROTOZOALS

TYPE	*ACTION AND MECHANISM*	*TOXICITY*	*USE*	*EXAMPLES*
Alkaloids	Active vs. vegetative forms Inhibit protein synthesis by interfering with transfer of amino acids to ribosomes	Cardiac depression	Initial in amebiasis and in hepatitis	Emetine hydrochloride
Halogenated hydroxy-quinolines	Uncertain	Local irritation	Intestinal amebiasis Locally for bacterial and trichomonas infections	Iodochlor-hydroxyquin

(cont.)

SUMMARY: AMEBICIDES AND OTHER ANTIPROTOZOALS (cont.)

TYPE	*ACTION AND MECHANISM*	*TOXICITY*	*USE*	*EXAMPLES*
Antimalarial quinolines	Directly amebicidal Mechanism probably DNA attachment	See Antimalarials	Amebic hepatitis	Chloroquine phosphate
Pentavalent arsenicals	Directly amebicidal by —SH inactivation	Minor	Intestinal amebiasis	Carbarsone
Antibiotics	Indirectly amebicidal by inhibiting food bacteria	Variable	Intestinal amebiasis	Tetracycline
Benzylamine group	Probably directly amebicidal	Diarrhea, dermatitis, agranulocytosis	Acute amebiasis	Bialamicol hydrochloride
Nitroimidazole group	Active vs. trichomonas, giardia, amebae Mechanism uncertain	Drowsiness, blurred vision, leukopenia	Trichomonas vaginitis, giardiasis, amebiasis	Metronidazole
Arsenicals	Active vs. protozoa and spirochetes Mechanism based on affinity for SH groups	Nitritoid, Herxheimer reactions, jaundice, neuritis, marrow depression, encephalitis, purpura, optic atrophy	Trypanosomiasis	Tryparsamide
Bismuth and mercury	Probably similar	Liver and kidney damage	Obsolete	Bismuth subsalicylate
Suramin	Active vs. trypanosomes	Hemolysis, agranulocytosis, dermatitis	African trypanosomiasis	Suramin
Aromatic diamidines	Active vs. trypanosomes	Light sensitivity, paresthesias, CNS damage	Trypanosomiasis	Stilbamidine isethionate

Reviews

Clark, D., Solomons, E., and Siegal, S. Drugs for vaginal trichomoniasis. Obstet. Gynec., 20:615, 1962.

Steigman, F., and Skloes, W. Treatment of amebiasis. Med. Clin. N. Amer., 48:159, 1964.

Thompson, P. E. Parasite Chemotherapy. Ann. Rev. Pharmacol., 7:77, 1967.

Anon. Drugs for parasitic infections. The Medical Letter, H. Aaron, ed. 11:21, 1969.

Scott, F., and Miller, M. Trials with metronidazole in amebic dysentery. J.A.M.A., 211: 118, 1970.

11. Anthelmintics and Other Agents for Metazoal Diseases

Vermifuges are among the most ancient of medicines, and they are still of great importance as it is estimated that even in the United States about one fourth of the population is infested. Both flatworms and roundworms are responsible.

I. AGENTS AGAINST FLATWORMS (CESTODES)

A. Quinacrine

1. History and Chemistry. See Antimalarials.

2. Action. Effective against *Taenia solium*, *T. saginata*, and *Diphyllobothrium latum;* repeated treatment necessary for *Hymenolepis nana*.

3. Mechanism. Mechanism unknown; worms stained bright yellow.

4. Uses. Has replaced all the older, more toxic agents in the therapy of tapeworm, except for the dwarf tapeworm, *H. nana* (see Hexylresorcinol).

5. Preparation

QUINACRINE HYDROCHLORIDE (Atabrine)

Dose: 0.8 gm by mouth (may be given in divided doses to reduce nausea). Patient prepared by omission of supper and administration of magnesium sulfate or an enema on preceding evening (omitted by some physicians); 2 hours after administration of vermifuge, saline purge is given, followed 2 hours later by an enema if the head has not appeared.

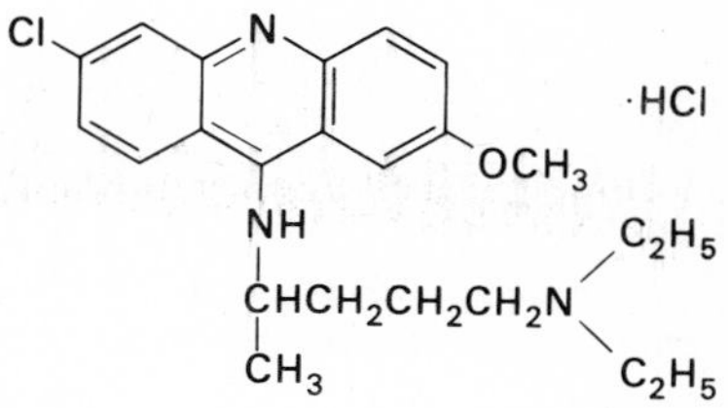

Cl N ·HCl OCH_3 NH $CHCH_2CH_2CH_2N(C_2H_5)_2$ CH_3

B. Others

Oleoresin of aspidium; pelletierine tannate, pumpkin seed; spigelia; tin compounds.

II. AGENTS AGAINST ROUNDWORMS (NEMATODES)

A. Chlorinated Hydrocarbons (Tetrachloroethylene)

1. History. a. Carbon tetrachloride and tetrachloroethylene introduced by Hall (1921).

b. Extensive use by Lambert (*A Yankee Doctor in Paradise*).

2. Chemistry. Chlorinated hydrocarbons derived from chloroform.

3. Action. Effective against hookworms; *Necator americanus* more sensitive than *Ancyclostoma duodenale*.

4. Mechanism. Mechanism uncertain, but drugs may enter and depress hypoderm muscle cells, or neighboring nerve structures.

5. Pharmacodynamics. Mild local irritants, ordinarily not absorbed. When absorbed, excreted in expired air.

6. Toxicity. If absorbed, dizziness, staggering, narcosis; later hepatitis.

7. Uses. a. Tetrachloroethylene is the drug of choice in hookworm infestation, having largely replaced the more toxic carbon tetrachloride.

b. If ascaris also present, it should be removed first (piperazine), according to tradition, but this is probably unnecessary. (Brown, Clin. Pharmacol. Ther., 1:87, 1960.)

8. Preparation

TETRACHLOROETHYLENE

Dose: 5 ml by mouth; administered in the morning, in the fasting state, without attendant purgation. Several treatments may be required.

$$Cl_2C{=}CCl_2$$

B. Phenol Derivatives (Hexylresorcinol)

1. History. Hexylresorcinol introduced by Lamson (1932) as the most desirable of the phenols, replacing thymol.

2. Chemistry. Potency increases with length of side chain until the compound becomes insoluble; thus hexylresorcinol is more potent than thymol.

3. Action and Mechanism. Directly vermicidal on hookworms, ascaris, trichuris.

4. Pharmacodynamics. After oral administration (hexylresorcinol) about 30% absorbed. Excretion rapid.

5. Toxicity. Local irritants, but ordinarily without systemic toxicity because of rapid excretion.

6. Uses. a. Generally less effective than piperazine on ascaris, and tetrachloroethylene on hookworm, but occasionally used when both infestations are present.

b. Moderately effective against dwarf tapeworm.

c. Bithionol may be useful in paragonomiasis.

7. Preparations

DICHLOROPHEN (Anthiphen)

Used in Europe; macerates worms.
Dose: 6 gm by mouth on 2 successive mornings.

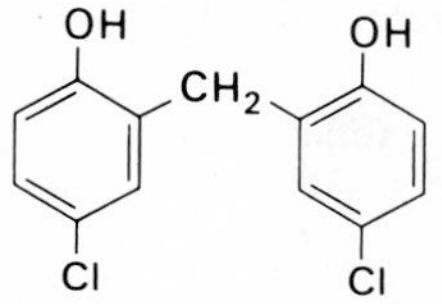

OH OH CH_2 Cl Cl

HEXYLRESORCINOL

Dose: 1 gm by mouth, given to the fasting patient in the morning (tablets must be swallowed whole to avoid burning mouth), and followed in 2 hours by a saline purge.

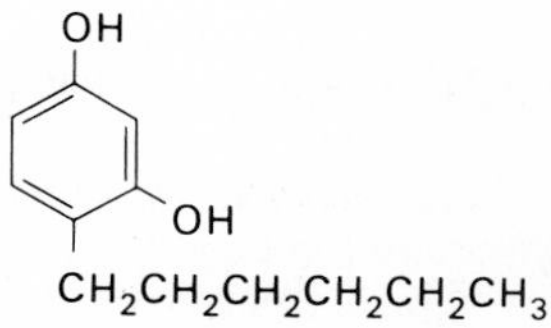

OH OH $CH_2CH_2CH_2CH_2CH_2CH_3$

NICLOSAMIDE (Yomesan)

May be effective in tapeworm infestation refractory to other agents (Lloyd, Practitioner, 187:679, 1961).
Dose: 2 gm by mouth.

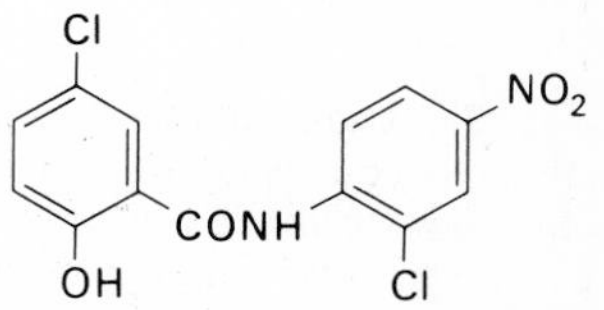

Cl NO_2 CONH OH Cl

OTHERS

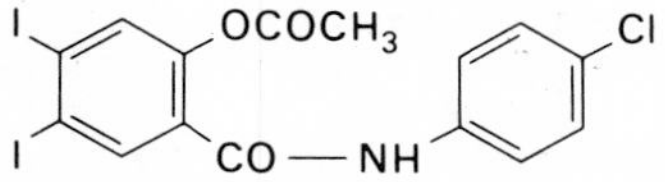

I $OCOCH_3$ Cl I CO — NH

clioxanide (Tremerad)

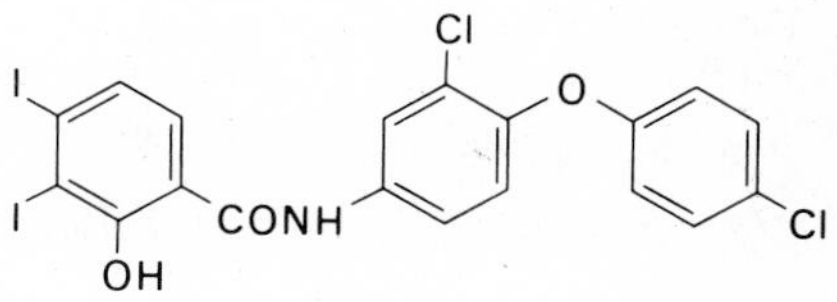

Cl I O I CONH Cl OH

rafoxanide

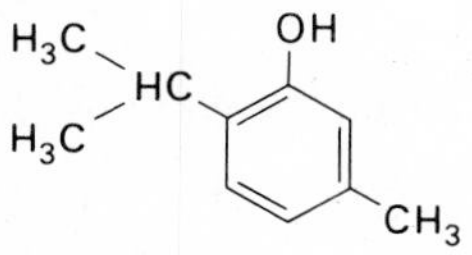

H_3C OH HC H_3C CH_3

thymol

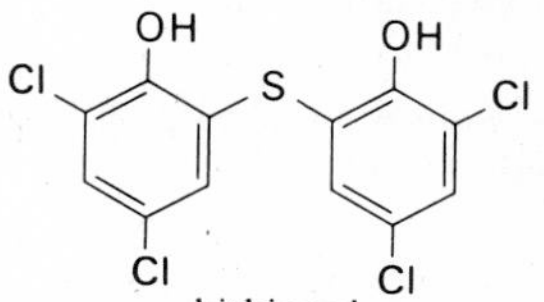

OH OH Cl S Cl Cl Cl

bithionol

C. Cyanine Dyes (Dithiazanine)

1. **History.** McCowan (1957) developed the series during the search for antifilarial compounds during World War II.

2. **Chemistry.** a. Cyanine derivatives derived from dyes used in color photography.

b. Systems in which a quaternary N is separated from a trivalent N by a resonating chain of alternating double and single bonds, each N being incorporated in a heterocyclic ring.

3. **Action.** Effective against a variety of helminths, including strongyloides, trichocephalus, hookworm, ascaris, pinworms.

4. **Mechanism.** In low concentration, inhibit oxygen uptake of parasites. In higher concentration, inhibit anaerobic metabolism of parasites.

5. **Pharmacodynamics.** Relatively poorly absorbed by mouth.

6. **Toxicity.** a. Frequent nausea, vomiting, and other gastrointestinal symptoms (up to 30%).

b. Nephrotoxic if absorbed; rare fatal reactions of undetermined mechanism.

c. Pyrvinium turns stools red; dithiazanine blue.

7. **Uses.** a. Dithiazanine is the only effective agent for strongyloides, and the only convenient one for trichocephalus. Less desirable than tetrachloroethylene for hookworm, and piperazine for ascaris and pinworms.

b. Pyrvinium is used against pinworms.

8. **Preparations**

DITHIAZANINE IODIDE (Delvex)

Dose: 200 mg 3 times a day by mouth for 5 or more days; withdrawn from market.

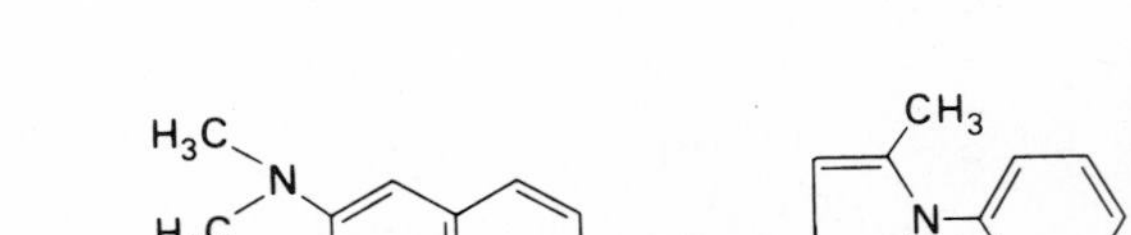

S, $\overset{+}{N}$, C_2H_5 —CH=CH—CH=CH—CH= S, N, C_2H_5 $\cdot I^-$

PYRVINIUM PAMOATE (Povan)

Dose: 5 mg per kg by mouth; repeat 1 week later.

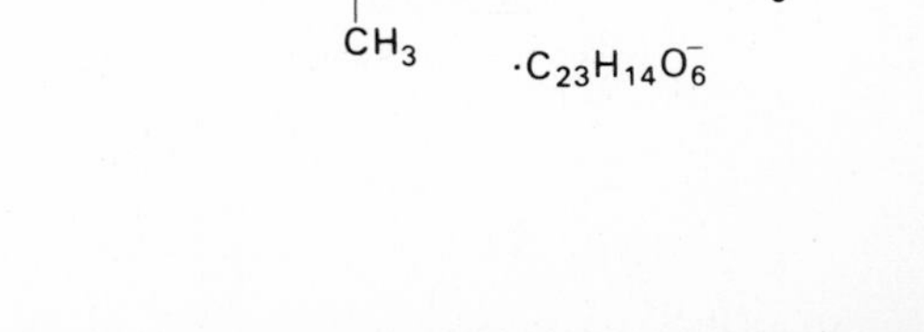

H_3C, N, H_3C, $\overset{+}{N}$, CH_3, CH=CH, CH_3, N, CH_3 $\cdot C_{23}H_{14}O_6^-$

STILBAZIUM IODIDE (Monopar)

Dose: 300 mg twice daily by mouth for 3 days.

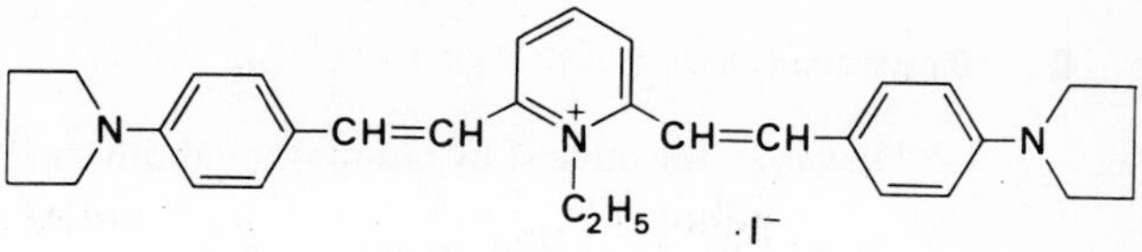

N—C6H4—CH=CH—(pyridinium, N^+—C_2H_5)—CH=CH—C6H4—N · I^-

D. Piperazines

1. **History.** Fayard (1949) introduced piperazine as an anthelmintic.

2. **Chemistry.** Piperazine salts.

3. **Action.** Inhibit ascaris and pinworms (enterobiasis or oxyuriasis).

4. **Mechanism.** a. Block acetylcholine at ascaris myoneural junction, paralyzing worms, which then wash out.

b. Also decreases production of succinate in worm.

5. **Pharmacodynamics.** Absorption minimal.

6. **Toxicity.** a. Piperazine causes infrequent nausea, vomiting, headache, abdominal cramps, and rare urticaria.

b. Excessive doses may give neurological disturbances such as vertigo, tremor, and memory defects.

7. **Uses.** a. Piperazine salts are the present therapy of choice in ascaris and pinworm infestations.

b. In pinworm infestation the whole family usually needs to be treated.

8. **Preparations**

PIPERAZINE CITRATE (Antepar, Multifuge, and others)

Dose: 1 gm by mouth daily for 7 days (pinworms); 3 gm by mouth daily for 2 days (ascariasis).

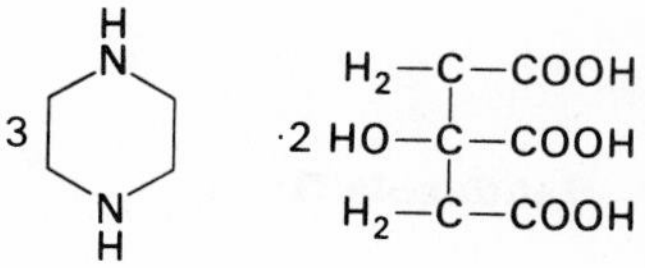

3 (piperazine, HN—NH) ·2 H_2—C—COOH / HO—C—COOH / H_2—C—COOH

Piperazine calcium edetate (Perin), *piperazine tartrate* (Piperat), *piperazine hexahydrate*, *phosphate*, *adipate*, *trichlorophenate*. Other salts of piperazine.

OTHERS

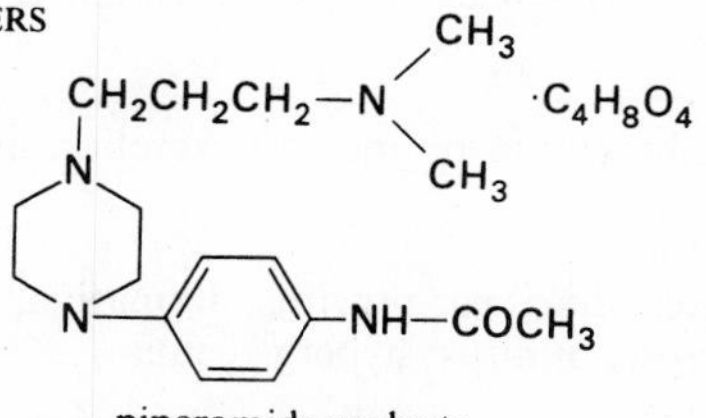

$CH_2CH_2CH_2$—$N(CH_3)_2$ · $C_4H_8O_4$; piperazine N—C6H4—NH—$COCH_3$

piperamide maleate

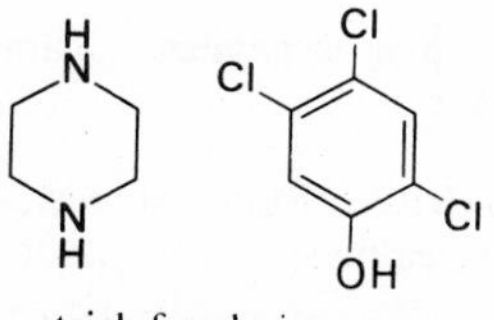

piperazine (HN—NH) ; Cl, Cl, Cl, OH (trichlorophenol)

triclofenol piperazate (Ranestol)

E. Bephenium

1. **History.** Introduced by Goodwin and others (1958).

2. **Chemistry.** A quaternary ammonium.

3. **Action and Mechanism.** a. Active against hookworm and ascaris; not against whipworm.
b. Reported to inhibit glucose transport and aerobic glycolysis in parasite.

4. **Pharmacodynamics.** Poorly absorbed; absorbed drug excreted in urine.

5. **Toxicity.** Relatively nontoxic, but slight nausea, vomiting, and soft stools have been reported.

6. **Uses.** Effective against *Ancylostoma duodenale* and ascaris; less effective against *Necator americanus* (Hsieh, Amer. J. Trop. Med. Hyg., 9:496, 1960).

7. **Preparation**

BEPHENIUM HYDROXYNAPHTHOATE (Alcopara)

Dose: 2.5 gm twice a day by mouth for 1 to 3 days.

$$C_6H_5-O-CH_2CH_2-\overset{+}{N}(CH_3)_2-CH_2-C_6H_5 \cdot C_{11}H_7O_3^-$$

THENIUM CLOSYLATE (Bancaris)

Anthelmintic for canine hookworm.

$$C_4H_3S-CH_2-\overset{+}{N}(CH_3)_2-CH_2CH_2O-C_6H_5 \cdot C_6H_4O_3SCl^-$$

F. Bendazole Group

1. **Chemistry.** Benzimidazole derivatives.

2. **Action and Mechanism.** a. Broad-spectrum anthelmintics, active especially against roundworms in animals and man, including pinworms, strongyloides, hookworm, whipworm, and cutaneous larva migrans.
b. Mechanism assumed to be interference with an essential, unidentified metabolic pathway in the parasite.

3. **Pharmacodynamics.** Rapid absorption by mouth; excretion in 24 to 48 hours in urine.

4. **Toxicity.** May produce nausea, diarrhea; pruritus, dermatitis; headache, drowsiness, weakness, numbness, collapse, tinnitus; hyperglycemia.

5. **Uses.** Promising agents for the treatment of roundworm infestations.

6. Preparations

THIABENDAZOLE (Mintezol)

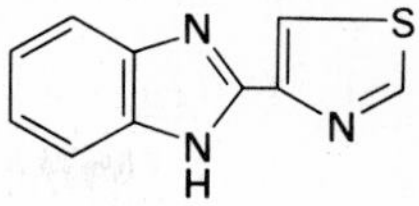

Dose: 25 to 50 mg per kg twice daily for 1 to 2 days.

OTHERS

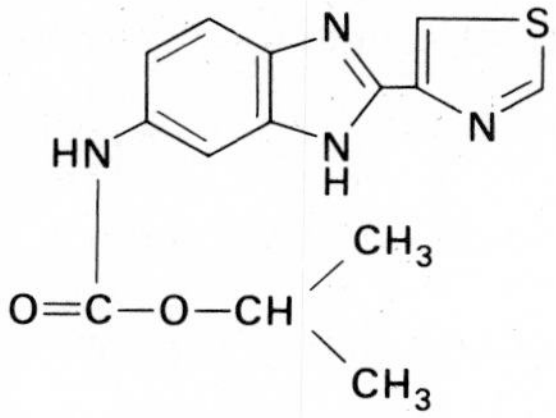

cambendazole

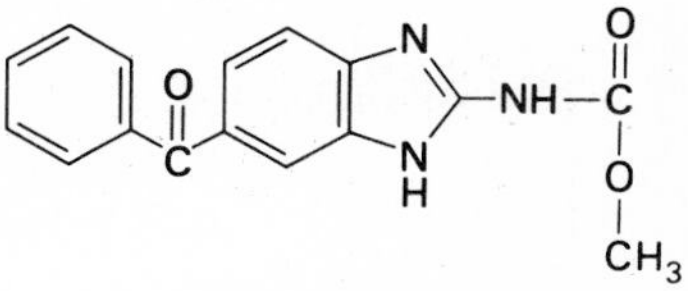

mebendazole

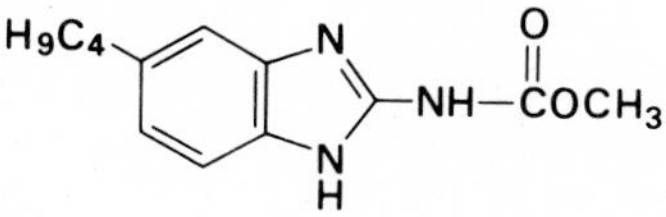

parabendazole

G. Other Anthelmintics

IMIDAZOTHIAZOLES

LEVAMISOLE HYDROCHLORIDE (Tramisol)

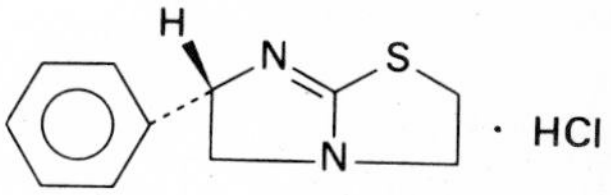

TETRAMISOLE HYDROCHLORIDE (Ripercol and others)

Both are also under investigation as immunostimulants.

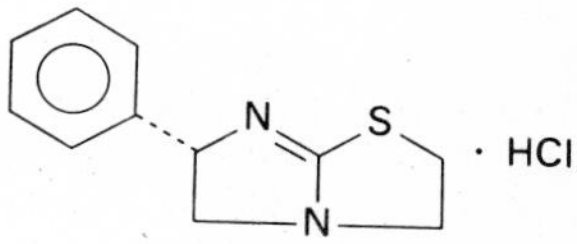

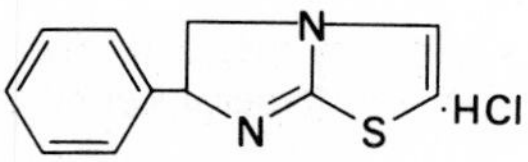

antafenite HCl

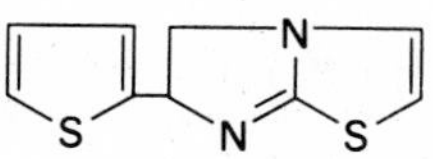

antiente

THIENYLPYRIMIDINES

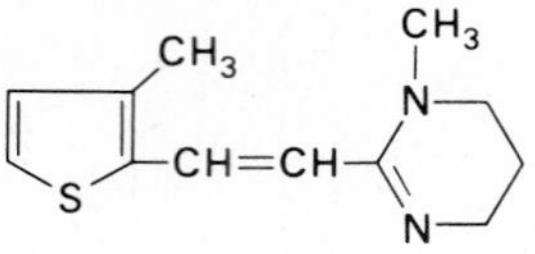

$\cdot C_4H_6O_6$

morantel tartrate

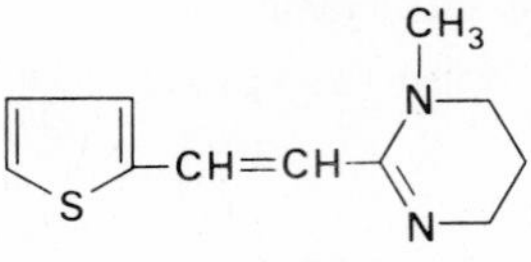

$\cdot C_{23}H_{16}O_6$

pyrantel pamoate

MISCELLANEOUS

BITOSCANATE

Has been tried in hookworm infestation.

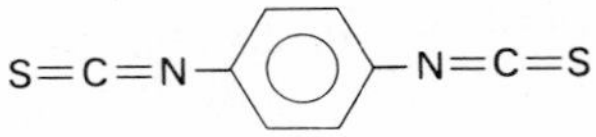

S=C=N–C_6H_4–N=C=S

Beta-methoxyethylpyridine (Promintic), dichlorvos, dymanthine (DODA), haloxon, imidocarb HCl.

H. Older Anthelmintics

A number of older compounds once used in roundworm infestations now have little but historical interest.

METHYLROSANILINE CHLORIDE (gentian violet)

Synthetic dye formerly used in pinworm infestations; relatively nontoxic, but may cause some local irritation.

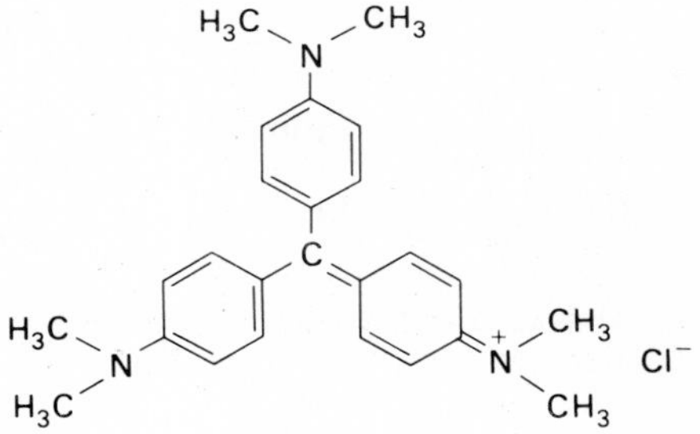

gentian violet

OIL OF CHENOPODIUM

Oil distilled from American wormseed; active constituent ascaridole, one of the few natural peroxides. Effective against roundworms, presumably by direct paralysis. Absorption produces nausea, vomiting, deafness, renal damage, and rare fatalities.

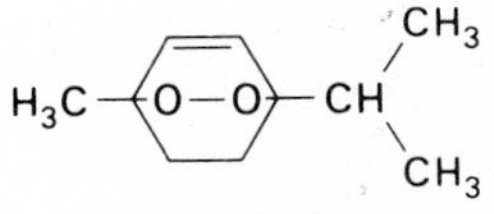

ascaridole

SANTONIN

Anciently used naphthalene compound from wormwood (absinthe); moderately effective against roundworms but may be absorbed giving vomiting, diarrhea, hematuria, convulsions, and collapse.

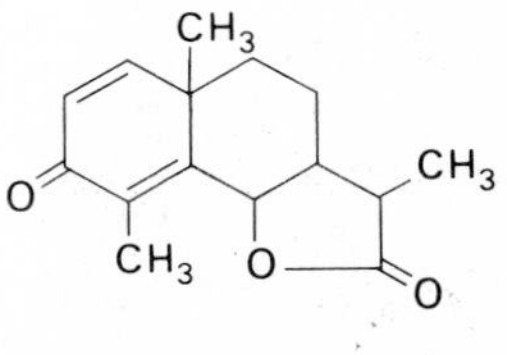

III. SCHISTOSOMIASIS

Three trematodes cause the human disease schistosomiasis (bilharziasis): the blood flukes *Schistosoma haematobium*, *S. mansoni*, and *S. japonicum*. Ova are passed in the stool, undergo development to cercariae in a snail, which reinfect man or other host animals through the skin.

A. Antimonials

1. History. a. Antimonials have been used as medicines and cosmetics since 4000 B.C. They were the basis for much of the fame of Paracelsus (1493–1541).

b. Vianna (1912) discovered the effectiveness of tartar emetic in leishmaniasis and so introduced the use of antimonials in tropical diseases.

2. Chemistry. As with the arsenicals, which the antimonials resemble in many respects, both trivalent and pentavalent organic antimonials have been used.

3. Action. a. Antimonials inhibit the organisms of granuloma inguinale, schistosomiasis, filariasis, and leishmaniasis.

b. They may also produce a local caustic action, or emesis, the latter being the result of both local and central effects.

4. Mechanism. a. The antiparasitic action probably is similar to that of arsenic, residing in sulfhydryl inhibition, with pentavalent forms being reduced to trivalent forms to become active.

b. Or may inhibit phosphofructokinase, which is involved in anaerobic breakdown of glucose by schistosomes (Bueding, Pharmacol. Rev., 9:329, 1957).

5. Pharmacodynamics. a. Most preparations are poorly absorbed, in part because of their irritant nature.

b. After injection, excretion is moderately rapid (three days) through the kidneys.

6. Toxicity. a. Generally similar to arsenicals.

b. Trivalent forms are more toxic than pentavalents and may produce coughing, vomiting, pneumonitis, arthralgia, bradycardia.

c. Pentavalent forms may produce emesis, hepatitis, anaphylactoid reactions late in the course of injections.

7. Uses. Antimonials are still important drugs in the treatment of schistosomiasis, furnishing alternatives to the new lucanthone; also used, but decreasingly, in leishmaniasis and filariasis.

8. Preparations

ANTIMONY POTASSIUM TARTRATE (tartar emetic)

Dose: 40 mg intravenously repeated in gradually increasing doses on alternate days.

```
COO—Sb=O
|
CHOH
|
CHOH
|
COOK
```

STIBOPHEN (Fuadin)

Preferred to tartar emetic as less toxic, but is less effective.

Dose: 1.5 ml of 6.3% solution intramuscularly in gradually increasing doses on alternate days in courses lasting 2 weeks; up to a total of 100 to 150 ml.

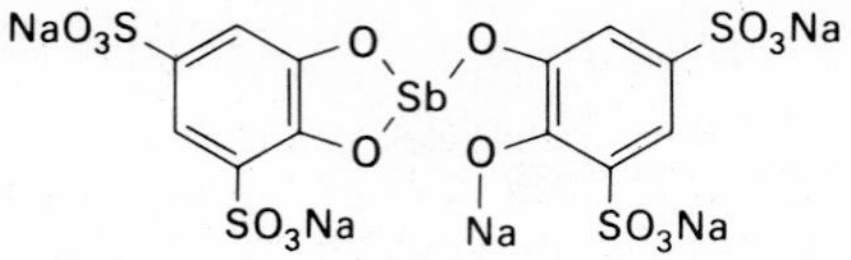

STIBAMINE GLUCOSIDE (Neostam)

Representative of pentavalent antimonials, no longer marketed.

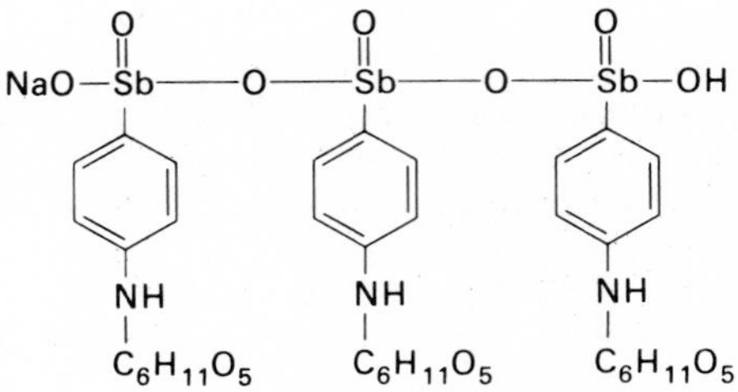

OTHERS: Antimony dimercaptosuccinate (Astiban), stibogluconate

B. Thioxanthones (Lucanthone)

1. **History.** Developed by Kikuth during World War II.

2. **Chemistry.** Thioxanthone derivatives.

3. **Action.** Inhibit *Schistosoma haematobium*, *S. mansoni* less, and *S. japonicum* least. Also bacteriostatic and carcinostatic.

4. **Mechanism.** Reported to combine with DNA.

5. **Pharmacodynamics.** Absorbed by mouth. Largely metabolized in the body.

6. **Toxicity.** May produce prostration, insomnia, yellow skin, tremor, convulsions, psychoses, especially in adults.

7. **Uses.** a. Administered orally in schistosomiasis.
b. A satisfactory alternative to antimony compounds in children.

8. **Preparations**

BECANTHONE

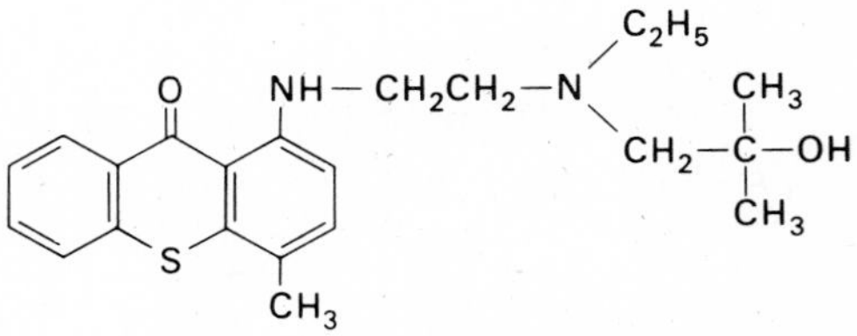

HYCANTHONE

Dose: 3 to 3.5 mg per kg body weight once intramuscularly.

Hycanthone mesylate (Etrenol)

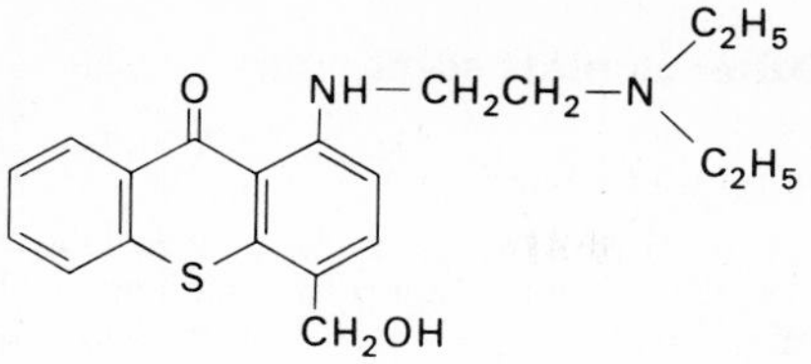

C_2H_5
O NH—CH_2CH_2—N
C_2H_5
S
CH_2OH

LUCANTHONE HYDROCHLORIDE (Miracil D; Nilodin)

Dose: 10 to 20 mg per kg body weight daily by mouth for 8 to 20 days.

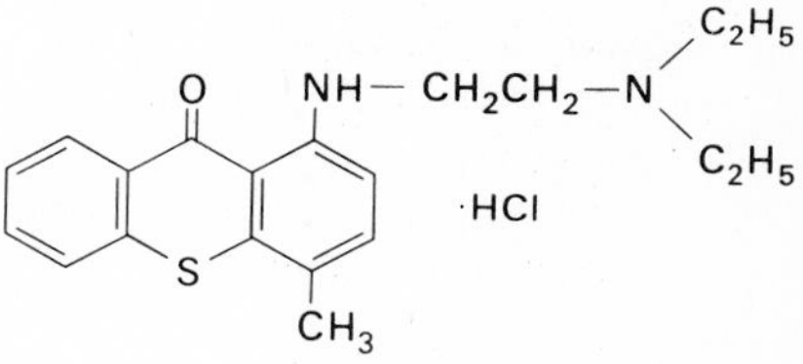

C_2H_5
O NH—CH_2CH_2—N
C_2H_5
·HCl
S
CH_3

C. Triphenylmethane Dyes

PARAROSANILINE PAMOATE

1. Chemistry. A triphenylmethane dye.

2. Action and Mechanism. Inhibits acetylcholinesterase of schistosomes. Removes glycogen from specific areas of schistosomes.

3. Uses. Recent use shows promise in schistosomiasis.

4. Preparation

PARAROSANILINE PAMOATE (fuchsin)

Under investigation.

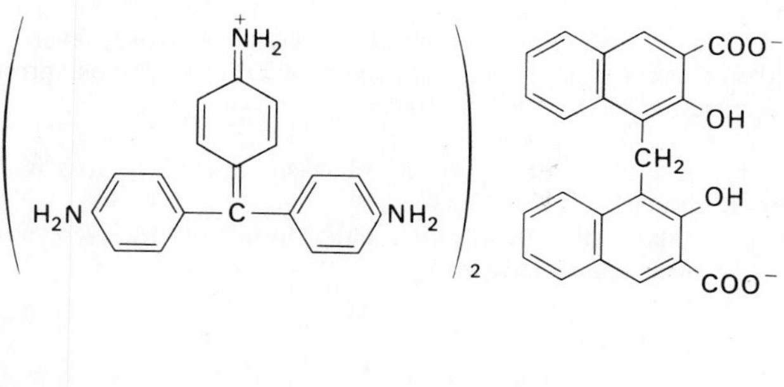

$\overset{+}{N}H_2$
H_2N C NH_2
2
COO^-
OH
CH_2
OH
COO^-

D. Other Schistosomacides

NIRIDAZOLE (Ambilhar)

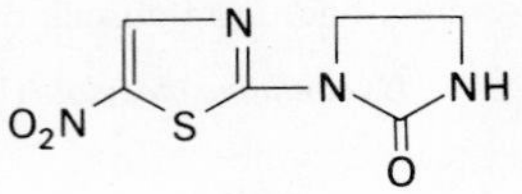

A nitrothiazole. Stops egg laying, then kills adult flukes. Depletes glycogen stores by inhibiting of phosphorylation enzymes of the worm. May produce nausea, confusion, convulsions, inhibition of spermatogenesis.

Dose: 25 mg per kg body weight daily by mouth for 5 to 7 days.

TEROXALENE

A piperazine derivative.

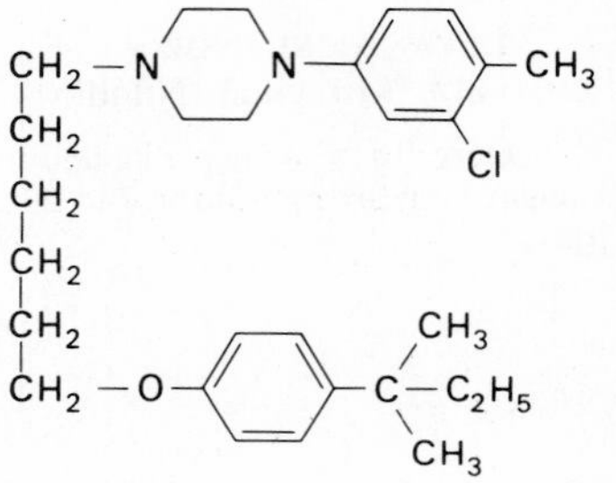

IV. FILARIASIS

DIETHYLCARBAMAZINE

1. History. Developed by Hewitt and others (1947) in search for antifilarial agents.

2. Chemistry. Piperazine carbamate derivative.

3. Action. a. Leads to destruction of microfilaria.
b. Little effect on adult worms (which give the symptoms).

4. Mechanism. May act by altering the surface so that antibodies can have access.

5. Pharmacodynamics. Absorbed by mouth.

6. Toxicity. a. May produce dermatitis, headache, nausea, fever.
b. In onchocerciasis may produce severe allergic reactions, presumably from massive destruction of the microfilariae.

7. Uses. a. Useful in all types of filariasis, including loiasis, calabar swelling, and onchocerciasis.
b. The microfilaria disappear, and usually do not return, even though the death of the adult worms is problematical.

8. Preparations

DIETHYLCARBAMAZINE *Diethylcarbamazine citrate* (Hetrazan)

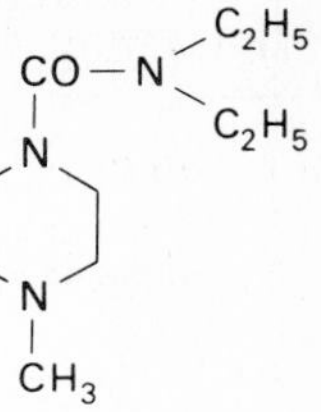

Dose: 100 mg by mouth 3 times a day for 3 weeks.

$$\mathrm{CO{-}N(C_2H_5)_2}$$
$$\text{piperazine ring: } \mathrm{N} \cdots \mathrm{N{-}CH_3}$$

OTHER ANTIFILARIAL AGENTS: Melarsonyl (Mel W) (see Trivalent Organic Arsenicals).

SUMMARY: ANTHELMINTICS AND OTHER AGENTS FOR METAZOAL DISEASES

TYPE	*ACTION AND MECHANISM*	*TOXICITY*	*USE*	*EXAMPLES*
Quinacrine	Active vs. flatworms Mechanism unknown	Mental symptoms, yellow skin	Flatworm infestation	Quinacrine hydrochloride
Chlorinated hydrocarbons	Active vs. roundworms Mechanism uncertain	Hepatitis	Hookworm and ascaris	Tetrachloro-ethylene
Phenol derivatives	Active vs. hookworm, ascaris	Minor	Hookworm, ascaris	Hexylresorcinol
Cyanine dyes	Active vs. many roundworms Metabolic inhibitor	Nephrotoxicity	Various roundworm infestations	Pyrvinium pamoate
Piperazines	Active vs. ascaris, pinworms Block acetylcho-line in worm	Urticaria, vertigo	Ascaris and pinworm infestations	Piperazine citrate
Bephenium group	Active vs. hookworm and ascaris Metabolic inhibitor	Minor	Ascaris and hookworm	Bephenium hydroxynaph-thoate
Bendazole group	Active vs. many roundworms	Dermatitis, numbness, tinnitus	Roundworm infestations	Thiabendazole
Antimonials	Active vs. schistosomiasis, leishmaniasis Sulfhydryl inhibition	Arthralgia, hepatitis	Schistosomiasis	Stibophen

(cont.)

SUMMARY: ANTHELMINTICS AND OTHER AGENTS FOR METAZOAL DISEASES (cont.)

TYPE	*ACTION AND MECHANISM*	*TOXICITY*	*USE*	*EXAMPLES*
Thioxanthones	Active vs. schistosomiasis	Tremor, convulsions, psychoses	Schistosomiasis	Lucanthone HCl
Triphenylmethane dyes	Active vs. schistosomiasis Affects glycogen	Minor	Schistosomiasis	Pararosaniline pamoate
Diethyl-carbamazines	Kills microfilaria	Fever, allergic manifestations	Filariasis	Diethylcar-bamazine

Reviews

Wolstenholme, G. E. W. (ed.). Bilharziasis. Boston, Ciba Foundation, 1962.

Hoskins, D., and Kean, B. Drugs for travelers. Clin. Pharmacol. Ther., 4:673, 1963.

Most, H. Treatment of the more common worm infections. J.A.M.A., 185:874, 1963.

Brown, H., and Belding, D. Basic Clinical Parasitology, 2nd ed. New York, Appleton-Century-Crofts, 1964.

Thompson, P. Parasite chemotherapy. Ann. Rev. Pharmacol., 7:77, 1967.

Douglas, J., and Baker, N. Chemotherapy of animal parasites. Ann. Rev. Pharmacol., 8:213, 1968.

Bueding, E., and Fisher, J. Pharmacologic and chemotherapeutic properties of niridazole and other antischistosomal compounds. N.Y. Acad. Sci., 160:536, 1969.

Jucker, E. (ed.) Progress in Drug Research, Vol. 19, Basel, Birkäuser, 1975.

12. Insecticides, Repellents, and Rodenticides

A. Insecticides

CHLORINATED HYDROCARBONS

1. History. a. Chlorphenothane (DDT) synthesized (1875).
b. Müller (1939) recognized insecticidal properties.

2. Chemistry. Chlorinated phenyls (DDT, methoxychlor); cyclohexanes (lindane); indanes (chlordane); camphenes (aldrin).

3. Action. a. In insects: Produce instability and stimulation of the nervous system, especially peripheral sensory structures.
b. In mammals: Abnormal function of the CNS, especially the cerebellum and motor cortex.

4. Mechanism. a. Lethal effect (DDT) in insects appears to be partly owing to a physical mechanism, in which a "charge transfer complex" is made with a component of the axon reducing its ability to carry impulses, and partly to liberation of butyrobetaine or acetylcholine (Rothschild, Nature, 192:283, 1961); oxidative enzymes also rise. Camphenes inhibit excretory processes of Malpighian tubules.
b. In some organisms, but not man, competitive antagonism with inositol has been observed (lindane).
c. Resistance may be induced in insects (DDT) and is accompanied by increased alanine content (Micke, Science, 131:1615, 1960).

5. Pharmacodynamics and Toxicity. a. DDT, lindane, and chlordane infrequently cause poisoning in man, but ingestion, or absorption through the skin, may produce irritability, numbness and tingling, tremors, and later convulsions and death (fatal dose of DDT about 10 gm); stored in fat.
b. Toxaphene group easily absorbed through the skin of mammals with resultant convulsions and death.

6. Uses. a. DDT, besides its principal use as an insecticide, is used in medicine in pediculosis and scabies, where the insects are ordinarily still susceptible.
b. Lindane is used similarly to DDT as an insecticide, but is active against a somewhat wider range of insects.
c. Chlordane (roaches) and the toxaphene group are not used medicinally.

7. Preparations

CHLOROPHENOTHANE (DDT)

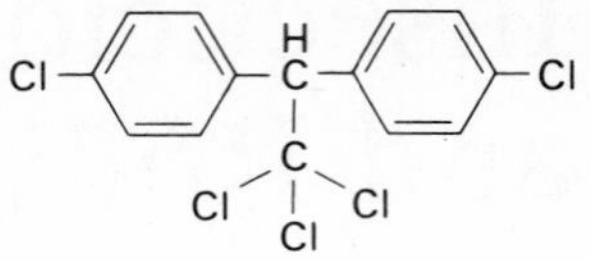

Dose: Applied locally in a 1 to 10% solution in kerosene; or 2% to 5% in a dusting powder.

Benzyl benzoate-chlorophenothane-ethyl amino benzoate:

Mixture used in emulsions or ointment as a scabicide.

LINDANE (hexachlorocyclohexane, gammexane)

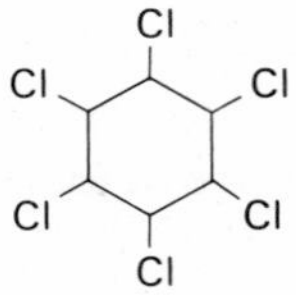

(Incorrectly called "benzene hexachloride")
Dose: Applied locally in 1% ointment or lotion.

Nonmedicinal:

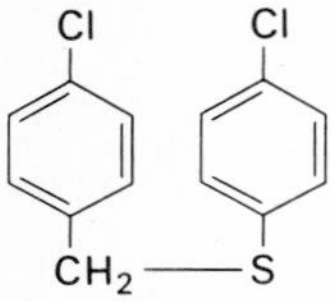

mitox

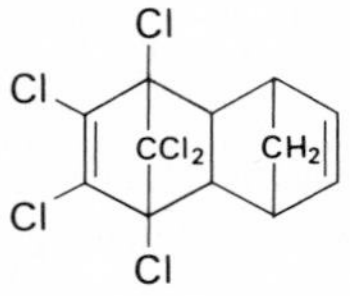

aldrin

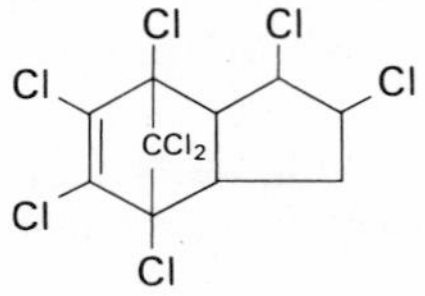

chlordane

BENZYL BENZOATE AND OTHER SCABICIDES

BENZYL BENZOATE LOTION

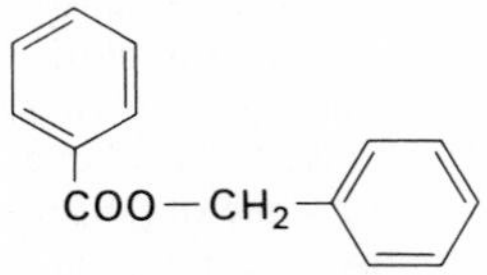

Widely used scabicide.

Dose: Applied locally; contains 25% of the agent.

CROTAMITON (Eurax)

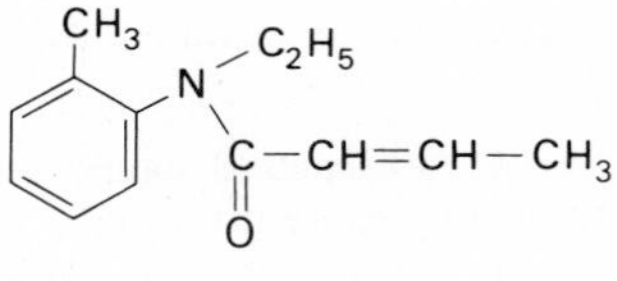

Dose: 30 gm of 10% ointment or lotion to entire body except head; repeat in 24 hours.

ORGANOPHOSPHORUS COMPOUNDS

1. **Chemistry.** Esters of phosphoric acid (see Myoneural Agents).

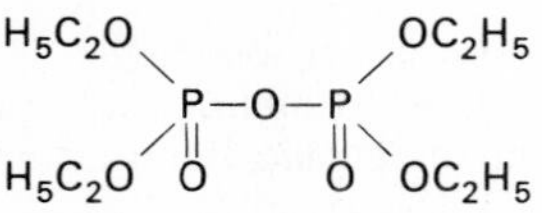

tetraethyl pyrophosphate

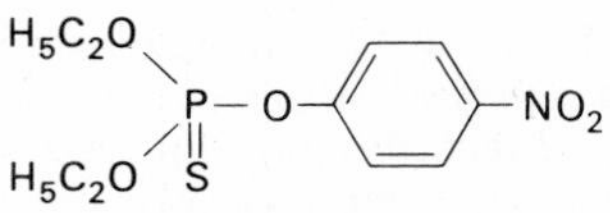

parathion

2. Action and Mechanism. Insecticides of varying potency acting through inhibition of acetylcholinesterase; also may inhibit phosphorylation of other enzymes.

3. Pharmacodynamics and Toxicology. a. Poisoning produces symptoms of extreme cholinergic stimulation: headache, blurred vision, nausea, diarrhea, constriction in the chest, salivation, muscle twitching, convulsions (see Myoneural Agents for treatment).

b. Highly toxic members include tetraethyl pyrophosphate (TEPP) and parathion; less toxic members include Malathion, Chlorthion, Dipterex, and Trolene.

4. Uses. As a veterinary insecticide.

5. Preparation

CRUFOMATE (Ruelene)

For livestock; to kill internal and external parasites.

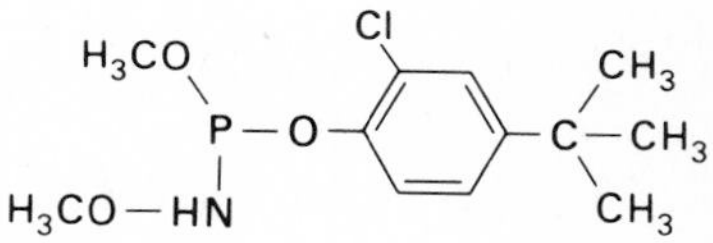

H_3CO, H_3CO-HN, P—O, Cl, $C-CH_3$, CH_3, CH_3

NATURAL PRODUCTS

1. Chemistry. a. Rotenone is the active ingredient of derris root, cubé, and other natural products.

b. Pyrethrins are active ingredients from pyrethrum flowers.

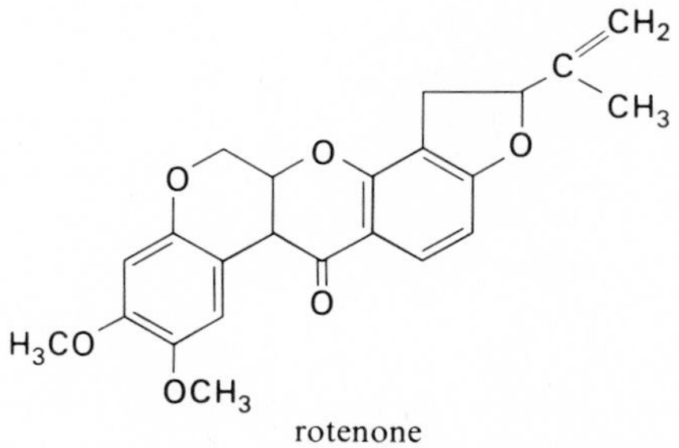

CH_2, C, CH_3, O, O, O, O, H_3CO, OCH_3

rotenone

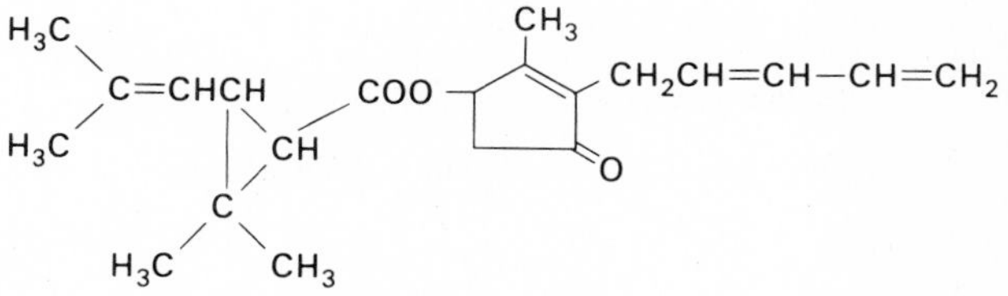

H_3C, H_3C, C=CHCH, COO, CH, C, H_3C, CH_3, CH_3, $CH_2CH=CH-CH=CH_2$, O

a pyrethrin

2. Actions. Produce immediate knockdown of flies and other insects, in contrast to the slow effect of DDT.

3. Mechanism. a. Rotenone inhibits glutamic acid oxidation, but the essential action may be cardiac depression; blocks electron transport system at diaphorase level in mitochondria and decreases oxygen uptake (Lindahl, Exp. Cell. Res., 23:228, 1961).

b. Pyrethrins cause a toxin to appear in the insect's blood; this may cause release of acetylcholine and interfere with neuromuscular function.

4. Pharmacodynamics and Toxicity. a. Poisoning infrequent in man, but respiratory stimulation, hyperexcitability, incoordination, and convulsions may be produced.

b. Patients allergically sensitive to chrysanthemums may be cross sensitive to pyrethrins.

5. Uses. Not used medicinally.

OTHER INSECTICIDES

A number of other insecticides are not used medicinally, but may cause poisoning:

DICHLOROBENZENE (*para- or ortho-*)

Moth repellents; low toxicity.

FLUORIDES

Used as roach poisons. Act as enzyme poisons in the conversion of glyceric acid to pyruvic acid by enolase in aerobic glycolysis.

FLUOROSILICATES

Used to impregnate cloth against moths; toxic.

NAPHTHALENE

Moth repellent; more toxic than the dichlorobenzenes. May produce hepatic and CNS damage with stimulation, then depression; may cause cataracts.

NICOTINE (see Ganglionic Agents)

SODIUM PENTACHLOROPHENATE (Sanobrite)

Not an insecticide, but used to kill snails in streams.

THIRAM

Methyl analogue of disulfiram. Used as an antibacterial and antifungal agent as well as an insecticide.

B. Insect Repellents and Attractants

REPELLENTS

Ideal insect repellents would be effective, odorless, and nontoxic. Much progress was made in developing such agents during World War II.

1. Chemistry. Various types of organic molecules.

2. Action and Mechanism. Deter the approach of insects; little known about mechanism.

3. Uses. To discourage or prevent approach and biting by mosquitoes, flies, and other insects.

4. Preparations

BUTOPYRONOXYL (Indalone)

Ineffective against mosquitoes but good against flies.

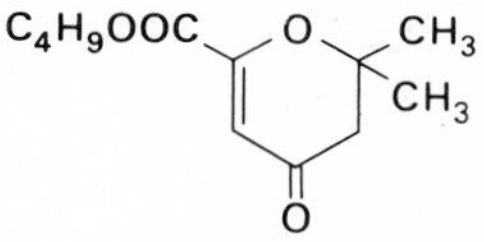

C_4H_9OOC, O, CH_3, CH_3, O

DIETHYLTOLUAMIDE (*m*-Delphene; Off)

Best repellent at present. Nontoxic. Is replacing *Dimethylphthalate Compound*, which contains butopyronoxyl, ethohexadiol and dimethylphthalate.

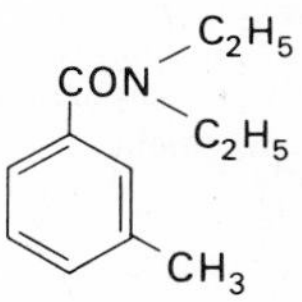

$CON(C_2H_5)_2$, CH_3

DIMETHYLPHTHALATE

One of the older compounds. May be irritating to the skin.

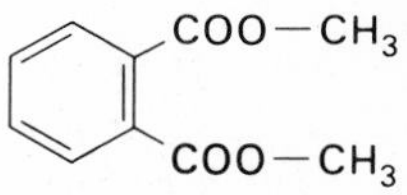

$COO-CH_3$, $COO-CH_3$

DIBUTYLPHTHALATE

ETHOHEXADIOL (Rutgers 612)

Effective and popular agent.

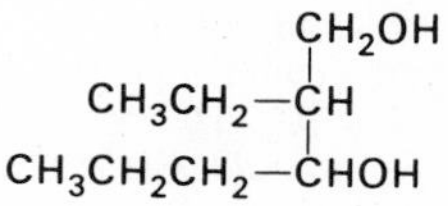

CH_2OH
CH_3CH_2-CH
$CH_3CH_2CH_2-CHOH$

ATTRACTANTS

4-(*p*-ACETOXYPHENYL)-2-BUTANONE

Synthetic lure for melon fly. Example of attractant for agricultural use. (Science, 131:1044, 1960).

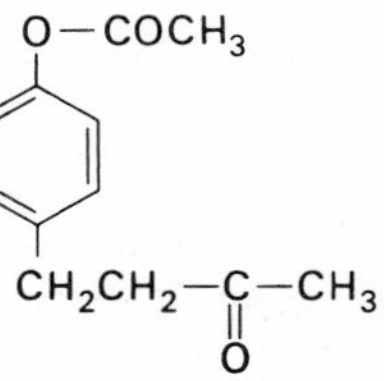

$O-COCH_3$
$CH_2CH_2-C(=O)-CH_3$

C. Rodenticides and Fumigants

RODENTICIDES

Rodenticides of great potency are now available. For the most part they are also toxic to man.

1. Preparations

ALPHA-NAPHTHYLTHIOUREA (ANTU)

Relatively effective though some rats are resistant; produces pleural effusion.

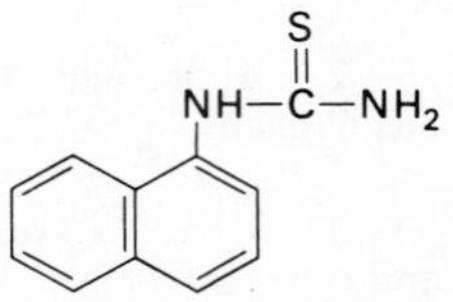

S
||
NH—C—NH₂

PHOSPHORUS

Highly toxic to man. Antidote: copper salts when material is still in the stomach (produces CuP_2 coating on the phosphorus particles).

RED SQUILL

Contains scillaren and other glycosides. Produces convulsions and respiratory failure in rats (as digitalis does); not dangerous to larger mammals which can vomit because it acts as an emetic.

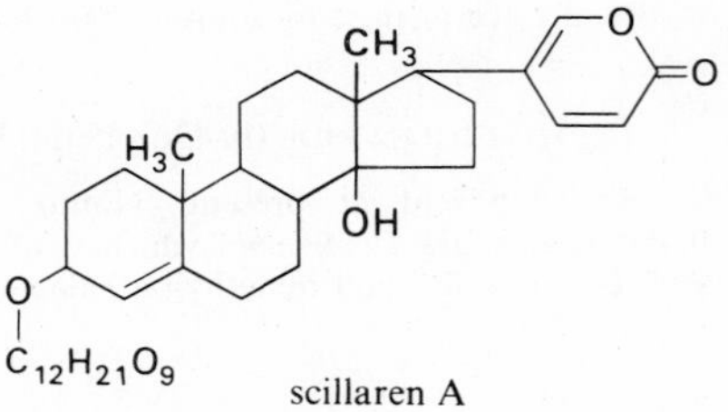

CH_3 H_3C OH O $C_{12}H_{21}O_9$ O O

scillaren A

SODIUM MONOFLUORACETATE (1080)

Replaces acetate in energy production (lethal synthesis of fluorocitrate poisons enzyme aconitase); highly lethal to man.

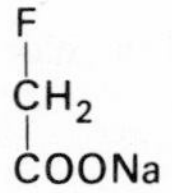

F—CH_2—COONa

Antidote: *glyceryl monoacetate* (monacetin): Furnishes 2C moieties which reduce the amount of fluorocitrate formed.

Dose: 0.1 to 0.5 mg per kg body weight intramuscularly every hour for several hours.

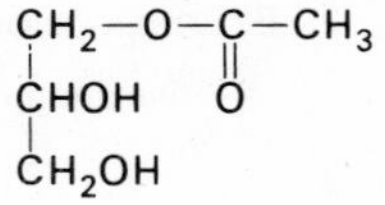

CH_2—O—C(=O)—CH_3, CHOH, CH_2OH

THALLIUM

Rat and ant poison; may produce acute and chronic poisoning in man. BAL not an efficient antidote.

WARFARIN

Acts by inhibiting blood clotting (see Anticoagulants). Unlikely to poison man as repeated intake needed.

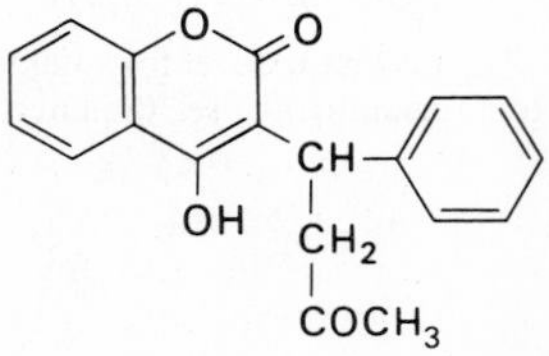

O O OH CH CH_2 $COCH_3$

ZINC PHOSPHIDE (Zn_3P_2)

HCl of stomach releases phosphine gas (PH_3).

FUMIGANTS

Fumigants have been used since medieval times as agents to render articles safe which have been in contact with sick persons. Thus letters were "sterilized" with vinegar and smoke as early as the 1300's. Present use of fumigants is largely to kill rodents and insects, rather than microorganisms.

1. Preparations

HYDROGEN CYANIDE (HCN)

Used in ships and empty buildings; highly toxic. The mechanism of toxicity is through combination with cytochrome oxidase, rendering it unavailable for cellular respiration.

Antidotes:

Methylene blue: Forms methemoglobin, then cyanmethemoglobin, sparing cytochrome oxidase; relatively ineffective against cyanide.

More valuable as an antidote for methemoglobinemia (reverse effect) caused by aniline, nitrobenzene, chlorates, nitrates, and others.

Dose: 1 to 2 mg per kg body weight intravenously (as 1% to 2% solution); repeat if necessary in 1 to 2 hours.

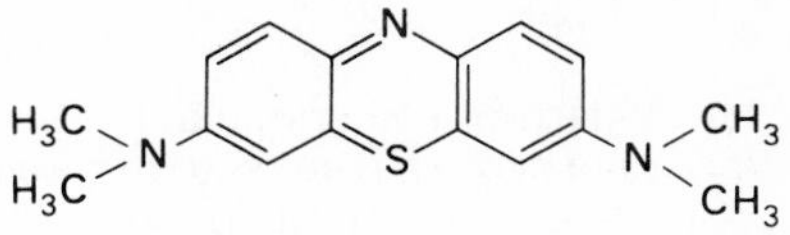

H3C N N S N CH3 H3C CH3

Sodium nitrite ($NaNO_2$): Forms methemoglobin better than methylene blue; may produce severe hypotension.

Dose: 2.5 to 5 ml per min of 3% solution intravenously up to a total of 10 to 15 ml; or amyl nitrite inhalation for 15 to 30 sec.

Sodium thiosulfate ($Na_2S_2O_3$): Favors conversion of cyanide to harmless thiocyanate. Dose: 12.5 gm (50 ml of 25% solution) intravenously.

OTHER FUMIGANTS

CARBON BISULFIDE (CS_2) Soil fumigant.

CARBON TETRACHLORIDE (CCl_4) Veterinary vermifuge.

METHYL BROMIDE (CH_3Br) Highly toxic, causes pulmonary irritation.

ETHYLENE OXIDE (C_2H_4O) General fumigant and sterilizer.

FORMALDEHYDE (HCHO) General disinfectant.

CHLORPICRIN ($CCl_3 \cdot NO_2$) Strong lacrimator and pulmonary irritant. Used as an insecticide and parasiticide to disinfect grains and cereals.

SULFUR DIOXIDE (SO_2) Used as an insecticide and to blanch fruits.

SULFURYLFLUORIDE (SO_2F_2) (Vicane) Fumigant for termites and other insects.

D. Herbicides and Other Plant Factors

AUXIN ANALOGUES

1. Chemistry. Analogues of the plant growth hormone, 3-indolyl acetic acid (auxin).

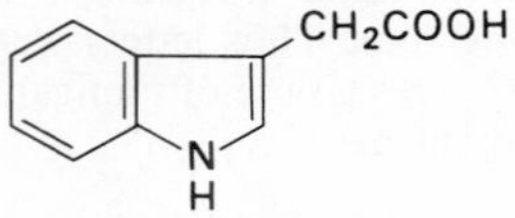

CH_2COOH N H

indole-3-acetic acid

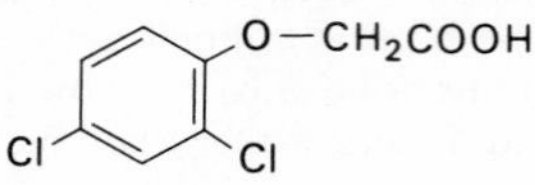

$O-CH_2COOH$ Cl Cl

2,4-D

2. Action and Mechanism. Analogues act as competitive antagonists, or by producing excessive growth.

3. Toxicity. May produce a myotonic-like condition in mammals, responding to quinidine.

4. Examples

BETA-NAPHTHOXY ACETIC ACID
BETA-CHOLORONAPHTHOXY ACETIC ACID
2,4-DICHLOROPHENOXYACETIC ACID (2,4-D)
2,4,5-TRICHLOROPHENOXYACETIC ACID (2,4,5-T)

GIBBERELLINS

1. History. Kurosawa (1926) derived as fungus extracts.

2. Chemistry. Gibberellic acid best known of four types.

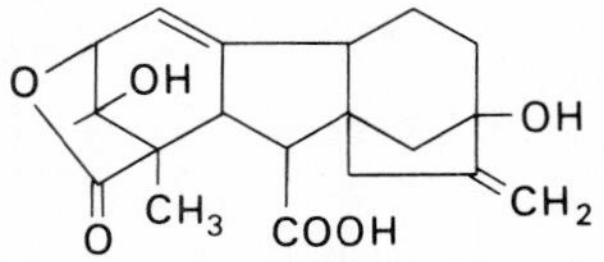

O OH OH O CH_3 COOH CH_2

gibberellic acid

3. Action and Mechanism. Induces height and flowering in plants. Inhibits an oxidase of indole acetic acid which would otherwise act as an inhibitor of auxin-induced growth.

4. Toxicity. Apparently not toxic in animals.

NITROPHENOLS

1. Chemistry

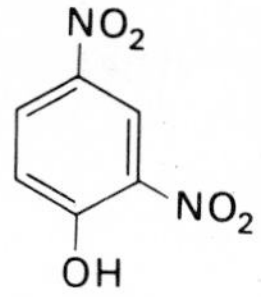

2,4-dinitrophenol 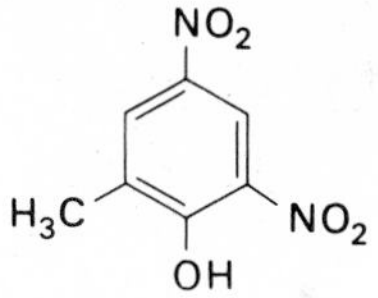 4,6-dinitro-*o*-cresol

2. Action and Mechanism. Effective weed killers. Act by uncoupling phosphorylation, which allows excessive oxidation.

3. Toxicity. In animals produce increased metabolism and fever; cataracts. Use in obesity obsolete.

2,2-DICHLOROPROPIONIC ACID

1. Action and Mechanism. Weed killer. Competes with pantoate in synthesis of pantothenic acid. Action reversible by pantoate or pantothenic acid.

2. Example

2,2-DICHLOROPROPIONIC ACID (Dalapon)

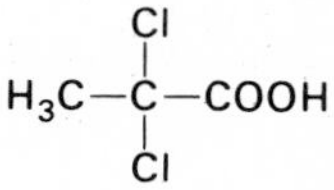

$$H_3C-CCl_2-COOH$$

METALS

Numerous metals, mostly highly toxic to man, are used to kill plants: salts of As, Pb, Hg, Cu, B.

OILS

Various oils and solvents are also used as herbicides; most are not highly toxic to man: crude oil, kerosene.

OTHER HERBICIDES

Other weed and brush killers include aminotriazole and sodium ammate.

PENTACHLOROPHENOL

Used to control algae.

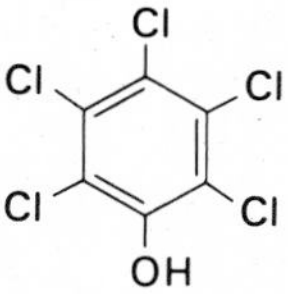

E. Human Repellents

CHLORACETOPHENONE

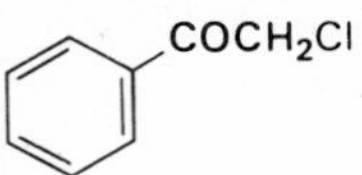

"Mace" is a 1% solution in kerosene, with Freon propellant. Disabling tear gas. Direct contact with eyes may damage from solid crystals which may stick into the cornea.

SUMMARY: INSECTICIDES, REPELLANTS, AND RODENTICIDES

TYPE	*ACTION AND MECHANISM*	*TOXICITY*	*USE*	*EXAMPLES*
Chlorinated hydrocarbons	Instability in CNS; mechanism complex	Numbness, tremors, convulsions	Insecticide	Chloropheno-tane (DDT)
Benzyl benzoate	Scabicide	Minor	Scabicide	Benzyl benzoate
Organophos-phorus compounds	Insecticide by acetylcholine inhibition	Cholinergic stimulation	Insecticide	Cruformate
Natural products	Paralysis, possibly by cardiac depression	Hyperexcitability, convulsions	Insecticide	Rotenone
Repellents	Repel insects	Minor	Insect repellant	Diethyltolu-amide
Rodenticides	Kill rodents by various mechanisms	Various and usually severe	Rodenticides	Warfarin
Fumigants	Kill all forms of pests	Highly toxic to man	Fumigation vs. roaches, mice, rats	Sulfurylfluoride
Herbicides	Various	Vary in toxicity to man	Killing weeds	Dinitrophenol

Reviews

Barnes, J. M. Toxicity of Pesticides. Bull. Hygiene, 34:1205, 1959.

Done, A. K. Clinical pharmacology of systemic antidotes. Clin. Pharmacol. Ther., 2:750, 1961.

Jacobson, M., and Beroza, M. Chemical insect attractants. Science, 140:1367, 1963.

Hayes, W. Review of the metabolism of chlorinated hydrocarbon insecticides especially in mammals. Ann. Rev. Pharmacol., 5:27, 1965.

Gilbert, I. Evaluation and use of mosquito repellants. J.A.M.A., 196:163, 1966.

Frazer, A. Pesticides. Ann. Rev. Pharmacol., 7:319, 1967.

13. Cancer Chemotherapy

It is at present impossible to propose any thoroughly satisfactory hypothesis to explain cancer. The fundamental change is most commonly thought of as a mutation, the result of an alteration of genetic material of a cell by a physical or chemical agent, or a virus. The virus may be an RNA virus, either harbored inside the cell and derepressed by a carcinogen, radiation, or other influences, or entering from the outside. It has been suggested that cancer RNA viruses may induce the formation of new DNA in the host cell, which redirects the nature of the cell.

Chemotherapy of cancer has followed these conceptions of causation and has been directed particularly at providing for the incorporation of false DNA in the cancer cells or at antiviral effects.

A. Alkylating Agents

NITROGEN MUSTARDS

1. History. a. Sulfur mustard was used as a poison gas in World War I, and the related nitrogen mustards studied for the same purpose during World War II.

b. They were found to cause atrophy of lymphoid tissue and bone marrow and were therefore tried in lymphosarcoma and other tumors.

2. Chemistry. Highly reactive, bifunctional compounds in which the chlorines may be replaced by groups from one or two other molecules; the latter are thus alkylated with the residue from the nitrogen mustard.

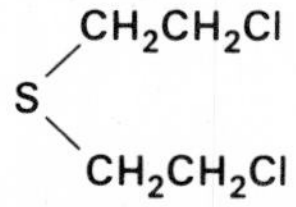

$$S(CH_2CH_2Cl)_2 \qquad H_3C{-}N(CH_2CH_2Cl)_2 \longrightarrow H_3C{-}N\begin{matrix} CH_2CH_2{-}R' \\ CH_2CH_2{-}R'' \end{matrix}$$

sulfur mustard 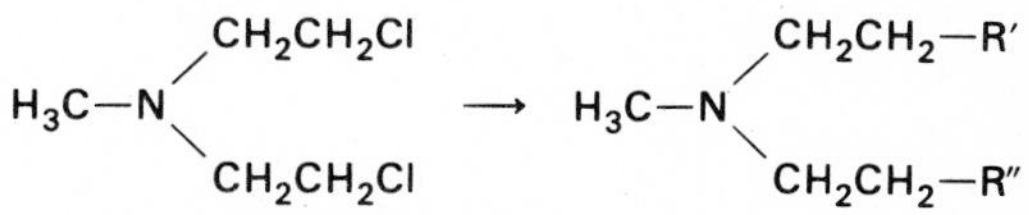 — nitrogen mustard

An ethyleneimmonium ring may be formed as an intermediate, as in the following example of the alkylation of a phosphate group:

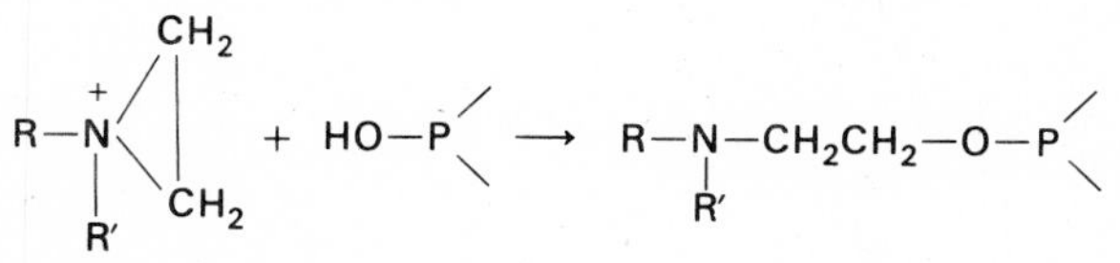

$$R{-}\overset{+}{N}(R')\!<\!\begin{matrix} CH_2 \\ | \\ CH_2 \end{matrix} + HO{-}P\!<\; \longrightarrow\; R{-}N(R'){-}CH_2CH_2{-}O{-}P\!<$$

3. Action. Cytotoxic to all tissues, especially rapidly renewed tissues, such as intestinal mucosa, corneal epithelium, germinal tissues, lymphatic and hematopoietic tissues.

4. Mechanism. a. Antineoplastic action is based on the alkylating power of the compounds.

b. Alkylation may interfere with synthesis or cross-linking in a number of places. Thus an attachment at the 7 position of guanine may prevent H bonding between the chains of DNA, arresting proper replication.

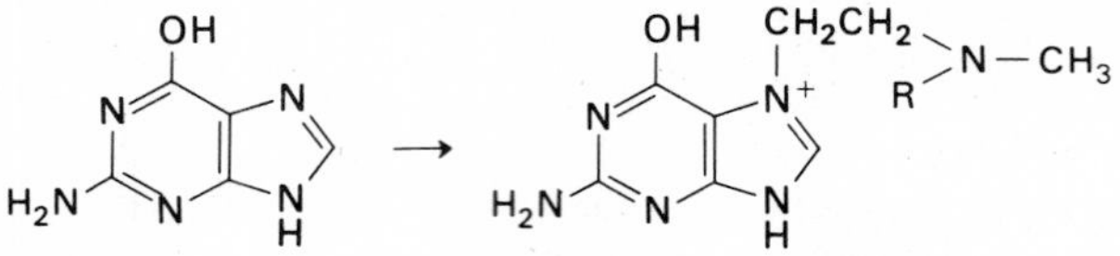

5. Pharmacodynamics. a. May be too irritating for oral administration, but chlorambucil satisfactory and well absorbed.

b. All are quickly distributed in the body, and hydrolyzed in the tissues.

6. Toxicity. a. Nitrogen mustards: Local vesicants and necrotizing agents. Abdominal pain, diarrhea, nausea, muscular paralysis, convulsions, damage to bone marrow.

b. Chlorambucil: Not irritating, and relatively nontoxic in therapeutic doses; cyclophosphamide may cause temporary alopecia and occasionally severe cystitis.

7. Uses. a. Palliative in neoplasms of lymphatic and hematopoietic tissues, including lymphosarcoma, chronic lymphatic leukemia, Hodgkin's disease, mycosis fungoides, and at times bronchogenic, ovarian, breast, and testicular carcinoma and other epithelial tumors.

b. Intensity of therapy is limited by bone marrow depression.

8. Preparations

CARMUSTINE

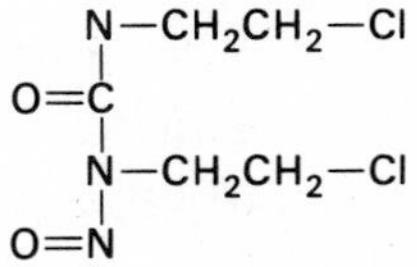

Used in Hodgkin's disease and lung cancer. Skin contact may cause pigmentation.

Dose: 100 mg per sq m per day intravenously.

CHLORAMBUCIL (Leukeran)

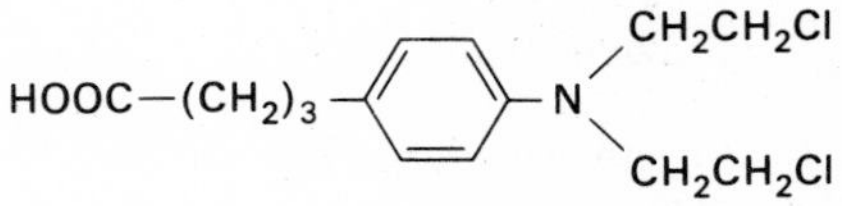

Dose: 0.1 to 0.2 mg per kg body weight by mouth daily for 3 to 6 weeks.

$HOOC-(CH_2)_3-C_6H_4-N(CH_2CH_2Cl)_2$

CYCLOPHOSPHAMIDE (Cytoxan; Endoxan)

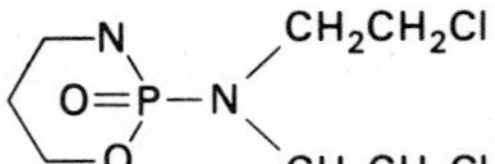

Dose: 2 to 3 mg per kg body weight intravenously daily for 6 days (lymphoma, leukemia, Hodgkin's disease); 4 to 8 mg per kg similarly (solid tumors).

MECHLORETHAMINE HYDROCHLORIDE (Mustargen; nitrogen mustard)

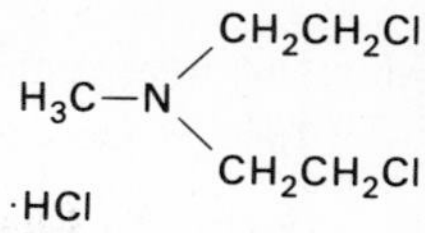

Dose: 0.1 mg per kg body weight intravenously daily for 4 days, in a dilute infusion.

$$H_3C{-}N(CH_2CH_2Cl)_2 \cdot HCl$$

MELPHALAN (Alkeran; sarcolysin)

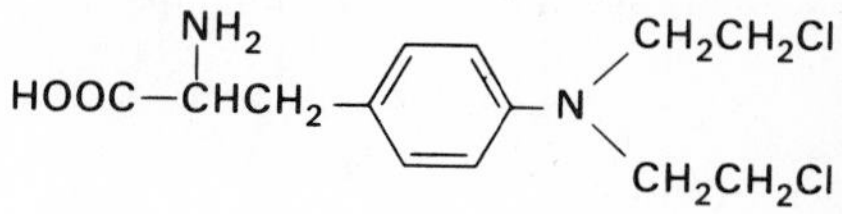

Phenylalanine nitrogen mustard. Used against multiple myeloma.

Dose: 6 mg daily by mouth in 2- to 3-week courses.

$$HOOC{-}CH(NH_2)CH_2{-}C_6H_4{-}N(CH_2CH_2Cl)_2$$

URACIL MUSTARD

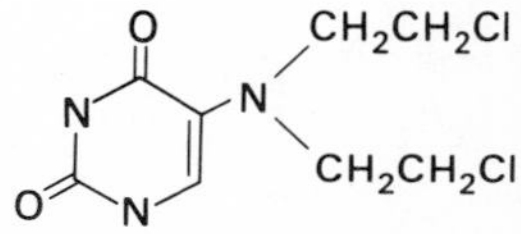

Used in leukemias and lymphomas.
Dose: 1 to 2 mg daily by mouth.

DACARBAZINE

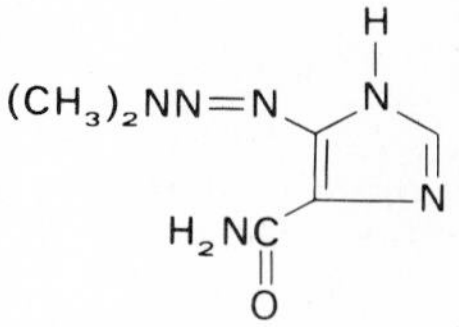

$$(CH_3)_2NN{=}N{-}\text{(imidazole ring)}{-}CONH_2$$

ETHYLENEIMINES

1. **Chemistry.** Similar to the nitrogen mustards except that the ethyleneimine ring is already present in the compound; conversion to the reactive quaternary ethyleneimmonium form in the body.

2. **Action and Mechanism.** Same as nitrogen mustards.

3. **Pharmacodynamics and Toxicity.** a. Well absorbed by mouth.
b. Not local vesicants; somewhat more prolonged in action than the nitrogen mustards, and produce less anorexia, nausea, and vomiting.

4. **Uses.** Same as for nitrogen mustards.

5. **Preparations**

TRIETHYLENE MELAMINE (TEM)

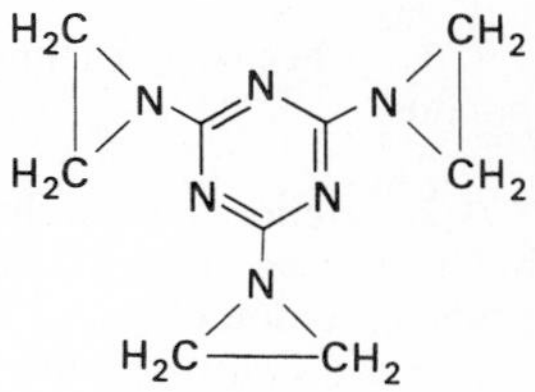

Dose: 2.5 mg by mouth daily for 2 or 3 days, then maintenance with 0.5 to 1 mg every 1 to 2 weeks.

THIOTEPA (Triethylene thiophosphoramide)

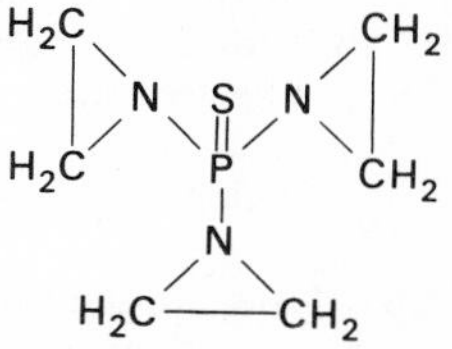

Dose: 0.2 mg per kg body weight by any parenteral route daily for 3 to 5 days.

URedepa (Avinar)

Tried in mammary cancer, leukemias, melanoma.

Dose: 2 to 3 mg per kg body weight intravenously, intraperitoneally, or intrapleurally.

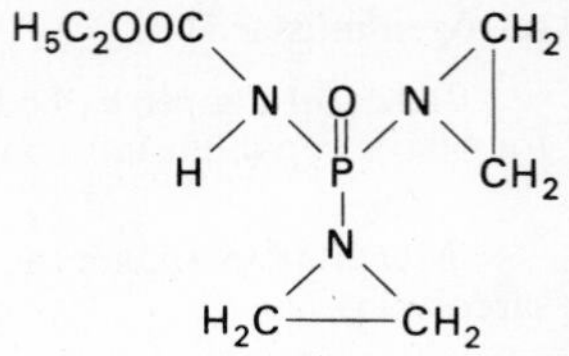

H_5C_2OOC N O N CH_2 H P CH_2 N H_2C CH_2

Others

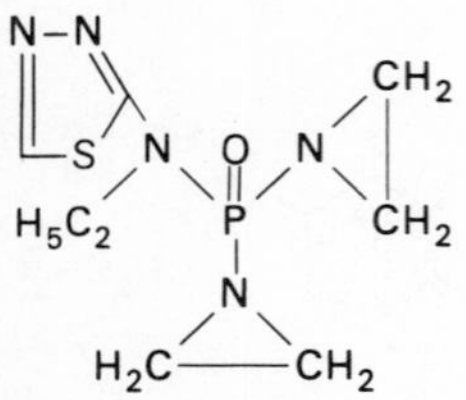

N–N S N O N CH_2 H_5C_2 P CH_2 N H_2C CH_2

azetepa

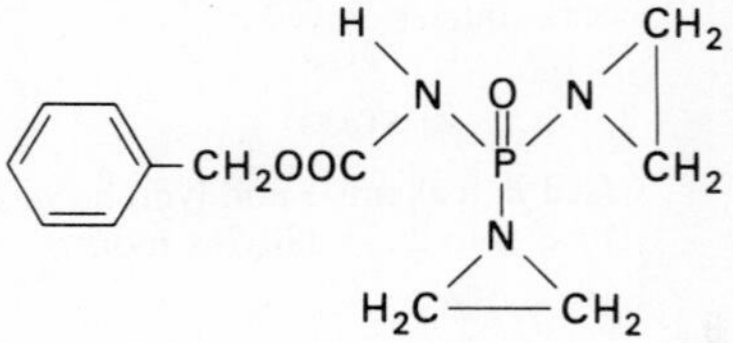

H N O N CH_2 CH_2OOC P CH_2 N H_2C CH_2

benzodepa

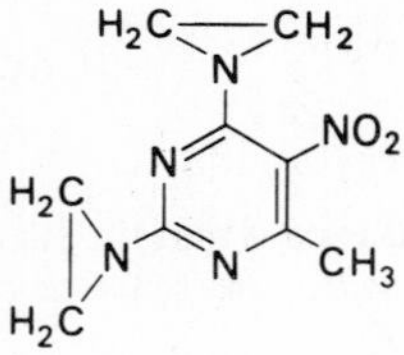

H_2C CH_2 N N NO_2 H_2C N N CH_3 H_2C

Elderfield pyrimidine mustard

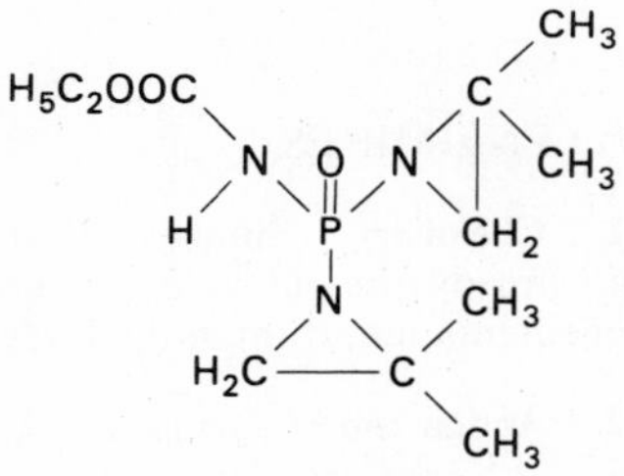

H_5C_2OOC CH_3 C N O N CH_3 H P CH_2 N CH_3 H_2C C CH_3

maturedepa

METHYLSULFONATE ESTERS

1. Chemistry. Dimethanesulfonoxybutanes and allied bifunctional compounds.

2. Action and Mechanism. a. Probably similar to other alkylating agents but it has been suggested that they may also interfere with utilization of sulfur amino acids by complexing with the sulfur.

b. Cytotoxic effect largely limited to the bone marrow.

3. Pharmacodynamics. a. Well absorbed from the intestinal tract.

b. Metabolic fate unknown.

c. Partly excreted as tetrahydrothiophene.

4. Toxicity. Thrombocytopenia and general bone marrow depression.

5. Uses. Used principally in chronic myelogenous leukemia; also in myelofibrosis, polycythemia vera.

6. Preparations

BUSULFAN (Myleran)

Dose: 2 to 6 mg daily by mouth.

$$\begin{matrix} CH_2CH_2-O-SO_2-CH_3 \\ | \\ CH_2CH_2-O-SO_2-CH_3 \end{matrix}$$

PIPOBROMAN (Vercyte)

Dose: 1 mg per kg body weight daily by mouth (polycythemia vera), to 1.5 to 2.5 mg (granulocytic leukemia).

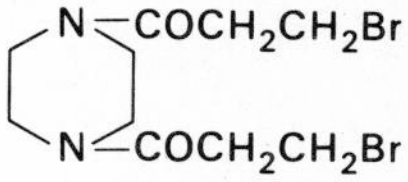

N—$COCH_2CH_2Br$ / N—$COCH_2CH_2Br$ (piperazine ring)

PIPOSULFAN (Ancyte)

N—$COCH_2CH_2-O-SO_2-CH_3$ / N—$COCH_2CH_2-O-SO_2-CH_3$ (piperazine ring)

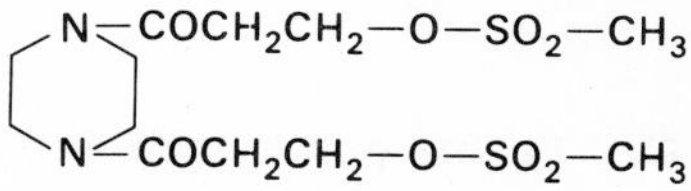

B. Folic Acid Antagonists

1. History. Farber (1948) introduced aminopterin, the first of a large number of folic acid antagonists.

2. Chemistry. Derivatives of folic acid.

3. Action and Mechanism. a. The folic acid antagonists exert their cytotoxic effect by competitively interfering with the conversion of folic acid into folinic acid (by inhibiting dihydrofolate reductase).

b. Folinic acid is a normal carrier of one-carbon moieties in many reactions, especially those concerned with the formation of purines for nucleic acids, and in its deficiency this manufacture cannot proceed.

c. Resistance after continued therapy is probably due to increased dihydrofolate reductase.

4. Pharmacodynamics. Well absorbed by mouth.

5. Toxicity. Damage to rapidly growing tissues, especially alimentary epithelium and bone marrow; may cause ulceration of buccal mucosa, bleeding gums, diarrhea, purpura, ecchymoses.

6. Uses. a. Used for acute leukemia in children and choriocarcinoma of women; also for psoriasis.

b. As aminopterin is highly cytotoxic to embryonic tissue it has been misused to produce early miscarriage, but is too dangerous for this purpose.

7. Preparations

AMINOPTERIN SODIUM

Dose: 0.25 to 0.5 mg 3 to 6 times weekly by mouth for 3 or more weeks. Not marketed in the United States.

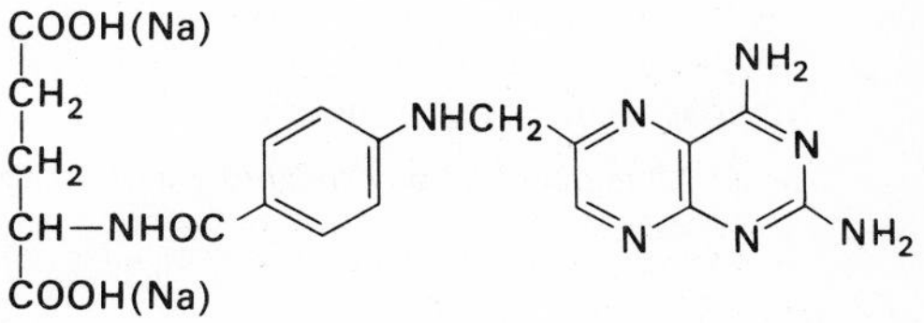

COOH(Na)—CH_2—CH_2—CH(COOH(Na))—NHOC—(benzene ring)—$NHCH_2$—(pteridine ring with N, N, N, N; NH_2, NH_2)

METHOTREXATE (Amethopterin)

Dose: 1.5 to 5 mg daily by mouth for 3 to 8 weeks for acute leukemia in children; daily doses as high as 25 mg daily in adults.

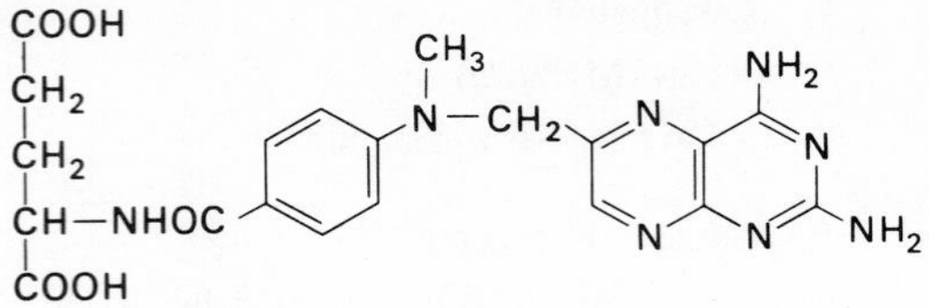

C. Purine and Pyrimidine Antagonists

PURINE ANTAGONISTS

1. History. a. The observation that 8-azaguanine would inhibit *Tetrahymena* (Kidder, 1941) led to interest in purine antimetabolites as growth inhibitors.

b. Hitchings and Elion (1952) synthesized 6-mercaptopurine; since then a large number of purine analogues have been made for anticancer trial.

2. Chemistry. Analogues of purine bases.

3. Action and Mechanism. a. The formation of both adenine and hypoxanthine may be interfered with, either by inhibition of formation, or by fraudulent construction.

b. May have immunosuppressive action.

4. Pharmacodynamics. Absorbed orally; pharmacologically relatively inert.

5. Toxicity. Nausea, vomiting, marrow depression; leucopenia, thrombocytopenia, bleeding.

6. Uses. a. Used to induce temporary remissions in acute leukemia and, less effectively, in chronic myelogenous leukemia.

b. Used (azathioprine) as immunosuppressives in organ transplantation.

7. Preparation

AZATHIOPRINE (Imuran)

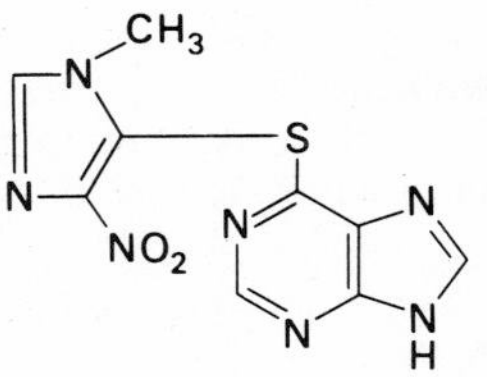

Antileukemic; to suppress rejection of transplanted tissue.

Dose: 2 mg per kg body weight intravenously every 24 hours.

MERCAPTOPURINE (Purinethol)

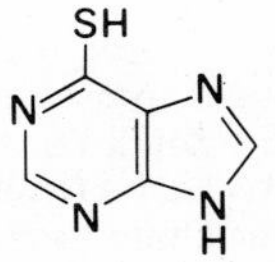

Dose: 2.5 mg per kg body weight by mouth daily.

THIAMIPRINE (Guaneran)

Antileukemic agent.
Dose: Under investigation.

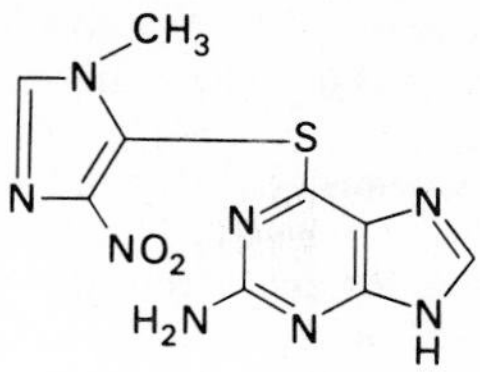

THIOGUANINE (6-TG)

Under trial in nephrosis and leukemias.
Dose: 2 mg per kg body weight per day by mouth.

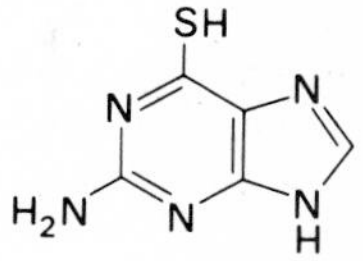

PURINE GLYCOSIDES

Adenosine analogues, largely investigational. Puromycin inhibits protein synthesis at assembly stage on ribosome; is added at growing carboxyl end of the peptide chain, stopping further additions, and causing release of incomplete or fraudulent chain from the ribosome. Cordycepin prevents elongation of nucleotide chain.

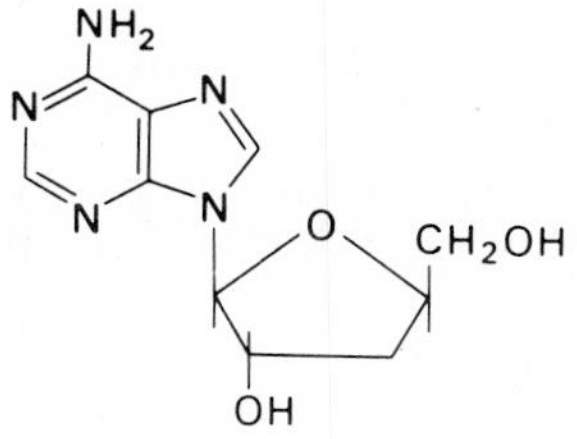

cordycepin

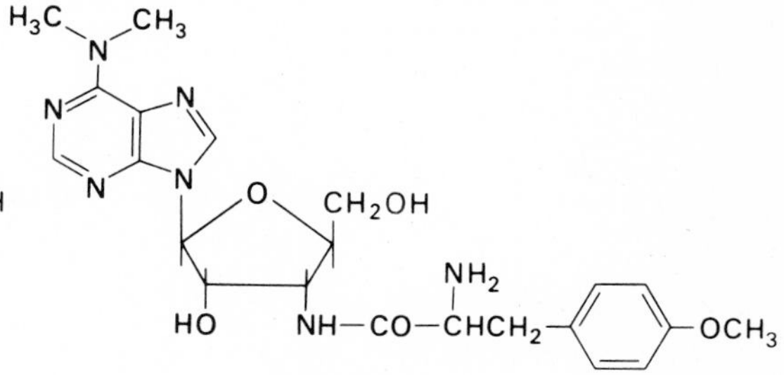

puromycin

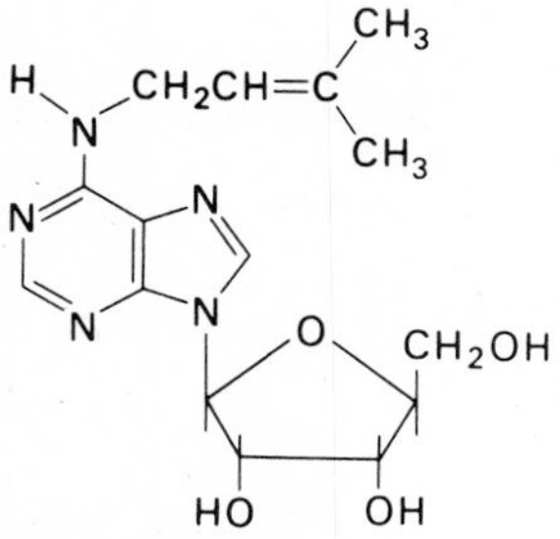

riboprine

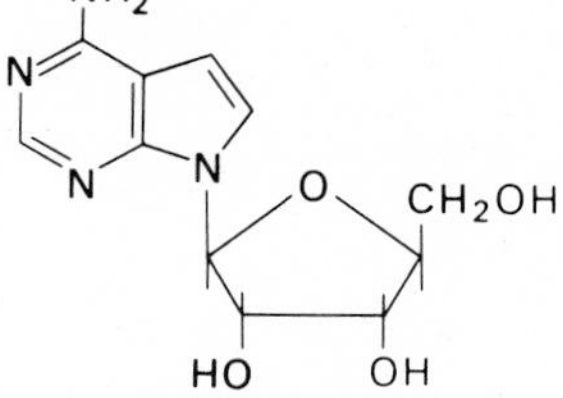

tubercidin

PYRIMIDINE ANTAGONISTS

1. History. a. Pyrimidine derivatives have been studied with the same rationale as the purines.

b. Of the large number of compounds tried, the fluorinated pyrimidines (Heidelberger) have been among the most interesting.

2. Chemistry. Pyrimidine analogues.

3. Action and Mechanism. Azauridine inhibits orotidylic decarboxylase; fluorouracil and fluorodeoxyuridine inhibit thymidylic synthetase; both thus interfere with DNA synthesis.

4. Pharmacodynamics and Toxicology. a. Pharmacology incompletely studied; given intravenously.

b. Toxicity includes stomatitis, diarrhea, and marrow depression.

5. Uses. a. May be tried in carcinoma of stomach, colon, breast, liver.

b. May show local antiviral activity.

6. Preparations

AZARIBINE (Triazure)

In severe psoriasis.

Dose: 45 mg per kg body weight 3 times a day by mouth.

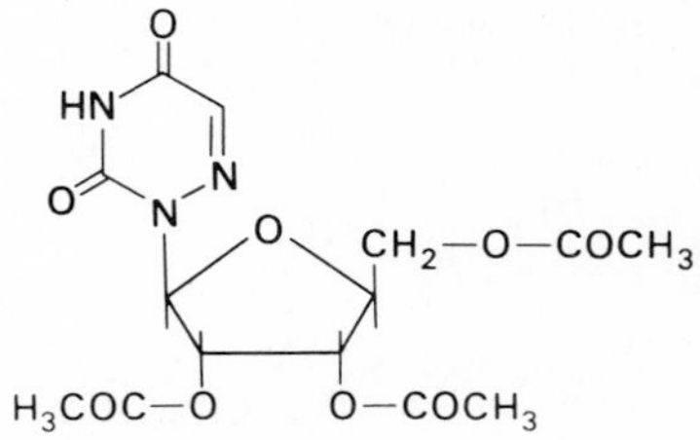

O
HN
N
O
N
O
$CH_2—O—COCH_3$
$H_3COC—O$
$O—COCH_3$

AZAURIDINE (AZUR)

Under trial in leukemias.
Dose: 60 to 600 mg per kg body weight daily intravenously.

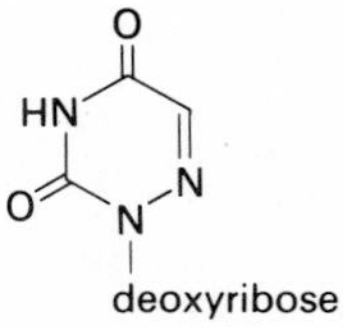

O
HN
N
O
N
deoxyribose

CYTARABINE (cytosine arabinoside; Cytosar)

Tried in acute leukemias and against viral infections.

Dose: 2 mg per kg body weight intravenously daily for 10 days.

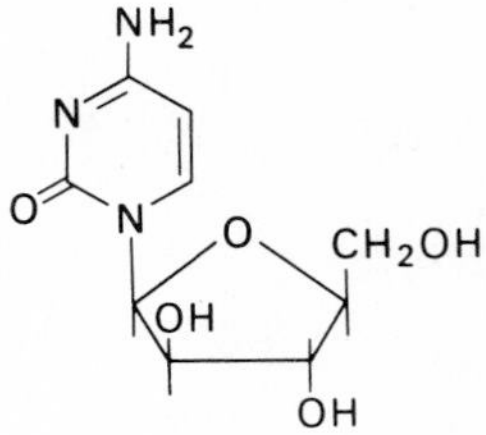

NH_2
N
O
N
O
CH_2OH
OH
OH

FLOXURIDINE (5-FUDR)

Inhibits thymidylic synthetase and also uracil phosphatase, inhibiting utilization of uracil in RNA.

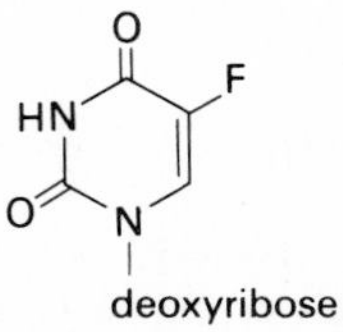

O
F
HN
O
N
deoxyribose

FLUOROURACIL (5-FU; Efudex; Fluoroplex)

Dose: 15 mg per kg body weight intravenously daily for 5 days, followed by reduced dosage on alternate days (experimental); 1% to 5% topically on actinic keratoses and skin cancer.

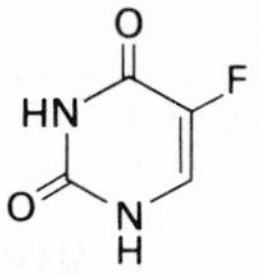

D. Antibiotics

ACTINOMYCINS

1. History. Waksman and others have isolated a number of actinomycins from *Streptomyces antibioticus*.

2. Chemistry. Derivatives of phenoxazone differing in type and sequence of amino acids in peptide side chains.

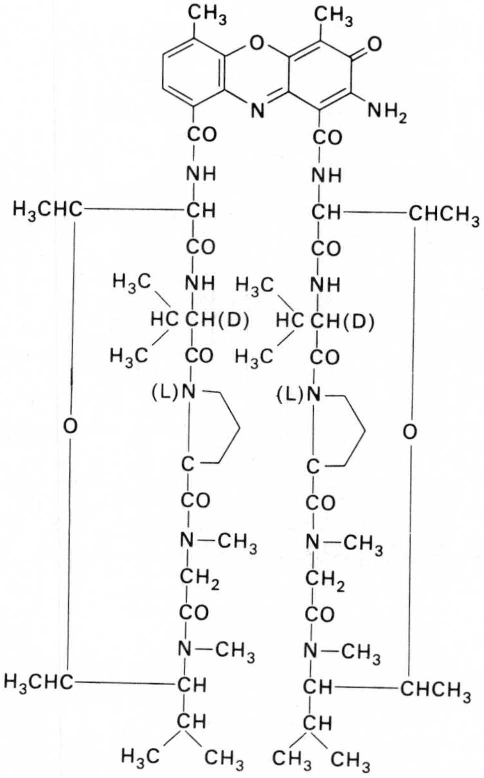

dactinomycin (actinomycin D)

3. Action and Mechanism. a. Combine with and inactivate the DNA specifically needed for RNA synthesis (RNA polymerase is DNA dependent); do not combine with genetic DNA; attachment to DNA may be at a guanine base, fitting between sugar-phosphate chains and stiffening the bases on either side, thus preventing the DNA from acting as a complete template for RNA.

b. Do not inhibit DNA synthesis or protein synthesis (from preformed RNA).

c. Experimentally inhibit DNA viruses by combining with them, but have no effect on RNA viruses because DNA not involved in their replication.

4. Pharmacology and Toxicity. Highly irritating and corrosive to tissues; may produce nausea, vomiting, stomatitis, diarrhea, skin eruptions, bone marrow depression.

5. Uses. Used against Wilms's tumor in children and trophoblastic disease in women.

6. Preparation

DACTINOMYCIN (Actinomycin D; Cosmegen)

Dose: 500 mcg intravenously daily for 4 or 5 days.

CACTINOMYCIN (Actinomycin C; Sanamycin)

From *Streptomyces chrysomallus;* mixture of cactinomycin C_2, C_3, etc.

MITOMYCIN C

1. Chemistry. A mitosane; from *Streptomyces caespitosus.*

2. Action and Mechanism. Depolymerizes DNA; bacteria enlarge without dividing; no effect on RNA.

3. Pharmacodynamics. Disappears rapidly from plasma; no localization.

4. Toxicity. Marrow depression: leukopenia, thrombocytopenia, bleeding, infection.

5. Uses. Under trial in lymphomas, leukemias, some solid tumors.

6. Preparations

MITOMYCIN C

Dose: 1 mg per kg body weight intravenously daily for 4 to 10 days.

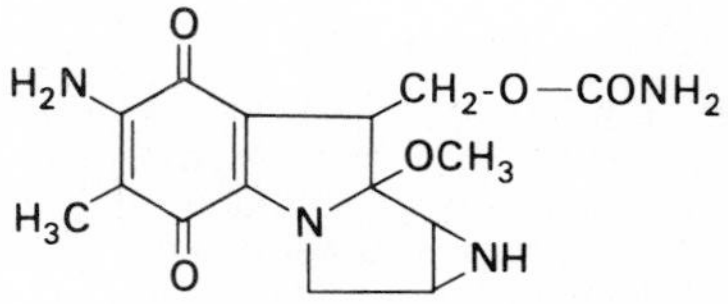

DAUNAMYCIN

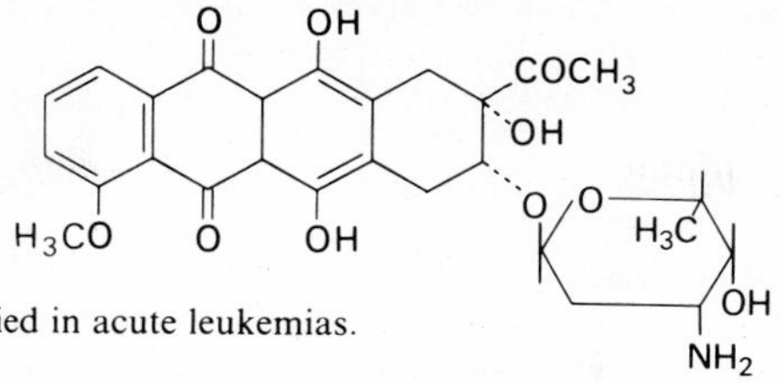

From *Streptomyces pencetius.* Complex of daunamycinone plus daunosamine. Binds DNA, inhibiting DNA and RNA polymerases. Vesicant, marrow depressant, cardiac toxin. Tried in acute leukemias.

Dose: 1 mg per kg body weight daily for 4 or 5 days, and in repeated courses.

MITHRAMYCIN (Mithracin)

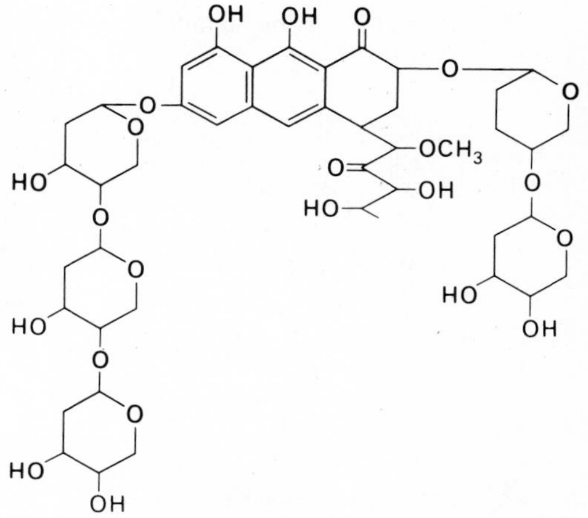

From *Streptomyces plicatus.* Probably complexes with RNA, inhibiting RNA and enzymatic synthesis. Mg needed for activity. May cause thrombocytopenia and bleeding. Used in germinal neoplasm of testis to reduce hypercalcemia in malignancy and to suppress Paget's disease.

Dose: 25 to 50 mcg per kg body weight daily for 5 days intravenously.

DOXORUBICIN (formerly Adriamycin)

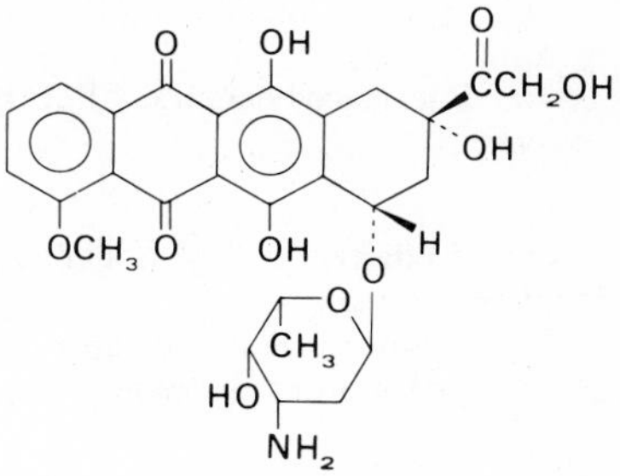

OTHER ANTIBIOTICS

Acetoxycycloheximide, ambomycin, anthramycin, asperlin, azotomycin, bleomycin, carzinophilin, chromomycin A_3 (Toyomycin), cirolemycin, cycloheximide, duazomycin, hadacin, mitocarm, mitocromin, mitogillin, mitomalcin, mitorubrin, mitosper, nogalomycin, peliomycin, porfiromycin, rhodamycin, sparsomycin, spiramycin, streptoazotacin, streptonigrin (Nigrin), streptovitacin A.

There is special interest in N-demethylrifampin, which can inhibit the RNA-dependent DNA polymerase found in a number of tumors associated with viruses.

E. Alkaloids

VINCA ALKALOIDS

1. History. a. Johnson and others (1957) observed antineoplastic activity of the periwinkle plant (*Vinca rosea*).

b. Noble (1958) isolated "vincaleukoblastine."

2. Chemistry. Dimeric indole-dihydroindole alkaloids.

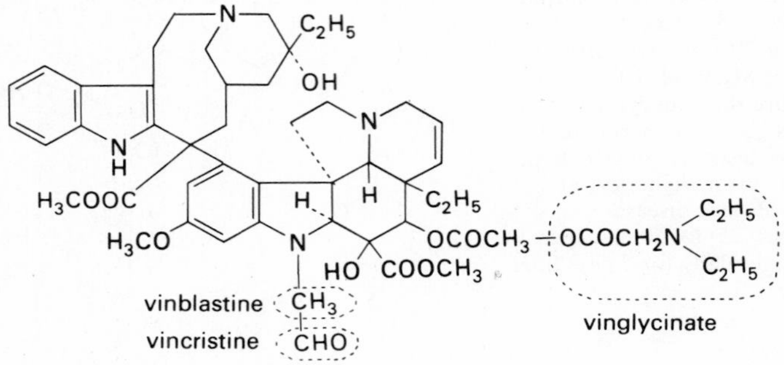

N
C_2H_5
OH
N
N
H
H
H
H_3COOC
C_2H_5
H_3CO
N
$OCOCH_3$
$OCOCH_2N$
C_2H_5
C_2H_5
HO
$COOCH_3$
vinblastine CH_3
vincristine CHO
vinglycinate

3. Action and Mechanism. a. Arrest mitosis in metaphase; vincristine more active than vinblastine.

b. Vinblastine, but not vincristine, exerts antimetabolic action (interference with glutamic acid utilization?).

4. Pharmacodynamics. Poorly absorbed by mouth. Mostly broken down in the liver.

5. Toxicity. a. Minor: nausea, vomiting, diarrhea, constipation; alopecia; muscle pain; malaise.

b. Severe: leukopenia, usually reversible; thrombophlebitis; paresthesias, sensory then motor; jaw pain; visual defects.

6. Uses. Under investigation for Hodgkin's disease, choriocarcinoma resistant to other agents, acute lymphocytic leukemia, and various carcinomas.

7. Preparations

VINBLASTINE SULFATE (Velban)

Dose: 0.1 to 0.15 mg per kg body weight intravenously (initial); then 0.1 to 0.2 mg per kg every 1 to 2 weeks if white count over 4,000 per cu mm.

VINCRISTINE SULFATE (Oncovin)

Dose: 0.05 to 0.15 mg per kg body weight intravenously once weekly.

VINDESINE

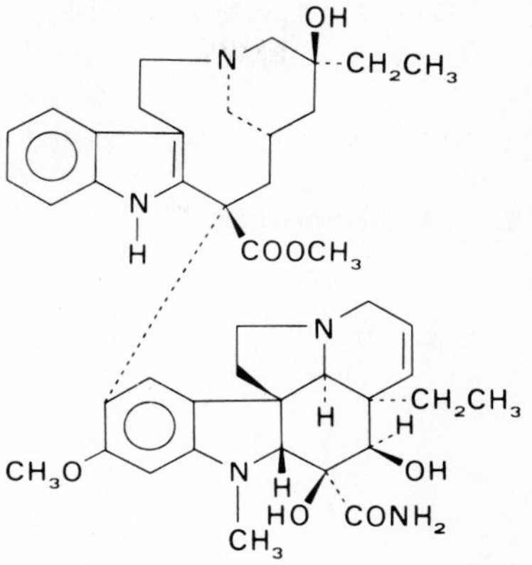

VINROSIDINE SULFATE

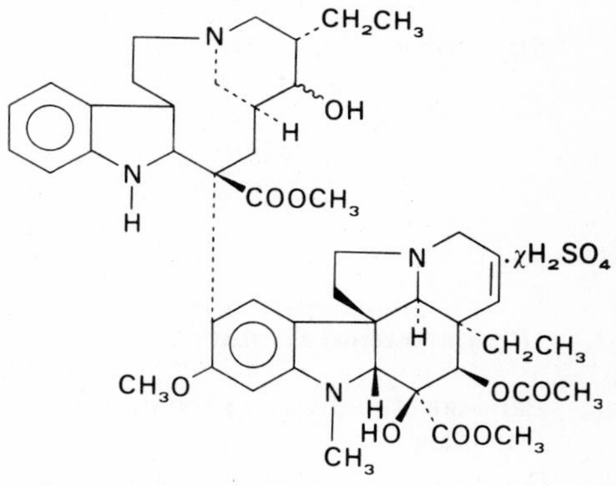

OTHERS

Vinglycinate sulfate; vinleurosine; vincathine; vincloline; perivine.

F. Other Alkaloids from Higher Plants

Aristolochic acid, camptothecin, euparotin acetate.

G. Urea Derivatives

HYDROXYUREA (Hydrea)

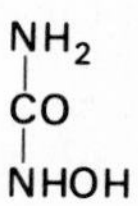

Interferes with DNA synthesis. Used in leukemias.
Dose: 40 mg per kg body weight per day; later reduced to 20 mg.

NH_2
|
CO
|
NHOH

URETHANE

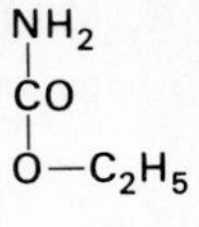

NH_2–CO–O–C_2H_5

Formerly used as a palliative in chronic myeloblastic leukemia and in multiple myeloma. Carcinogenic in mice.

Dose: 2 to 4 gm by mouth daily.

H. Nitrosoureas

LOMUSTINE

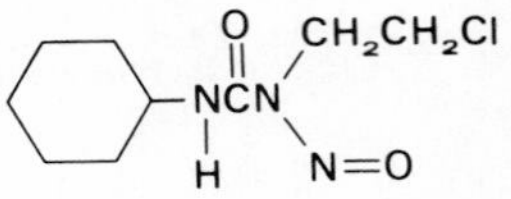

STREPTOZOCIN (Zanosar)

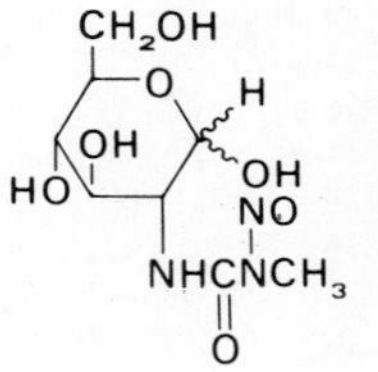

I. Procarbazine Group

PROCARBAZINE HYDROCHLORIDE (Matulane)

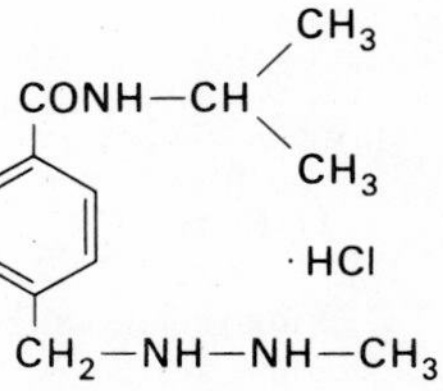

Degrades DNA, possibly by liberating H_2O_2. Is both a carcinogen and a potent immunosuppressive as well as an anticancer agent. Marrow depressant. Used in Hodgkin's disease.

Dose: 50 mg 2 times a day by mouth.

J. Enzymes

ASPARAGINASE

Asparagine is needed by all cells; some make it with asparagine synthetase; others require it from the outside. The latter die in the presence of L-asparaginase, which destroys circulating asparagine. Asparaginase may cause side effects: confusion, hypoproteinemia, impaired liver function, azotemia, and marrow damage. Used in acute lymphocytic leukemia and melanoma.

Dose: 1,000 iu per kg body weight, 3 to 7 times a week for 1 month.

K. Hormones

Cortisone

Cortisone and other corticoids may be useful in emergencies in acute leukemia, and in episodes of hemolytic anemia and thrombocytopenia (see The Adrenal).

Sex hormones

Androgens and estrogens are extremely useful in prostatic carcinoma and moderately useful in breast carcinoma (see Androgens; Estrogens).

L. Other Anticancer Agents

Enpromate, mitotane (Lysodren) (see Adrenal), simtrazene.

Laetrile

A substance prepared from apricot kernels, most likely containing laevomandelonitrile beta-glucuronosides. In the body it can break down to cyanide (HCN), which is a highly toxic substance; in near lethal doses it retards growth of experimental tumors in animals. Laetrile is promoted for palliative and curative treatment and prevention of cancer. Its clinical effectiveness is not yet substantiated; it is potentially toxic. In the U.S. Laetrile is not approved by the Food and Drug Administration, but its sale is legitimate in several states.

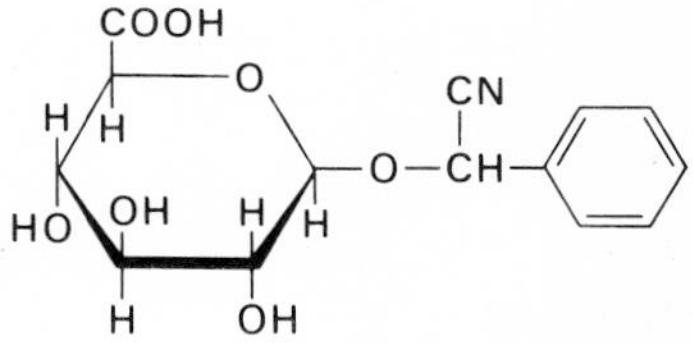

SUMMARY: CANCER CHEMOTHERAPY

TYPE	*ACTION AND MECHANISM*	*TOXICITY*	*USE*	*EXAMPLES*
Nitrogen mustards	Cytotoxic by alkylation of base components of DNA	Most are vesicants; diarrhea, marrow damage	Lymphomas, lymphatic leukemia Bronchogenic, ovarian, breast, and other carcinomas	Mechlorethamine HCl
Ethyleneimines	Same	Not vesicant; otherwise similar	Same	Triethylene melamine
Methylsulfonate esters	Same	Marrow depression	Chronic myelogenous leukemia	Busulfan
Folic acid antagonists	Antagonists to folic acid in synthesis of bases for nucleic acid synthesis	Alimentary tract damage, marrow depression	Acute leukemia, choriocarcinoma	Methotrexate

(cont.)

SUMMARY: CANCER CHEMOTHERAPY (cont.)

TYPE	*ACTION AND MECHANISM*	*TOXICITY*	*USE*	*EXAMPLES*
Pyrimidine and purine antagonists	Compete in synthesis of nucleic acids	Same	Leukemias and solid tumors, immunosuppression	Mercaptopurine, fluorouracil
Antibiotics	Most bind to and inactivate DNA, which then cannot form RNA polymerase	Same	Wilms's tumor, choriocarcinoma	Dactinomycin
Vinca alkaloids	Arrest mitosis Mechanism uncertain	Same	Hodgkin's disease, choriocarcinoma, acute lymphocytic leukemia, carcinomas	Vincritine sulfate
Procarbazine	Degrades DNA	Marrow damage	Hodgkin's disease	Procarbazine HCl

Reviews

Southam, C. M. The complex etiology of cancer. Cancer Res., 23:1105, 1963.

Dustin, P., Jr. New aspects of the pharmacology of antimitotic agents. Pharmacol. Rev., 15:449, 1963.

Darken, M. Puromycin inhibition of protein synthesis. Pharmacol. Rev., 16:223, 1964.

Fairly, G., and Simister, J. Cyclophosphamide. Baltimore, The Williams & Wilkins Co., 1965.

Cromwell, N. Chemical carcinogens, carcinogenesis, and carcinostasis. Amer. Sci., 33:213, 1965.

Oliverio, V., and Zubrod, C. Clinical pharmacology of the effective antitumor drugs. Ann. Rev. Pharmacol., 5:335, 1965.

Tatum, E. L. Molecular biology, nucleic acids, and the future of medicine. Perspec. Biol. Med., p. 19, 1966.

Shimkin, M. Cancer chemotherapy. Topics Med. Chem., 1:79, 1967.

Heidelberger, C. Cancer chemotherapy with purine and pyrimidine analogues. Ann. Rev. Pharmacol., 7:101, 1967.

Sartorelli, A., and Creasey, W. Cancer chemotherapy. Ann. Rev. Pharmacol., 9:51, 1969.

14. Virus Chemotherapy

A. Chemotherapy

Virus chemotherapy at the clinical level is still extremely limited, except in localized infections, such as keratitis, where it may be highly effective.

As reproduction is the principal enterprise of viruses, its various steps offer perhaps the most likely places for chemotherapeutic approach.

The cycle starts with the free particle, which first attaches to a prospective host cell. The virus then enters the cell and loses its structural identity during an eclipse phase. After an interval new nucleic acid is synthesized, then coated with protein to make complete virus, and finally released for transit to a new host cell.

B. Agents Acting on the Free Particle

In this stage the virus is inert, being simply in transit to the next cell. It is immune to subtle mechanisms, but may be damaged by various forms of energy: heat, UV or x-ray irradiation, radiomimetics (nitrogen mustards, kethoxal, beta-propiolactone), which are of importance in extinguishing hepatitic virus from blood products. Antibodies presumably act during this phase by direct combination with the virus particles.

C. Agents Affecting Attachment or Entry

The principal early chemotherapeutic trials were based on interrupting the attachment phase concerned with the influenza type of attachment mechanism. A number of substances can intercept the virus by mimicking the neuraminic acid moiety of the receptor, or at least this is a suggested mechanism. These substances include various polysaccharides, pectin, and possibly certain polysulfonic acids. Other substances, called receptor destroying enzymes (RDE), found in extracts from *Vibrio cholerae* and other microorganisms, presumably fit and enter the receptors and thereby prevent attachment of the virus particle, or induce it to discharge the neuraminic acid necessary for the initiation of attachment. As with virus chemotherapy generally, however, the results are modest, and it is difficult to demonstrate any definite dose-response relationship.

AMANTADINE

1. Chemistry. Adamantine derivative introduced by Hoffman and others in 1964.

2. Action and Mechanism. a. Inhibits influenza and rubella viruses in vitro; pretreatment reduces serological evidence of influenza A_2 (Asian) in man.

b. Presumed to inhibit attachment of the virus particle to the cell or its penetration into, or uncoating in, the cell.

c. May release dopamine from storage sites.

3. Pharmacodynamics. Absorbed easily. Excreted slowly in the urine; cumulation may occur.

4. Toxicity. Toxicity low at therapeutic level, but severe CNS symptoms may be produced at twice this level: nervousness, insomnia, blurred vision, ataxia, depression, hallucinations, convulsions.

5. Uses. Prophylactically in influenza A_2 (Asian). Against parkinsonism alone or preferably in combination with levodopa.

6. Preparations

AMANTADINE HYDROCHLORIDE (Symmetrel)

Dose: 200 mg per day by mouth.

NH_2 ·HCl

RIMANTADINE HYDROCHLORIDE

Dose: 200 mg twice daily by mouth.

NH_2 | $CH-CH_3$ ·HCl

D. Agents Acting During Eclipse and Nucleic Acid Replication

1. Eclipse. No inhibiting agents are recognized to act during the eclipse phase, but the complex steps involved suggest that this might be a likely time for interference.

2. Replication of Nucleic Acid. It is at this mechanism that the most intense chemotherapeutic attack has been directed. A great number of purine and pyrimidine antagonists have been examined for antiviral effect, with a considerable yield of positive results.

PURINE AND PYRIMIDINE DERIVATIVES

1. History. Kaufman (1962) introduced idoxuridine (2-deoxy-5-iodouridine) into the treatment of virus keratitis.

2. Chemistry. Idoxuridine (iododeoxyuridine) and other members of a series of pyrimidine analogues.

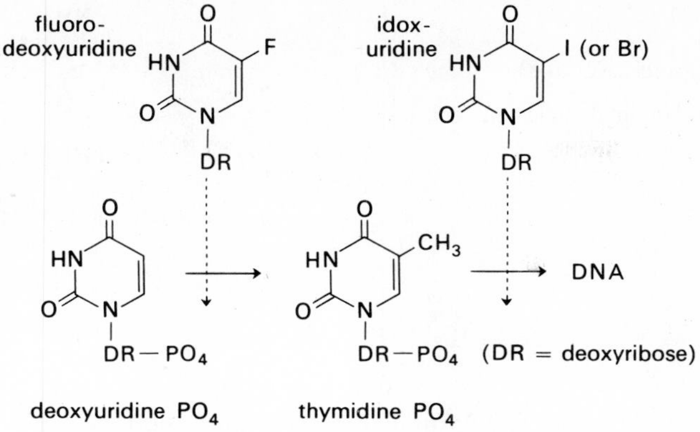

fluoro-deoxyuridine

idox-uridine I (or Br)

DNA

$DR-PO_4$ (DR = deoxyribose)

deoxyuridine PO_4 thymidine PO_4

3. Action and Mechanism. a. The pyrimidine derivatives produce both antiviral (DNA virus) and anticancer effects by interference with DNA synthesis.

b. Fluorodeoxyuridine inhibits thymidylic synthetase.

c. Idoxuridine inhibits thymidylic phosphorylase and the specific DNA polymerase necessary for synthesis of viral DNA (Kaufman, Chemotherapia, 7:1, 1963).

d. Cytosine arabinoside blocks synthesis or utilization of deoxycytidine.

4. Pharmacodynamics and Toxicity. Systemic use generally toxic, but adapted to local application.

5. Uses. Used locally in the eye in keratitis from herpes simplex or vaccinia.

6. Preparations

IDOXURIDINE (5-IUDR; Stoxil)

Dose: 0.1% solution topically to conjunctiva every 1 to 2 hours for 4 days.

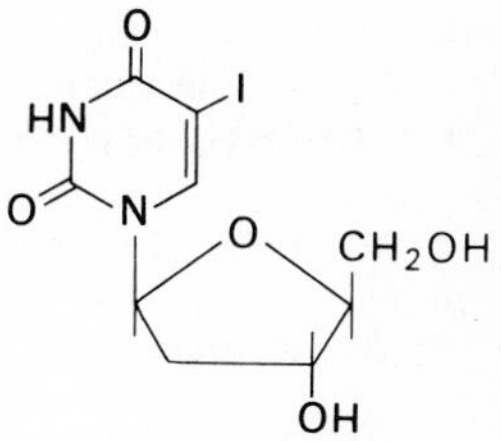

RIBAVIRIN (Virazole)

Dose: 100 mg 3 times daily.

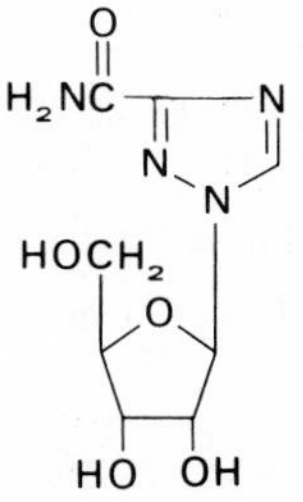

VIDARABINE (Vira-A)

Dose: 3% ophthalmic ointment.

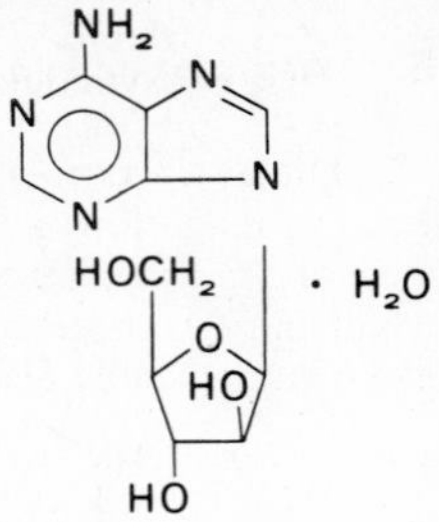

NH_2 N N N N HOCH₂ O HO HO · H_2O

OTHERS

See also cytarabine and floxuridine under Cancer Chemotherapy.

INTERFERON

1. **History.** Natural antiviral factor discovered by Lindenmann and Isaacs (1957).

2. **Chemistry.** A protein; 20,000 to 160,000 mol. wt.

3. **Action and Mechanism.** a. Produces an antiviral action in virus infected cells: appears before antibodies and may be a normal mechanism of resistance to virus infection. Not virus specific, but relatively species specific.

b. Interferon is formed in cells in response to the presence of virus, nucleic acid, and even such other substances as polyanionic copolymers.

c. Interferon, in turn, probably induces the formation of a second protein that is the active antiviral agent.

d. The second protein appears to inhibit virus replication at the ribosomal level, probably be preventing incorporation of mRNA into the ribosome apparatus.

4. **Use.** Clinical use not yet established.

5. **Preparations (Interferon inducers)**

STATOLON

A natural double-stranded RNA produced in cultures of *Penicillium stoloniferum*.

POLY I–C

A double-stranded complex of polyriboinosinic acid and polyribocytidylic acid.

TILORONE HYDROCHLORIDE

(Mayer, *Science*, 169:1214, 1970).

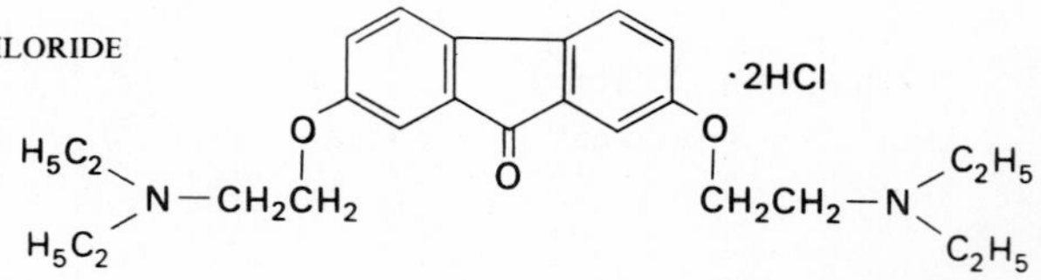

·2HCl O O O H_5C_2 H_5C_2 N—CH_2CH_2 CH_2CH_2—N C_2H_5 C_2H_5

E. Agents Affecting the Protein Coat

Dietary, amino acid, and vitamin deficiency have each been reported to inhibit virus propagation, and it is logical to suppose that in at least some instances the mechanism lies in a resultant deficiency of the protein formation. Chloramphenicol, which inhibits protein formation, limits the growth of phage, but not of other viruses; canavanine, which may compete with arginine, has also been noted to be inhibitory.

ISATIN THIOSEMICARBAZONES

1. History. Thompson (1953) showed that isatin thiosemicarbazones were active against vaccinia in mice.

2. Chemistry. Isatin thiosemicarbazones with substitutions principally on the isatin N or on the peripheral amino:

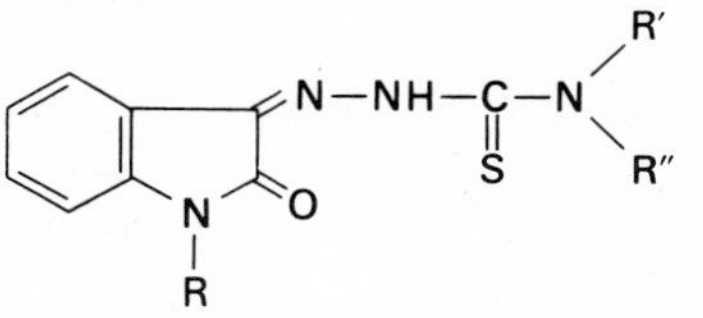

isatin-beta-thiosemicarbazone (R's = H)

3. Action. a. Principal therapeutic activity against pox viruses.
b. N-methyl derivative active against vaccinia and smallpox.
c. Dimethyl active against mouse pox; dibutyl against poliovirus.

4. Mechanism. Produces a defect in protein incorporation into the virus and in late assembly of the particle, probably by interfering with attachment of mRNA to ribosome; virus DNA increases and host cell is damaged, but infectious virus is not produced.

5. Pharmacodynamics and Toxicity. Absorbed orally. Nausea and vomiting may be severe.

6. Uses. a. Prophylactic against smallpox.
b. May be of value in vaccinia gangrenosa or disseminata.

7. Preparation

METHISAZONE (Marboran)
Dose: 1.5 to 3 gm twice daily by mouth.

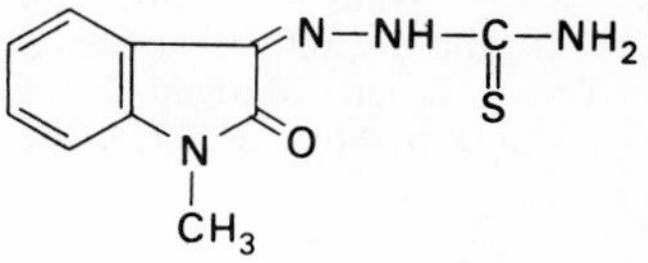

F. Agents Affecting Release or Energy Production

Experimentally the release of phage may be partially inhibited by 5-methyltryptophan, but no clinically useful agents are known.

The total energy production of the host cell is little altered in viral reproduction, and no agents have been found which would alter it in virus-infected cells (possibly excepting interferon).

G. Other Agents Under Study Against Viruses

Dihydroisoquinoline acetamide, flumidin (Virugon), famotine, memotine, xenazoic acid (Xenalamine), steffimycin, rifampin.

SUMMARY: VIRUS CHEMOTHERAPY

TYPE	*ACTION AND MECHANISM*	*TOXICITY*	*USE*	*EXAMPLES*
Amantadine	Impairs entry or attachment	CNS symptoms	To prevent influenza A	Adamantine HCl
Purine and pyrimidines	Interfere with virus DNA synthesis	Minor, locally	Keratitis from vaccinia or herpes simplex	Idoxuridine
Interferon	Inhibits viral replication at ribosomal level	Undetermined	Experimental	Poly I–C
Isatin thiosemicarbazones	Inhibit protein incorporation into virus	Vomiting	Smallpox, disseminated vaccinia	Methisazone

Reviews

Sadler, P. W. Chemotherapy of virus diseases. Pharmacol. Rev., 15:407, 1963.

Wagner, R. R. The interferons. Ann. Rev. Microbiol., 17:285, 1963.

Bauer, D., St. Vincent, L., Kempe, C., and Downie, A. Prophylactic treatment of smallpox contacts with N-methylisatin-β-thiosemicarbazone. Lancet, 2:492, 1963.

Thompson, R. L. Chemoprophylaxis—chemotherapy of viral diseases. Advances Chemother., 1:85, 1964.

Stuart-Harris, C., and Dickenson, L. The Background to Chemotherapy of Virus Diseases. Springfield, Ill., Charles C Thomas, 1964.

Merigan, T. Interferons of mice and men. New Eng. J. Med., 276:913, 1967.

Prusoff, W. Recent advances in chemotherapy of viral diseases. Pharmacol. Rev., 19:209, 1967.

Osdene, T. Antiviral agents. Topics Med. Chem., 1:137, 1967.

Goz, B., and Prusoff, W. Pharmacology of viruses. Ann. Rev. Pharmacol., 10:143, 1970.

De Clercq, E., and Merigan, T. Current concepts of interferon and interferon induction. Ann. Rev. Med., 21:17, 1970.

15. Topical Antiinfectives

Antiseptics are agents designed to kill microbes on exposed surfaces. They are used to prepare the skin for minor and major surgical procedures, to sterilize inanimate articles, and the like, but have long since been replaced by aseptic practice in surgery, and by systemic chemotherapy in most infections.

Antiseptics applied to animate bodies are called antiseptics, bactericides, or bacteriostats; those applied to inanimate bodies are called disinfectants or germicides.

A. Phenol and Derivatives

1. History. The applications of bacteriology to medicine began in 1867 when Lister used antiseptic mists of carbolic acid in the operating room.

2. Chemistry. Phenol and derivatives.

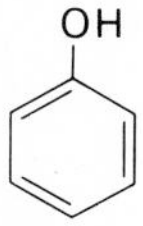

phenol

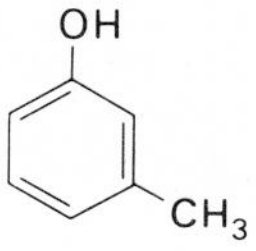

cresol

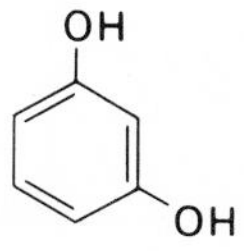

resorcinol

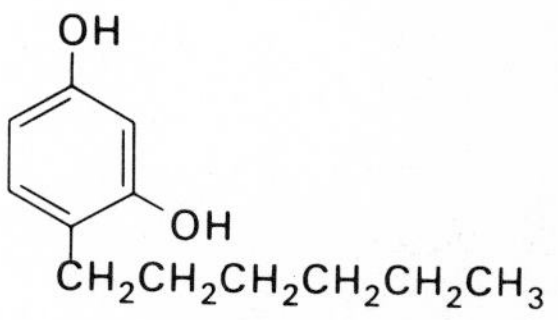

hexylresorcinol

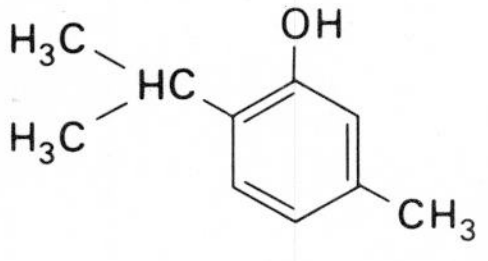

thymol

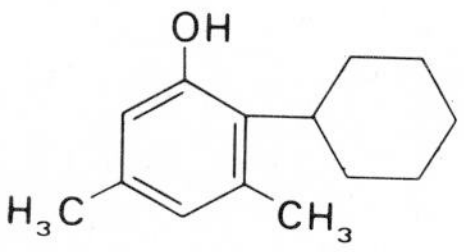

dimethylcyclohexyl phenol

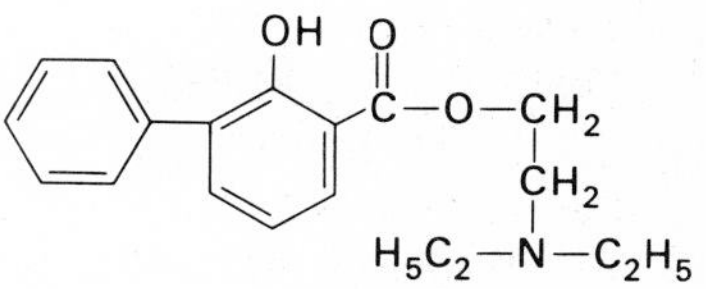

biphenamine

3. Action and Mechanism. a. Traditionally described as protoplasmic poisons; this is the result of protein precipitation, possibly both physical and enzymatic.

b. The agents have high surface activity because of containing both lipophilic and lipophobic moieties.

4. Pharmacodynamics and Toxicology. If absorbed through massive application, or use on abraded surfaces, may cause convulsions and renal damage.

5. Uses. Antiseptics, caustics, antipruritics, anthelmintics.

6. Preparations

CRESOL; META-CRESYL ACETATE; SAPONATED SOLUTION OF CRESOL (Lysol)

More potent antiseptic (phenol coefficient = 5) and more useful disinfectant than phenol.

HEXYLRESORCINOL

Vermifuge (phenol coefficient = 50).

PHENOL (carbolic acid); Liquefied phenol

Caustics for appendiceal stumps, to open boils.

PARACHLOROPHENOL

More potent than phenol.

RESORCINOL

Used in psoriasis (phenol coefficient = 0.4).

THYMOL; THYMOL IODIDE

Used as dusting powders (phenol coefficient = 30).

OTHERS

Biphenamine HCl, dimethylcyclohexyl phenol. Bacteriostats in shampoos for seborrhea of scalp.

B. Metallic and Metalloid Compounds

1. History. a. Koch (1881) showed the antiseptic activity of mercuric chloride.

b. Geppert (1889) showed it to be bacteriostatic, reversed by sulfide.

2. Action and Mechanism. Bacteriostatic through denaturation of protein; inactivate –SH groups.

3. Pharmacodynamics and Toxicology. Relatively nontoxic unless ingested; systemic effects include particularly renal tubular damage.

4. Uses. All-purpose antiseptics, but penetrate poorly and are quickly inactivated by protein.

5. Preparations

a. Mercurials

AMMONIATED MERCURY ($Hg\text{-}NH_2\text{-}Cl$)

5% ointment locally on the skin.

MERCURIC CHLORIDE ($HgCl_2$)

Sterilizes dishes in 1:1,000 concentration.

YELLOW MERCURIC OXIDE (HgO)

1% ointment locally in the eyes.

OTHERS

Acetomeroctol, meralein (Merodicein), merbromin (Mercurochrome), mercocresols, nitromersol (Metaphen), phenylmercuric borate, phenylmercuric picrate, thiomerfonate, thiomersol (Merthiolate). Organic mercurials of minor interest formerly used on cuts and abrasions.

b. Silver preparations

SILVER NITRATE ($AgNO_3$)

Used by Credé (1881) to prevent ophthalmia neonatorum; 0.1 ml of 1% solution.

OTHERS

Silver sulfadiazine, mild silver protein (Argyrol; Neosilvol), silver picrate, strong silver protein. Organic silver compounds formerly used on mucous membranes but of little value.

c. Other agents

Bismuth tribromphenate (Xeroform), boric acid, zinc sulfanilate (Nizin). Of no particular advantage and may be toxic.

C. Halogen Compounds

1. Chemistry. Inorganic and organic halogen compounds.

2. Action and Mechanism. Interfere with enzymes and coagulate protein. More potent than most local antiseptics.

3. Uses. Antiseptics and disinfectants; water sterilizers.

4. Preparations

a. Long established

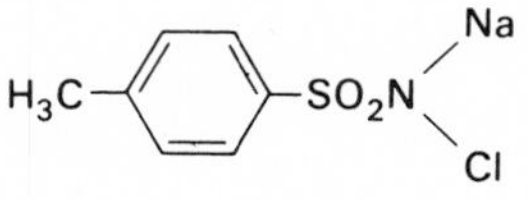

H3C—C6H4—SO2N(Na)(Cl)

chloramine T

Cl—N=C(H2N)—N=N—C(NH2)=N—Cl

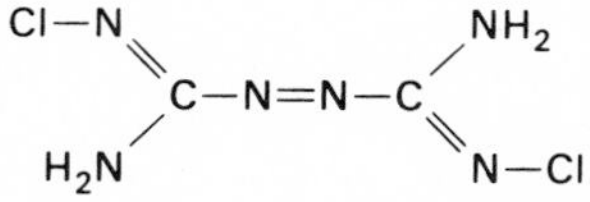

chloroazodin

IODOFORM (HCI_3)

Organic iodide dusting powder.

TINCTURE OF IODINE

Common antiseptic (2% iodine) for use on the skin before surgical procedures; should not replace simple cleansing for cuts and scratches.

OTHERS

Chloroazodin (Azochloramid), chloramine T, sodium hypochlorite (NaClO). Slowly liberate Cl; used to dissolve dead tissue.

b. Chlorophenes

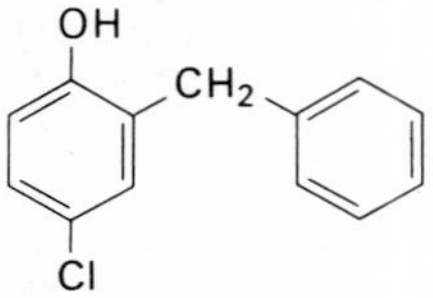

chlorophene

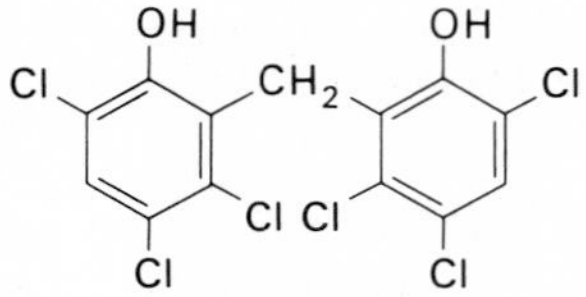

hexachlorophene

CHLOROPHENE (Santophen); HEXACHLOROPHENE (Gamophen; Hexosan; G11)

Incorporated in soaps and creams.

c. Halocarbans

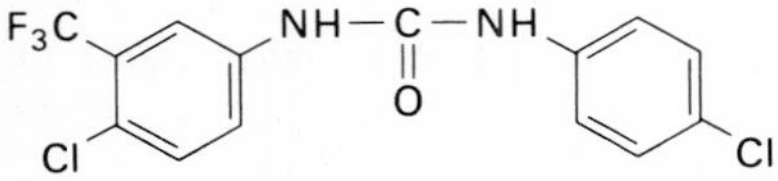

cloflucarban

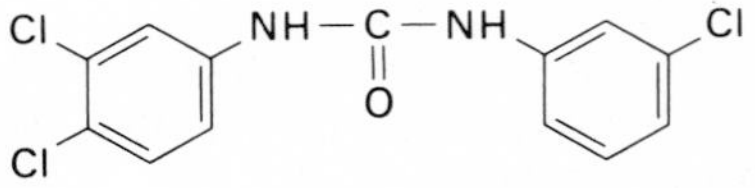

triclocarban

CLOFLUCARBAN (Irgosan CF3); HALOCARBAN; TRICLOCARBAN (TCC):

Bacteriostats in soaps and deodorants.

d. Salans

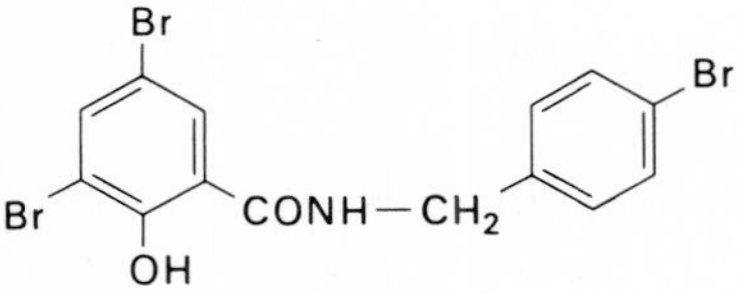

bensalan

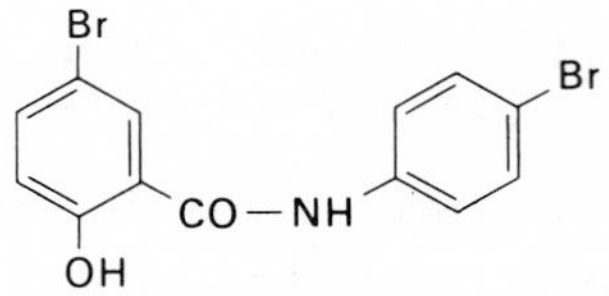

dibromsalan

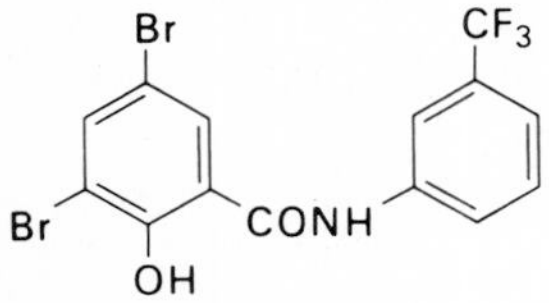

fluorosalan

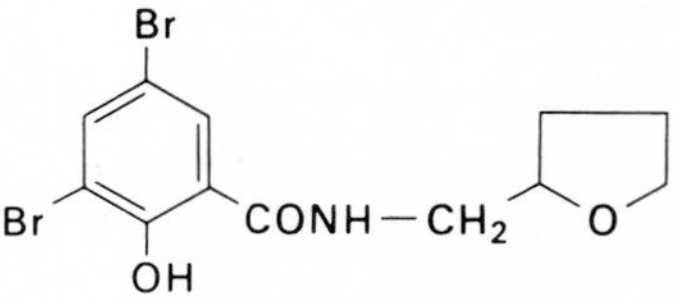

fursalan

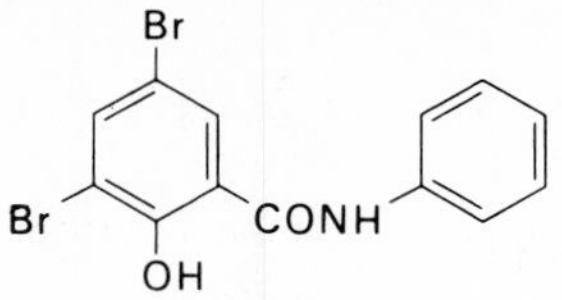

metabromsalan

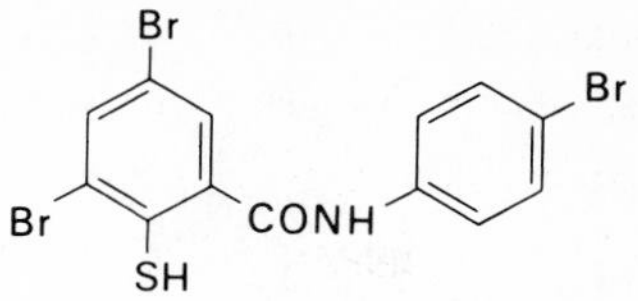

thiosalan

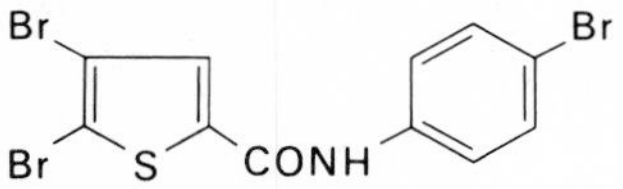

tibrofan

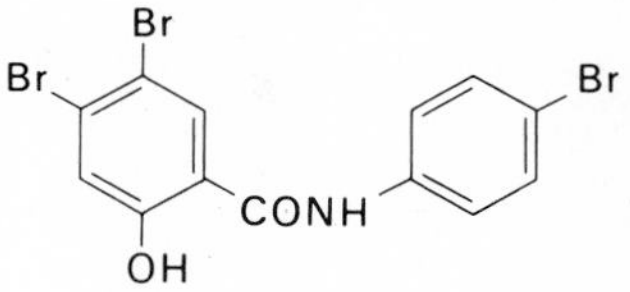

tribromsalan

BENSALAN; DIBROMSALAN; FLUOROSALAN (Fluorophene); FURSALAN; MIXED BROMSALANS (Diaphene); METABROMSALAN; THIOSALAN; TIBROFAN; TRIBROMSALAN

Antiseptics for soaps and lotions.

e. Disinfectants for drinking water

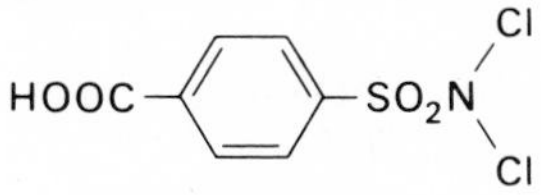

halazone

DIGLYCOCOLL HYDRIODIDE-IODINE (Bursoline); HALAZONE; TETRAGLYCINE HYDROPERIODIDE $[(NH_2—CH_2—COOH)_4 \cdot HI$ plus I_2, 1:25] (Globaline)

For disinfection of drinking water.

f. Bithionol group

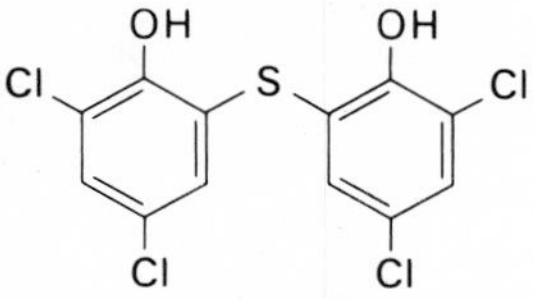

bithionol

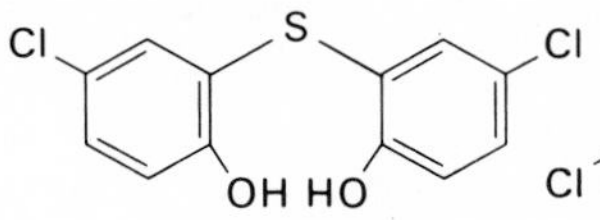

fenticlor

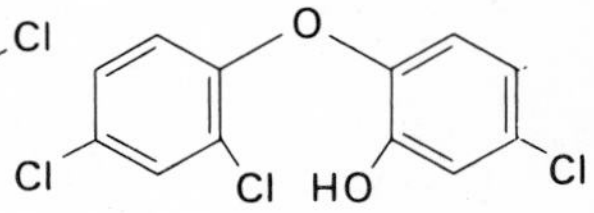

irgasan DB300

BITHIONOL (Actamer); FENTICLOR; IRGASAN DB300

Local antiseptics; bacteriostats for soaps and detergents.

g. Others

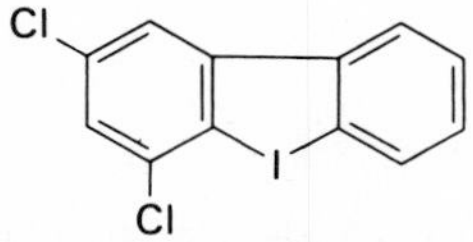

dichlorindolene

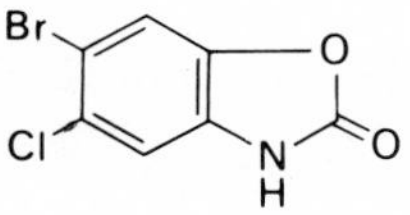

bromochlorenone

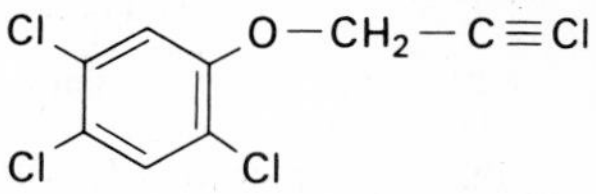

haloprogin

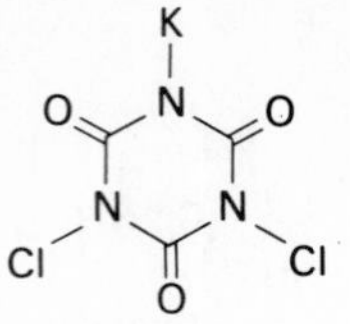

potassium troclosene

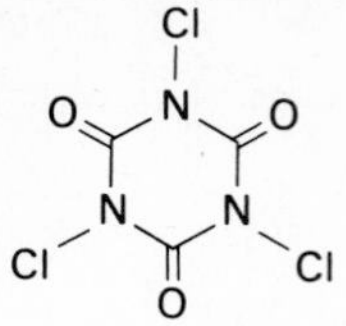

symclosene

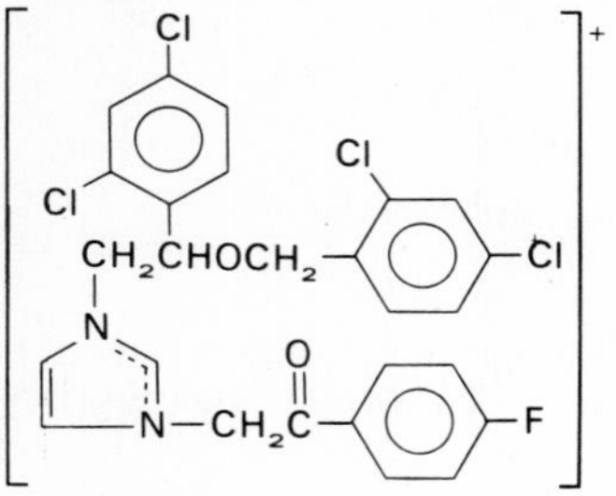

fludazonium chloride

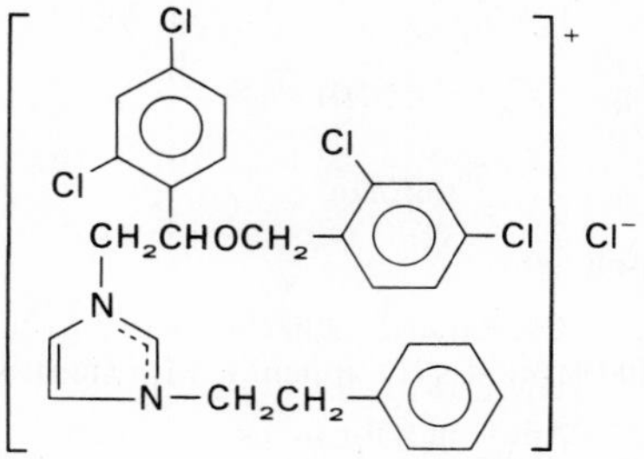

sepazonium chloride

BROMCHLORENONE (Vinyzene); DICHLORINDOLENE LACTATE; HALOPROGIN (Halotex); POTASSIUM TRICLOSENE; POVIDONE-IODINE; SYMCLOSENE

Local antiinfectives.

D. Oxidizing Agents

1. Chemistry. Compounds liberating oxygen.

2. Action. Strong oxidizers of organic matter, mostly transient in effect.

3. Preparations

HYDROGEN PEROXIDE (H_2O_2)

3% solution may cleanse a wound by bubbling out foreign material; practically obsolete.

POTASSIUM PERMANGANATE ($KMnO_4$)

Used in antiseptic washes, irrigations, and douches in concentrations up to 1:5,000; practically obsolete.

PROPIOLACTONE ($\overbrace{CH_2-CH_2-C}^{O}=O$)

For sterilization of vaccines, blood products, tissue grafts.

SODIUM PERBORATE ($NaBO_3$)

Used as paste in wounds containing anaerobes and in mouthwashes; practically obsolete.

ZINC PEROXIDE, MEDICINAL (ZnO_2)

Has been used on exposed, infected neoplasms.

E. Alcohols and Aldehydes

1. **Action.** Protein precipitants and enzyme inhibitors.

2. **Preparations**

ETHYL ALCOHOL (C_2H_5OH)

70% solution used as an antiseptic on the skin.

FORMALDEHYDE ($H{-}CHO$)

Used to sterilize instruments and as a fumigant. Formalin is a 40% formaldehyde solution.

GLUTARAL $OCH(CH_2)_3CHO$

Glutaraldehyde

ISOPROPYL ALCOHOL $[(CH_3)_2CHOH]$

50% solution used on the skin as an alternative for ethyl alcohol.

PROPYLENE GLYCOL $[CH_3CH(OH)CH_2OH]$

Largely used as a solvent.

F. Essential Oils

OILS OF CLOVE; EUCALYPTUS; MENTHOL

Mildly anesthetic and antiseptic.

G. Dyes

1. **Chemistry.** Acridine and triphenylmethane dyes.

2. **Action.** Enzyme inhibitors of brief action.

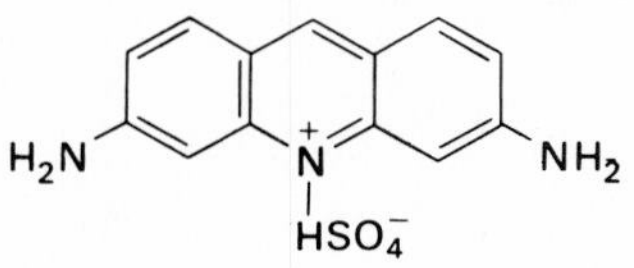

H_2N NH_2 $\overset{+}{N}$ HSO_4^-

proflavine

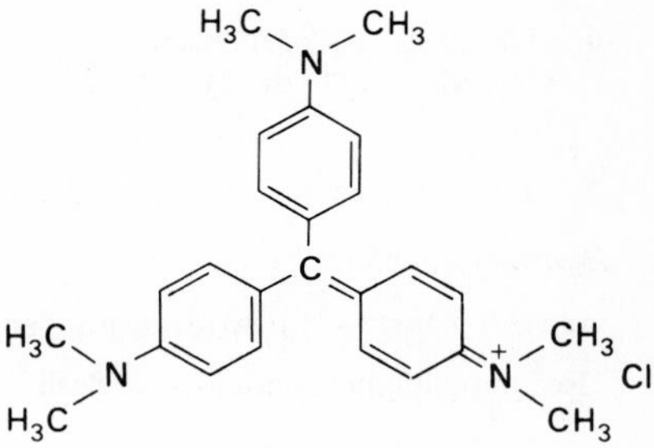

H_3C CH_3 N C H_3C N H_3C $\overset{+}{N}$ CH_3 CH_3 Cl^-

gentian violet

3. Preparations

ACRIFLAVINE; PROFLAVINE

Acridine dyes which are active when ionized and denature protein; slow and transient; not much used.

AMINACRINE HYDROCHLORIDE

BRILLIANT GREEN; CARBOL FUCHSIN; GENTIAN VIOLET; METHYL VIOLET; PARAROSANILINE (Fuchsin)

Triphenylmethane dyes; practically obsolete.

SCARLET RED

An azo dye formerly thought to promote wound healing.

H. Quinolines and Related Compounds

1. History. Mühlens and Merck (1920) first used chiniofon in amebiasis; synthesized in 1892.

2. Chemistry. Quinolines, hydroxyquinolines, quinoxalines, and related compounds.

3. Action and Mechanism. a. Directly antimicrobial; tend to be polyvalent against bacteria, protozoa, and fungi.

b. Mechanism may be based on chelation.

4. Pharmacodynamics. Absorption generally poor from mouth, skin, or vagina.

5. Toxicity. a. Relatively nontoxic, but may cause local irritation of the skin, vagina, or bowel.

b. Chiniofon and related compounds may rarely produce iodism.

6. Uses. a. Widely used as topical antiseptics on the skin and in the vagina.

b. Iodinated hydroxyquinolines used in intestinal amebiasis (see Amebiasis).

7. Preparations

a. Hydroxyquinolines

ACTINOQUINOL SODIUM (Sodium Tequinol)

Used in ophthalmic ointment for flash burns.

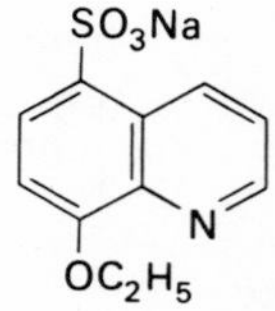

SO_3Na

N

OC_2H_5

BENZOXIQUINE

Used as a gastrointestinal antiseptic to treat parasites and amebae.

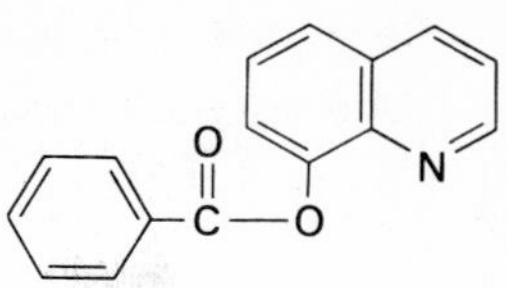

CHINIOFON (Yatren)

Dose: 0.5 gm by mouth twice daily for 10 days (amebiasis).

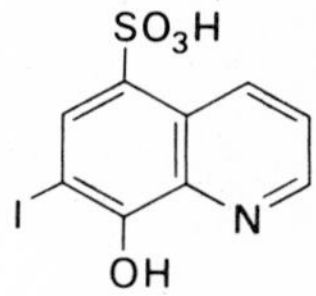

CHLORQUINALDOL (Sterosan)

Fungicide, bactericide, keratoplastic; 3% topically.

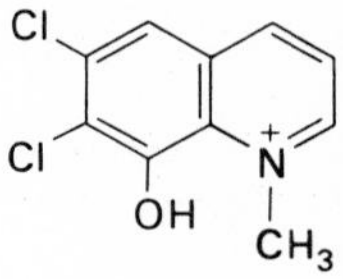

CLAMOXYQUIN HYDROCHLORIDE

Dose: Under investigation (amebiasis).

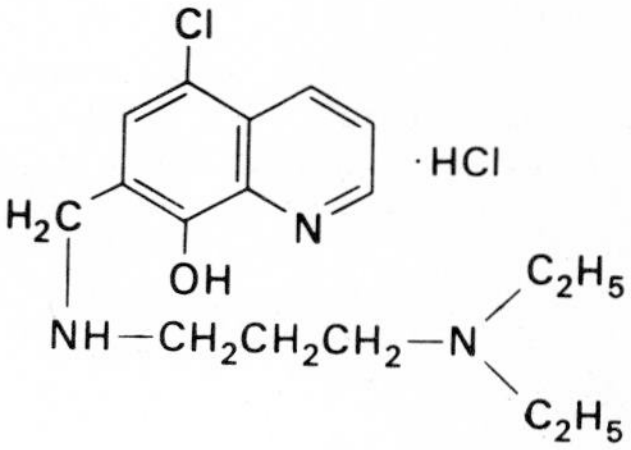

DIIODOHYDROXYQUIN (Diodoquin)

Dose: 0.5 gm 4 times daily by mouth (amebiasis); locally in powders or suppositories.

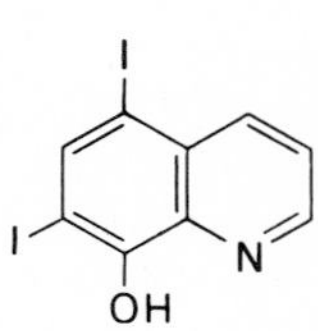

HALQUINOLS (in Quinolor)

Mixture of various derivatives.

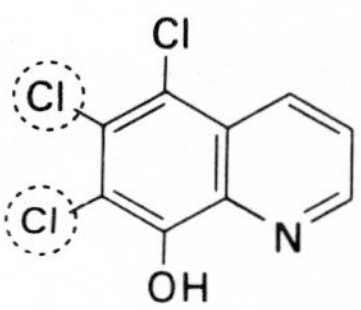

IODOCHLORHYDROXYQUIN (Vioform)

Dose: 0.5 gm twice daily by mouth (amebiasis); locally in 3% creams, ointments, and lotions; by suppository.

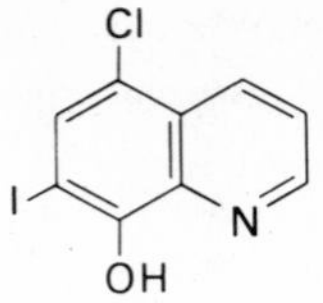

OCTOQUIN METHYLSULFATE

Dose: Used locally as an ophthalmic ointment.

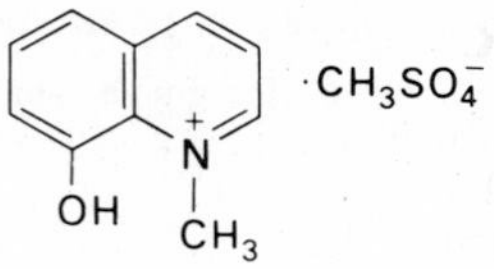

OXYQUINOLINE BENZOATE

Dose: Used as a fungistat.

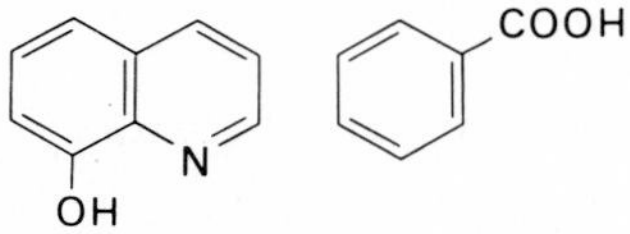

b. Quinolates. Mostly poultry coccidiostats

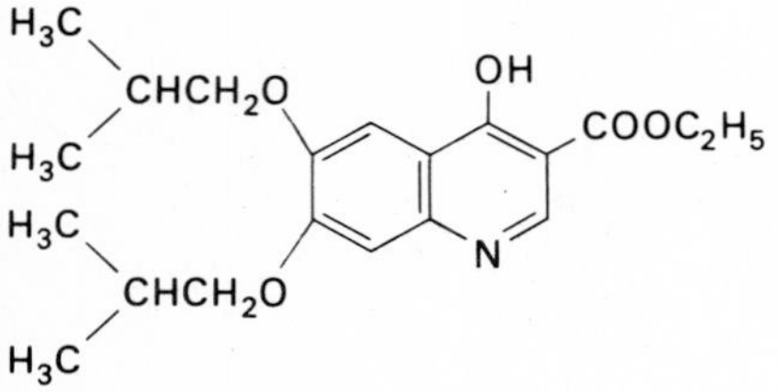

buquinolate

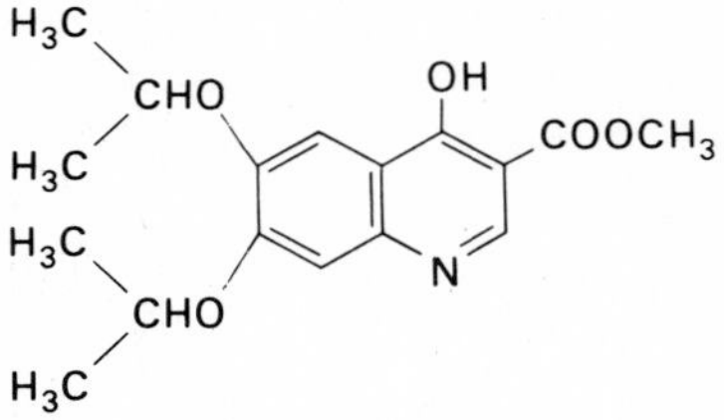

proquinolate

OTHERS

Amquinate; cyproquinate; decoquinate; nequinate.

c. Quinoxalines. Antibacterials

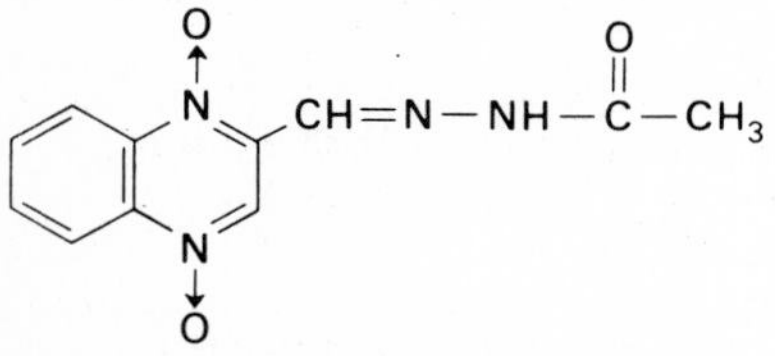

carbadox

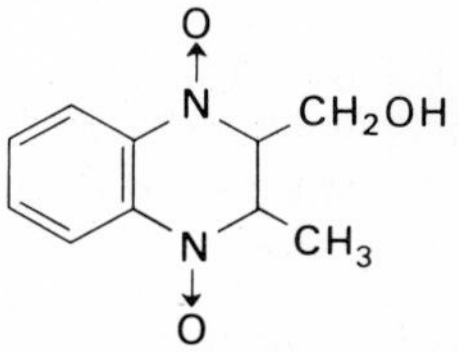

mequidox

d. Other quinolines and related compounds. Antiseptics

Hexidine (in Sterisol); quindecamine acetate; ticlatone (Landromil).

I. Nitrofurans (See Other Antibacterials)

J. Local Fungicides (See Antifungal Agents)

K. Contraceptives

Spermicidal creams, jellies, and suppositories for use with or without mechanical devices. The active agents include phenylmercuric acetate, oxyquinoline sulfate, sodium borate, lactic acid, ricinoleic acid, hexylresorcinol, sodium lauryl sulfate, sodium chloride, chlorindanol, nonoxynol, and others.

CHLORINDANOL (in Lanesta)

Dose: 0.1%.

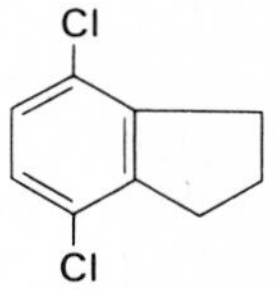

LAURETH 9 (in Lanettes)

Nonionic surfactant emulsifier.
Dose: 15% with 0.1% chlorindanol.

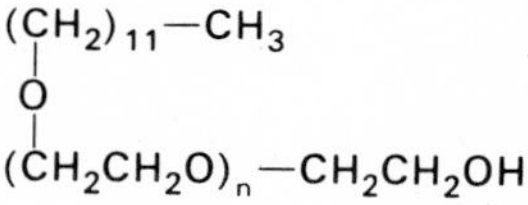

$(CH_2)_{11}-CH_3$
O
$(CH_2CH_2O)_n-CH_2CH_2OH$

NONOXYNOL 9 (in Delfen, Ortho-Creme)

Dose: 8% with 0.2% benzethonium.

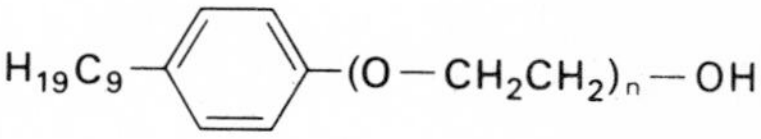

$H_{19}C_9-C_6H_4-(O-CH_2CH_2)_n-OH$

CYOXYLATE

COOH
C_2H_5 CH_3

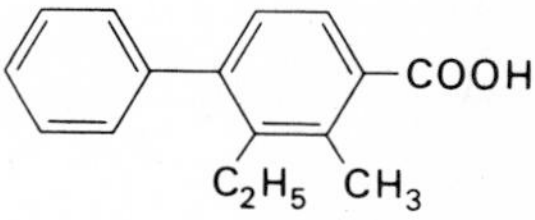

L. Surface-Active Compounds

As the traditional antiseptics have decreased in importance they have been replaced for many uses by surface-active bactericides.

1. Chemistry. a. Surface-active compounds characteristically have hydrophobic (fat-soluble) and hydrophilic (water-soluble) groups in each molecule.

b. These groups lead to orientation of the compounds at interfaces.

2. Action and Mechanism. The surface-active compounds damage or disrupt cell membranes by inactivation of the enzymes which maintain the membranes, or by physical disorganization of the membranes.

ANIONIC TYPE

1. Chemistry. Each molecule contains:

a. Hydrophobic group: paraffinic chain, alkyl substituted benzene, naphthalene.

b. Hydrophilic group: carboxyl, sulfate, sulfonate, phosphate (negative charge).

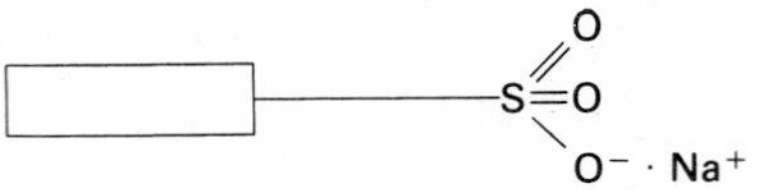

prototype

2. Uses. a. Detergents. Have been used in toothpastes, shampoos, dish-washing and washing machine powders.

b. Have been tried as inhibitors of alimentary enzymes.

c. Antibacterials, mostly active on gram-positives; sclerosing agents (varicose veins).

3. Preparations

SODIUM TETRADECYL SULFATE

Detergent.

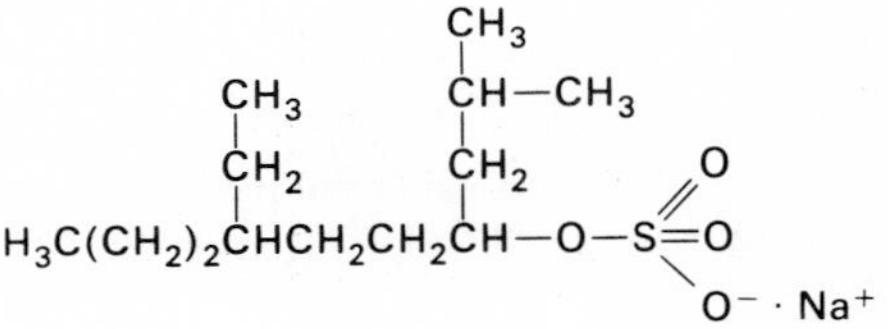

$$H_3C(CH_2)_2CH(CH_2CH_3)CH_2CH_2CH(CH_2CH(CH_3)CH_3)-O-SO_2-O^- \cdot Na^+$$

SODIUM LAURYL SULFATE

Detergent.

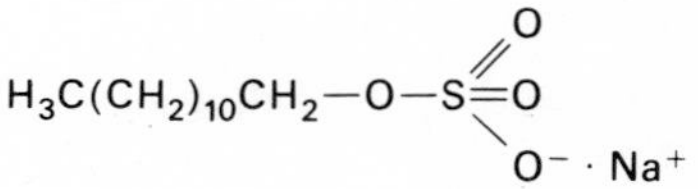

$$H_3C(CH_2)_{10}CH_2-O-SO_2-O^- \cdot Na^+$$

SODIUM ETHASULFATE (in Tergemist)

Mucolytic in bronchiectasis.

Dose: 3 ml of 0.1% solution by aerosol. Preparations withdrawn from market.

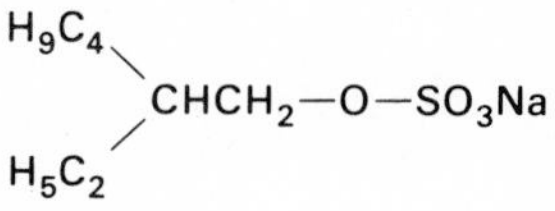

$$(H_9C_4)(H_5C_2)CHCH_2-O-SO_3Na$$

CATIONIC TYPE

1. Chemistry. Each molecule contains:

a. Hydrophobic group: same as anionic type.

b. Hydrophilic group: quaternary ammonium, sulfonium, phosphonium, iodonium (positive charge).

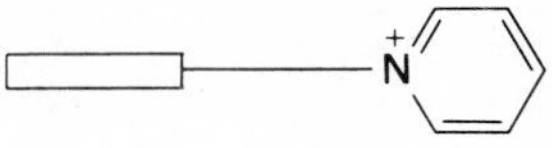

prototype

2. Uses. Detergents. Antibacterials, active on both gram-positives and gram-negatives; nonantibiotic type less effective against pseudomonas; inactivated by soap; pH influences activity.

3. Preparations

BENZALKONIUM CHLORIDE (Zephiran)

Antiseptic.

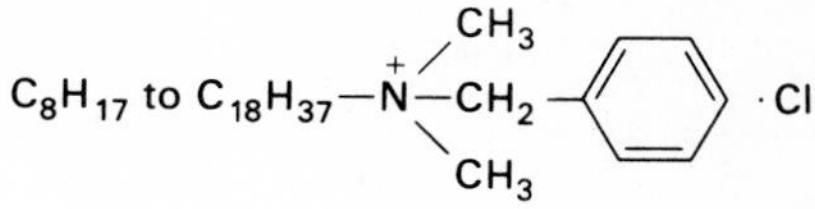

C_8H_{17} to $C_{18}H_{37}—\overset{+}{N}(CH_3)_2—CH_2—C_6H_5 \cdot Cl^-$

CENTRIMONIUM CHLORIDE

Antiseptic.

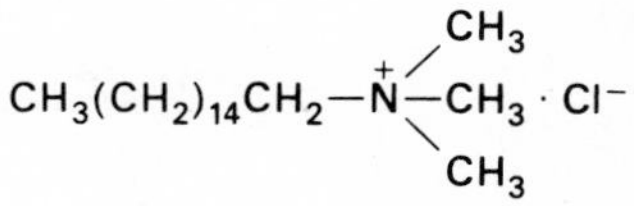

$CH_3(CH_2)_{14}CH_2—\overset{+}{N}(CH_3)_3 \cdot Cl^-$

CETALKONIUM CHLORIDE (Zettyn)

Antiseptic.

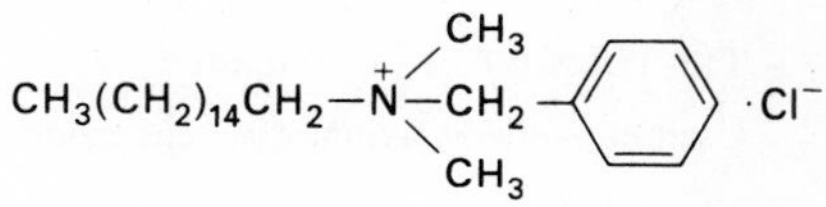

$CH_3(CH_2)_{14}CH_2—\overset{+}{N}(CH_3)_2—CH_2—C_6H_5 \cdot Cl^-$

CETYL PYRIDINIUM CHLORIDE (Ceepryn)

Antiseptic.

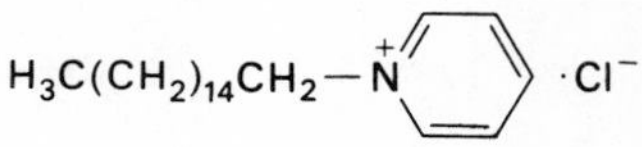

$H_3C(CH_2)_{14}CH_2—\overset{+}{N}C_5H_5 \cdot Cl^-$

DENATONIUM BENZOATE (Bitrex)

Denaturant for alcohol.

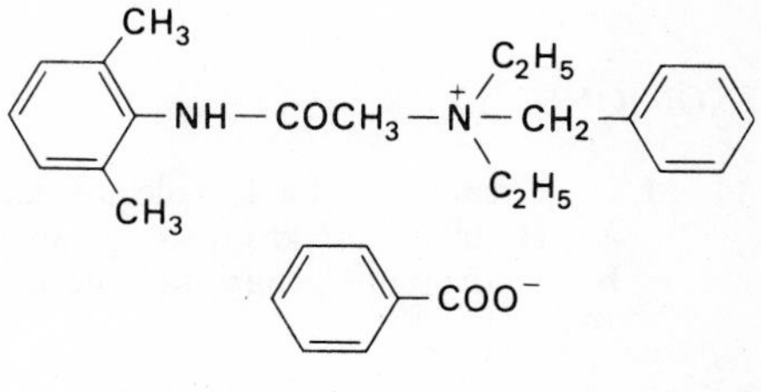

$2,6\text{-}(CH_3)_2C_6H_3—NH—COCH_3—\overset{+}{N}(C_2H_5)_2—CH_2—C_6H_5$

$C_6H_5—COO^-$

DOMIPHEN BROMIDE (Bradosol)

Bacteriostatic, fungistatic.

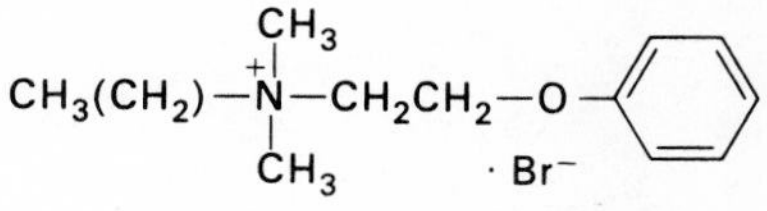

$CH_3(CH_2)—\overset{+}{N}(CH_3)_2—CH_2CH_2—O—C_6H_5 \cdot Br^-$

IMIDECYL IODINE (Amphodyne)

Antiseptic for skin and hair.

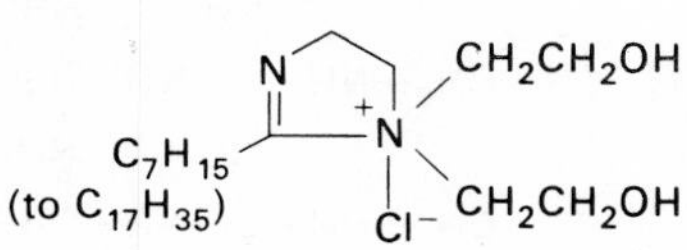

C_7H_{15} (to $C_{17}H_{35}$) imidazolinium ring, $\overset{+}{N}(CH_2CH_2OH)_2$, Cl^-

$C_{13}H_{27}O—(CH_2CH_2O)_{12}—CH_2CH_2OH \cdot I$

METHYLBENZETHONIUM CHLORIDE (Diaparene)

Diaper rinse.

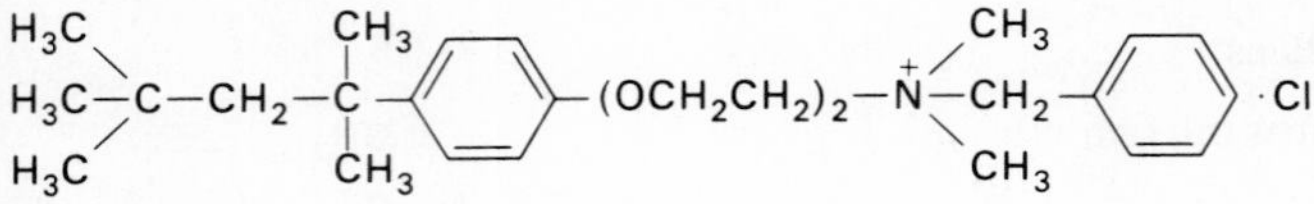

$(H_3C)_3C-CH_2-C(CH_3)_2-C_6H_4-(OCH_2CH_2)_2-\overset{+}{N}(CH_3)_2-CH_2-C_6H_5 \cdot Cl^-$

THONZONIUM BROMIDE (Thonzide)

Detergent.

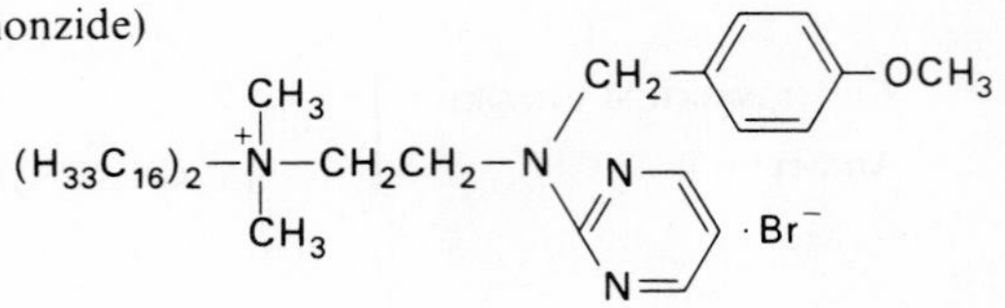

$(H_{33}C_{16})_2-\overset{+}{N}(CH_3)_2-CH_2CH_2-N(CH_2-C_6H_4-OCH_3)(C_4H_3N_2) \cdot Br^-$

TRICLOBISONIUM (Triburon)

Used in pyodermias; may be sensitizing.

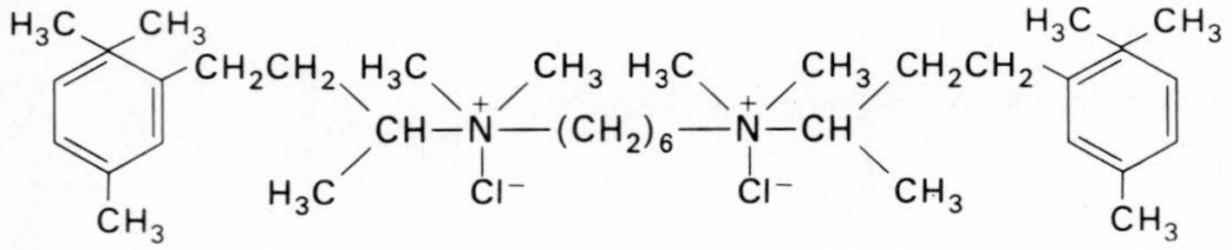

$[C_6H_3(CH_3)(C(CH_3)_2)-CH_2CH_2-CH(CH_3)-\overset{+}{N}(CH_3)_2]_2(CH_2)_6 \cdot 2Cl^-$

NONIONIC TYPE

1. **Chemistry.** Each molecule contains:
   a. Hydrophobic group: same as ionic types.
   b. Hydrophilic group: polymerized ethylene oxide; polyhydro alcohols.

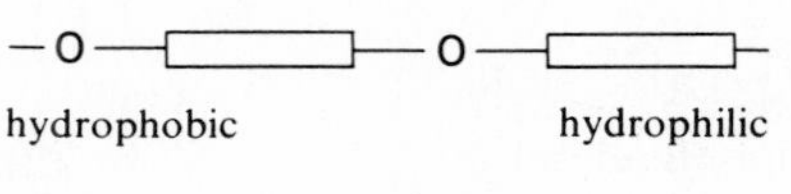

prototype

2. **Uses.** To lower surface tension; minor antibacterials; to wet, thin, and loosen mucus in bronchioles.

3. **Preparations**

ALEXIDINE (Bisguadine)

Antimicrobial.

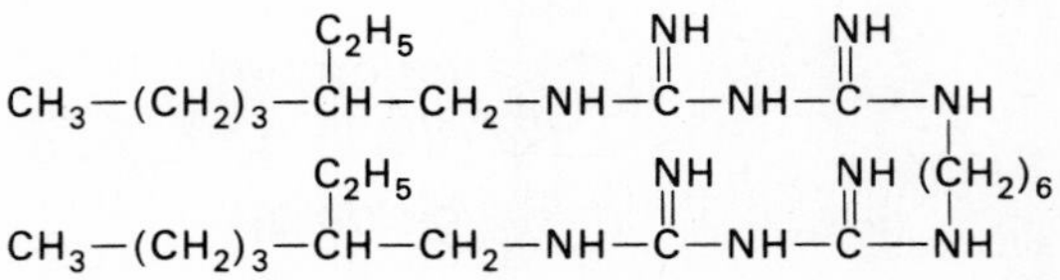

$[CH_3-(CH_2)_3-CH(C_2H_5)-CH_2-NH-C(=NH)-NH-C(=NH)-NH]_2(CH_2)_6$

CHLORHEXIDINE HYDROCHLORIDE (Hibitane)

Bactericidal agent used in lozenges and for handwashing in hospitals.

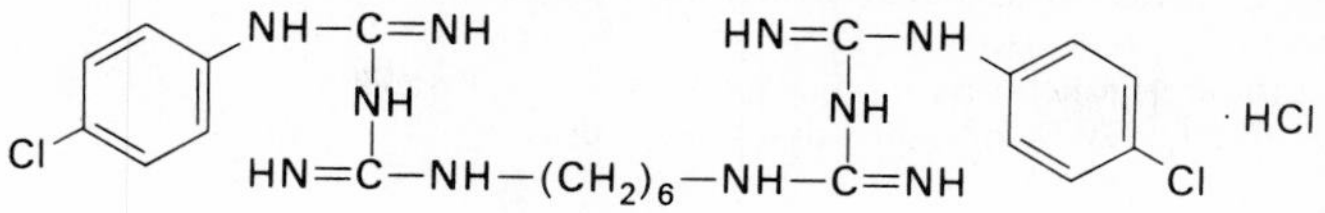

$$\text{Cl}-C_6H_4-NH-\underset{\underset{\displaystyle HN=C-NH-(CH_2)_6-NH-C=NH}{|}}{\overset{}{C}}(=NH)\ldots$$

NH—C=NH HN=C—NH
NH NH · HCl
Cl HN=C—NH—$(CH_2)_6$—NH—C=NH Cl

OTHERS

DEXTRANOMER (Debrisan)

For cleaning and debriding secreting wounds.

NONOXYNOL 9

Spermicide. (See Contraceptives.)

POLOXALENE (Bloat Guard)

Veterinary surfactant.

POLYSORBATE 80 (Tween 80)

Promotes dispersed growth of tubercle bacilli in culture; can be metabolized by these organisms.

TRIETHANOLAMINE POLYPEPTIDE OLEATE (Cerumenex)

To dissolve cerumen from ears.

TYLOXAPOL: (See Mucolytic Agents.)

M. Detergents

Detergents are surface-active agents which reduce surface tension and so allow particles of dirt to be surrounded and loosened. Lawrence (Nature, 183:1491, 1959) proposed that a principal component of the action was the formation of liquid crystals which penetrated dirt particles by cryoscopic forces.

1. Preparations

SOAP

Salts of fatty acids and alkalies.

MEDICINAL SOFT SOAP

A potassium soap made with vegetable oils and without the removal of glycerin.

SYNTHETIC DETERGENTS: (See preceding section.)

N. Mucolytic Agents

Wetting agents to liquefy mucus and promote easier breathing; of questionable value.

ACETYLCYSTEINE (Mucomyst; Respaire)

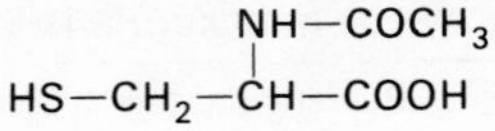

$HS-CH_2-CH(NH-COCH_3)-COOH$

Mucolytic agent; given by aerosol.

SH of drug may interchange with S—S of mucoprotein, giving lessened viscosity.

May produce bronchospasm in asthmatics.

Dose: 10 ml of 20% solution 3 or 4 times a day.

METHYL CYSTEINE HYDROCHLORIDE

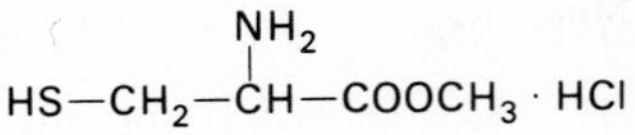

$HS-CH_2-CH(NH_2)-COOCH_3 \cdot HCl$

Similar to acetylcysteine.

Not marketed in the U.S.

TYLOXAPOL (Superinone; WR1339) (in Alevaire)

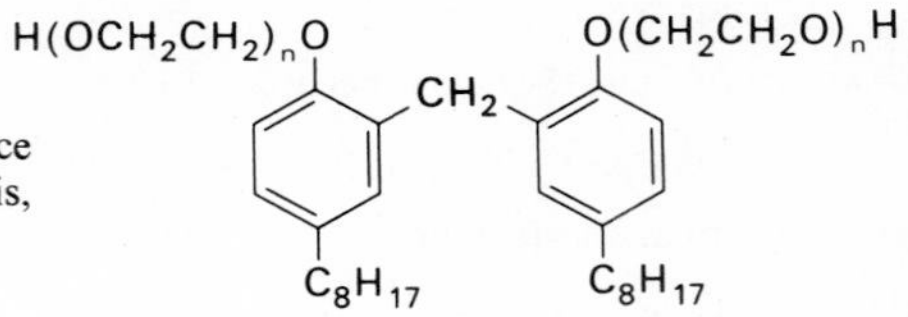

$H(OCH_2CH_2)_nO$, $O(CH_2CH_2O)_nH$, CH_2, C_8H_{17}, C_8H_{17}

Loosens secretions by surface detergent action; used in bronchitis, bronchiectasis, asthma.

3 times a day through a mechanical nebulizer.

SUMMARY: TOPICAL ANTIINFECTIVES

TYPE	*ACTION AND MECHANISM*	*TOXICITY*	*USE*	*EXAMPLES*
Phenol group	Protein precipitation, physical and enzymatic	Convulsions, renal damage	Antiseptic anthelmintic	Cresol
Metallic group	Same	Renal tubular damage	Antiseptic	Silver nitrate
Halogens	Same	Local irritation	Same	Iodine
Oxidizing agents	Oxidation of organic matter	Same	Same	Hydrogen peroxide
Alcohols	Protein precipitants and enzyme inhibitors	Same	Same	Ethyl alcohol
Quinolines	Antimicrobial; mechanism not clear	Same	Antiseptic amebicides	Chiniofon
Contraceptives	Spermicidal in various ways, especially by lowering surface tension	Same	Contraception	Nonoxynol

SUMMARY: TOPICAL ANTIINFECTIVES (cont.)

TYPE	*ACTION AND MECHANISM*	*TOXICITY*	*USE*	*EXAMPLES*
Surface-active compounds	Disrupt or dislodge by lowering surface tension	Same	Detergents	Sodium lauryl sulfate
Mucolytic agents	Facilitate airway by mobilizing and moving mucus	May produce broncospasm in asthmatics	Bronchitis	Acetylcysteine

16. Local Irritants, Protectives, and Cosmetics

A. Irritants

The category of irritants is an ancient one in medicine and one in which change is not rapid. In general the agents are comforting rather than curative.

COUNTERIRRITANTS

1. Actions. a. Counterirritants may lessen pain by distracting the patient's attention; any reflex vasodilatation is more incidental than therapeutic.

b. Classified as rubefacient, vesicant, and pustulant, in increasing order of severity.

c. The basic mechanism is irritation which produces warmth, redness, and even blistering.

2. Uses. a. Counterirritants are nearly obsolete except in such conditions as psoriasis where they are still used.

b. Used as solutions, plasters, ointments, and liniments.

3. Preparations

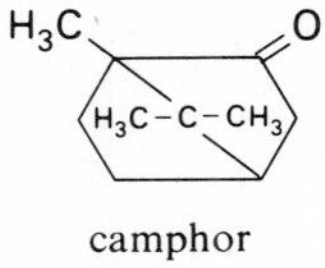

camphor

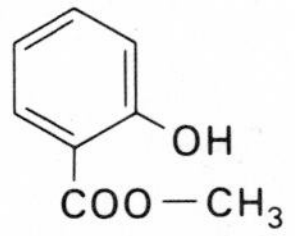

methyl salicylate

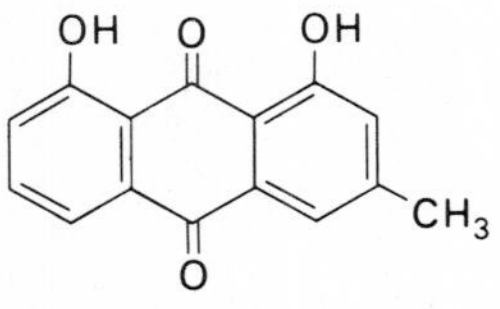

chrysophanic acid

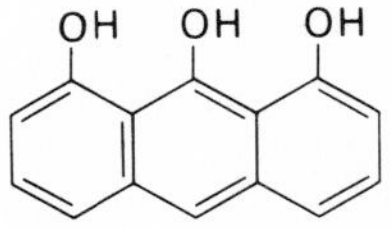

anthralin

CAMPHOR LINIMENT

Formerly rubbed on the chest or joints as a rubefacient.

CHLOROFORM LINIMENT

Rubefacient.

CHRYSAROBIN OINTMENT; ANTHRALIN; COAL TAR OINTMENT or SOLUTION

Of current use in psoriasis.

METHYL SALICYLATE

Old favorite rubefacient for painful joints.

MUSTARD PLASTER

Formerly used on the chest in bronchitis.

CAUSTICS AND STYPTICS

1. **Action.** Coagulate protein, corrosive.

2. **Uses.** a. To remove granulation tissue, excessive growths, warts.
   b. To destroy noxious agents such as snake venom and rabies virus.
   c. To stop bleeding.

3. **Preparations**

ALUM [$Al_2(SO_4)_3$]

Formerly used on aphthous ulcers, but probably more harmful than useful.

CARBON DIOXIDE (CO_2)

Solid form used as a caustic and irritant.

NITRIC ACID (HNO_3)

Highly caustic (rabies).

PODOPHYLLUM

Effective in removing venereal warts.

SILVER NITRATE, TOUGHENED ($AgNO_3$)

Styptic and to remove granulation tissue.

TETRAQUINONE (Kelox)

Used locally for keloids.

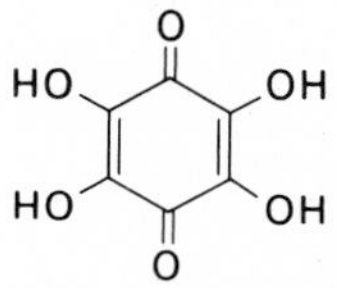

TRICHLORACETIC ACID (Cl_3CCOOH); BICHLORACETIC ACID ($Cl_2CHCOOH$)

Styptic and to remove warts.

ASTRINGENTS

1. **Action.** Produce mild coagulation of tissue proteins.

2. **Uses.** To dry, harden, and protect the skin.

3. **Preparations**

ACETPYROGALL

Astringent.

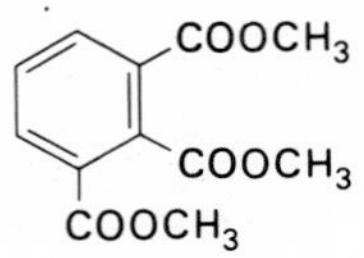

$COOCH_3$ $COOCH_3$ $COOCH_3$

ALCLOXA

Astringent; keratolytic.

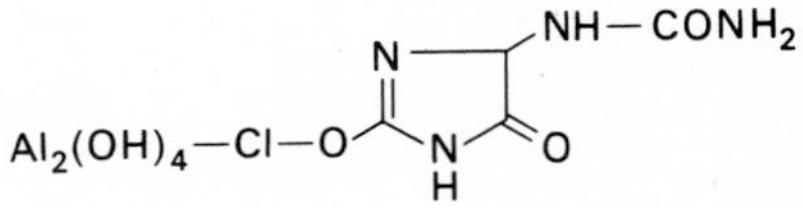

$Al_2(OH)_4-Cl-O$ N NH—$CONH_2$ N H O

ALDIOXA

Astringent; for treatment of diaper dermatitis.

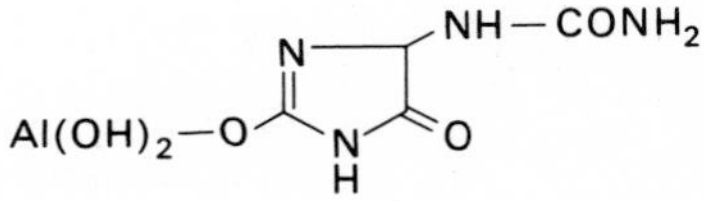

$Al(OH)_2-O$ N NH—$CONH_2$ N H O

ALUMINUM SUBACETATE SOLUTION (Burow's solution) $[Al(OH)(CH_3CO_2)_2]$

Used on weeping eczema.

CADMIUM SULFIDE CAPSEBON (CdS)

Used as a shampoo in seborrheic dermatitis of the scalp in 1% suspension; odorless.

CALAMINE LOTION (contains ZnO)

Widely used protective.

COMPOUND TINCTURE OF BENZOIN

Mixture of benzoic and cinnamic acids with resins and essential oils. Protective.

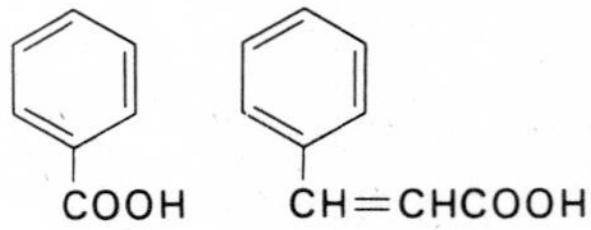

COOH CH=CHCOOH

CUPRIC CITRATE

Sparingly soluble astringent.

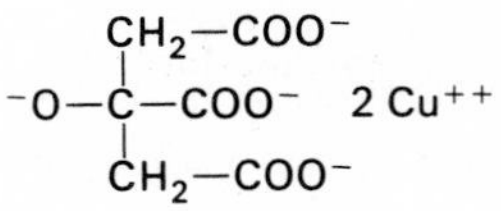

CH_2-COO^-
$^-O-C-COO^-$ $2\,Cu^{++}$
CH_2-COO^-

SELENIUM SULFIDE LOTION (SELSUN) (SeS)

Used as a detergent lotion and shampoo in seborrheic dermatitis of the scalp (dandruff).

SILVER NITRATE ($AgNO_3$)

Astringent and antiseptic in 1:1,000 solutions.

WHITE LOTION (Lotio Alba)

Contains sulfurated potash and zinc sulfate; drying lotion in eczema and seborrhea.

ZINC OXIDE (ZnO)

Powder and ointment mild astringents and protectives.

KERATOLYTICS

1. Action. Dry the skin and produce exfoliation.

2. Uses. In various dermatoses; epidermaphytosis.

3. Preparations

BENZOIC and SALICYCLIC OINTMENT (Whitfield's ointment)

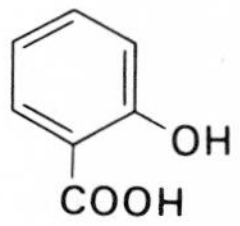

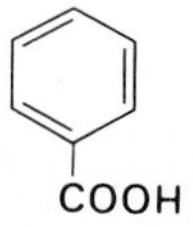

Contains 12% and 6% of the respective acids; traditional exfoliative agent to expose fungi in epidermophytosis.

COOH COOH OH

ICHTHYOL

Used in 2% to 10% concentrations.

Ictasol (Sodium ichthyol light)

RESORCINOL

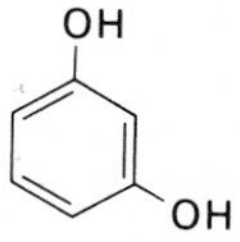

Used in 2% to 6% concentrations.

OH OH

SULFUR, PRECIPITATED

Used in 2% to 10% concentrations.

ANTIPRURITICS

1. Actions. Soothe itching by protecting the skin and perhaps by distracting the attention.

2. Uses. In itching, best where the skin has not been excoriated. (See Antihistamines; also Tranquilizers, for drugs with systemic antipruritic action.)

3. Preparations

CALAMINE LOTION (contains $ZnCO_3$)

Drying and protective; often used with menthol (0.25% to 1%) or phenol (0.5% to 1%) to increase the cooling, analgesic effect.

COAL TAR SOLUTION

Used in baths, 100 ml in a tub of water.

THYMOL; RESORCINOL; CAMPHOR

Any of these may be helpful in low concentrations (usually less than 1%).

ANTIPERSPIRANTS

1. Actions. a. Mild astringents which coagulate secretion and debris in the mouths of sweat glands, thus temporarily occluding the openings.
b. Major effect of most is probably antimicrobial.

2. Uses. To limit sweating and odor, especially in axillae.

3. Preparations

ALUMINUM SULFAMATE [$Al(SO_3NH_2)_3$]

25% in lotions or ointments.

ALUMINUM SULFATE [$Al_2(SO_4)_3$]

25% in lotions or ointments.

SCLEROSING AGENTS

1. Actions. Destroy the endothelium locally in varicose veins, obliterating the lumen.

2. Uses. To obliterate varicose veins by intravenous injection into the vein.

3. Preparations

SODIUM MORRHUATE

5% solution.

SODIUM PSYLLIATE (Sylvasol)

5% solution.

SODIUM RICINOLEATE (Soricin)

2% solution.

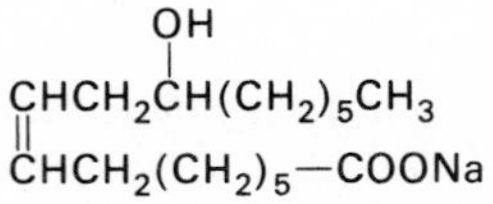

$$\begin{array}{l} \quad\;\; OH \\ \quad\;\; | \\ CHCH_2CH(CH_2)_5CH_3 \\ \| \\ CHCH_2(CH_2)_5{-}COONa \end{array}$$

SODIUM TETRADECYL SULFATE (Sotradecol)

1% to 5% solution.

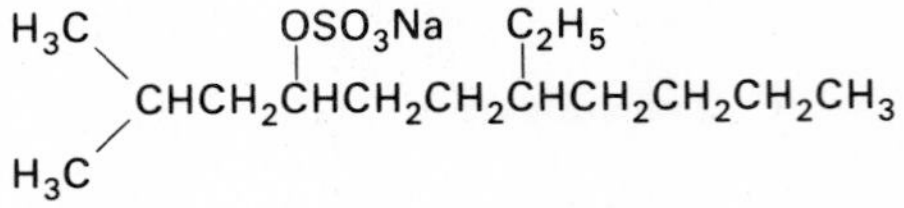

$$(CH_3)_2CHCH_2CH(OSO_3Na)CH_2CH_2CH(C_2H_5)CH_2CH_2CH_2CH_3$$

TRIBENOSIDE (Glyvenol)

$$C_6H_5{-}CH_2{-}O{-}CH_2{-}CH{-}O{-}CH_2{-}C_6H_5 \text{ (furanoside ring with } OC_2H_5, OH, \text{ and } O{-}CH_2{-}C_6H_5)$$

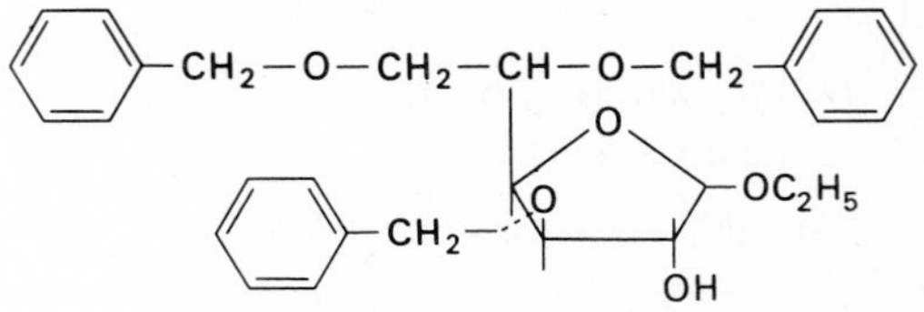

B. Protectives

Protectives are agents that smooth, soften, or otherwise protect the skin. They are perhaps most used as ingredients in pharmaceutical powders, ointments, and dressings.

POULTICES, DRESSINGS, AND BATHS

1. Actions. Comforting, analgesic; may hasten necrosis ("pointing") in boils.

2. Preparations

LINSEED; and CATAPLASM OF KAOLIN

Used as poultices; practically obsolete.

MAGNESIUM SULFATE; SODIUM CHLORIDE; ALUMINUM SUBACETATE; POTASSIUM PERMANGANATE

Solutions used on dressings as cleansing, soothing vehicles and for the application of heat; antipruritic and analgesic; may assist the escape of inflammatory exudates.

TAR; OATMEAL; STARCH

Used in baths as soothing, antipruritic, or anti-inflammatory agents.

DEMULCENTS

1. Actions. Soothe and protect the skin by providing extra surface covering or lubrication.

2. Preparations

ACACIA; TRAGACANTH

Polysaccharide gums used as vehicles and lubricating jellies.

FLEXIBLE COLLODION (cellulose tetranitrate in ether and alcohol); PARAFFIN; ADHESIVE TAPE

Protective coverings.

STARCH; PURIFIED TALC (magnesium trisilicate)

Lubricating powders.

EMOLLIENTS AND PHARMACEUTICAL NECESSITIES

1. Action. a. Soften and lubricate the skin and mucous membranes, usually as ingredients of ointments.
b. Pharmaceutical necessities.

2. Preparations

OINTMENT BASES

Anhydrous lanolin (wool fat), benzoinated lard, dimethicone (Silicote), hydrophilic ointment (water removable), hydrophilic petrolatum (water absorbing), petrolatum (petroleum jelly), white wax.

PLASTICIZERS (for spray-on surgical dressings)

Cellaburate, plastofen (TM Santicizer 141).

SOLVENTS

Carbitol, carbomer (Carboprol) (suspending agent), dipropyleneglycolmethylether (to remove adhesive tape), glycerin, liquid petrolatum, olive oil (enema), polyethylene glycols (carbowaxes), propylene glycol, povidone (emulsifying agent).

SUPPOSITORY BASE

Theobroma oil (cocoa butter).

TABLET DISINTEGRATORS

Dextrates (Celutab), polacrilin potassium (Amberlite IRP-88).

PROSTHETICS AND RELATED MATERIALS

1. Action. Provide supporting or adhesive materials, particularly in surgery.

2. Preparations. Arterial graft (bovine origin); flucrylate (tissue adhesive): mecrylate and ocrylate (in Coapt Tissue adhesives); polyglycotic acid (suture), polymacon (hydrophilic contact lens); polytef (paste for injection); polyurethane foam (for intramedullary fixation of bone).

C. Cosmetics

Cosmetics are agents used to enhance beauty. For the most part they employ agents of protective and decorative nature.

CREAMS

Creams are ointments used as emollients, lubricants, and vehicles.

1. Chemistry

a. Creams: water-in-oil and oil-in-water.
b. Bleaches: creams containing peroxide.
c. Antiseptics: creams containing boric acid.
d. Deodorants: creams containing perfume.
e. Antiperspirants: creams containing astringent aluminum salts.
f. Pomades: water-free creams.

2. Preparations

ROSEWATER OINTMENT (cold cream)

Water-in-oil, contains beeswax, water, oils, borax.

VANISHING CREAM

Oil-in-water, contains petroleum, liquid petrolatum, stearic acid, glycerin, triethanolamine, carbitol, water, potassium hydroxide.

LOTIONS

Lotions are astringent alcoholic solutions.

1. Preparations

AFTER-SHAVE LOTIONS

Similar to alcohol rubs.

ALCOHOL RUB

Alcohol and volatile oils.

CALAMINE LOTION

Zinc oxide gives drying and astringency.

HAND LOTIONS

Contain karaya gum and glycerin for softness and consistency.

POWDERS

Powders are blends of white pigment, suitably tinted and perfumed.

1. Chemistry

a. Body: titanium dioxide, starch, kaolin (adhesiveness), chalk (adsorbency), zinc oxide, magnesium oxide.
b. Slip: talc, metallic soaps.
c. Color: synthetic, vegetable, or mineral (ochre, brilliant pink lake).
d. Perfume: essential or volatile oils.
e. Orris root: texture (may be sensitizing).

2. Preparations

COMPACT POWDER

Talcum powder and tragacanth pressed into a cake.

LIQUID FACE POWDER

Talcum powder in water and alcohol or glycerin.

TALCUM POWDER

MAKE-UP

Make-up products are colored preparations to increase attractiveness.

1. Preparations

EYE SHADOW, EYEBROW PENCIL, MASCARA

Preparations of blue or black (or other) pigments mixed with fats or waxes.

LIPSTICK

Color agent in fatty base with flavor and perfume. Color: fluorescein salts; dibromfluorescein for indelibility. Base: wax, mineral oil, lanolin, castor oil, petroleum.

LIQUID LIPSTICK

Color in plastic mixture, ethyl cellulose plus plasticizer plus alcohol.

ROUGE

Iron oxide or lake colors in high melting fat base, pressed into a cake.

MISCELLANEOUS

BLEACHES

Hydrogen peroxide in creams or lotions.

BRUSHLESS SHAVING CREAM

Stabilized soap foam and a wetting agent.

DEPILATORIES

Wax-resin mixtures applied melted and pulled off when cold; soluble sulfides (of Ca or Ba) cause the hairs to swell and soften, after which they can be scraped off; thioglycolic acid similarly used.

HAIR DYES

Vegetable dyes including henna; para-phenylene diamine dangerous.

HAIR WAVING FLUIDS

Vegetable gums (karaya) with a glycol in water and alcohol.

LIQUID STOCKINGS

Talcum powder in water and alcohol or glycerin.

NAIL LACQUER

Nitrocellulose in acetone or ethyl acetate, with a plasticizer, resin, and color. Remover: acetone or ethyl acetate.

SHAMPOOS

Soap or other detergent in water (and often alcohol); selenium or cadmium sulfide for dandruff.

SHAVING CREAM

Soap or a wetting agent in glycerin or a glycol.

D. Suntan Preparations; Pigmenting Agents

PERMEABLE

1. Actions. Allow some penetration of UV light; lessen probability of burning.

2. Preparations

OLIVE OIL and OTHER VEGETABLE OILS

OBSCURING

1. Action. Screen out tanning wavelengths.

2. Preparations

a. Impenetrable to all wavelengths

TITANIUM DIOXIDE

b. Absorb short, ultraviolet rays that burn

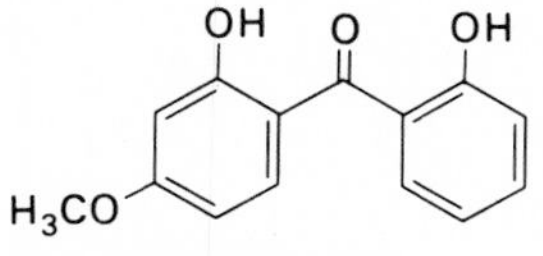

dioxybenzone (Spectra-Sorb UV 24)

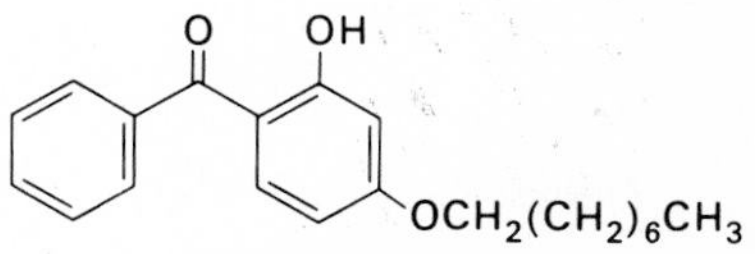

octabenzone (Spectra-Sorb UV 531)

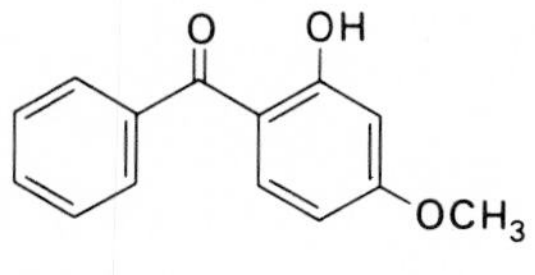

oxybenzone (Spectra-Sorb UV 9)

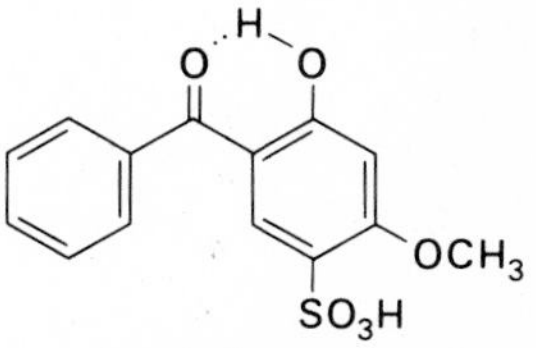

sulisobenzone (Spectra-Sorb UV 284)

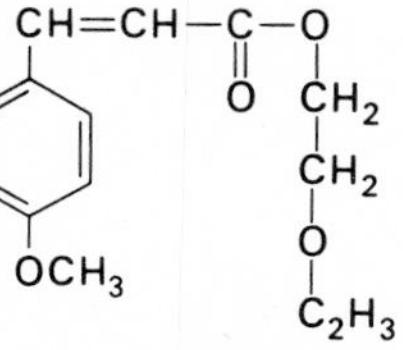

cinoxate (Givaudan)

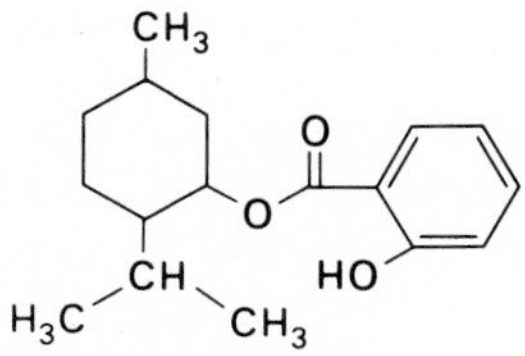

menthyl salicylate

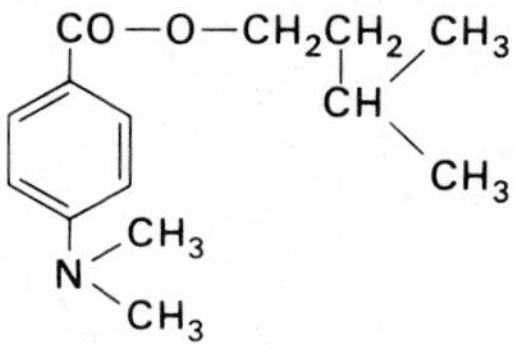

padimate (Escalol 500)

OTHERS: Methyl umbelliferone, red petrolatum, salicoylaminophenol.

METHOXSALEN

1. History. For centuries the Arabians have used the Egyptian plant *Ammi majus* for vitiligo; the active principle is 8-methoxypsoralen (methoxsalen).

2. Chemistry. Methoxypsoralen derivatives.

3. Action and Mechanism. a. Photosensitizer which increases the responsiveness of the skin to light, including the longer wave lengths (above 3,200 Å).

b. The result is increased production of melanin in the skin which causes tanning and protection from burning. The melanin is formed only when the skin is exposed to light. (Becker, J.A.M.A., 173:1483, 1960).

4. Pharmacodynamics and Toxicity. a. Absorbed orally.

b. May produce severe erythema and blistering in vitiligo when applied locally.

c. Systemic administration may cause hepatic damage.

5. Uses. Used in vitiligo and as a tanning agent.

6. Preparations

METHOXSALEN (Meloxine; Oxosoralen)

Dose: 10 to 20 mg by mouth 2 hours before exposure; topically in 1% lotion.

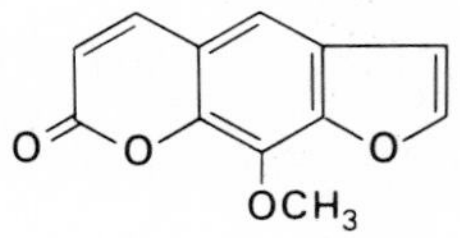

O O O
OCH_3

TRIOXSALEN (Trisoralen)

Suntan screen in lotions.

Dose: 10 mg 2 to 4 hours before exposure, by mouth daily.

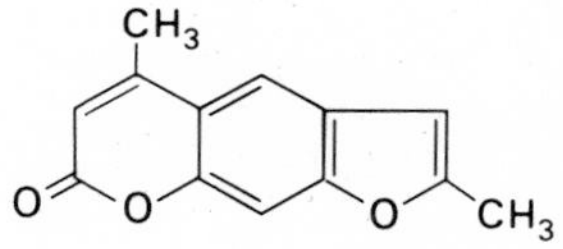

CH_3
O O O CH_3

DIOXYACETONE

1. Chemistry. Dioxyacetone.

2. Action and Mechanism. a. Produces a yellow color in the keratin layer of the skin.

b. Mechanism unknown. Is a normal intermediate in the Krebs cycle.

3. Pharmacology and Toxicity. May make acne worse.

4. Uses. Used to produce a yellow-tan color of the skin; not protective against sunburn. Color may be imperfect (splotchy and too yellow).

5. Preparation

DIOXYACETONE (Man-Tan; Tan-o-Rama)

Applied locally.

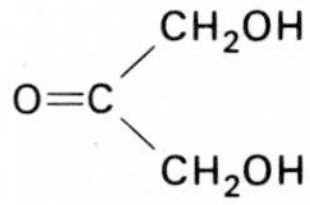

CH_2OH
$O{=}C$
CH_2OH

E. Depigmenting Agents

BENZONES

1. Chemistry. Derivatives and relatives of monobenzone.

2. Action and Mechanism. a. Produces depigmentation of the skin.
b. Mechanism is through inhibition of tyrosinase which prevents melanin formation.

3. Pharmacodynamics and Toxicity. Local application may produce skin irritation.

4. Uses
a. Applied in severe freckling and melasma to depigment the skin.

5. Preparation

MONOBENZONE (Benoquin)
Dose: 10% to 20% topically as a lotion.

$HO-C_6H_4-OCH_2-C_6H_5$

OTHERS

CAPTAMINE HYDROCHLORIDE
Cutaneous depigmenter.

$HS-CH_2CH_2-N(CH_3)_2 \cdot HCl$

HYDROQUINONE (Eldoquin)
Cutaneous depigmenter.
Dose: 2% cream every 12 hours topically.

$HO-C_6H_4-OH$

SUMMARY: LOCAL IRRITANTS, PROTECTIVES, AND COSMETICS

TYPE	*ACTION AND MECHANISM*	*TOXICITY*	*USE*	*EXAMPLES*
Counterirritants	Irritants producing warmth	Blistering	Obsolete except for psoriasis	Coal tar ointment
Caustics	Destroy tissue	Corrosive	To remove granulation tissue and warts	Podophyllum
Astringents	Harden skin by protein coagulation	Minor	Eczema to protect skin	Calamine lotion

(cont.)

SUMMARY: LOCAL IRRITANTS, PROTECTIVES, AND COSMETICS (cont.)

TYPE	*ACTION AND MECHANISM*	*TOXICITY*	*USE*	*EXAMPLES*
Keratolytics	Exfoliation	Minor	Fungal infections	Benzoic and salicylic ointment
Antipruritics	Allay itching	Minor	Itching	Calamine lotion with 1% menthol
Antiperspirants	Coagulate secretions and antimicrobial	Minor	To limit sweating and odor	Aluminum sulfate
Sclerosing agents	Coagulation in veins	Minor	Varicose veins	Sodium morrhuate
Poultices, dressings	Local warmth	Minor	Local infection	Magnesium sulfate
Demulcents	Lubricate skin	Minor	Reduce friction	Talcum powder
Emollients	Soften skin	Minor	Ointment vehicles	Petrolatum
Cosmetics	Adornment	Minor	Cosmetic	Rosewater ointment (cold cream)
Suntan preparations	Control UV access to skin	Minor	To prevent or control tanning	Methoxsalen
Depigmenting agents	Reduces pigmentation by inhibiting tyrosinase or other means	Minor	Freckles	Monobenzone

17.
Antidotes

Most drugs are toxic in overdose; some are toxic at ordinary dosage for particular people—for instance, those with allergic hypersensitivity, genetic defect, unsuitable environment, or disease.

The toxic manifestations of most individual drugs are noted, in this book, in the general consideration of the drug in question, along with any specific antidotal measure. However, some antidotes have broader application and are described in this chapter.

I. METAL-BINDING AGENTS

A. Chelation and Complexing

Metals are usually involved in physiological processes by the chemical mechanism of chelation or complexing. These are reactions between a metal ion and an organic compound in which the metal unites in a ring structure with the complexing agent, forming a definite geometric pattern.

1. Chemistry. a. Chelation. Requires a free H (as —OH, —NH, —SH); a free pair of electrons (as N:, O:, S:); spacing so that a five- or six-membered ring can be formed with a metal, usually a transitional element such as copper.

b. A simple example of chelation is that of 8-hydroxyquinoline with copper:

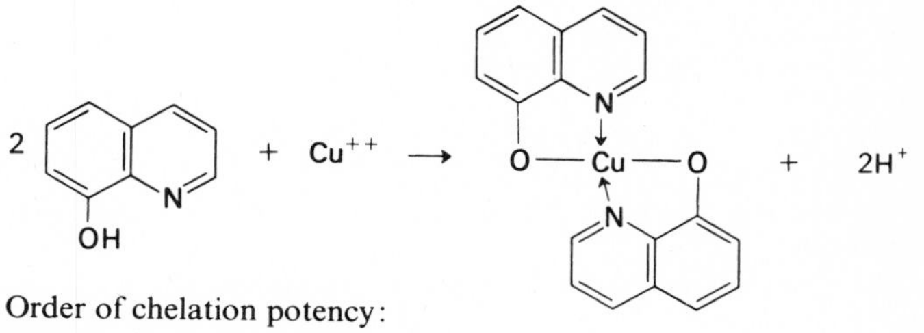

2 (8-hydroxyquinoline: N, OH) + Cu^{++} ⟶ (O—Cu—O, N → Cu ← N) + $2H^{+}$

c. Order of chelation potency:

Strong → Pb > Cu > Ni > Co > Zn > Ca > Fe > Mn > Mg → Weak

2. Toxicity of Metals. Some extraneous metals may replace the normal metals of physiological complexes and thus act as poisons.

3. Metal-Binding Antidotes. A toxic metal may at times be removed from the body by introducing another compound (antidote) with which the metal will chelate even more strongly. That harmful metal may then be excreted in the complex or held so tenaciously that the tissues are inaccessible.

B. Thiols and Related Compounds

DIMERCAPROL

1. History. Stocker and Peters at Oxford, during the early years of World War II, followed the older knowledge that thiol compounds combined with metals to develop the more effective diol, dimercaprol, as an antidote for the poison gas, lewisite, that contains arsenic.

2. Chemistry. Example of binding of Hg by dimercaprol:

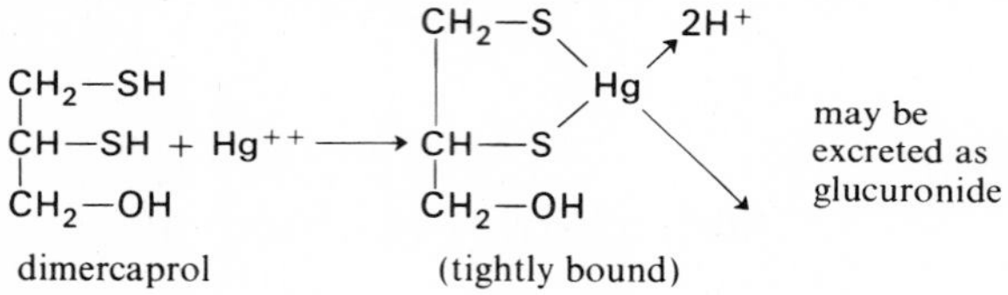

```
                              CH2—S         2H+
                              |     \      ↗
CH2—SH                        |      Hg
|                             |     /      \          may be
CH—SH + Hg++ ———————→         CH—S          \         excreted as
|                             |              ↘        glucuronide
CH2—OH                        CH2—OH

dimercaprol                   (tightly bound)
```

3. Action and Mechanism. a. BAL can form complexes as shown, with As, Sb, Au, Hg, Cu, and Te. Results are less satisfactory with Fe, Cd, or Pb.

b. The combination may then be permanently and harmlessly bound in the tissues, may be excreted, may dissociate, or may itself be toxic.

4. Pharmacodynamics. a. BAL produces little pharmacological effect on the subject in low doses.

b. It does not enter cells; excretion is rapid enough so that there is no cumulation with 4-hour intervals of administration.

5. Toxicity. a. Massive symptoms may follow large, though not necessarily extratherapeutic, doses. These may include unrest, weakness, fatigue, paresthesias, lacrimination, perspiration, salivation, vomiting, and increased heart rate and blood pressure.

b. Local application may sensitize.

6. Uses. a. The most important agent in arsenic, mercury, antimony, and gold poisoning.

b. Clinical effectiveness against other metals less regular.

7. Preparation

DIMERCAPROL (British anti-lewisite; BAL)

Dose: 3 mg per kg body weight 4 to 6 times daily for 2 days intramuscularly; 3 mg 2 to 4 times on third day; then 1 to 2 mg daily for 10 days.

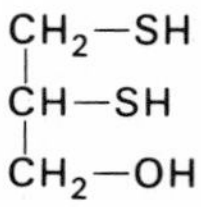

```
CH2—SH
|
CH—SH
|
CH2—OH
```

DISULFIRAM (Antabuse)

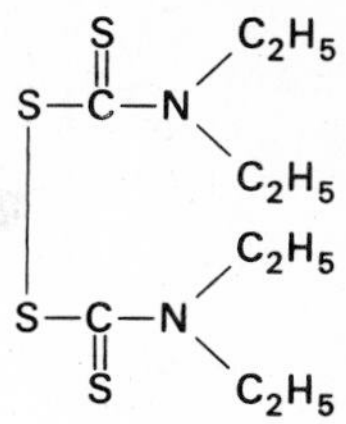

Effective chelator in Ni and Cu poisoning (Sunderman, J. New Drugs, 4:154, 1964).

Dose: 30 mg per kg body weight by mouth, or 10 mg per kg intravenously.

$$\begin{array}{l} S{-}C({=}S){-}N(C_2H_5)_2 \\ | \\ S{-}C({=}S){-}N(C_2H_5)_2 \end{array}$$

C. Edetic Acid Derivatives

EDETATE SODIUM

1. Chemistry. Edetate sodium is the soluble disodium salt of edetic acid (EDTA; ethylenediamine-tetra-acetic acid).

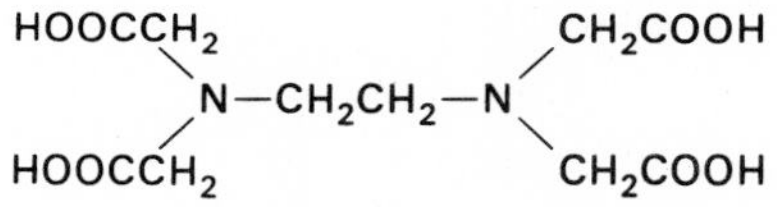

$$(HOOCCH_2)_2N{-}CH_2CH_2{-}N(CH_2COOH)_2$$

edetic acid (EDTA)
(insoluble)

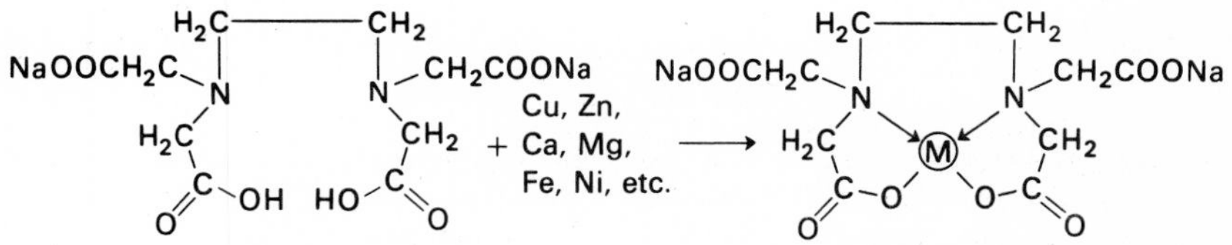

$$\text{disodium EDTA (soluble)} + \text{Cu, Zn, Ca, Mg, Fe, Ni, etc.} \longrightarrow \text{chelated metal}$$

disodium EDTA
(soluble)

chelated metal

2. Action and Mechanism. a. Chelates metals, as noted above, to make three rings, a highly stable structure.

b. Will remove Ca from normal blood or tissues.

3. Pharmacodynamics. Administered by injection. Not metabolized in the body.

4. Toxicity. a. Principal toxicity results from withdrawal of calcium from tissues and blood with the danger of hypocalcemia and deposit of calcium in the kidneys.

b. Also may give mucocutaneous lesions from chelation of zinc (?).

c. Too irritating for local application to remove stones from urinary tract.

5. Uses. a. Still relatively experimental, but has been tried in hypercalcemia and atherosclerosis, in corneal calcification, and in digitalis poisoning for the removal of calcium.

b. In vitro it has been a satisfactory anticoagulant by binding the calcium.

6. Preparation

EDETATE DISODIUM
(Edathamil; Sodium versenate; Sequestrene; Endrate)

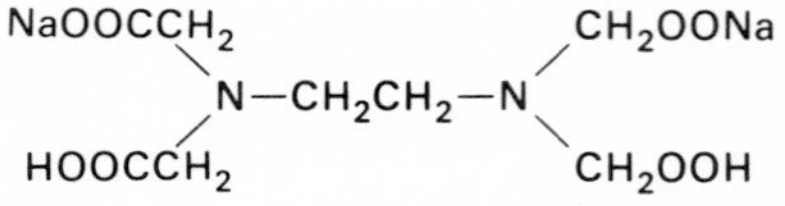

$$\begin{matrix} NaOOCCH_2 & & CH_2OONa \\ & N{-}CH_2CH_2{-}N & \\ HOOCCH_2 & & CH_2OOH \end{matrix}$$

Dose: 50 mg per kg body weight (to a maximum of 3 gm) in 500 ml of a 5% dextrose solution infused intravenously over 3 to 4 hours.

OTHERS

Edetate tetrasodium (in Vagesic), edetate trisodium (pharmaceutical necessity).

EDETATE CALCIUM DISODIUM

1. Chemistry

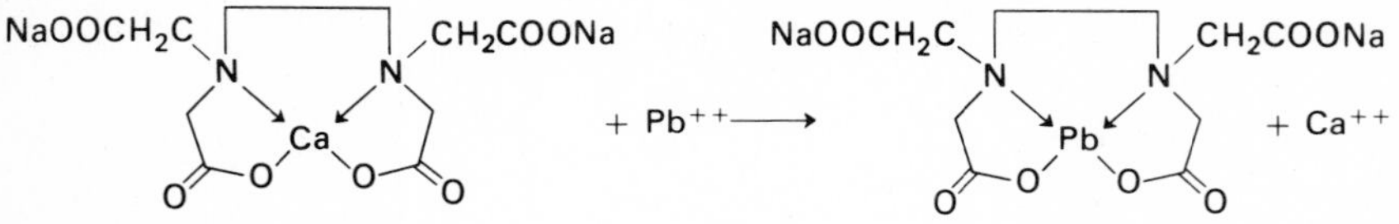

$$\begin{matrix} NaOOCH_2C\diagdown & & \diagup CH_2COONa \\ N & Ca & N \\ O{=}C{-}O & & O{-}C{=}O \end{matrix} \; + Pb^{++} \longrightarrow \; \begin{matrix} NaOOCH_2C\diagdown & & \diagup CH_2COONa \\ N & Pb & N \\ O{=}C{-}O & & O{-}C{=}O \end{matrix} \; + Ca^{++}$$

edetate calcium disodium — chelated metal (soluble)

2. Action and Mechanism. a. Chelated Ca is easily exchanged for lead, and the combination then promptly excreted in the urine.

b. It may remove: Sr, Pu, Y, Cd; it will not remove: Mg, Ba, Fe; results inconclusive: Cr, Ni, Cu.

3. Pharmacodynamics. Not metabolized in the body.

4. Toxicity. Therapeutic margin wide; appears not to produce blood or kidney damage, except with prolonged administration.

5. Uses. a. Used to mobilize lead for excretion in a soluble form.

b. Has been tried in chrome skin ulcers, in nickel and copper eczemas, in kidney stones.

6. Preparation

EDETATE CALCIUM DISODIUM (calcium disodium edathamil, EDTA, or versenate)

Dose: 0.04 gm per kg body weight per hour in 3% saline by intravenous drip; total not to exceed 0.45 gm per kg and best given in interrupted courses.

PENTETATE CALCIUM TRISODIUM
(penthamil; DTPA)

Affinity for lead; also for Cu, Co, Fe, Mn, Pu, Sc, U, Yt.

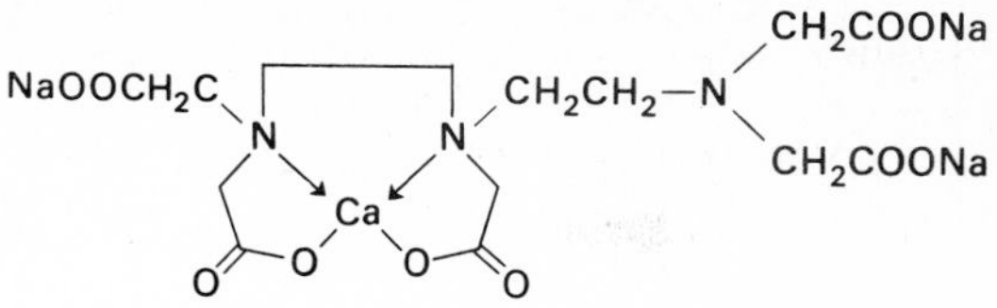

$$NaOOCH_2C{-}N(\text{—}CH_2COO\text{—})\rightarrow Ca \leftarrow N(\text{—}CH_2COO\text{—})CH_2CH_2{-}N(CH_2COONa)_2$$

D. Penicillamines

1. Chemistry. Dimethylcysteines.

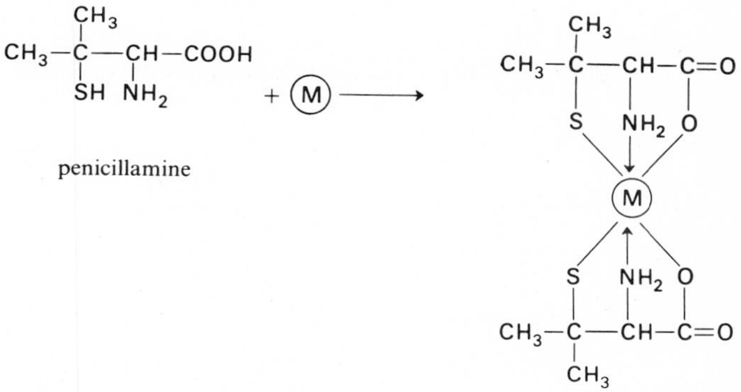

$$CH_3{-}C(CH_3)(SH){-}CH(NH_2){-}COOH + \text{(M)} \longrightarrow [CH_3{-}C(CH_3)(S){-}CH(NH_2){-}C(=O)O]_2\text{(M)}$$

penicillamine

2. Action and Mechanism. a. Can chelate with Cu, Hg, Pb, Fe, and probably other metals.

b. Can react with cystine to form a more soluble mixed disulfide.

3. Pharmacodynamics. a. Absorbed by mouth.

b. The acetyl derivative is more stable, presumably because the acetyl protects the amino group from degradation, and also penetrates better (Hirschman, New Eng. J. Med., 269:889, 1963).

4. Toxicity. a. Toxicity from D form seldom severe, but may cause rash, ecchymoses, fever, lymphadenopathy, leukopenia, thrombocytopenia, nephrotic syndrome, possibly cataracts.

b. L (and DL) form may induce pyridoxine deficiency, including optic atrophy.

5. Uses. a. Used to remove Cu, including that in hepatolenticular degeneration (Wilson's disease); should be prescribed with K_2S, 25 mg with meals, to precipitate Cu in food and water (Scheinberg, J. Chron. Dis., 17:293, 1964), and 25 to 50 mg of pyridoxine daily.

b. Tried in macroglobulinemia (dissociates macroglobulin); in cystinuria; in Hg, Pb, Fe, and Au poisoning; in scleroderma and other types of fibrosis.

c. May replace BAL in some instances, even though generally less potent, because of the advantage of oral administration.

6. Preparation

PENICILLAMINE (D-penicillamine, Cuprimine)
Dose: 250 mg daily by mouth, increasing to 250 to 500 mg 4 times a day.

E. Deferoxamine

1. History. Discovered by Bickel (1960).

2. Chemistry. a. Ferrioxamine B is a siderochrome isolated from *Streptomyces griseus;* contains iron in an octahedral complex; is not antibacterial.

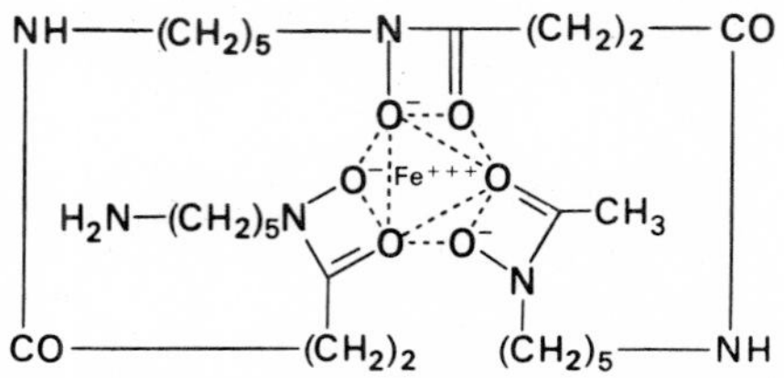

NH—$(CH_2)_5$—N—$(CH_2)_2$—CO
$H_2N—(CH_2)_5N$ Fe^{+++} —CH_3
CO—$(CH_2)_2$ $(CH_2)_5$—NH

ferrioxamine B (suggested formula)

3. Action and Mechanism. a. Desferrioxamine B binds the iron in transferrin and ferritin, not hemoglobin.

b. Promotes renal excretion of Fe and may block absorption of Fe.

c. Does not remove other metals (Moeschlin, New Eng. J. Med., 269:57, 1963; Jacobs, New Eng. J. Med., 273:1124, 1965).

4. Pharmacodynamics. a. Soluble, but not absorbed by mouth.

b. Excreted easily with or without Fe by the kidneys.

5. Toxicity. Apparently of low toxicity.

6. Uses. a. Used in polycythemia, hemochromatosis (primary and secondary), porphyria cutanea tarda, cirrhosis of the liver.

b. Can remove 1 to 3 mg of Fe daily (7 to 18 gm per year).

c. Continuous therapy shows little advantage over intermittent, and may be block Fe absorption (Bannerman, Brit. Med. J., 2:1573, 1962).

d. Used by mouth in acute iron poisoning.

7. Preparation

DEFEROXAMINE (desferrioxamine B; Desferal)

```
     CH3          (CH2)2                 (CH2)2
    /            /      \               /      \
  OC           OC        CO           OC        CO
   |            |         |            |         |
   N            NH        N            NH        N          NH2
  / \          /         / \          /         / \         /
HO   (CH2)5          HO   (CH2)5            HO   (CH2)5
```

Dose: 400 to 600 mg once or twice daily intravenously; in acute iron poisoning, 8 to 12 mg by gastric tube plus 2 gm intramuscularly or intravenously.

F. Phosphates

1. Action. Certain organic phosphate compounds may complex with calcium.

2. Preparations

SODIUM PHYTATE (Rencal)

Reported to form unabsorbable complex with Ca and Mg ions, thus reducing their alimentary absorption and renal excretion. Given with a low Ca diet to reduce calciuria in renal stone; therapeutic value undetermined. May cause diarrhea.

Dose: 3 gm in 200 ml ice water three times a day by mouth.

```
              OPO3=
               |
=O3PO  /\  OPO3=
      |  |             (H3Na9)12+
=O3PO  \/  OPO3=
               |
              OPO3=
```

EDITRONIC ACID

```
          O   OH
          ||/
          P
        /   \
             OH
H3C—C—OH
        \    OH
          \ /
          P
          ||\
          O   OH
```

II. ADSORBENTS

Action. Adsorb suspended or dissolved substances, gases, bacteria, and toxins.

Uses. For internal use as general antidotes (see Alimentary Tract Agents).

CHARCOAL ACTIVATED

In specially prepared devices for hemoperfusion to remove from the blood drugs and other toxic substances (Hill, J. B., et al. Clin. Chem., 22:754, 1976).

III. RADIOPROTECTANTS

A. Radiation Damage

There are two current theories of the mechanism of radiation damage.

1. Direct or Target Theory. X-ray, heat, or electrical discharge can break a strong double electron bond to give particles with lone electrons, high energy, and no charge, called free radicals.

Examples:

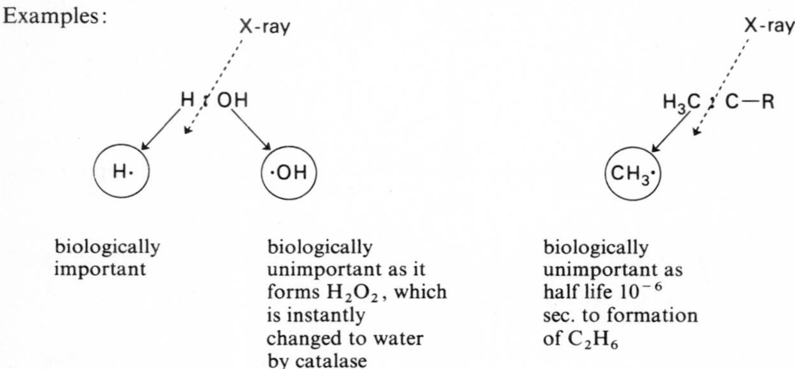

Free radicals are unstable and must liberate their energy quickly, as heat, or as mechanical energy in collisions with other atoms. (Enzymatic oxidation-reductions use a less violent free radical mechanism.) The fragments formed after a compound is struck by a free radical have low energy and may combine, producing cross-linking, as in the example:

(H·)

$$2\ H{-}S{-}CH_2CH(NH_2){-}COOH \longrightarrow \begin{array}{l} S{-}CH_2CH(NH_2){-}COOH \\ | \\ S{-}CH_2CH(NH_2){-}COOH \end{array}$$

H

cysteine cystine

2. Indirect or Ionization of Water Theory. a. Radiation creates water ions, which then unite to form peroxide and other compounds.

b. The peroxide inactivates catalase and other enzymes by damaging SH groups.

c. This mechanism appears to apply more to living organisms; the direct mechanism applies more to completely dehydrated structures.

B. Aminothiols

1. History. 2-Aminoethyl-iso-thiuronium (AET) was the first compound to come into general interest as an antiradiation drug.

2. Chemistry. a. Most effective compounds related to cysteamine: $HS{-}CH_2CH_2{-}NH_2$.

b. AET is itself inactive as an —SH group is not available, but is changed in the body to an active derivative, as well as to a toxic compound.

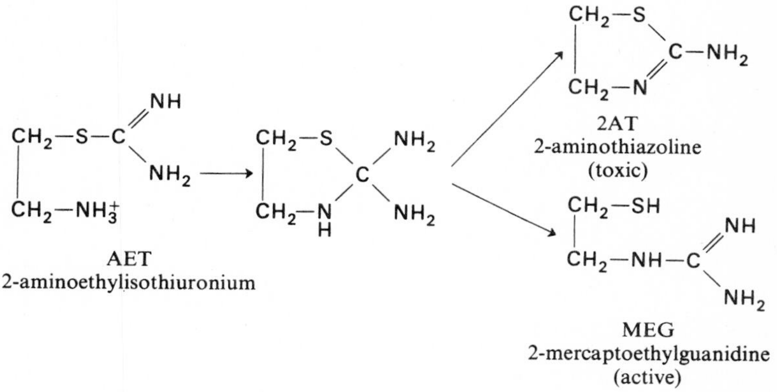

$CH_2{-}S{-}C(=NH){-}NH_2$ / $CH_2{-}NH_3^+$

AET
2-aminoethylisothiuronium

→ $CH_2{-}S$ / $CH_2{-}NH$ — $C(NH_2)_2$

→ $CH_2{-}S{-}C(-NH_2){=}N{-}CH_2$ (ring)

2AT
2-aminothiazoline
(toxic)

→ $CH_2{-}SH$ / $CH_2{-}NH{-}C(=NH){-}NH_2$

MEG
2-mercaptoethylguanidine
(active)

3. Action and Mechanism. a. Several theories have been proposed:

b. May provide —SH groups, which combine with peroxide, thus protecting the —SH groups of catalase and other enzymes.

c. May chelate metals, such as copper, which promote the longevity of free radicals.

d. May exhaust free radicals by furnishing accessible and unstable —SH groups.

e. May bind and stabilize parts of the DNA helix not covered by histones; this reduces damage and DNA replication rate is decreased, so that repairs can be accomplished before alterations are replicated.

4. Pharmacodynamics. AET penetrates quickly to liver, kidney, spleen, and marrow after injection; evanescent in action.

5. Toxicity. AET may produce apnea, hypotension, bradycardia, gut contractions; higher doses block ganglia; convulsions in guinea pigs; toxicity at least in part due to 2AT.

6. Uses. a. Used experimentally to protect against x-rays and other radiation.

b. Must be given almost simultaneously with exposure to radiant energy.

c. 2-Mercaptoethylamine has been tried in macroglobulinemia; by forming S—S linkages, large protein molecules may be broken into smaller units.

7. Preparations

$$\begin{array}{l} CH_2{-}S{-}C(=NH){-}NH_2 \\ | \\ CH_2{-}\overset{+}{N}H_3 \end{array}$$

2-aminoethylisothiuronium (AET)

$$\begin{array}{l} CH_2{-}SH \\ | \\ CH_2{-}NH_2 \end{array}$$

2-mercaptoethylamine

SUMMARY: ANTIDOTES

TYPE	*ACTION AND MECHANISM*	*TOXICITY*	*USE*	*EXAMPLES*
Thiols	Complex with metals, then excreted	Weakness, paresthesias, salivation, tachycardia	Antidotes for As, Hg, and other metals	Dimercaprol
Edetic acid group	Same	Hypocalcemia (with disodium salt)	Antidotes for Pb, and others; decalcifying agents	Edetate calcium disodium
Penicillamine group	Same	Rash, fever, leukopenia, nephrotic syndrome	To remove Cu; macroglobulin-emia	Penicillamine
Ferrioxamine derivatives	Same	Minor	To remove Fe in polycythemia; hemo-chromatosis	Deferoxamine
Aminothiols	Exhaust free radicals from irradiation	Apnea, brady-cardia, convulsions	Radiation excess (experimental)	Aminoethyliso-thiuronium

Reviews

Done, A. K. Clinical pharmacology of systemic antidotes. Clin. Pharmacol. Ther., 2:750, 1961.

Haley, T. New aspects in the development of radioprotectant drugs. G. Ital. Chemiother., 6–9:213, 1962.

Furst, A. Chemistry of Chelation in Cancer. Springfield, Ill., Charles C Thomas, 1963.

Ambrus, J., et al. Selective protection of gastrointestinal tract against radiation injury by perfusion with MEG. Cancer Res., 25:609, 1965.

Gosselin, R., and Smith, R. Trends in the therapy of acute poisonings. Clin. Pharmacol. Ther., 7:279, 1966.

Shubert, J. Chelation in medicine. Sci. Amer., 214:40, 1966.

Brown, P. E. Mechanism of action of aminothiol radioprotectors. Nature, 213:363, 1967.

Wieland, T. Poisonous principles of mushrooms of the genus *Amanita*, Science, 159:946, 1968.

Chenoweth, M. Clinical uses of metal binding drugs, Clin. Pharmacol. Ther., 9:365, 1968.

Dreisbach, R. Handbook of Poisoning, 5th ed. Lange, Los Altos, 1969.

18.
Cardiac Glycosides

1. History. a. Ebers papyrus (ca.1500 B.C.) mentions squill; Fuchs (Fuchsius; 1542) named *Digitalis purpurea* (and the fuchsia); London Pharmacopeia (1722) included foxglove in a salve.

b. Withering (1785) used foxglove in dropsy; Ferriar (1799) ascribed the action of foxglove to cardiac effects.

c. Homolle and Quevenne (1840), Nativelle (1869), Arnaud (1888) separated increasingly pure glycosidal preparations from digitalis.

d. Kraft, Cloeta, Windaus, DeVry, Fraser, Karrer, Smith, Stoll, Ruzika, Reichstein (1900 to present) furnished chemical clarification of various cardiac glycosides.

e. Cushny, Mackenzie, Lewis, Hatcher, Eggleston, McMichael (1900 to present) clarified the actions of digitalis.

2. Chemistry. a. Classical cardiac glycosides are composed of three portions: a sugar (hence glycoside), a steroid nucleus, and a lactone, as shown in the following structural formula for digitoxin.

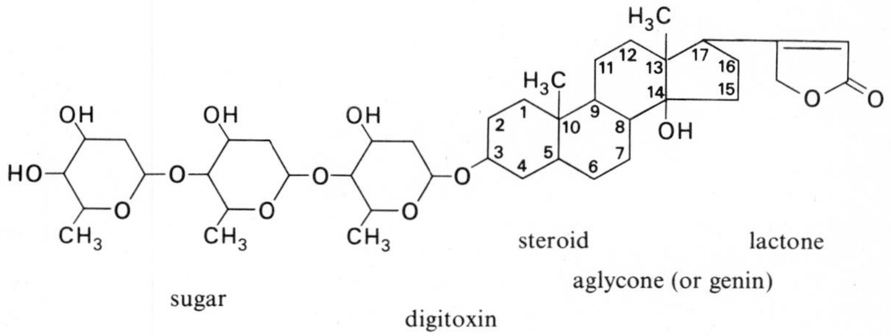

steroid lactone

aglycone (or genin)

sugar

digitoxin

b. Compounds of this type are found widely in nature, from both plant and animal sources. Example sources:

Digitalis purpurea, *D. lanata:* Foxgloves; sources of the majority of medicinal preparations.

Strophanthus gratus, *S. kombe:* The ouabaio tree.

Scilla maritima (*Urginea maritima*): Squill—red, white, Indian.

Thevita neriifolia, *Nerium oleander*, *Convallaria majalis*.

Bufo toad poisons, and others not ordinarily used in medicine.

c. The following formulas give examples of the different general structures, i.e., with varying types of glycosidal side chains, steroid substitutions, and lactones.

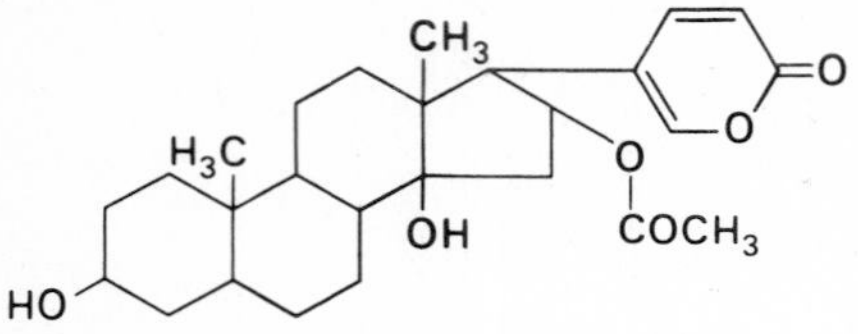

bufotalin

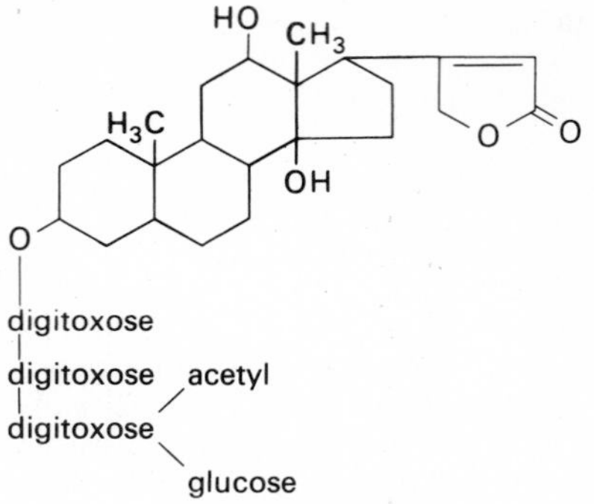

lanatoside C

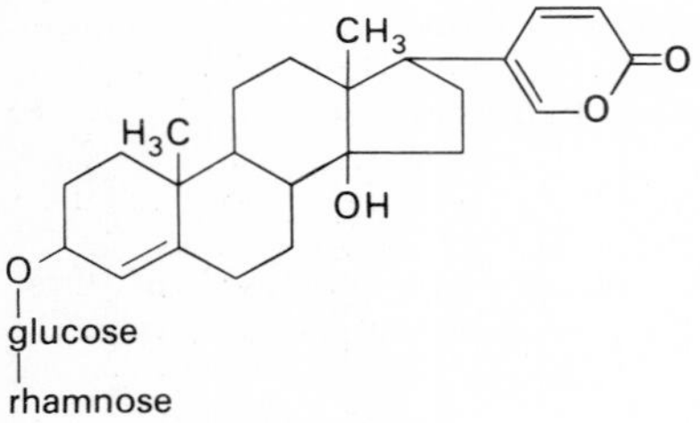

scillaren A

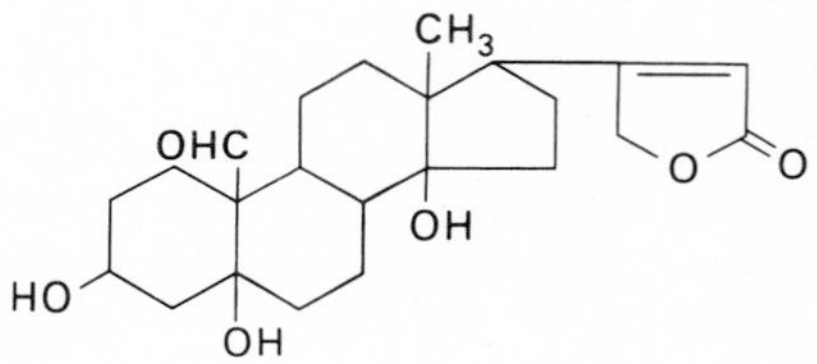

strophanthidin

d. It is possible to make certain correlations between portions of the molecule and activity:

a′. Aglycone (glycoside minus the sugar): Activity usually less than that of the glycoside.

b′. Steroid nucleus: May be substitutions at 1,5,10,12,13,14,16; usually of CH_3, OH, and CHO; OH at 14 usually necessary for activity; spatial isomerism important. Semisynthetic derivatives may be made by substitutions on the steroid. Squill derivatives may have double bond at 5=6. Lantosides also have an OH at C12.

c′. Lactone ring: Essential to action; lactones alone give cardiac depression. Synthetic coupling to other steroids unsuccessful. Ring unsaturated; may be five or six membered.

d′. Sugar: Attached at 3 by glycosidal linkage. May be usual sugars (glucose, rhamnose, arabinose, xylose, lyxose), or unusual (digitoxose, digitalose, cymarose, antiarose, oleandrose, sarmentose, thevitose). Sugars usually increase activity by modifying solubility, absorption, permeability, or distribution. Sugars, or acetyl groups, may be removed in steps giving intermediates between the glycoside and the aglycone.

e. The intermediates formed by the hydrolysis of *Digitalis lanata* and *purpurea*, and their relationships to each other, are shown in the following diagram; acetyl hydrolyses are by gentle alkali, glucose by enzyme, and digitoxose by acid (after Stoll, J. Pharm. Pharmac. 1:849, 1949).

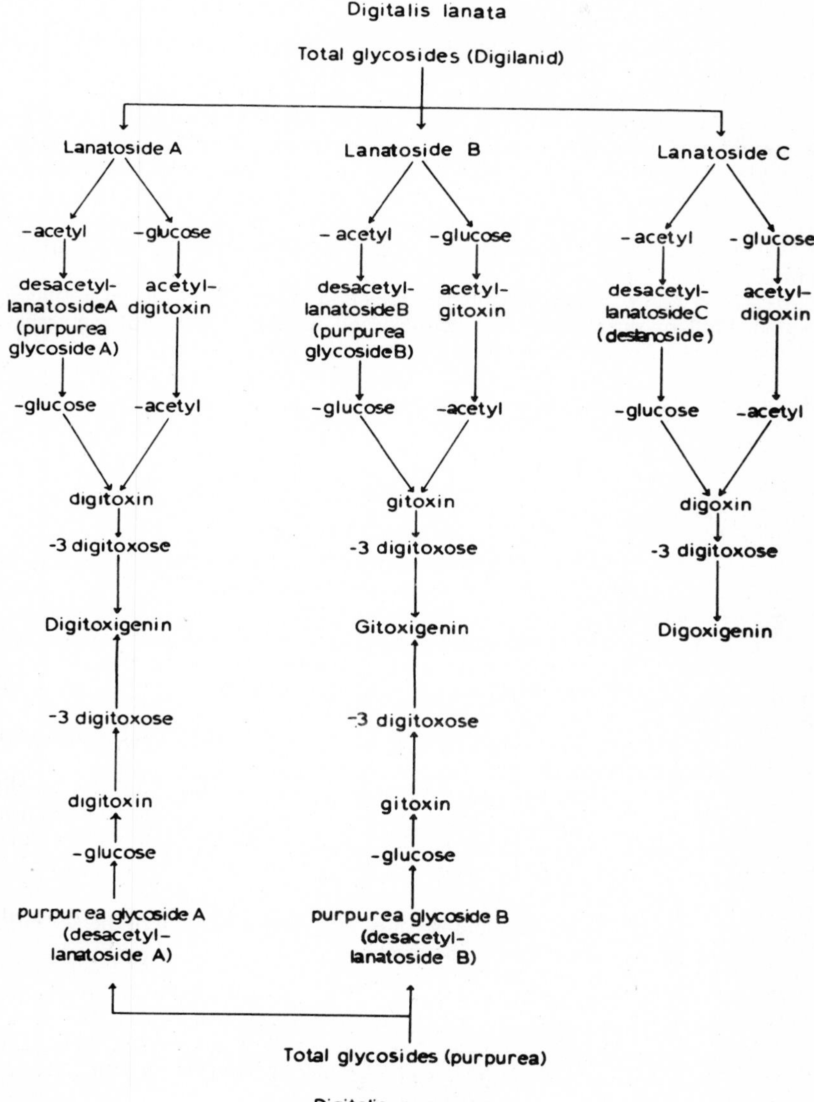

3. Action

a. In normals: Tends to increase contractility, but effects counteracted by reflex adjustments with no significant change in cardiac output.

b. In heart failure: Improves function by increasing the force and efficiency of the heart muscle without corresponding increase in O_2 consumption; called positive inotropic action. Results include:

a′. Increased cardiac output.

b′. Slower rate; reflexly, via the vagus.

c′. Lower venous pressure.

d′. Diuresis; increased renal circulation gives less time for Na reabsorption.

e′. Improved ventilation; from relief of hypoxia in lungs.

c. In arrhythmias: Slows the heart rate in atrial fibrillation and flutter by depressing conduction at the AV node. Flutter may pass through fibrillation, and then revert to normal; paroxysmal atrial tachycardia may be terminated. These effects, which may occur with or without heart failure, are characterized by:

a′. Atrium: Shortened refractory period (reflex) but lengthened (direct).

b′. AV node: Impaired conduction from a lengthened refractory period, both by direct and reflex actions (and probably peripheral sympathetic inhibition; Mendez, J. Pharmacol. Exp. Ther., 131:199, 1961).

c′. Ventricle: Shortened refractory period, reduced excitability, increased automatism; no interference in conduction.

4. Mechanism

a. In heart failure: The mechanism of the effect on the heart muscle has received much attention, but is not as yet well understood. The following appear to be relevant factors:

a′. Heart failure in which energy is produced defectively is little helped by digitalis (beri-beri, thyrotoxicosis); that in which energy is used (converted to work) defectively is greatly helped (heart failure of valvular disease or hypertension).

b′. There has been no dearth of suggestion as to how digitalis acts on the contractile apparatus of the heart. Present thought is that it increases available intracellular Ca^{++}, both by release from intracellular binding and by increased entry from the cell membrane; the Ca^{++} then facilitates excitation-contraction coupling, the mechanism by which the impulse gives rise to contraction.

c′. Other suggested mechanisms, some of which may provide minor effects, include:

a″. Effects on Na^+ and K^+ flux, especially inhibition of the K^+ pump that returns K^+ into the cells after contraction.

b″. Effects on contractile protein (actomyosin).

c″. Release of catechol amines.

d″. Direct effects on smooth muscle in vessels.

b. In arrhythmias: It is assumed that the mechanism of the impairment of conduction through the AV node, and the effects on the atria, are related to the effect on muscle contraction, but the explanations are incomplete.

5. Pharmacology. a. The fundamental actions of all the digitalis group are probably identical, but different preparations vary in solubility, absorption, presence of irritating material, rapidity of effect, and the like.

b. Absorption after oral administration varies from nil to nearly 100%, but rapidity of action depends also on the degree of protein binding. After intravenous injection ouabain, digoxin, and lanatoside C act almost immediately; the effect of digitoxin is delayed for 10 to 20 minutes because of this binding effect.

c. Distribution is widespread.

d. There is slow degradation in the liver, with about 75% final excretion in the urine, mostly as metabolic products.

e. The pharmacological characteristics of a number of cardiac glycosides are given in the following table:

Table of Digitalis Preparations

NAME	*SOURCE*	*ABSORPTION %*	*ONSET**	*DURATION*	*DOSAGE INITIAL ORAL*	*DOSAGE INITIAL IV*	*MAINTENANCE*
digitalis	*Digitalis purpurea*	0.1 ±	med.	long	1.5 gm	—	0.1 gm
digitoxin	*Digitalis purpurea*	90	slow	long	1.2 mg	1.2 mg	0.1 mg
acetyl-digitoxin	*Digitalis lanata*	75	med.	med.	1.8 mg	—	0.15 mg
digoxin	*Digitalis lanata*	65	fast	med.	2–4 mg	1 mg	0.5 mg
deslanoside	*Digitalis lanata*	40	fast	med.	8 mg	1.4 mg	1.0 mg
ouabain	*Stroph. gratus*	0	fast	short	—	0.5 mg	—

* After oral administration (except ouabain).

f. Digitalis glycosides are standardized by biological tests (dose to kill a frog, cat, or pigeon; or dose to make a pigeon vomit) or by chemical estimation (available for digitoxin and digoxin).

6. Toxicity

a. Overdosage may give a variety of toxic manifestations:

a′. Alimentary. Anorexia, nausea, diarrhea, vomiting (with crude preparations partly from saponins).

b′. CNS: Weakness; yellow figures dancing before the eyes (Purkinje).

c′. Heart: Premature beats, bigeminal rhythm, paroxysmal atrial tachycardia with AV block, paroxysmal atrial fibrillation or flutter, paroxysmal ventricular tachycardia.

d′. Endocrine: Rare gynecomastia.

b. Antidotes: K can overcome certain aspects of digitalis toxicity (arrhythmias) and clinical use now common; EDTA forms CaEDTA which lowers Ca and reciprocally raises K; propranolol is effective against arrhythmias.

7. Uses

a. Of great value in certain types of congestive heart failure; of greater value in "low output" failure, as from valvular disease, than in "high output" failure, as in hyperthyroidism; of no value in shock (see 4.b.a'.).

b. Also of great value in the control of atrial fibrillation, atrial flutter, and paroxysmal atrial tachycardia, especially by slowing the ventricular rate in the first two, less dependably in preventing or terminating the third.

c. The principle of therapy is to digitalize the patient (saturate to the therapeutic level), and then to maintain this level.

a'. Initiation: Give large digitalizing doses over hours or a day or two, until the patient improves (or until initial signs of toxicity, especially anorexia, have barely appeared); or if fibrillation is present, until there is a slowing of the cardiac rate below 70 or the appearance of bigeminal rhythm. In emergency may give the initial dose intravenously. In any case, caution if a digitalis preparation has been taken within the previous two weeks.

b'. Maintenance: Give daily dose just adequate to maintain digitalis effect without toxicity.

c'. Outpatient: Give intermediate doses over days or weeks; i.e., powdered leaf, 0.2 gm daily until digitalized (about two weeks), then maintenance as above.

8. Preparations

ACETYLDIGITOXIN (Acylanid)

Similar to digilanid but slightly more rapidly and briefly acting.

Dose: 1.8 mg (initial), 0.15 mg (maintenance) daily by mouth.

CH_3 H_3C OH O H O

$C_{18}H_{30}O_8-COCH_3$

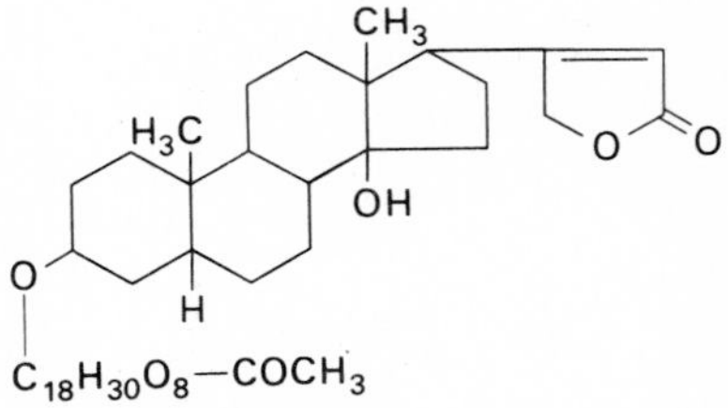

DESLANOSIDE (Cedilanid D)

Similar to digoxin, both acting promptly intravenously.

Dose: 1.4 mg intravenously.

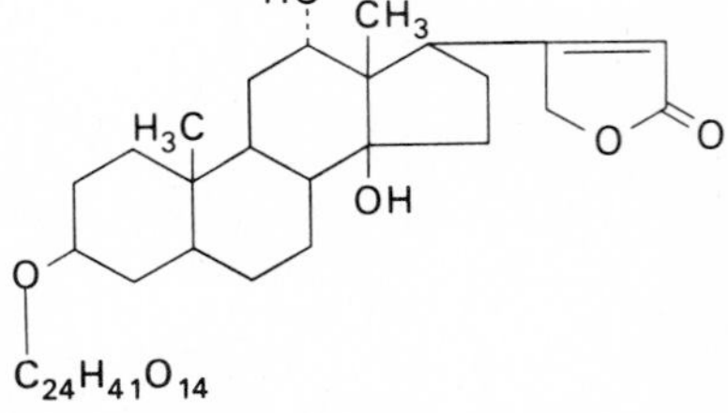

HO CH_3 H_3C OH O O O

$C_{24}H_{41}O_{14}$

DIGITALIS (Whole leaf)

The traditional preparation, still entirely satisfactory. May produce more gastrointestinal irritation than refined preparations.

Dose: 1.5 gm in divided doses (initial), 0.1 gm (maintenance) daily by mouth.

DIGITOXIN

Similar to digitalis but at 1/1,000 dose; nearly completely absorbed and long acting.

Dose: 1.2 mg (initial), 0.1 mg (maintenance) daily by mouth; 1.2 mg intravenously.

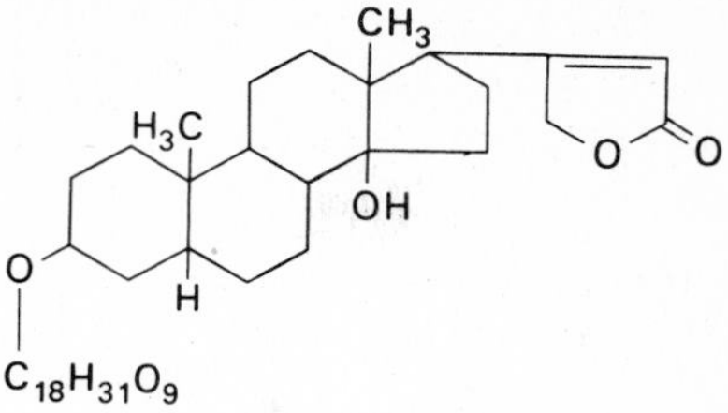

DIGOXIN (Lanoxin)

More briefly acting than preceding (purpurea) preparations.

Dose: 2 to 4 mg (initial), 0.5 mg (maintenance) daily by mouth; 1 mg intravenously.

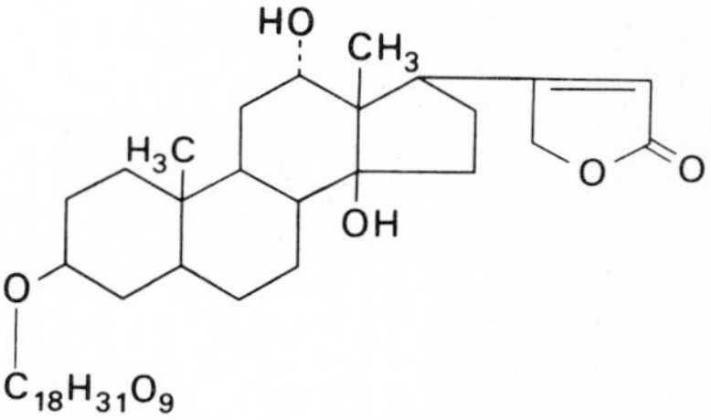

GITALIN, AMORPHOUS (Gitalgin)

Intermediate between digitoxin and digoxin.
Dose: 6 mg (initial), 0.5 mg (maintenance), daily by mouth.

LANATOSIDE C (Cedilanid)

Dose: 8 mg (initial), 1.0 mg (maintenance) daily by mouth.

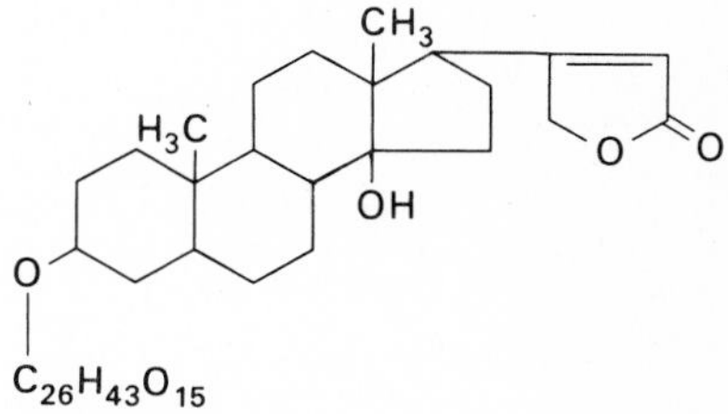

OUABAIN (G-strophanthin)

Rapid onset; for emergency use
Dose: 0.25 to 0.5 mg intravenously.

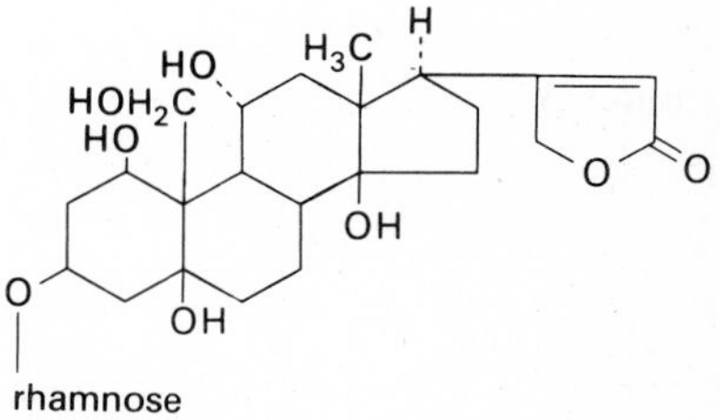

ACTODIGIN

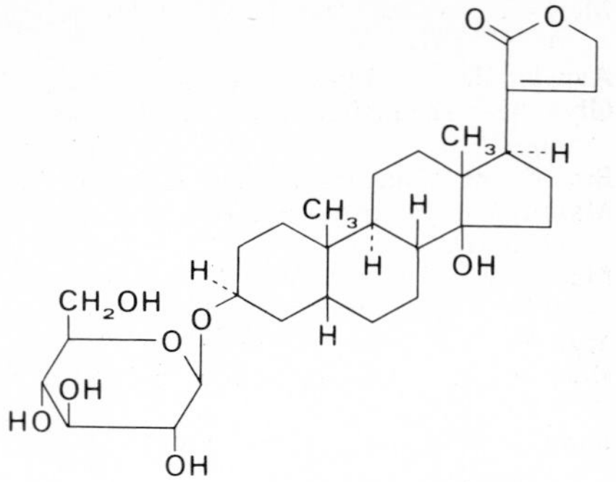

PROSCILLARIDIN (Talusin)

Derived from squill; rapid onset and excretion.

Dose: 0.75 mg 3 times a day by mouth (initial); 0.65 mg daily (maintenance); 0.125 mg intravenously.

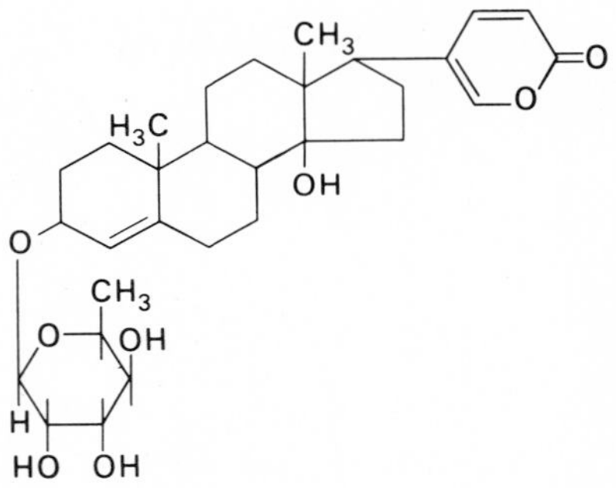

SUMMARY: CARDIAC GLYCOSIDES

TYPE	*ACTION AND MECHANISM*	*TOXICITY*	*USE*	*EXAMPLES*
Digitalis ouabain, squill group	Increase efficiency of heartbeat, plus slow heart by AV depression in atrial fibrillation Increase available intracellular Ca	Anorexia, diarrhea, Purkinje figures, premature beats, arrhythmias	Heart failure, atrial fibrillation and other arrhythmias	Digitoxin

Reviews

Dimond, E. G. (ed.). Digitalis. Springfield, Ill., Charles C Thomas, Publisher, 1957.

Hajdu, S., and Leonard, E. Cellular basis of cardiac glycoside action. Pharmacol. Rev., 11:173, 1960.

Cotten, M., and Moran, N. Cardiovascular pharmacology. Ann. Rev. Pharmacol., 1:261, 1961.

Fawaz, G. Cardiovascular pharmacology. Ann. Rev. Pharmacol., 3:57, 1963.

Marks, B. Effect of drugs on the inotropic property of the heart. Ann. Rev. Pharmacol., 4:155, 1964.
Aviado, D. Cardiovascular pharmacology. Ann. Rev. Pharmacol., 4:139, 1964.
Glynn, I. The action of cardiac glycosides on ion movements. Pharmacol. Rev., 16:381, 1964.
Bing, R. J. Cardiac metabolism. Physiol. Rev., 45:171, 1965.
Mason, D. T. Cardiovascular effects of digitalis in normal man. Clin. Pharmacol. Ther., 7:1, 1966.
Modell, W. Pharmacologic basis of the use of digitalis in congestive heart failure. Physiol. Pharmacol. Phys., 1:1, 1966.
Myerson, R. Digitalis. Topics Med. Chem., 1:303, 1967.
Koch-Weser, J. Mechanism of digitalis action on the heart. New Eng. J. Med., 277:469, 1967.
Thorp, R. H., and Cobbin, L. B. Cardiac Stimulant Substances. New York, Academic Press, 1967.
Jewell, B., and Blinks, J. Drugs and the mechanical properties of heart muscle. Ann. Rev. Pharmacol., 8:113, 1968.

19. Quinidine and Antiarrhythmia Agents

A. Quinidine

Quinidine is representative of a group of much studied drugs, the cardiac depressants.

1. History. Wenckebach (1914) noted benefit in paroxysmal atrial fibrillation from quinine. Frey (1918) found quinidine more effective.

2. Chemistry. An isomer of quinine; the quinuclidine portion is necessary for action, which is probably related to the dialkylaminoethyl group (also present in procainamide).

3. Action

a. In normal hearts, therapeutic doses produce no obvious effect, but in arrhythmias the abnormal rhythm may be terminated, usually after some degree of slowing.

b. The sequence in arrhythmias may be summarized as follows:

a′. In atrial fibrillation and flutter: First, the atrial rate slows (Prinzmetal, Scherf: depression of ectopic foci; Circus: depression of conduction). Second, conversion to flutter. Third, conversion to sinus rhythm (Prinzmetal: further depression of ectopic foci; Circus: refractory time becomes relatively more lengthened than the conduction is slowed, and so the circus is extinguished).

b′. In paroxysmal atrial or ventricular tachycardia: Atrial or ventricular rate slows; sinus mechanism then appears abruptly, from suppression of ectopic focus (?).

4. Mechanism. a. General depression of the heart.

b. The primary effect appears to be an increase in the effective refractory period; both depolarization and repolarization are lengthened.

c. Other effects include decreased conduction velocity; pacemaker depression.

d. Effects probably the result of impaired permeability of the cell membrane; Na^+ influx and K^+ efflux inhibited.

5. Pharmacodynamics. Absorption by mouth rapid. Distribution wide. About 75% metabolized; balance excreted in 12 hours.

6. Toxicity. a. Nausea, vomiting, diarrhea, tinnitus, and other signs of cinchonism.

b. Sensitivity phenomena, especially thrombocytopenia.

c. Occasional paroxysmal ventricular tachycardia; also rapid ventricular rates may appear as the fibrillating or fluttering atria slow and more impulses pass the AV node, preventable by prior digitalization.

7. Uses. a. The principal indication is probably to prevent or terminate paroxysmal ventricular tachycardia, except when this complicates complete AV block. Formerly used to control supraventricular tachycardia, but digitalis now more commonly used.

b. May be used for the prevention or termination of atrial fibrillation or flutter, as after myocardial infarction.

c. May be used after electrical conversion of arrhythmias to maintain normal rhythm.

d. May also be used to terminate atrial fibrillation when this persists or appears after correctional cardiac surgery, but is less effective in terminating chronic atrial fibrillation in the presence of mitral insufficiency or whenever the underlying cardiac disease cannot be removed.

e. Quinidine should be avoided in complete AV block, and, less urgently, in incomplete AV block or bundle branch block.

8. Preparations

QUINIDINE

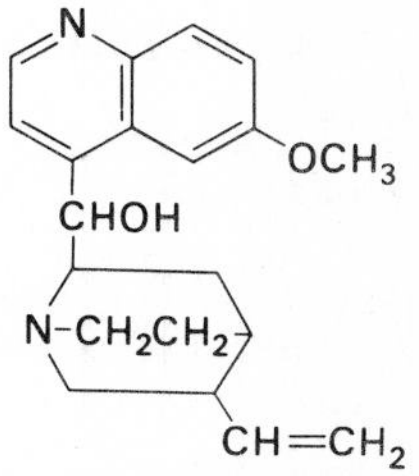

Dose: 0.2 to 0.4 gm by mouth with an additional 0.2 gm every 4 hours until success or toxicity.

Quinidine gluconate
Dose: 0.2 gm (prepared solution contains 0.8 gm per 10 ml) intramuscularly, or diluted intravenously (emergency).

Quinidine polygalacturonate (Cardioquin)
Nonirritating as sparingly soluble.
Dose: 275 to 825 mg every 4 hours by mouth for 3 to 4 doses (275 mg = 200 mg quinidine).

QUINDONIUM BROMIDE

Resembles quinidine; action probably similar.

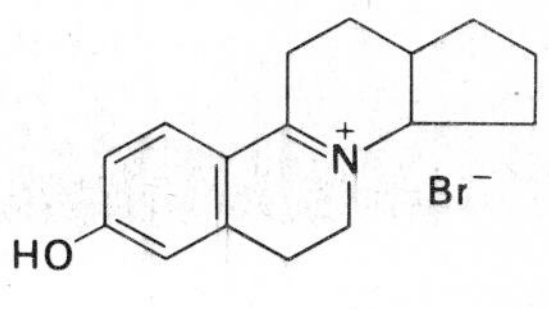

B. Procainamide and Local Anesthetics

1. History. Kayden (1951) used procainamide in clinical arrhythmias.

2. Chemistry. Amide analogue of procaine, the amide being less quickly hydrolyzed than the ester.

3. Action. a. Effect in arrhythmias similar or identical to that of quinidine.

b. The excitability of the heart muscle is decreased, conduction slowed, refractory period may be lengthened, sinus activity depressed.

c. Also an atropinelike action; not strongly anesthetic.

4. Mechanism. Not clear, but presumably similar to that of quinidine.

5. Pharmacodynamics. a. Rapid absorption: peak levels in one hour after oral administration; 15 minutes after intramuscular.

b. Distributed widely. Small amount converted to PABA. Effect apparently not proportional to blood level.

6. Toxicity. a. Hypotension after intravenous administration. Granulocytopenia.

b. Occasional paroxysmal ventricular tachycardia; also rapid ventricular rates may appear as the fibrillating or fluttering atria slow and more impulses pass the AV node, preventable by prior digitalization.

c. CNS stimulation as with local anesthetics.

d. Syndrome resembling chronic lupus erythematosus.

7. Uses. Primary use is in paroxysmal ventricular or atrial tachycardia, as an alternative to quinidine.

8. Preparation

PROCAINAMIDE HYDROCHLORIDE (Pronestyl)

$H_2N-C_6H_4-CO-NH-CH_2CH_2-N(C_2H_5)_2 \cdot HCl$

Dose: 1 gm by mouth, followed by 0.5 to 1 gm every 4 hours as needed; in emergency, 1 gm intramuscularly or intravenously (grave; at rate of not over 0.1 gm per minute).

LIDOCAINE HYDROCHLORIDE (Xylocaine) (See Local Anesthetics, p. 534.)

Used in ventricular arrhythmias, especially after cardiac infarction. Action rapid and transient after intravenous administration, allowing continuous control. If convulsions should appear, treat with intravenous barbiturate.

Dose: 50–100 mg bolus followed by infusion of 2–4 mg per minute intravenously.

DISOPYRAMIDE (Norpace)

Decreases myocardial contractility; does not block beta receptors.

Dose: 400 to 800 mg daily by mouth in divided doses.

$H_2N-C(=O)-C(C_6H_5)(C_5H_4N)-CH_2CH_2-N[CH(CH_3)_2]_2$

C. Other Agents

PHENYTOIN (Dilantin) (See Anticonvulsants) Previous name Diphenylhydantoin.

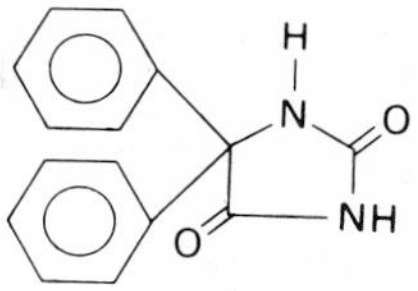

Improves AV and interventricular conduction. Used in paroxysmal atrial tachycardia and ventricular arrhythmias.

Dose: 1 gm (initial), then 0.4 to 0.6 gm daily thereafter by mouth; 50 to 100 mg intravenously, repeated several times at 15-minute intervals if needed (caution).

PROPRANOLOL HYDROCHLORIDE (Inderal)

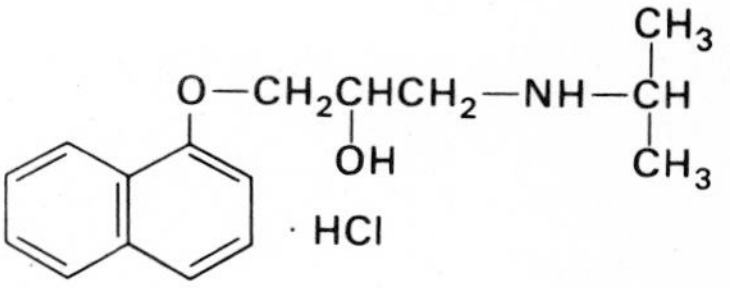

Blocks beta-adrenergic action of sympathetic nerves to heart. This prevents arrhythmias, augmented by a direct quinidine-like action (used for atrial arrhythmias only). Also decreases angina pectoris, presumably as the result of the slowed rate and decreased blood pressure. May be combined with nitrites.

Dose: 10 to 20 mg 3 times a day by mouth.

METOPROLOL

Dose: 50 mg 3 times a day.

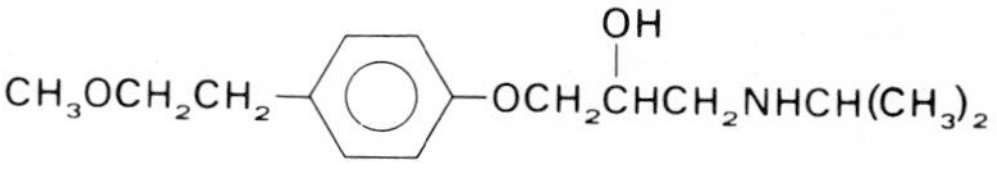

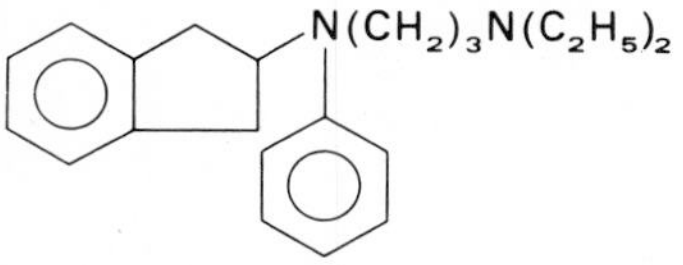

aprindine

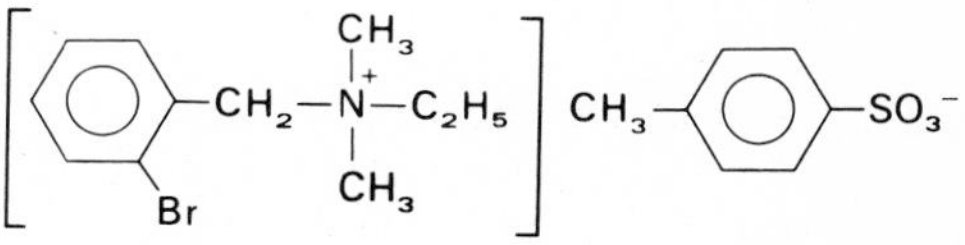

bretylium tosylate

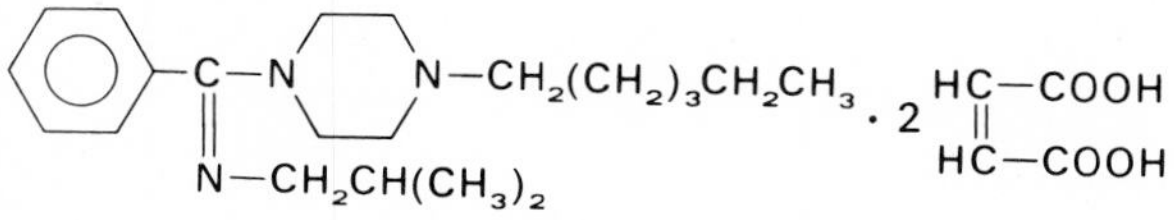

bucainide maleate

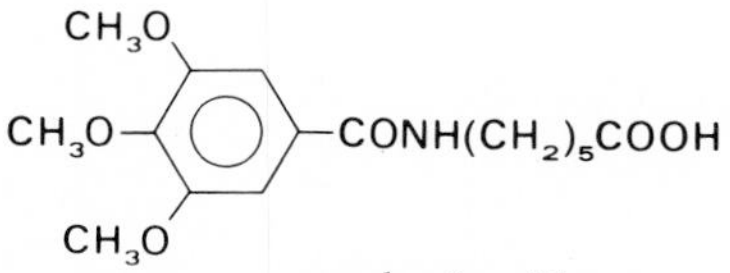

capobenic acid

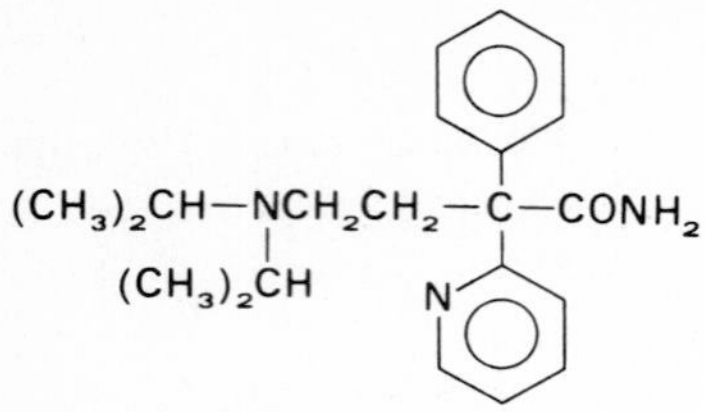

$(CH_3)_2CH-N(CH(CH_3)_2)CH_2CH_2-C(C_6H_5)(C_5H_4N)-CONH_2$

disopyramide

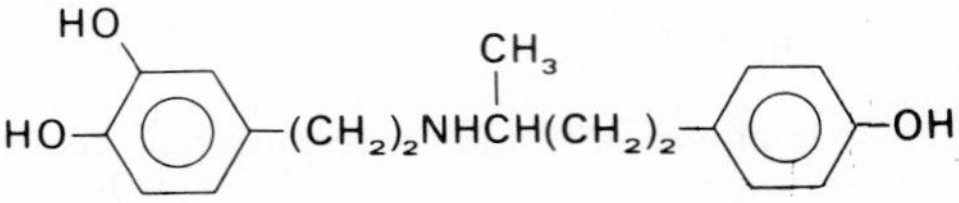

HO, $HO-C_6H_3-(CH_2)_2NHCH(CH_3)(CH_2)_2-C_6H_4-OH$

dobutamine (Dobutrex)

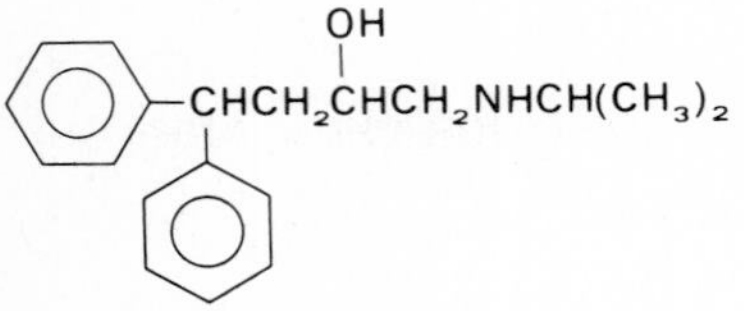

$C_6H_5-CH(C_6H_5)CH_2CH(OH)CH_2NHCH(CH_3)_2$

drobuline

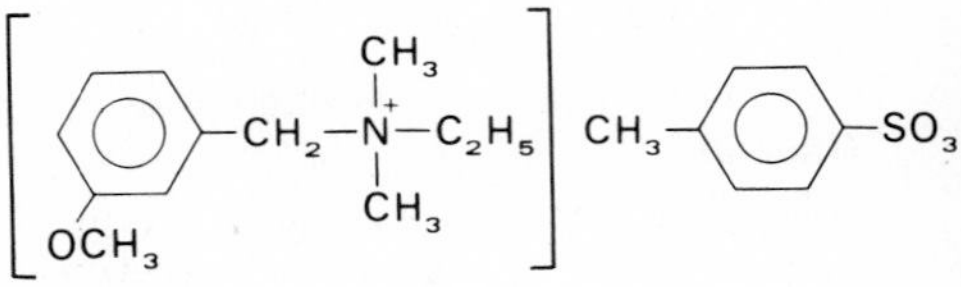

$[CH_3O-C_6H_4-CH_2-N^+(CH_3)_2-C_2H_5]\ CH_3-C_6H_4-SO_3^-$

emilium tosylate

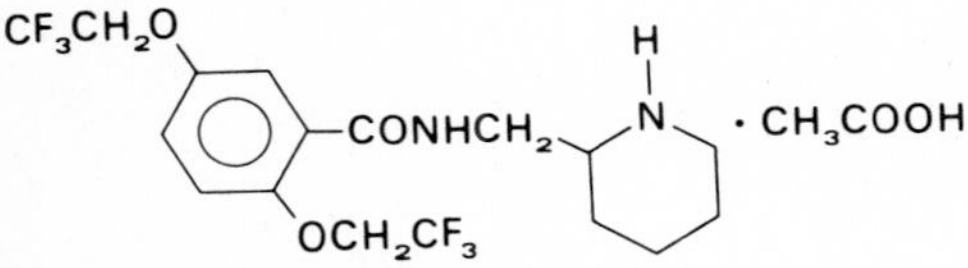

CF_3CH_2O, OCH_2CF_3 $-CONHCH_2-$(piperidin-2-yl, N–H) $\cdot CH_3COOH$

flecainide acetate

$OCOCH_2Cl$, CH, OH, $N-CH_3$, C_2H_5 $\cdot HCl$

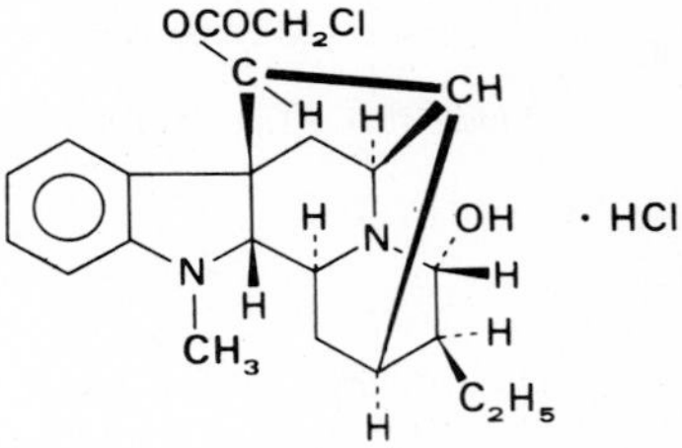

lorajmine hydrochloride

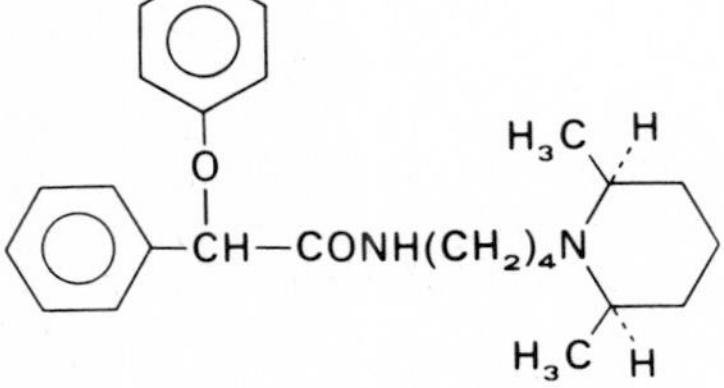

$C_6H_5-O-CH(C_6H_5)-CONH(CH_2)_4N$ (2,6-dimethylpiperidine, H_3C, H)

oxiramide

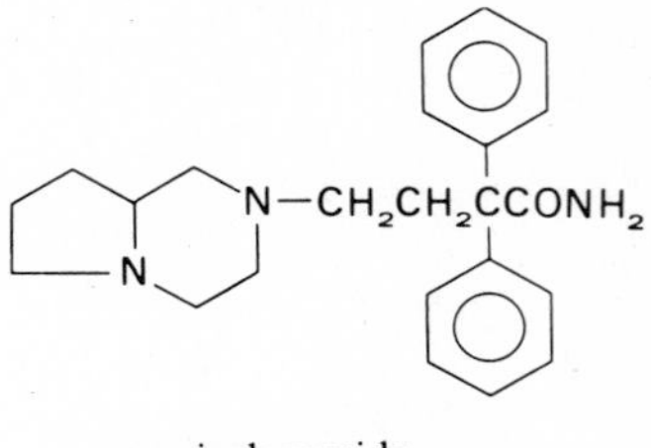

(pyrrolo-pyrazine)$N-CH_2CH_2C(C_6H_5)_2CONH_2$

pirolazamide

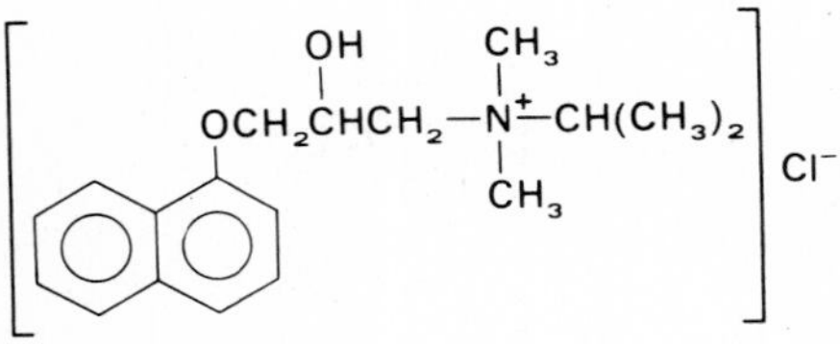

$[C_{10}H_7-OCH_2CH(OH)CH_2-N^+(CH_3)_2-CH(CH_3)_2]\ Cl^-$

pranolium chloride

(2-pyridyl)$_2$C(OH)–(cyclohexadienylidene)=C(2-pyridyl)$_2$

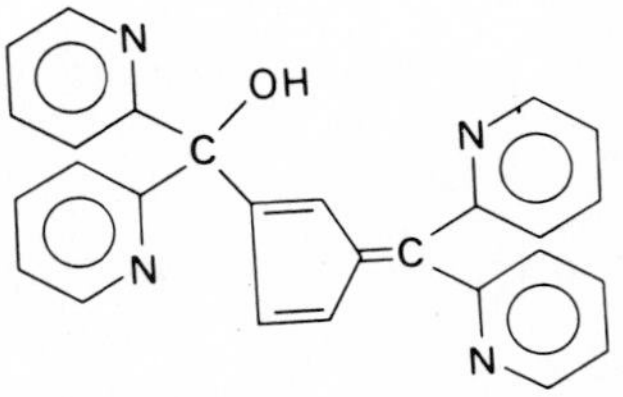

pyrinoline (Surexin)

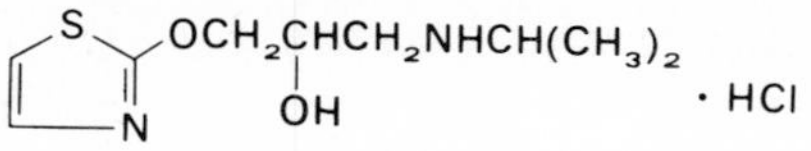

$OCH_2CHCH_2NHCH(CH_3)_2 \cdot HCl$ (S, N, OH)

tazolol hydrochloride

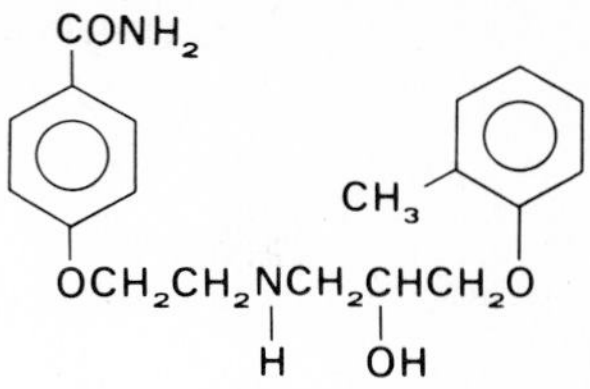

$CONH_2$, CH_3, $OCH_2CH_2NCH_2CHCH_2O$ (H, OH)

tolamolol

D. Agents in Heart Block

The sympathomimetic amines may increase heart rate in complete heart block, and may prevent Stokes-Adams seizures from ventricular standstill (see Sympathetic Stimulants).

ISOPROTERENOL

1. Action. Isoproterenol resembles epinephrine in its effects on the heart, but is less likely to cause paroxysmal ventricular tachycardia. It is probably the most satisfactory drug in complete heart block.

2. Preparation

ISOPROTERENOL HYDROCHLORIDE (Isuprel)

Dose: 10 to 20 mg sublingually every 2 to 3 hours; 0.2 mg subcutaneously every 6 hours; by intravenous drip in emergency.

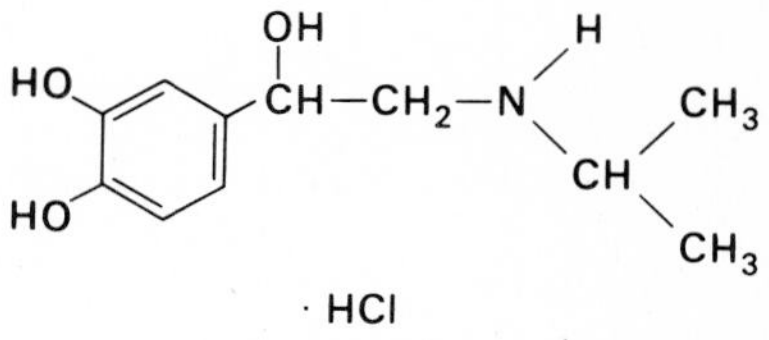

HO, HO, OH, $CH-CH_2-N$, H, CH, CH_3, CH_3 $\cdot HCl$

SUMMARY: QUINIDINE AND ANTIARRHYTHMIA AGENTS

TYPE	*ACTION AND MECHANISM*	*TOXICITY*	*USE*	*EXAMPLES*
Quinidine	Conversion of arrhythmias General depression of the heart, primarily increase of refractory period	Cinchonism, thrombocytopenia	Ventricular tachycardia and other arrhythmias	Quinidine
Procainamide group	Same	Hypotension arrhythmia, CNS stimulation	Same	Procainamide

(cont.)

SUMMARY: QUINIDINE AND ANTIARRHYTHMIA AGENTS (cont.)

TYPE	*ACTION AND MECHANISM*	*TOXICITY*	*USE*	*EXAMPLES*
Diphenyl-hydantoin	Improves AV and inter-ventricular conduction	Sensitivity	Atrial tachy-cardia, ventric-ular arrhythmias	Diphenyl-hydantoin
Beta blocker	Blocks β-adrener-gic sympathetic nerves, slowing arrhythmias and improving angina pectoris	Hypotension	Arrhythmias and angina pectoris	Propranolol HCl
Sympatho-mimetics	Increase heart rate	Tachycardia	Complete heart block	Isoproterenol

Reviews

Bellet, S. Clinical pharmacology of antiarrhythmic drugs. Clin. Pharmacol. Ther., 2:345, 1961.

Szekeres, L., and Vaughan-Williams, E. M. Antifibrillatory action. J. Physiol., 160:470, 1962.

Trautwein, W. Generation and conduction of impulses in the heart as affected by drugs. Pharmacol. Rev., 15:277, 1963.

Stanzler, R. Cardiac arrhythmias. New Eng. J. Med., 274:1307, 1966.

Mason, D., Spann, J., Zelis, R., and Amsterdam, E. The clinical pharmacology and therapeutics of the antiarrhythmic drugs. Clin. Pharmacol. Ther., 11:460, 1970.

Selzer, A., and Cohn, K. Treatment of ventricular extrasystoles and tachyarrhythmias in acute myocardial infarction. Ann. Rev. Med., 21:47, 1970.

20.
Diuretics and Renal Tubule Inhibitors

Diuretics are agents which increase the rate of urine flow. Although this could theoretically be the result of either increased glomerular filtration or decreased tubular reabsorption, the latter appears to be the chief action with most diuretics.

The most effective diuretics influence primarily the excretion of sodium (or other ions) rather than of water itself. The mechanism of such diuresis is then an increased excretion of Na (naturesis), and with it an osmotic equivalent of water.

Diuretics are most helpful therapeutically in the edema of congestive heart failure where failure of the heart as a pump results in increased venous pressure and increased aldosterone production. In nephrosis, and cirrhosis, where there may also be the factor of decreased serum osmotic pressure, results are often less satisfactory, and in the edema of glomerular nephritis, nutritional deficiency, and pregnancy little may be expected.

The accompanying chart outlines the actions of diuretics.

A. Early Diuretic Measures

1. History. a. In the 1700's saline purgatives, blood letting, digitalis (1776), and inorganic mercurials were advised for diuretic effects.

b. In the late 1800's salt restriction and the xanthines came into use.

c. Acidifying salts (1918) were the last of old measures to precede the introduction of the highly effective organomercurials in 1920.

OSMOTIC DIURETICS

1. Action and Mechanism. Presence in the glomerular filtrate of any poorly reabsorbed material tends to carry its osmotic equivalent of water with it into the urine; reduces back diffusion of water and reabsorption of sodium.

2. Uses. May be useful in cerebral edema by mouth or intravenously. In acute oliguria may prevent concentration of toxic solutes in kidney.

3. Preparations

UREA

$$\begin{array}{c} NH_2 \\ | \\ C{=}O \\ | \\ NH_2 \end{array}$$

Nonthreshold molecule; rapid and nontoxic, but distasteful.

Dose: 15 to 20 gm 3 or 4 times a day as 50% solution by mouth; or 40 gm (Ureaphil) intravenously.

Actions of Diuretics

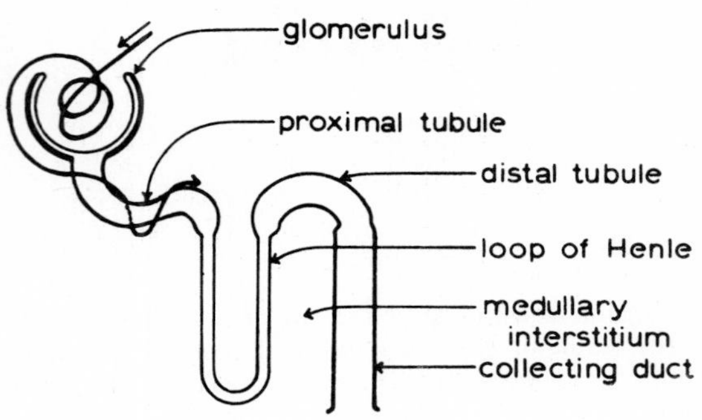

	FUNCTION	EFFECTS OF HORMONES AND DRUGS
Glomerulus	Filtration	Stimulated by thyroid, little affected by diuretics.
Proximal tubule	Reabsorption of Na and water (Na diffuses into cells as the result of active pumping of Na from the cells into the peritubular space; carries Cl and water passively; or less likely, Cl absorption is primary; alternate: bulk flow of fluid carries Na into cell; rise in Na stimulates outward transport).	Inhibited by most diuretics: xanthines, mercurials, carbonic anhydrase inhibitors, thiazides, phthalimidines.
Loop of Henle	Creation of hypertonicity in medullary interstitium (by acting with the interstitial tissues as a countercurrent multiplier system), allowing concentration of urine in collecting ducts.	Sodium reabsorption in ascending loop inhibited by mercurials, ethacrynic acid.
Distal tubule	Reabsorption of Na and water; excretion of K.	Reabsorption of Na facilitated by aldosterone; inhibited by spironolactone, triamterene. Reabsorption of water facilitated by antidiuretic hormone (ADH).
Collecting duct	Concentration and acidification of urine.	

Sorbitol, Mannitol, Sucrose, Isosorbide (Hydronol), and other nonmetabolized sugars

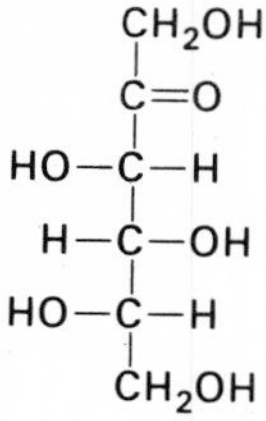

CH_2OH
C=O
HO—C—H
H—C—OH
HO—C—H
CH_2OH

sorbitol

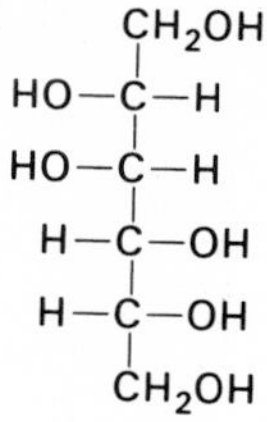

CH_2OH
HO—C—H
HO—C—H
H—C—OH
H—C—OH
CH_2OH

mannitol

CH_2
HO—C—H
O
H—C
C—H
O
HO—C—H
H_2C

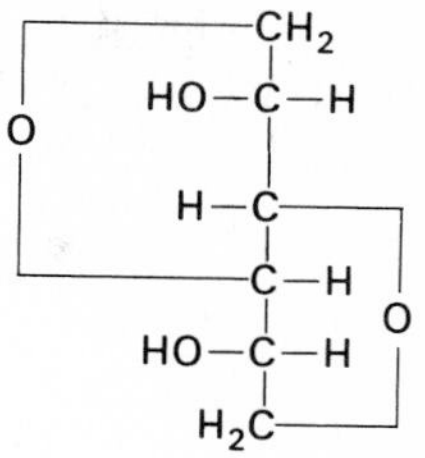

isosorbide

Dehydrate when given intravenously, but renal tubular damage may be produced by sorbitol; may precipitate heart failure.

Dose: (Mannitol) 12.5 gm intravenously over 3 to 5 min.; not over 200 gm in 24 hrs.

ACIDIFYING AND OTHER SALTS

1. Action. Acidifying salts may produce slight diuresis, but a more valuable action is enhancement of mercurial diuresis.

2. Mechanism. a. Mechanism of acidification is by dissipation of cation (poor absorption of Ca, or metabolism of NH_4), leaving excess of anion (Cl), giving acidosis.

b. Acidosis causes temporary (1 to 2 days) secondary excretion of sodium, and hence diuresis.

3. Uses. Useful to augment effect of mercurial diuretics, probably by maintaining available Cl in the blood.

4. Preparations

Ammonium chloride (NH_4Cl); Calcium chloride ($CaCl_2$)

Dose: 1 to 2 gm 4 to 6 times a day by mouth for 2 days.

L-Lysine monohydrochloride (Darvyl, Lyamine)

Acidifying agent for use with mercurial diuretics; more palatable than NH_4Cl.
Dose: 5 to 10 gm 4 times a day by mouth.

Potassium salts

Mechanism and effectiveness unclear. Replaced by newer agents because of relative ineffectiveness, and danger if renal function is impaired.

B. Xanthines

1. Chemistry. Methylated xanthines: caffeine, theobromine, theophylline.

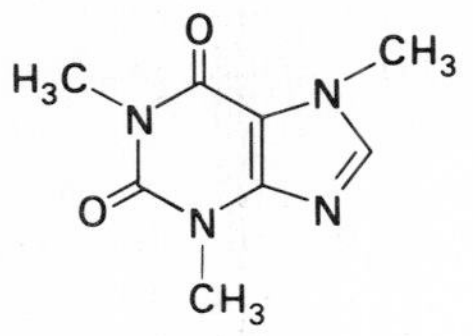

caffeine 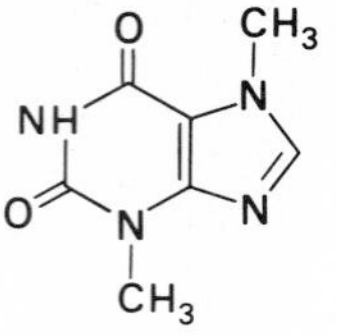 theobromine 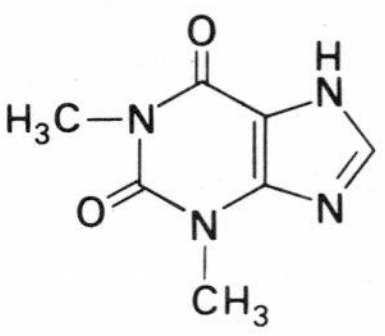 theophylline

2. Action and Mechanism. a. Increase (theophylline in particular) intracellular cyclic AMP by inhibiting the cyclic nucleotide phosphodiesterase (Butcher R. and Sutherland E., J. Biol Chem., 237: 1244, 1962).

b. Interference of reabsorption of sodium and chloride in proximal tubules; mechanism unknown. Increased glomerular filtration inconstant and less important (see Smooth Muscle Relaxants).

c. Chloride loss eventually halts diuresis, but concomitant NH_4Cl may sustain.

3. Uses. Theophylline most potent. Formerly used as a diuretic in congestive failure but newer diuretics more effective and less capricious. Principal use of caffeine is as a CNS stimulant; of theophylline as a bronchiolar dilator.

4. Preparation

AMINOPHYLLINE (Theophylline ethylenediamine)

Dose: 0.1 to 0.5 gm by mouth; intramuscularly, intravenously, or by suppository.

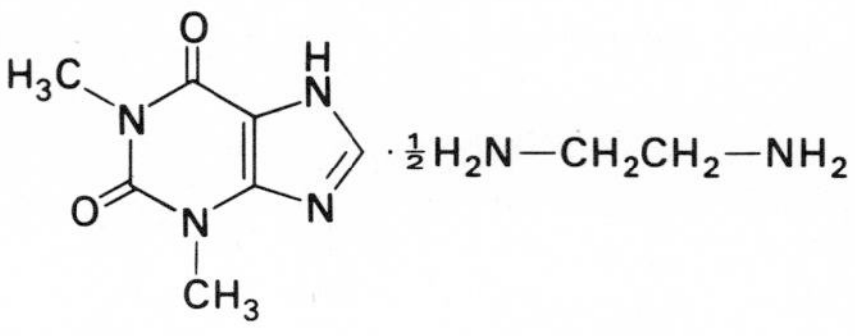

C. Mercurial Diuretics

1. History. Saxl and Heilig (1920) used the antisyphilitic agent merbaphen (Novasurol) as a diuretic.

2. Chemistry. Organic compounds, mostly methoxy-oxymercuripropylamides; combination with theophylline usual.

3. Action. a. Sodium excretion, with water and chloride following passively, may be increased by five times in edematous patients. The diuresis starts in about 3 hours, reaches a peak in 6 to 8 hours, and lasts up to 24 hours. A urinary output of 4 to 9 liters may occur during 24 hours.

b. Alternative theory: chloride excretion primary because chloride loss exceeds sodium loss, and hypochloremia inhibits diuresis.

4. Mechanism. a. Mercury is presumed to inhibit enzymes involved in the reabsorption of sodium throughout the nephron, maximally at the loop of Henle, by combination with sulfhydryl groups or in some other manner.

b. The enhancement of the action by salts such as ammonium chloride has been variously explained as the result of increased ionization of the Hg in the renal tubular cells, or as the result of increased plasma chloride concentration.

5. Pharmacodynamics. a. Most of the organic mercurials are poorly or irregularly absorbed by mouth, but mercumatilin and especially chlormerodrin are more satisfactorily absorbed.

b. The Hg is excreted in the urine, in combination with cysteine.

c. Preparations for injection are usually combined with theophylline which reduces local irritation, principally by speeding absorption.

6. Toxicity. a. Stomatitis, renal damage, hypersensitivity phenomena (fever, rash) uncommon.

b. Ventricular fibrillation may occur after rapid intravenous injection.

c. Sodium, potassium, or chloride deficiency may be produced, but less likely than with the thiazides.

7. Uses. a. Probably the most potent diuretics, but largely replaced by the thiazides because of the convenience of effective oral preparations of the latter.

b. Useful in cardiac decompensation; less useful in other forms of edema.

c. Should be avoided in acute nephritis, ventricular arrhythmias; caution in low sodium diets.

d. Administer following ammonium or calcium chloride if refractoriness results from hypochloremic acidosis.

8. Preparations

CHLORMERODRIN (Neohydrin)

Dose: 50 to 100 mg by mouth; about half as potent as meralluride.

$$NH_2-CONH-CH_2CH(OCH_3)CH_2-HgCl$$

MERALLURIDE SODIUM (Mercuhydrin)

Well tolerated and widely used.

Dose: 0.5 ml, later 1 to 2 ml, intramuscularly or intravenously.

$$CH_2-COONa$$
$$CH_2-CONH-CONH-CH_2CH(OCH_3)CH_2-HgOH \cdot \text{theophylline}$$

MERCAPTOMERIN SODIUM (Thiomerin)

Thioglycollate in place of theophylline.

Dose: 1 to 2 ml subcutaneously, intramuscularly, or intravenously.

$$H_3C, COONa, CH_3, CH_3 \text{ (cyclopentane ring)}$$
$$CONH-CH_2CH(OCH_3)CH_2-Hg-S-CH_2(COONa)$$

MERSALYL SODIUM and THEOPHYLLINE (Salyrgan theophylline)

Pioneer preparation.
Dose: 1 to 2 ml intramuscularly or intravenously.

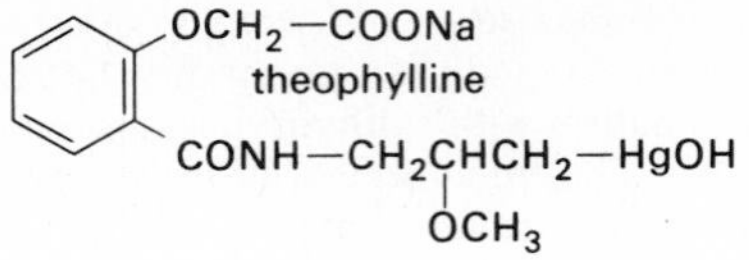

$OCH_2-COONa$
theophylline
$CONH-CH_2CH(OCH_3)CH_2-HgOH$

OTHERS (seldom used)
Mercurophylline,Mercumatilin.

D. Carbonic Anhydrase Inhibitors

1. History. Strauss and Southworth (1938) recognized that sulfanilamide produced acidosis; Mann and Keilin (1940) showed that sulfonamide acted as a carbonic anhydrase inhibitor.

b. Roblin (1950) introduced acetazolamide; Maren and others (1954) studied clinical effects.

2. Chemistry. Thiadiazole sulfonamides.

3. Action. General diminution in the formation of H_2CO_3 in the tissues results in:

a. Transient diuresis (6 to 7 hours and not immediately repeatable until metabolic acidosis clears).

b. Metabolic acidosis from increased urinary excretion of $NaHCO_3$.

c. Decreased formation of gastric HCl, but only in excessive doses.

d. Reduced rate of formation of aqueous humor and intraocular pressure.

4. Mechanism. a. Inhibition of carbonic anhydrase stops the formation of H^+, as H_2CO_3 not synthesized from CO_2 and H_2O.

b. In the kidney tubule the effects may be summarized as follows:

a′. Normal function: CO_2 and H_2O combine in the tubule cells with the assistance of carbonic anhydrase to form H_2CO_3, which dissociates to form H^+ and HCO_3^-; the H^+ enters the lumen and Na^+ is absorbed in its place; the Na^+ and HCO_3^- return to the blood, conserving base. Further, carbonic anhydrase facilitates reabsorption of filtered HCO_3^- from the lumen.

b′. Inhibition: H_2CO_3 is not formed and thus Na^+ is lost in the (alkaline) urine, carrying water osmotically. K^+ is also excreted as tubular excretion of K^+ is in competition with H^+, and when H^+ is removed, K^+ is excreted more easily. The principal effect, however, is probably inhibition of the reabsorption of HCO_3^- by the tubules; filtered HCO_3^- is then excreted in the urine with an osmotic equivalent of water. Transient because when HCO_3 lowered, enzyme has little substrate and inhibition inconsequential.

c′. These effects may be diagramed as follows:

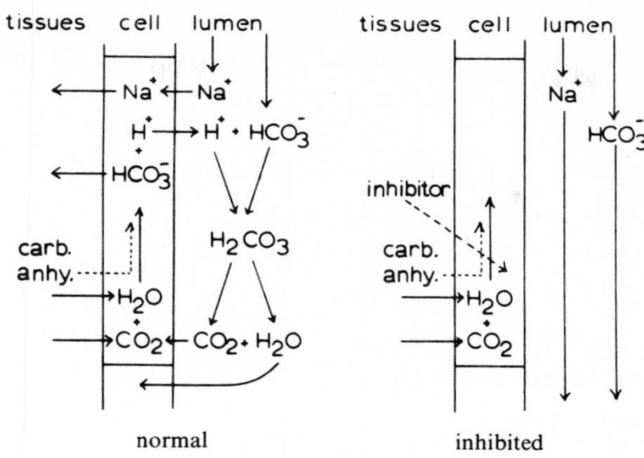

5. Pharmacodynamics. Absorption rapid, effects last about 8 hours. Excretion of unchanged drug in the urine over 12 to 24 hours.

6. Toxicity. a. Minor, but a number of side effects may be seen: anorexia, fatigue, drowsiness, tingling, leg pains.

b. Rare allergic manifestations and agranulocytosis; crystalluria, renal calculi.

7. Uses. a. Replaced by the chlorothiazides as diuretics, but helpful in glaucoma, used as adjuncts to conventional miotic therapy.

b. Also used in epilepsy in conjunction with usual anticonvulsants.

8. Preparations

ACETAZOLAMIDE (Diamox)

Dose: 250 mg by mouth every 4 hours (glaucoma).

DICHLORPHENAMIDE (Daranide)

Dose: 25 to 50 mg by mouth 1 to 4 times daily.

ETHOXZOLAMIDE (Cardrase)

Dose: 125 to 250 mg by mouth 2 to 4 times daily.

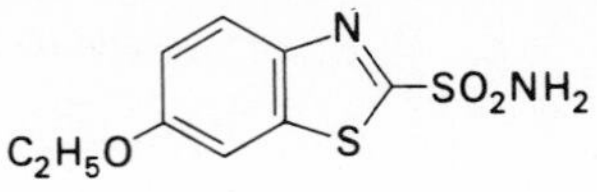

C_2H_5O — benzothiazole — SO_2NH_2

METHAZOLAMIDE (Neptazane)

May produce drowsiness, but less gastrointestinal disturbance and longer acting than acetazolamide.

Dose: 50 to 100 mg by mouth 2 to 3 times a day.

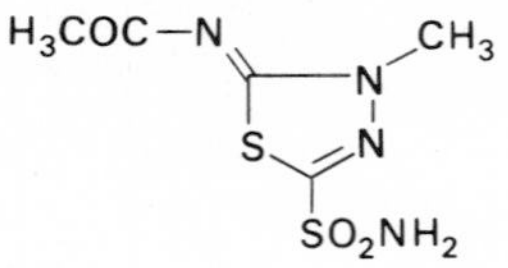

H_3COC-N ... CH_3 ... SO_2NH_2

E. Benzothiadiazines (Thiazides)

1. History. a. Novello (1957) synthesized chlorothiazide.

b. Beyer (1957) introduced clinically.

2. Chemistry. Group of highly modified sulfonamides derived from attempts at producing more potent carbonic anhydrase inhibitors by inclusion of two sulfonamide groups.

3. Action. a. Potent diuretics; preponderant action is saluresis.

b. Also hypotensive, particularly in enhancement of other agents.

4. Mechanism. a. Initially, Na^+ and Cl^- (and accompanying water) fail to be reabsorbed by the renal tubules by a mechanism similar to that of the mercurials, that is, by interference with the enzymatic mechanism for reabsorption. The nature of the enzymatic inhibition is unknown, but it is different from that effected by the mercurials since experimentally the effects are additive (Pitts, J. Pharmacol. Exp. Ther., 123:89, 1958). There is some uncertainty as to whether the effect is primarily proximal or distal to Henle's loop, and whether it is primarily naturetic or chloruretic. Latest evidence places it in the diluting part of the loop of Henle, or more distal.

b. Additionally, as the maximum action is approached, there is increased excretion of K^+ and HCO_3^- and the urine becomes alkaline, in part from carbonic anhydrase inhibition, and in part from Na-K exchange in the distal nephron.

c. Refractoriness is much less prominent than with acetazolamide, since the action is not dependent on normal acid-base balance and carbonic anhydrase inhibition is relatively unimportant.

d. The initial hypotensive effect is probably the result of a reduction of blood volume from sodium depletion; later, direct relaxation of arteriolar smooth muscle predominates (Rubin, J. Pharmacol. Exp. Ther., 140:46, 1963).

5. Pharmacodynamics. a. Absorption is prompt.

b. Distribution is in the extracellular fluids only, and not into RBC or the brain. The maximal diuretic effect develops in 4 hours and lasts 5 to 10 hours.

c. The drug is excreted by glomerular filtration and tubular excretion; the latter can be inhibited by probenecid.

6. Toxicity. a. There is no remarkable acute toxicity, except possibly minor nausea or vomiting.

b. The principal later toxic possibility is weakness from K loss, which may be prevented by a K supplement (KCl 1 to 3 gm daily). This is most likely to happen during aggressive therapy, as for nephrosis or cirrhosis. Muscle cramps from Na deficiency have been observed; also a rise in blood uric acid which may precipitate gout. Enteric-coated preparations of potassium should not be used, since they may cause erosion of the small bowel.

c. Other effects include rare agranulocytosis and thrombocytopenia, and unmasking of diabetes from a prodiabetic effect.

7. Uses. a. As potent and convenient diuretics in congestive heart failure and other types of edema.

b. As an adjunct in the treatment of hypertension.

8. Preparations

BENDROFLUMETHIAZIDE (Naturetin)

Longer action claimed.
Dose: 2 to 10 mg by mouth daily.

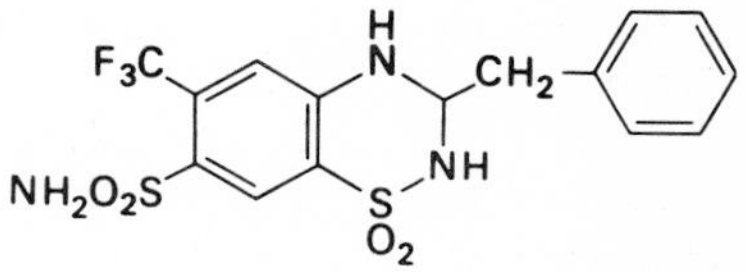

BENZTHIAZIDE (Exna; Na Clex)

Dose: 25 to 50 mg 1 or 2 times a day by mouth.

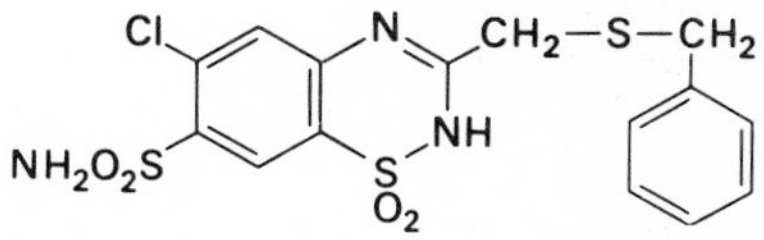

CHLOROTHIAZIDE (Diuril)

Dose: 0.5 to 1.0 gm by mouth 1 or 2 times a day.

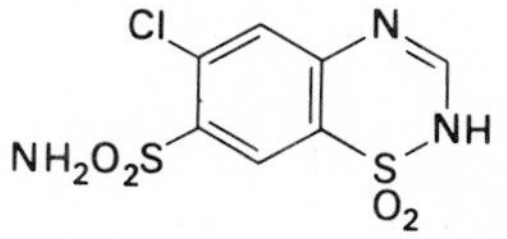

Chlorothiazide, sodium

Dose: 0.5 gm intravenously.

CYCLOTHIAZIDE (Anhydron)

Dose: 1 to 2 mg by mouth daily.

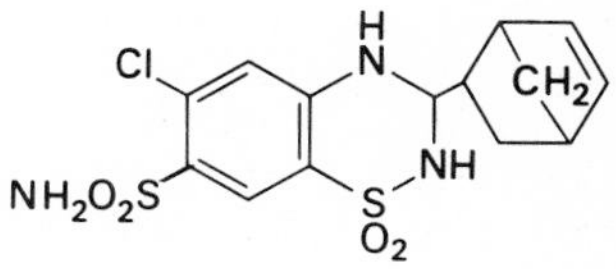

FLUMETHIAZIDE (Ademol)

Not essentially different from chlorothiazide.
Dose: 1 gm by mouth twice daily.

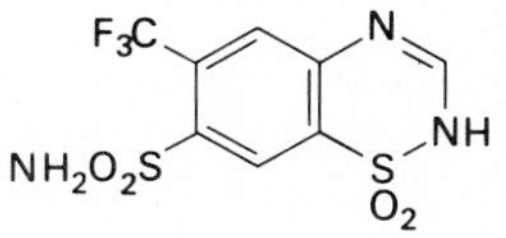

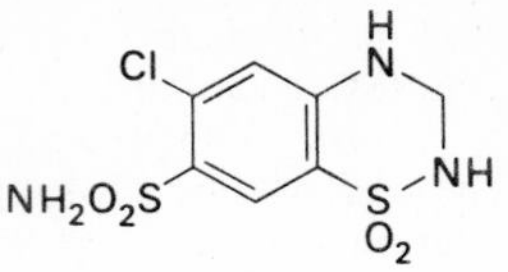

HYDROCHLOROTHIAZIDE (Hydrodiuril, Esidrix)

Dosage smaller than chlorothiazide but qualitative difference not great; considered by some to produce fewer side effects, especially less excretion of K, and to possess a longer action.

Dose: 50 to 100 mg 1 or 2 times a day (diuretic); 25 to 50 mg 1 or 2 times a day (hypertension; reduce dose of reserpine or ganglionic blockers if being given).

HYDROFLUMETHIAZIDE (Di-ademil)

Dose: 25 to 200 mg by mouth daily.

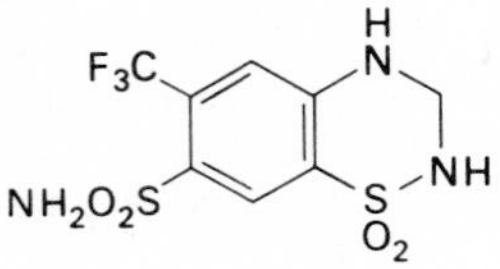

METHYCLOTHIAZIDE (Enduron)

Dose: 5 to 10 mg by mouth daily.

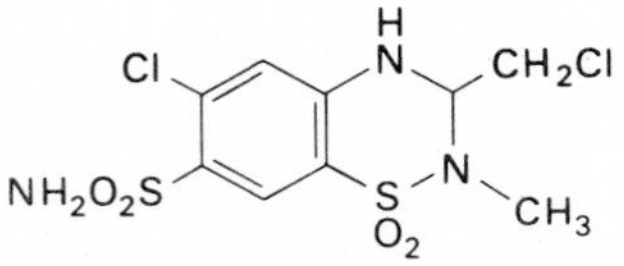

POLYTHIAZIDE (Renese)

Prolonged action.
Dose; 0.5 to 4 mg by mouth daily.

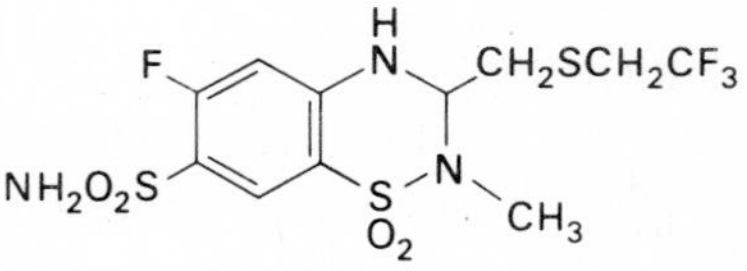

QUINETHAZONE (Hydromox)

Thiazide analogue. Rapid onset (2 hours).
Dose: 50 to 100 mg by mouth daily.

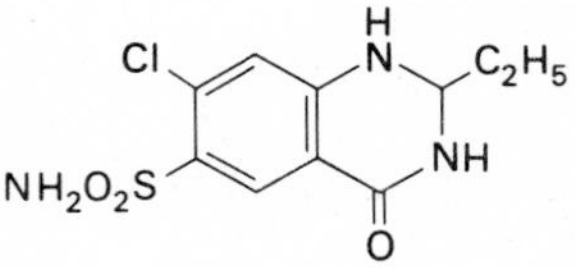

TRICHLOROMETHIAZIDE (Naqua)

Dose: 2 to 8 mg by mouth daily.

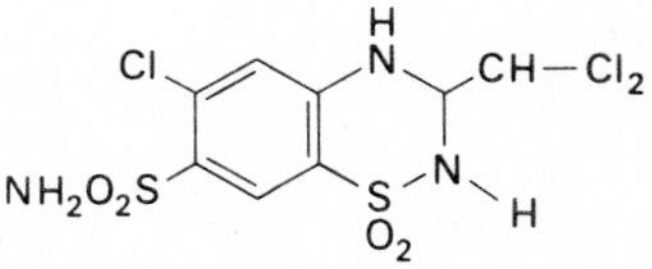

OTHERS

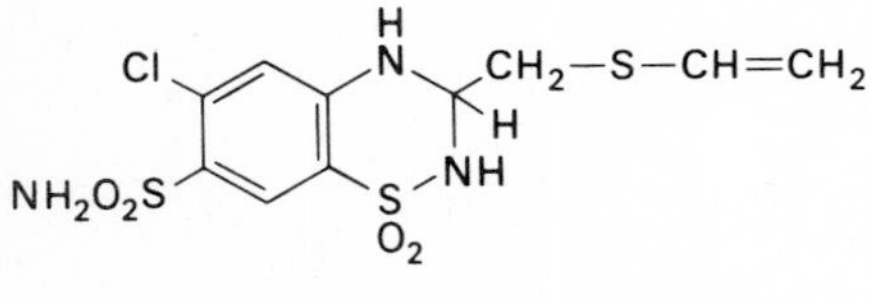

althiazide

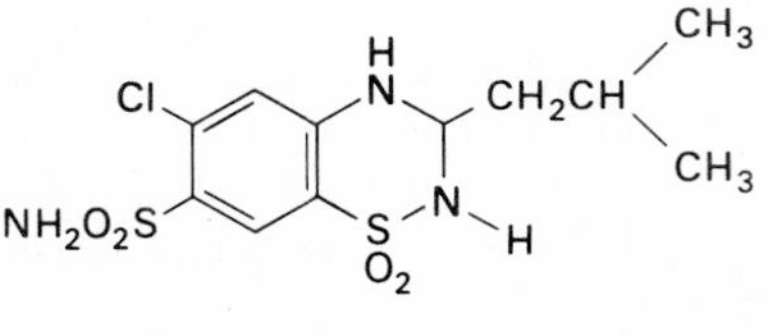

buthiazide

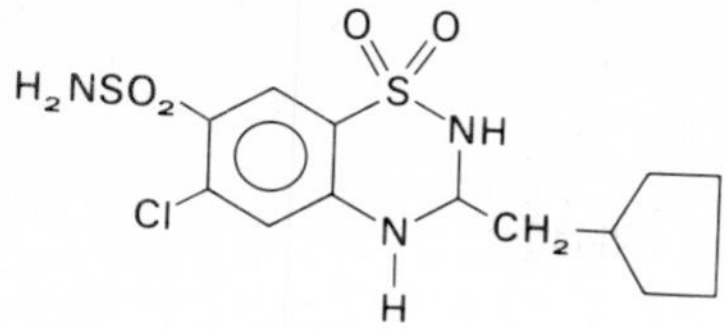

cyclopenthiazide

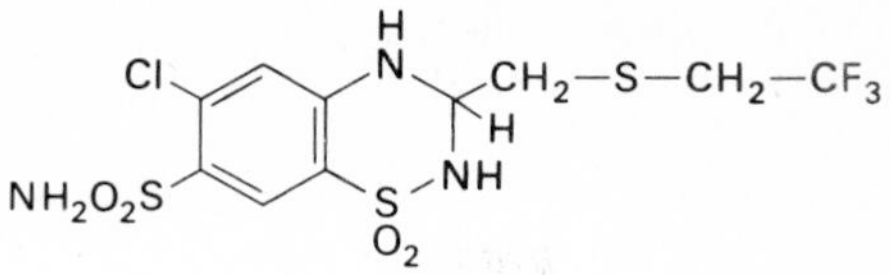

epithiazide

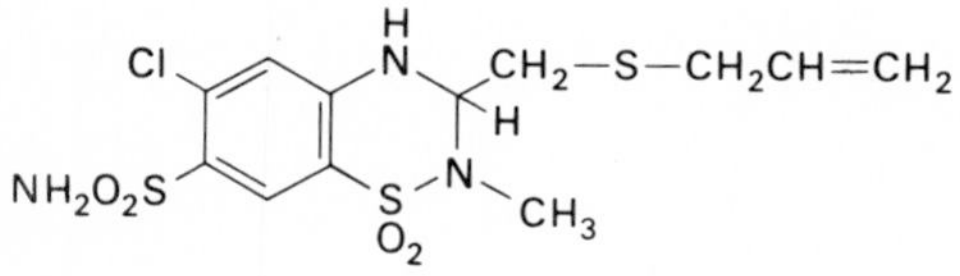

methalthiazide

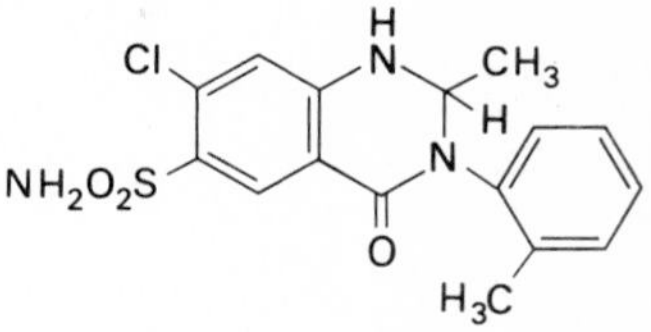

metolazone (Zaroxolyn)

F. Other Sulfonamide Derivatives

CHLORTHALIDONE

1. History. Stenger, Wirz, and Pulver (1959) introduced chlorthalidone in Switzerland.

2. Chemistry. Sulfamylated benzophenone; differs from other sulfonamide diuretics in the incorporation of a phthalimidine into the molecule.

3. Action and Mechanism. a. Produces a strong, protracted diuresis; also anti-inflammatory effects.

b. Mechanism probably similar to that of chlorothiazide, i.e., inhibition of enzyme system in tubule with promotion of Na^+ excretion; minimal K^+ loss because of lack of carbonic anhydrase inhibition; other evidence suggests the effect is like that of ethacrynic acid, primarily at the ascending loop of Henle.

4. Pharmacodynamics. a. Oral absorption practically complete.

b. Not metabolized; excreted in the urine. Diuretic effect sustained with infrequent dosage.

5. Toxicity. Infrequent headache, weakness, dizziness, and nausea. Elevation of serum uric acid.

6. Uses. a. To induce diuresis in congestive heart failure and other types of edema.

b. As an adjunct in the treatment of hypertension.

7. Preparation

ALIPAMIDE

Dose: 20 to 80 mg per day by mouth.

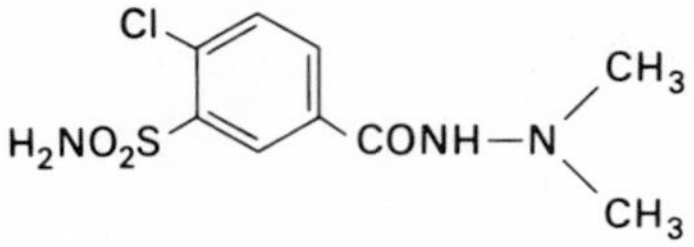

BUMETANIDE

Dose: 10 mg per day by mouth.

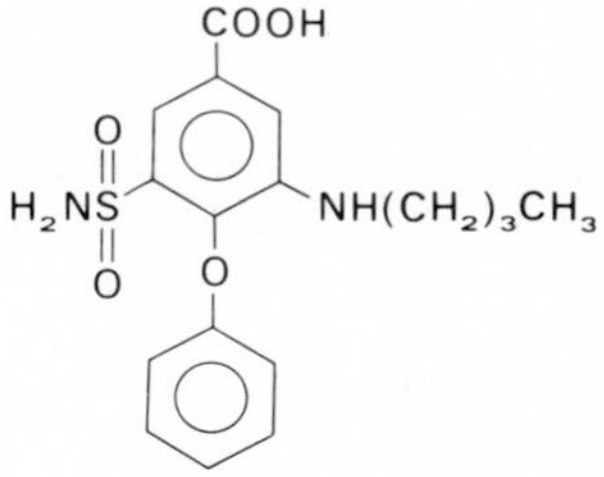

CHLOREXOLONE (Nephrolan)

Dose: 10 mg twice daily by mouth.

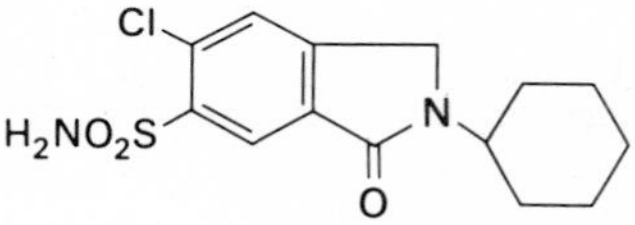

CHLORTHALIDONE (Hygroton)

Dose: 50 to 100 mg by mouth daily (initial); 200 mg 3 times a week (maintenance).

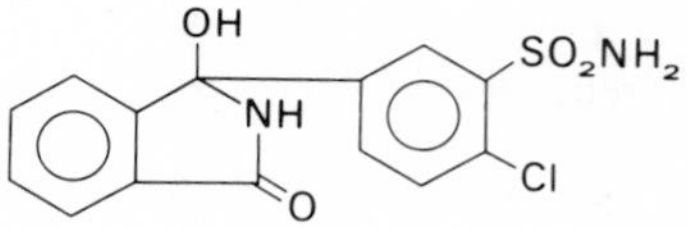

DIAPAMIDE

Dose: 10 mg per day by mouth.

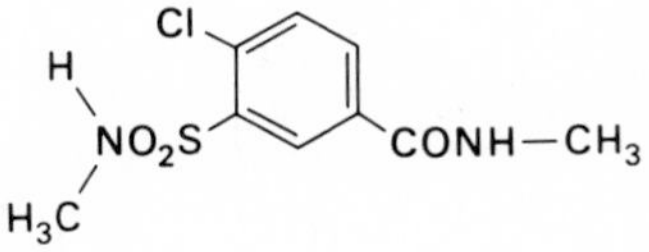

FUROSEMIDE (Lasix)

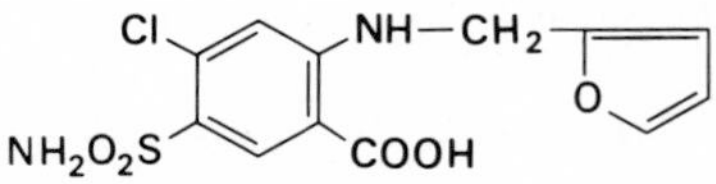

Highly effective. Fetal damage (animals), deafness reported.

Dose: 40 to 80 mg per day by mouth; 20 to 40 mg intravenously.

OTHERS

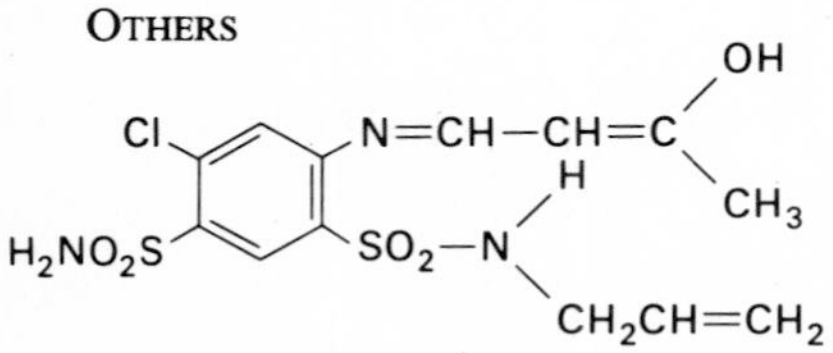

ambuside

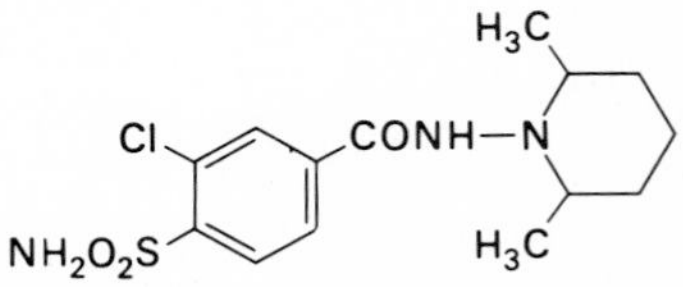

clopamide (Aquex; Brinaldix)

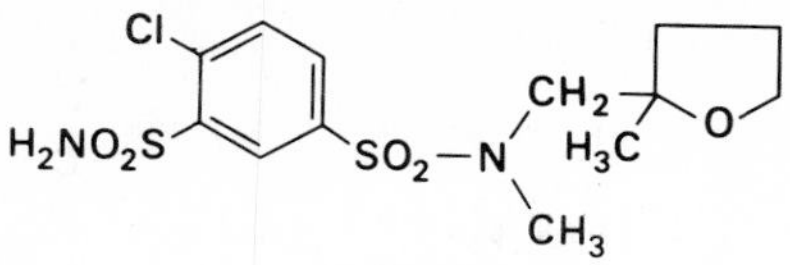

mefruside

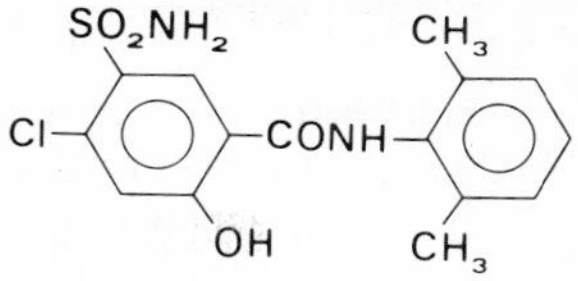

xipamide

G. Pteridines and Related Compounds

TRIAMTERENE

1. Chemistry. Pteridines or related compounds.

2. Action and Mechanism. a. Diuretic action about half as great as from mercurials; tolerance may develop.

b. Reduce reabsorption of Na in distal tubules (Ball, Proc. Soc. Exp. Biol. Med., 113:326, 1963); formerly considered possible aldolsterone antagonists.

c. Potentiate other diuretics; no K loss.

3. Pharmacodynamics and Toxicity. a. Ready oral absorption; effective about 12 hours.

b. Toxicity: nausea, vomiting; rise in blood urea; increase in uric acid excretion. Hyperkalemia may occur and be associated with cardiac irregularities.

4. Uses. Triamterene usefully combined with thiazides or ethacrynic acid; diuretic and hypotensive effects enhanced, K loss diminished.

5. Preparations

AMILORIDE HYDROCHLORIDE (Colectril)

Dose: 30 mg daily by mouth.

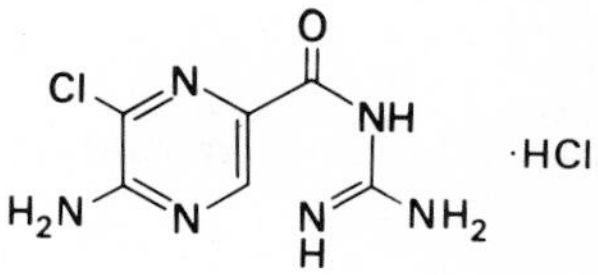

TRIAMTERENE (Dyrenium)

Dose: 100 to 200 mg by mouth daily.

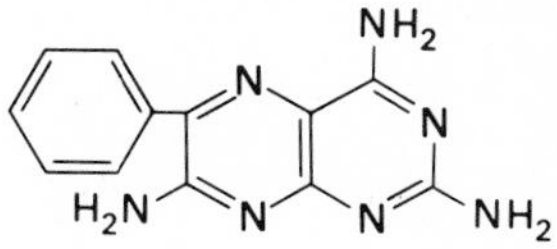

OTHERS

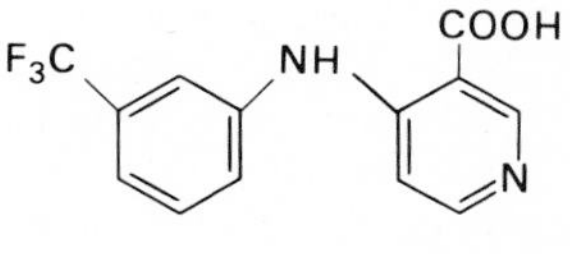

triflocin

H. Ethacrynic Acid

1. Chemistry. Unsaturated ketone derivative of aryloxyacetic acids.

2. Action and Mechanism. a. Potent diuretic; weak antihypertensive.

b. Inhibits Na reabsorption in ascending loop of Henle, and to some extent in both proximal and distal tubules. Increases K loss, but action not related to pH.

c. Mechanism may involve binding of sulfhydryl groups of renal cellular proteins.

3. Pharmacodynamics. Oral absorption satisfactory. Slower action than mercurials or thiazides.

4. Toxicity. a. Rapid electrolyte and fluid loss may result in excessive dehydration and hypokalemia.

b. Nausea, vomiting, diarrhea, deafness, vertigo; metabolic alkalosis; precipitation of gout; rise in blood urea in presence of renal damage; hepatic coma in presence of liver disease; gastrointestinal bleeding.

5. Uses. a. May be used in severe edema, as with patients with heart failure or cirrhosis. Probably should be reserved for use when other agents are ineffective.

b. May be used intravenously in acute pulmonary edema.

6. Preparation

ETHACRYNIC ACID (Edecrin)

Dose: 50 mg, increased to 100 or 200 mg daily by mouth for not more than 4 days (give also 3 to 6 gm of KCl daily); 25 to 50 mg intravenously.

Sodium ethacrynate (Lyovac Sodium Edecrin)

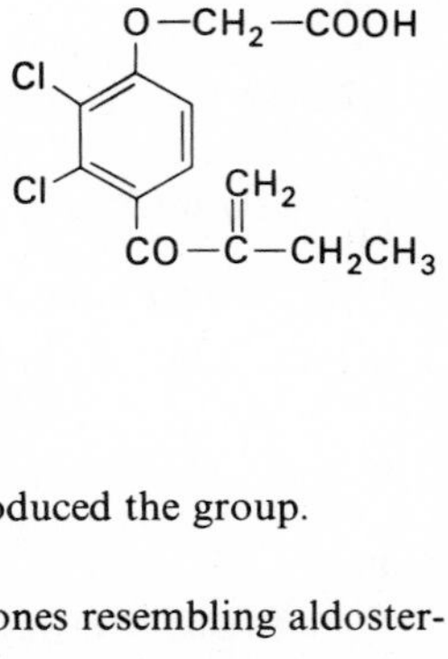

O—CH_2—COOH
Cl
Cl
CH_2
CO—C—CH_2CH_3

I. Aldosterone Antagonists (Spironolactone)

1. History. Kagawa (1957) and Liddle (1958) introduced the group.

2. Chemistry. Members of a group of 17-spirolactones resembling aldosterone in structure.

3. Action. a. Produce increased Na^+ excretion and diuresis (only when aldosterone present).

b. No increase in K^+ excretion, no tolerance.

4. Mechanism. Probably displace aldosterone competitively from receptors in the distal (and also proximal?) tubules (increases excretion of aldosterone), and thus interfere with the normal reabsorption of Na^+ in this region.

5. Pharmacodynamics. Absorbed orally; action develops slowly over two to three days.

6. Toxicity. Practically nontoxic; rare headache, drowsiness, abdominal pain, amenorrhea, gynecomastia.

7. Uses. a. Moderately effective, slowly acting diuretics. Used especially in edema resistant to other drugs.

b. Probably most effective in edema associated with excessive production of aldosterone, especially in nephrosis and cirrhosis.

c. Often given as a supplement to a thiazide or mercurial.

d. Under investigation in hypertension.

8. Preparation

SPIRONOLACTONE (Aldactone)

Dose: 25 to 50 mg 4 times a day by mouth.

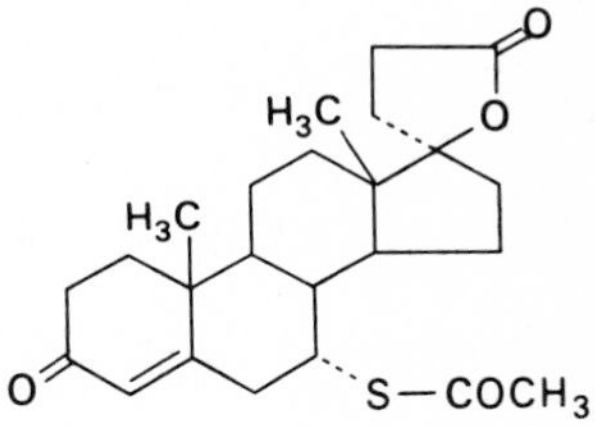

H₃C

H₃C

O

O

O

S—COCH₃

J. Cationic Exchange Resins

1. History. Introduced by Dock (1946).

2. Chemistry. Polycarboxylic or sulfonic resins; insoluble.

3. Action and Mechanism. Exchanges H^+ or NH_4^+ from the resin for Na^+ or K^+ from the intestine, thus reducing the fixed cation; or may exchange Na^+ from the resin for K^+ in the bowel (sodium polystyrene sulfonate).

4. Pharmacodynamics and Toxicity. a. Not absorbed.

b. May produce nausea from local irritation, constipation from bulk, or fecal impaction.

c. To prevent concurrent K^+ deficiency, K may be administered, or the resin given partly in the K cycle.

5. Uses. a. Formerly used as diuretics, but objectionable side effects limit use.

b. In hyperkalemia (as in anuria from acute tubular necrosis).

6. Preparations

CARBACRYLAMINE RESINS (Carbo-Resin)

Dose: 15 gm 3 times a day.

SULFONIC CATION EXCHANGE RESIN (Catonium; ammonium and potassium polystyrene sulfonate)

Dose: 15 gm 3 times a day.

AMMONIUM POLYACRYLIC CARBOXYLATE

Dose: 15 gm 3 times a day by mouth.

SODIUM POLYSTYRENE SULFONATE (Kayexalate)

Dose: 15 gm by mouth initially, then 5 gm 3 or 4 times a day (with 30 gm sorbitol to prevent constipation).

K. Salt Substitutes: Acidifying Agents

1. History. a. Low-sodium diets, e.g., Karrell milk diet (1866), the rice diet, and modern low-sodium diets are frequently prescribed to prevent or limit edema.

b. To make low-sodium diets more palatable (low-sodium diet contains only 1.5 to 2 gm of sodium, or 4 to 5 gm of NaCl), salt substitutes may be used.

2. Chemistry. a. Salt substitutes contain such salts as KCl, NH_4Cl, Ca_3PO_4, glutamic acid, ammonium glutamate, choline, K or Ca formate, magnesium citrate, or glycine.

b. Lithium salts, though effective, are toxic for this use.

3. Preparations

DIASAL; CO-SALT; NEOCURTASAL; GUSTAMATE

L. Other Inhibitors of Tubular Transport

During the early years of penicillin, when the drug was scarce, there was a desire to hinder its excretion and so prolong its tenure in the body. This led to the search for compounds which would block tubular excretion better than *p*-aminohippuric acid. As such compounds were developed it was found that they had two potential actions, first to block the excretory mechanism of the renal tubules and thereby reduce excretion of any drug eliminated by this mechanism, and second to block the same reabsorption mechanism and thereby increase the excretion of an agent normally resorbed. It is now the second function which is more useful, applied specifically to the elimination of uric acid.

BENZOIC ACID DERIVATIVES (PROBENECID)

1. History. a. Para-aminohippuric acid (PAH), used in renal function tests, was found to block renal excretion of penicillin by competition for a transport factor, but dose excessive (200 gm per day).

b. Carinamide an improvement, but nausea, fever, rashes, and a large dose (20 gm) made it undesirable.

c. Miller (1952) synthesized probenecid.

2. Chemistry. Organic acids.

3. Action and Mechanism. a. Inhibit excretion of penicillin, *p*-aminosalicylic acid, phenolsulfonphthalein, and other organic acids by the renal tubules.

b. Also inhibit the reabsorption of urates by the tubules.

c. The mechanism is competition for, and binding of, an essential factor in a shared enzymatic pathway between tubule cells and lumen.

4. Pharmacodynamics. a. Absorption is rapid; 90% is bound to plasma protein.

b. Excretion is also rapid, free drug by glomerular filtration, bound drug by tubular secretion, but then the drug is almost completely reabsorbed by the renal tubules. It is slowly metabolized in the body.

c. Salicylates antagonize the effect of probenecid.

5. Toxicity. a. Infrequent, but nausea and skin rashes have been noted. Attacks of gout may be precipitated.

b. A reducing substance giving a false positive for sugar may appear in the urine.

6. Uses. a. Used to promote the excretion of uric acid in gout, as interim treatment, not as an agent for acute attacks.

b. Occasionally used to obtain high blood level of penicillin when intensive therapy needed.

7. Preparation

PROBENECID (Benemid)

Dose: 0.5 gm 3 times a day by mouth.

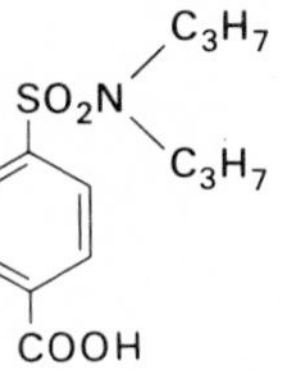

C_3H_7
SO_2N
C_3H_7
COOH

PYRAZOLON DERIVATIVES

1. Chemistry. Related to phenylbutazone and the pyrazolon analgesics (see Analgesics).

2. Action and Mechanism. a. Promotes the renal excretion of uric acid, probably by interfering with tubular reabsorption (lowers PAH clearance; no effect on inulin clearance); uric acid may fall somewhat.

b. Has only a weak analgesic effect.

3. Pharmacodynamics. a. Absorption rapid; one half excreted in 3 hours.

b. Salicylates antagonize; probenecid and phenylbutazone do not.

4. Toxicity. a. Danger of precipitation of acute gout; urolithiasis.

b. May cause epigastric distress and may activate a peptic ulcer.

c. Leukopenia; thrombocytopenia.

5. Uses. Alternative to probenecid in chronic gout; effects slow but tophi may recede. No relief in acute gout.

6. Preparation

SULFINPYRAZONE (Anturane)

Dose: 100 mg 4 times a day by mouth.

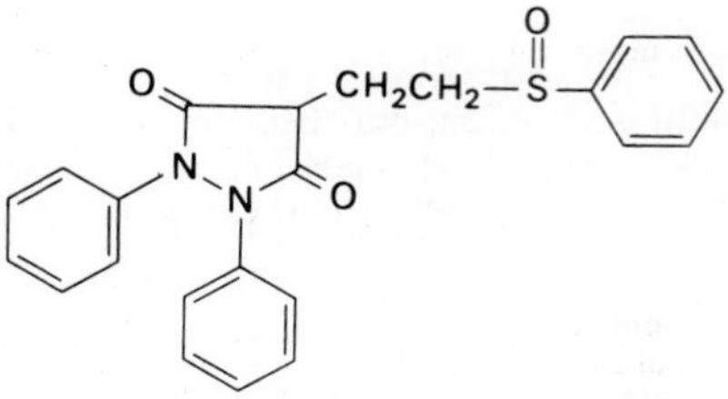

OTHERS

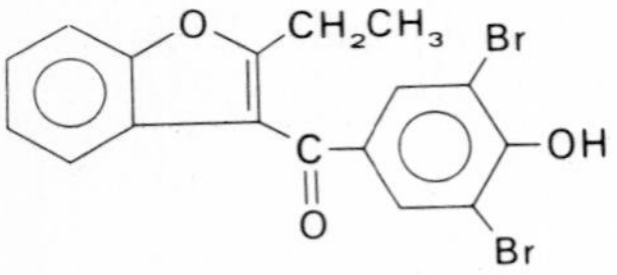

benzbromarone

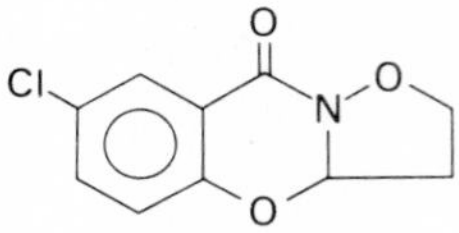

seclazone

OTHER URICOSURICS

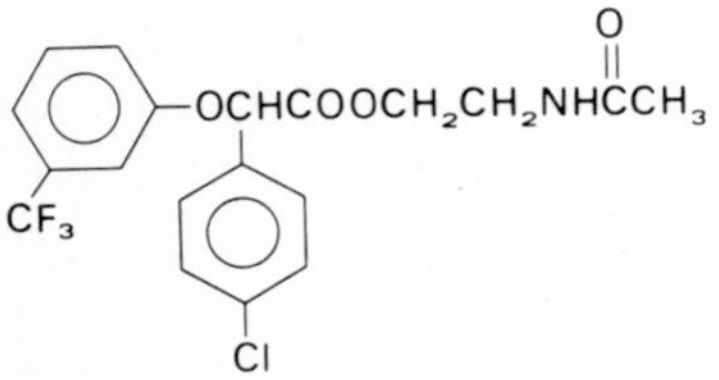

halofenate

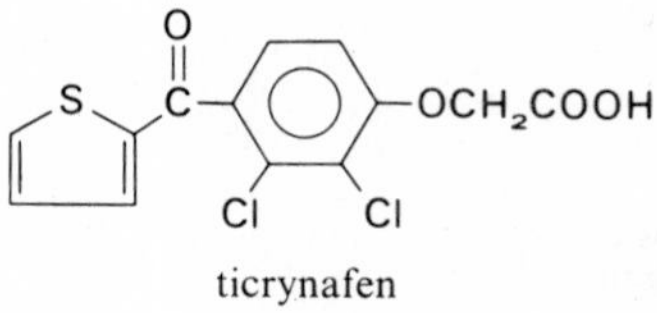

ticrynafen

SUMMARY: DIURETICS AND RENAL TUBULE INHIBITORS

TYPE	*ACTION AND MECHANISM*	*TOXICITY*	*USE*	*EXAMPLES*
Osmotic	Poorly absorbed materials carry water out in urine	Minor	Cerebral edema	Urea
Acidifying	Provide Cl ion	Same	Augment mercurial action	Ammonium chloride

SUMMARY: DIURETICS AND RENAL TUBULE INHIBITORS (cont.)

TYPE	*ACTION AND MECHANISM*	*TOXICITY*	*USE*	*EXAMPLES*
Xanthines	Uncertain	Same	Minor use as diuretics	Aminophylline
Mercurials	Enhance sodium excretion by inhibiting enzymes involved in reabsorption	Stomatitis renal damage, hypersensitivity, ventricular arrhythmia	Potent diuretics in heart failure	Meralluride sodium
Carbonic anhydrase inhibitors	Inhibition of reabsorption of HCO_3^-	Minor	Transient diuretics but useful in glaucoma	Acetazolamide
Thiazides	Similar to mercurials	Minor except for K loss	Potent and widely used in heart failure and other types of edema	Chlorothiazide
Other sulfonamides	Same	Same	Same	Chlorthalidone
Triamterenes	Reduce absorption of Na in distal tubules	May cause hyperkalemia	To potentiate thiazides and ethacrynic acid and counteract K loss	Triamterene
Ethacrynic acid	Inhibits Na reabsorption, especially in loop of Henle	Gout, bleeding, hepatic coma	Potent diuretic	Ethacrynic acid
Aldosterone antagonists	Limit reabsorption of Na by displacing aldosterone	Minor	Resistant edema as in cirrhosis and nephrosis	Spironolactone
Cationic exchange resins	Reduce available Na in intestine	Bad taste	Minor diuretics	Carbacrylamine resins
Salt substitutes	Reduce Na intake by replacing table salt	Minor	Low-salt diets	Lysine monoHCl
Tubule inhibitors	Block excretory and reabsorptive mechanisms for penicillin, uric acid	Rashes (probenecid), leukopenia (sulfinpyrazone)	Gout; to extend penicillin	Probenecid

Reviews

Pitts, R. Physiological Basis of Diuretic Therapy. Springfield, Ill., Charles C Thomas, Publisher, 1959.

Beyer, K., and Baer, J. Physiological basis for action of newer diuretic agents. Pharmacol. Rev., 13:517, 1961.

Milne, M. Renal pharmacology. Ann. Rev. Pharmacol., 5:119, 1965.

Mudge, G. Renal pharmacology. Ann. Rev. Pharmacol., 7:163, 1967.

Weiner, I. The renal excretion of drugs and related compounds. Ann. Rev. Pharmacol., 7:39, 1967.

Cafruny, E. Renal pharmacology. Ann. Rev. Pharmacol., 8:131, 1968.

Bank, N. Physiological basis of diuretic action. Ann. Rev. Med., 19:103, 1968.

21. Fluids: Blood Substitutes, Electrolytes

I. AGENTS USED IN SHOCK

The usual cause of shock is hemorrhage, trauma, or sepsis. The essential difficulty is a loss of blood volume: 15% to 20% in mild shock, and as much as 40% in severe shock. The decreased blood volume may result from loss of blood to the outside or into the venous bed, or from loss of plasma into the tissues.

Proper therapy includes all relevant measures to remove causative or aggravating factors as well as specific replenishment of the blood volume and electrolytes. Further trauma, however, which might include surgery or fracture repair, should be avoided until shock is controlled. Specific measures to restore the blood volume consist primarily of the intravenous administration of various fluids, supplemented at times by agents that may improve tissue perfusion (pressor or adrenolytic) and by corticoid hormones.

The logistic difficulties in procuring and administering whole blood, as well as the absence of any need for red cells in some cases, have made the use of substitutes of great importance.

A. Whole Blood and Blood Derivatives

WHOLE BLOOD

1. Uses. a. Transfusion with whole blood has the advantage of completely restoring the physiological deficiency, including the provision of oxygen transport. It is most desirable in shock from bleeding.

b. Disadvantages include difficulty of procurement, the need of typing and cross matching, and the danger of untoward reactions. These may include pyrogenic, hemolytic, or sensitization reactions, transfusion hemochromatosis, hemoglobinuric nephrosis, and the transmission of various infections, particularly hepatitis.

2. Preparation

CITRATED WHOLE BLOOD

Dose: Given intravenously in multiples of 500 ml. Various formulas used to determine the amount of blood needed.

HUMAN PLASMA

1. Uses. a. As a substitute for blood, plasma has both advantages and disadvantages. Advantages include facility of storage and transport and general effectiveness. It may be preferred in shock with little loss of blood because the red cells are not needed and their absence decreases the viscosity of the transfusion fluid.

b. Disadvantages are the lack of hemoglobin and the greater chance of homologous serum jaundice since plasma is obtained from pools rather than from single donors. Sterilization is difficult as the virus is highly resistant; among the agents used to inactivate any virus that may be present are ultraviolet irradiation, and the addition of nitrogen mustards or beta-propiolactone.

2. Preparation

NORMAL HUMAN PLASMA, whole or restored

Dose: Half the dose indicated for whole blood, intravenously.

HUMAN ALBUMIN

1. Chemistry. a. Serum albumin obtained by fractionation of human blood.
b. Molecular weight about 60,000.

2. Action. Albumin accounts for about 80% of the effective osmotic pressure of plasma, and acts as a satisfactory volume expander. It has the advantage of being stable, concentrated, and free of virus, but the disadvantage of being expensive.

3. Uses. As a plasma expander in shock. To raise the serum protein level in hypoproteinemia.

4. Preparations

ALBUMIN, NORMAL HUMAN SERUM

Dose: 2.2 ml of 25% solution per kg body weight, given intravenously in saline or dextrose solution.

PLASMA PROTEIN FRACTION, HUMAN (Plasmanate)

Contains a mixture of plasma proteins, including 88% albumin.
Dose: 1,000 ml of 5% solution intravenously.

OTHER BLOOD PRODUCTS

A number of other blood products, human and bovine, have been tried as sources of protein molecules which could expand the blood volume. These have included human hemoglobin, human globin, and bovine albumin and globulin. None has proved to be satisfactory.

B. Plasma Substitutes

The criteria for ideal plasma substitutes or expanders include an osmotic force, viscosity, and retention in the blood about equal to plasma; stability on storage and sterilization; nontoxicity and nonantigenicity; absence of unfavorable effects on cell structure and function. No present substitute meets these criteria completely, but some are reasonably satisfactory.

DEXTRAN

1. History. Originally developed in Sweden by Ingelman and Gronwall.

2. Chemistry. a. Inert polydispersoid isomers of glucose produced by the action of bacteria (*Leuconostoc mesenteroides*) on sucrose, with subsequent acid hydrolysis to smaller sizes.

b. Shape long and slender in comparison to albumin molecule (18 × 500 Å, compared to 36 × 150 Å).

3. Action and Mechanism. a. Expands blood volume comparably to albumin by osmotic effect.

b. Low mol. wt. dextran is stated to increase flow in the microcirculation.

4. Pharmacodynamics. a. Partly stored in RES; about half excreted in 24 hours; effective 12 to 24 hours.

b. Low mol. wt. dextran is rapidly excreted, about 60% appearing in the urine in 90 minutes.

5. Toxicity. a. Some preparations, especially those with particles of over 120,000 molecular weight, give a variety of allergic manifestations; bleeding time may be slightly prolonged.

b. Storage in tissues a potential danger with repeated use.

c. Quantities over 1.5 ml may interfere with clotting.

6. Uses. a. Useful in shock as a substitute for blood or blood products.

b. Low molecular weight dextran is an excellent hemodiluent in pump-oxygenators since less hemolysis occurs than with 5% dextrose in water as diluent. If it is demonstrated that it truly increases blood flow in small vessels by preventing intravascular red cell aggregation, the disadvantage of rapid excretion might be disregarded.

7. Preparations

DEXTRAN 40 (Gentran 40, Rheomacrodex, Rheotran) 10% Dextran, av. mol. wt.: 40,000, in 0.9% sodium chloride.

Dose: 500 ml.

DEXTRAN 70 (Hyskon, Macrodex) 6% Dextran, av. mol. wt.: 70,000, in 0.9% sodium chloride.

Dose: 500 ml.

DEXTRAN 75 (Gentran 75) av. mol. wt.: 75,000.

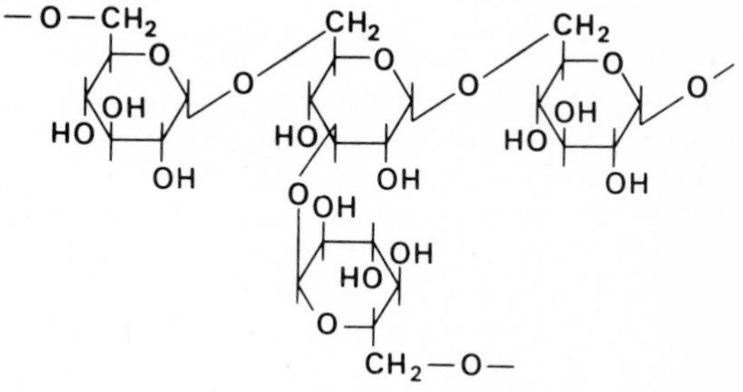

segment of dextran macromolecule

OTHER SUBSTITUTES

GELATIN

Obsolete.

HETASTARCH (Hydroxyethyl starch)

POVIDONE (Polyvinylpyrrolidone; PVP; Periston)

Little used.

SALT SOLUTIONS

1. Action and Uses. a. Although such solutions pass out of the bloodstream fairly rapidly, amounts of 2 or 3 times the volume of blood lost may be comparable in effect to plasma in moderate hemorrhage. Always useful as an initial or temporizing measure. May be combined with serum albumin for greater effect.

b. Adequate in burns involving less than 10% of the body surface; adjuvant to plasma in severe burns where extracellular fluids as well as plasma are lost through the wound.

2. Preparations

PHYSIOLOGICAL SALT SOLUTION (Saline)

LACTATED RINGER'S INJECTION

RINGER'S INJECTION

C. Pressor Agents (Sympathomimetic Amines)

1. Chemistry. Phenylethylamines (see Sympathetic Stimulants).

2. Action and Mechanism. Raise blood pressure by peripheral arteriolar vasoconstriction and in most instances by direct stimulation of the heart.

3. Toxicity. Excessive release of catechol amines may cause renal shutdown, and potentiation of bacterial toxins.

4. Uses. a. Of dubious or secondary value in traumatic or hemorrhagic shock; may possibly be of help in older patients. Elevation of blood pressure does not assure increased organ perfusion.

b. Widely used in shock from myocardial infarction, but true assessment of value difficult (Seltzer and Rytand, J.A.M.A., 168:762, 1958). Blood and expanders not used in myocardial shock.

c. Used to maintain blood pressure after spinal or epidural anesthesia.

5. Preparation

a. Both vasoconstrictor and cardiac effects

LEVARTERENOL BITARTRATE (Levophed)

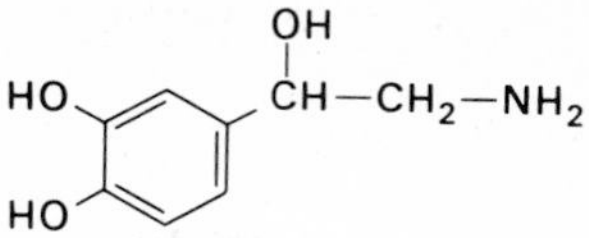

Most potent pressor; produces overall peripheral vasoconstriction and stimulates the heart directly. May cause ventricular arrhythmias.

Dose: 2 to 4 mcg per minute in 5% dextrose solution by intravenous drip, best through a polyethylene catheter. If extravasation should occur, phentolamine, 10 mg in 5 ml of saline locally, may prevent tissue damage.

METARAMINOL BITARTRATE (Aramine)

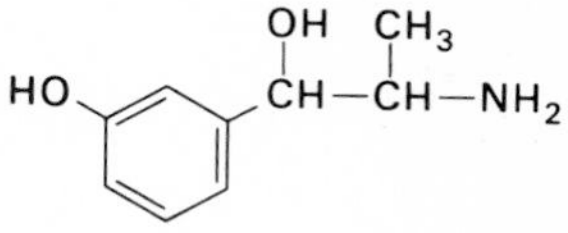

Similar to levarterenol; acts in part by releasing norepinephrine from vessel walls. Requires smaller volume of fluid than levarterenol; not irritating to veins.

Dose: 1 to 2 mg intravenously, repeated in 5 to 10 minutes if necessary. Later 2 to 10 mg subcutaneously or intramuscularly as needed to maintain blood pressure.

MEPHENTERMINE SULFATE (Wyamine)

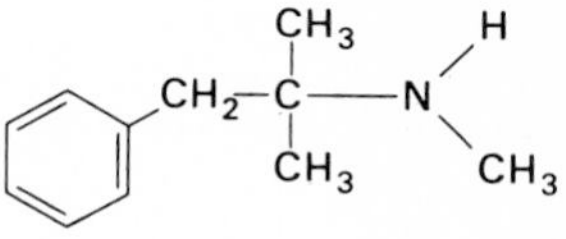

Similar to levarterenol but no danger of arrhythmia or vein damage.

Dose: 15 to 30 mg intravenously (slowly) or intramuscularly; effect lasts 4 hours.

b. *Principally vasoconstrictor effects*

METHOXAMINE HYDROCHLORIDE (Vasoxyl)

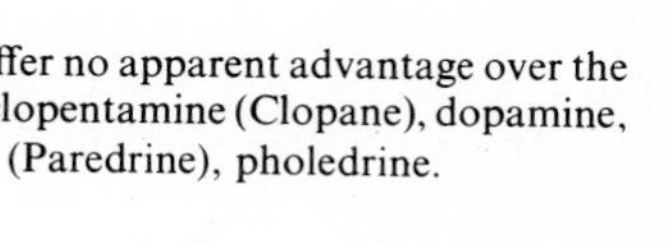

Primarily a vasoconstrictor; minimal CNS or cardiac effects.

Dose: 5 mg intravenously (slowly) or intramuscularly; effect lasts 4 hours.

OTHER SYMPATHOMIMETIC AGENTS

A number of other such agents have been used, but offer no apparent advantage over the generally more potent preceding agents. These include cyclopentamine (Clopane), dopamine, phenylephrine (Neo-Synephrine), hydroxyamphetamine (Paredrine), pholedrine.

ANGIOTENSIN

Potent vasoconstrictor (not a sympathomimetic amine) (see Smooth Muscle Stimulants).

D. Vasodilators (Sympatholytic Agents)

1. Chemistry. See Sympathetic Depressants.

2. Action and Mechanism. Block alpha receptors and produce peripheral vasodilatation which may improve visceral blood flow and mobilize interstitial fluid which has been derived from the vascular compartment by vasoconstriction (Fine, J.A.M.A., 188:427, 1964).

3. Toxicity. May produce local irritation; should be given in dilute solution.

4. Uses. a. May be used in shock accompanying hypovolemia from trauma, burns, or hemorrhage, from endotoxins, or from reduced cardiac output.

b. Should always be accompanied by replacement fluids.

5. Preparations

PHENOXYBENZAMINE HYDROCHLORIDE (Dibenzyline)

Dose: 1 mg per kg body weight intravenously, slowly.

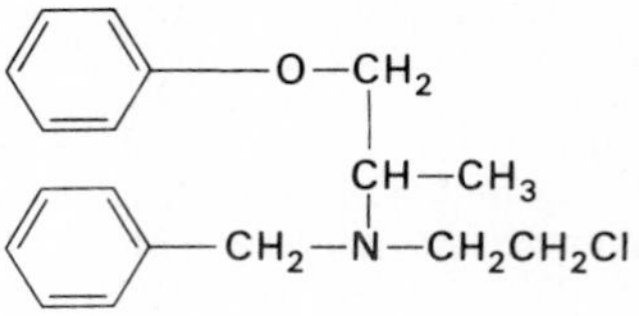

$C_6H_5-O-CH_2-CH(CH_3)-N(CH_2CH_2Cl)-CH_2-C_6H_5$

E. Other Agents

HYDROCORTISONE

Cortisone, other corticoids, and corticotropin ameliorate experimental shock, and are used clinically and as preoperative measures and as adjuncts in treatment. The mechanism of action is not clear, but blood vessels react poorly to vasopressors in cortisone deficiency, and hence it may act as a vasodilator. Cortisone has also been reported to have a positive inotropic effect on the heart and to inactivate fibrinolysin. Value doubted by some workers (Smith, New Eng. J. Med., 267:733, 1962).

Dose: 5 to 10 mg per hour intravenously in saline or dextrose (hydrocortisone).

II. WATER AND ELECTROLYTES

1. Chemistry. a. Body water comprises:

Extracellular water (plasma 5%; interstitial 11%)	16% of body weight
Intracellular water	30% to 50% body weight

b. Body electrolytes include:

	CATIONS (BASE, +)		ANIONS (ACID, −)	
Blood serum	sodium	142 mEq/L	HCO_3^-	28 mEq/L
	potassium	5	chloride	103
	calcium	5	organic acid	6
	magnesium	3	phosphate	1
			sulfate	1
			protein	16

Intracellular fluid	potassium	140	HCO_3^-	10
	magnesium	45	organic PO_4	100
	sodium	10	sulfate	20
			protein	65

Interstitial fluid: resembles serum, but with less protein and more chloride.

(1 mEq = mol. wt. in grams/valence × 1,000)

c. Daily basal requirements for adults: water, 1,800 ml; KCl, 30 to 60 mM; NaCl, 74 mM; Mg^{++}, 8 mM.

2. Action. Electrolytes are involved in three principal activities:

a. Osmotic activity, regulating the distribution of water between the extracellular and intracellular compartments. Na^+ is the principal extracellular cation; K^+ is the principal intracellular cation.

b. Buffer activity, regulating the pH of body fluids. The principal buffer is the system:

$$\frac{(H+)\quad(HCO_3^-)}{(Base+)\quad(HCO_3^-)}$$

c. Pharmacological activity, regulating membrane permeability, metabolic functions, neuromuscular activity, and others.

3. Uses. a. Dehydration: Normal daily water requirement (adult) is 1,500 to 2,000 ml. When intake is lowered, or need increased (fever), water may pass from the intracellular to the extracellular compartments, depleting cells. Treatment is with water made isotonic with glucose.

b. Overhydration: Excessive retention of water produces edema, sometimes rise in BP. Treatment is by abstinence from water plus indicated specific measures.

c. Sodium excess: Produces thirst, desiccation, oliguria. Treatment is with water (made isotonic with glucose if intravenous).

d. Sodium deficiency: Water moves into cells, producing hemoconcentration, lowered BP, shock. Treatment is with saline or hypertonic salt solution intravenously.

e. Potassium excess: From renal failure or overdosage with K salts; produces muscle weakness and paralysis, bradycardia, lowered BP, cardiac standstill.

f. Potassium deficiency: From decreased intake or absorption, as in sprue, diarrhea, or fistula; increased loss, as in diarrhea, burns, renal failure, thiazide diuretic administration, cortical hormone administration; familial periodic paralysis. Produces muscle weakness, lethargy, paralytic ileus, heart failure. Treatment is by replacing K cautiously.

g. Acidosis, respiratory: Increase in (H^+) (HCO_3^-) from retention of CO_2 in emphysema or decreased breathing. Body compensates by retention of $(base^+)$ (HCO_3^-) to increase pH to normal. Treatment is by facilitation of breathing; intravenous alkaline solutions.

h. Acidosis, metabolic: Decrease in $(base^+)$ (HCO_3^-) from loss of base in diarrhea, ingestion of NH_4Cl or other acid salts, retention of organic acids by kidney. Body compensates by blowing off CO_2 to elevate pH to normal. Treatment is by alkali by mouth or vein, and attention to the underlying condition.

i. Alkalosis, respiratory: Decrease in (H^+) (HCO_3^-) by hyperventilation. Body compensates by excreting (base$^+$) (HCO_3^-). Treatment is by inhalation of CO_2.

j. Alkalosis, metabolic: Increase in (base$^+$) (HCO_3^-) from excessive ingestion of alkali, loss of HCl. Body compensates by retention of (H^+) (HCO_3^-). Treatment is by administration of saline solution.

k. Renal failure: Kidney normally preserves fixed base (Na^+, Ca^{++}, K^+) by exchange for H^+ and NH_4^+.

4. Preparations

a. Solutions contributing fluid, sodium chloride, mixed electrolytes, potassium, and acidity or alkalinity are available for clinical use. Examples:

SOLUTION	ELECTROLYTE	gm/L	mEq/L Na^+	K^+	Ca^{++}	Cl^-	HCO_3^- or equivalent
Physiological saline	NaCl	9.0	155			155	
Ringer's	NaCl	8.6	145			145	
	KCl	0.3		4		4	
	$CaCl_2$	0.33			6	6	
Ringer-lactate (Hartmann's)	NaCl	6.0	102			102	
	Na lactate	3.0	27				27
	KCl	0.3		4		4	
	$CaCl_2$	0.2			4	4	
Darrow's	NaCl	4.0	70			70	
	Na lactate	6.0	53				53
	KCl	2.7		35		35	
KCl 0.2%	KCl	2.0		27		27	
NH_4Cl 0.9%	Cl(NH_4Cl)	9.0				170	
Sodium bicarbonate 5%	$NaHCO_3$	50.0	600				600
Sodium lactate 1/6 M	Na lactate	18.7	167				167

b. Dosage and frequency of administration vary according to the needs of the patient; the doses given are only indicative of a generally permissible minimum level.

a'. Preparations for general electrolyte replenishment:

PHYSIOLOGICAL SALT SOLUTION (Saline solution)

Dose: 500 ml, orally, subcutaneously, intravenously; (or NaCl tablets, 1 gm by mouth).

RINGER'S SOLUTION

Dose: 500 ml intravenously.

RINGER-LACTATE (Hartmann's)

Dose: 500 ml intravenously.

PERITONEAL DIALYSIS SOLUTION WITH DEXTROSE (Inpersol)

Contains:	Sodium	3.23 gm/l	Chloride	3.58
	Calcium	0.07	Lactate	3.96
	Magnesium	0.18	Dextrose	15 or 70
				(1.5% or 7%)

Dose: 2 liters, intraperitoneally.

b'. *Preparations for potassium replenishment:*

DARROW'S SOLUTION

Dose: 500 ml intravenously.

POTASSIUM CHLORIDE SOLUTION (0.2%)

Dose: 500 ml by mouth or intravenously (or KCl tablets, 1 gm by mouth).

POTASSIUM GLUCONATE

Dose: 9 gm by mouth (= 1.5 gm K) in solution (Kaon).

c'. *Preparations producing acidosis:*

AMMONIUM CHLORIDE SOLUTION (0.9%)

Dose: 500 ml intravenously; or tablets, 2 gm by mouth.

d'. *Preparations producing alkalosis:*

SODIUM LACTATE (1/6 M)

Dose: 500 ml intravenously.

SODIUM BICARBONATE SOLUTION (5%)

Dose: 500 ml intravenously (or tablets, 5 gm or more by mouth).

SHOHL'S SOLUTION (1 mEq Na per ml)

Contains: Citric acid 140 gm
Sodium citrate, hydrated 90 gm
Water to make final volume of 1 liter

Dose: As needed by mouth to replace sodium deficit.

TROMETHAMINE (TRIS; THAM)

$H_2N-C(CH_2OH)_3$

Buffers in the physiological range of the body.

$$(CH_2OH)_3C-NH_2 + HA \rightarrow (CH_2OH)_3C-NH_3^+ + A^-$$

Accepts a proton, usually from H_2CO_3. Thus titrates carbonic acid, correcting hypercapnia or metabolic acidosis. Increases urine and plasma pH. Produces diuresis. At pH 7 ionized to 70%; enters cells.

Used in CO_2 retention, salicylate in toxication, barbiturate poisoning. Increased excretion of barbiturates may be the result of ionization in an alkaline urine to a form not easily reabsorbed; or increased excretion of electrolytes may interfere with the reabsorption of barbiturate.

Dose: 0.5 to 1 liter of 0.3 M solution intravenously.

TRICINE

Aqueous solutions buffer at pH 5.2.

$$HOOC-CH_2-N(CH_2OH)_3$$

SUMMARY: FLUIDS: BLOOD SUBSTITUTES, ELECTROLYTES

TYPE	*ACTION AND MECHANISM*	*TOXICITY*	*USE*	*EXAMPLES*
Blood and derivatives	To restore blood volume	Minor except hepatitis	Shock	Human plasma
Blood substitutes	Same	Allergic manifestations	Same	Dextran
Pressor agents	Produce vaso-constriction and so raise blood pressure	Renal shutdown	Same	Levarterenol HCl
Vasodilators	Produce vasodilatation and so better tissue nourishment	Minor	Same	Phenoxybenz-amine HCl
Electrolyte solutions	Restore blood electrolytes	Minor	Dehydration, electrolyte abnormality	Physiological salt solution

Reviews

Nahas, G. Clinical pharmacology of THAM. Clin. Pharmacol. Ther., 4:784, 1963.

Lillehei, R., Longerbeam, J., Bloch, J., and Manax, W. Modern treatment of shock based on physiologic principles. Clin. Pharmacol. Ther., 5:63, 1964.

Couch, N. The clinical status of low molecular weight dextran; a critical review. Clin. Pharmacol. Ther., 6:656, 1965.

Bleich, H., and Schwarz, W. Tris buffer (THAM). New Eng. J. Med., 274:782, 1966.

Hodge, R. Clinical pharmacology of vasconstrictors. Clin. Pharmacol. Ther., 7:639, 1966.

Lefer, A., and Verrier, R. Role of corticosteroids in the treatment of circulatory collapse states. Clin. Pharmacol. Ther., 11:630, 1970.

22. Agents in Atherosclerosis

Atherosclerosis is characterized by deposits of cholesterol esters in the intima of arteries, followed by calcification. It appears to be due to a combination of injury to the arterial wall and a disturbance in lipid metabolism. It can be produced with uncertain fidelity in most animals.

Of the many suggested etiological factors—heredity, hypertension, obesity, masculinity, blood fibrin or elastase abnormalities, and cholesterol or lipid excess—only the last pair has been widely exploited in therapy. On the basis that high cholesterol or lipid blood levels are conducive to atherosclerosis attempts have been made to lower them in several ways. A cholesterol level over 300 mg% or a triglyceride level over 200 mg% suggests study and probable treatment. Drugs of the clofibrate group may reduce triglycerides; cholesterol may be reduced in three general ways:

a. Reduction of intake of cholesterol by low cholesterol diets or competitors of absorption (sitosterols);

b. Increase in metabolism or excretion of cholesterol, including biliary, and facilitation of transport (thyroid, linoleic acid, heparin);

c. Inhibition of synthesis of cholesterol (clofibrate; nicotinic acid).

Sites of drug action are shown in the following diagram:

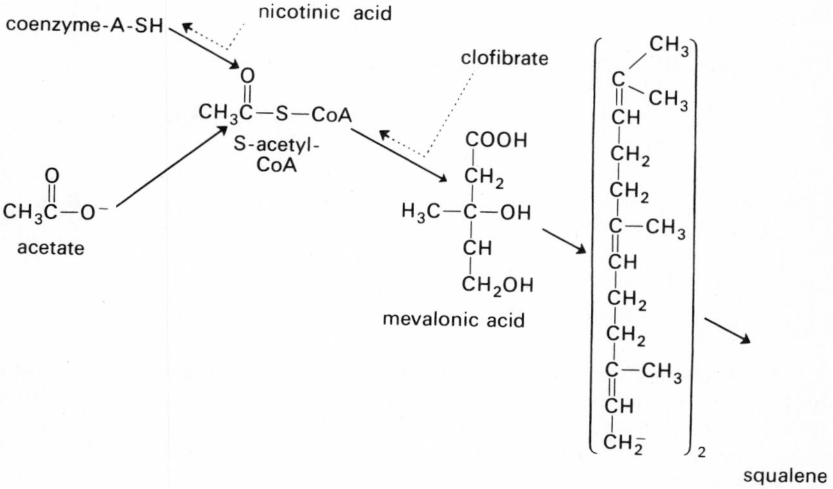

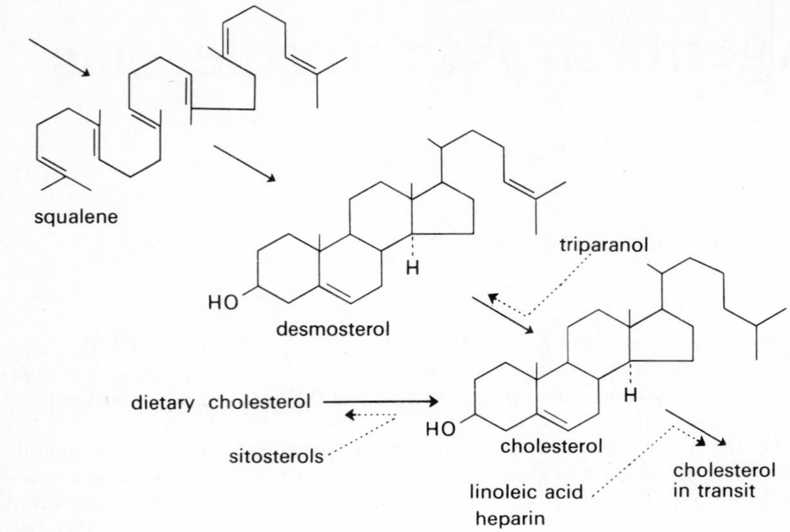

squalene

desmosterol

triparanol

dietary cholesterol

sitosterols

cholesterol

cholesterol in transit

linoleic acid

heparin

A. Agents Reducing Cholesterol Intake

LOW–CHOLESTEROL DIETS

The effectiveness of low-cholesterol or low-fat diets is limited because, if low enough to be effective, they have poor acceptance by the patient. Also, the body tends to compensate with increased synthesis when dietary cholesterol is reduced.

SITOSTEROLS

1. Chemistry. Plant sterols closely related to cholesterol.

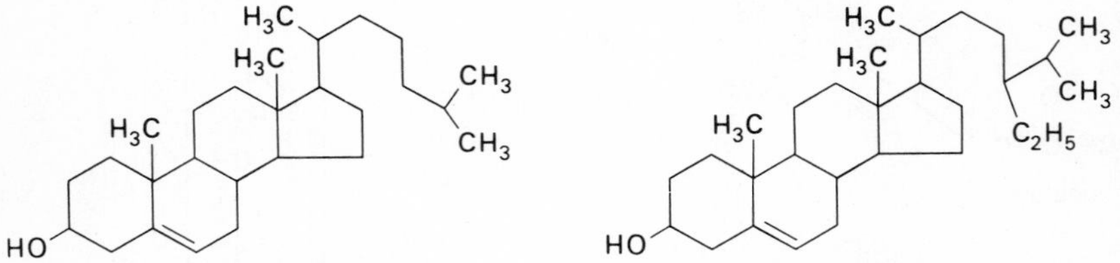

cholesterol

beta-sitosterol

2. Action and Mechanism. a. Interfere with cholesterol absorption competitively, both exogenous cholesterol from the diet, and endogenous cholesterol from the bile. Fecal cholesterol is increased.

b. May compete for esterification sites; may make nonabsorbable mixed crystals with cholesterol.

3. Pharmacodynamics and Toxicity. Presumably not absorbed. No toxic manifestations except occasional anorexia and diarrhea.

4. Uses. a. Tried in atherosclerosis and various hypercholesterolemic states: xanthomatosis, nephrosis, hypothyroidism, diabetes.

b. Still investigational.

5. Preparation

SITOSTEROLS (Cytellin)

Contains both beta- and dihydro-beta-sitosterol.

Dose: 3 gm or more 3 times daily by mouth at meal times in 20% suspension.

POLYMERS AND EXCHANGE RESINS

1. Chemistry. Tetraethylenepentamine polymer (colestipol); basic, anionic exchange resin (cholestyramine resin).

2. Action and Mechanism. Bind or complex bile acids in the intestine, thus promoting their excretion in the feces instead of their reabsorption from the bowel; the liver then presumably makes more bile acids instead of cholesterol. Blood cholesterol may be lowered 10% or more.

3. Pharmacodynamics and Toxicity. a. Generally insoluble and non-absorbable.

b. Large doses (cholestyramine resin) may cause nausea, vomiting, constipation, fecal impaction, steatorrhea, or deficiency of fat-soluble vitamins (A, D, and K).

4. Uses. a. Cholestyramine resin has been recommended for hypercholesterolemia, biliary cirrhosis, and jaundice with itching.

b. Colestipol is under trial in hypercholesterolemia and xanthomatosis.

5. Preparations

COLESTIPOL HYDROCHLORIDE (Colestid)

Dose: 10 gm twice daily.

CHOLESTYRAMINE RESIN (Cuemid; Questran)

Dose: 15 to 30 gm daily by mouth; admix with fluids.

B. Agents Facilitating Cholesterol Metabolism or Transport

UNSATURATED FATTY ACIDS

1. History. Byers (1952) reported that unsaturated fatty acids lower serum cholesterol, beta-lipoproteins, and other lipids.

2. Chemistry

a. Unsaturated acids have one or more double bonds:

Oleic acid	$CH_3-(CH_2)_7-CH{=}CH-(CH_2)_7-COOH$
Linoleic acid	$CH_3-(CH_2)_4-CH{=}CH-CH_2-CH{=}CH-(CH_2)_7-COOH$
Linolenic acid	$CH_3-(CH_2-CH{=}CH)_3-(CH_2)_7-COOH$

b. Various liquid vegetable oils (cottonseed, soya, safflower, corn) are rich in monounsaturated and polyunsaturated fatty acids. Thus safflower seed oil the richest, contains 75% of linoleic acid, a polyunsaturated fatty acid.

Values for fatty acid saturation in common cooking oils are as follows:

OIL	TOTAL UNSATURATION	POLYUNSATURATION
corn	84%	54%
cottonseed	71	50
Crisco	75	30
peanut	76	29
olive	84	7

c. Animal fats and solidified (hydrogenated) vegetable oils are in general low in unsaturated fatty acids.

3. Action and Mechanism. The mechanism is not clear, but the following have been suggested:

a. Polyunsaturated fatty acids may aid in the transport and elimination of cholesterol. Cholesterol is assumed to be normally transported as an ester of arachidonic acid, an unstable acid not contained in most foods, but made in the body from linoleic, linolenic, and other unsaturated precursors, catalyzed by pyridoxine.

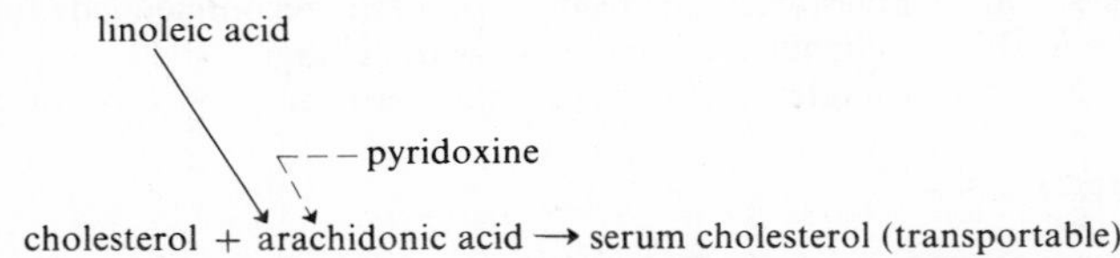

b. In a deficiency of such unsaturated fatty acids as linoleic acid, cholesterol is assumed to be esterified with saturated fatty acids, forming abnormal esters which are deposited in the tissues. It has also been thought that unsaturated fatty acids foster the formation of the more normal alpha-lipoproteins in place of beta-lipoproteins.

c. Polyunsaturated fatty acids also increase the excretion of bile acids.

4. Pharmacodynamics and Toxicity. a. The oils are well absorbed by mouth.

b. Aside from occasional mild diarrhea, and obesity when their caloric value is not appreciated, they are not toxic.

5. Uses. Unsaturated fatty acids are popularly given to patients with hypercholesteremia and to those who may have had cardiac infarctions. Their ultimate value is, however, conjectural. To cause a satisfactory lowering of serum cholesterol, ordinary fats must be highly restricted.

6. Preparations

SAFFLOWER OIL (Saff)

Dose: 75 ml of a 65% emulsion daily by mouth, given in divided doses and accompanied by simultaneous reduction of other fats (saturated fats should constitute less than ¼ of total).

"Lufa" contains pyridoxine and vitamin E (as an antioxidant) as well as safflower seed oil. There is no definite evidence that these additives increase the action.

LINOLEIC ACID

In such mixtures as "Linodoxine," which also contains pyridoxine.

COTTONSEED OIL and CORN OIL (Mazola)

As purchased for cooking; also corn oil margarine.

HEPARIN AND HEPARIN SUBSTITUTES

1. History. Hahn (1943) showed that heparin clarified lipemic serum in dogs.

2. Chemistry. See Anticoagulants.

3. Action. Heparin alters the physical state of the lipids in the blood, changing large, low-density lipoproteins into smaller, more physiological molecules, and thus reduces lipemia.

4. Mechanism. a. Heparin activates a clearing factor (lipoprotein lipase) in vivo (not in vitro) which hydrolyses the triglycerides of large fat particles (chylomicra, 0.5–1 microns) to fatty acids and glycerol. The fatty acids then form soluble complexes with plasma protein and leave the circulation at an increased rate. Heparin may also aid this complexing as a connecting link.

b. There is no evidence that the normal amounts of heparin in the body play this role, nor that the anticoagulant properties of heparin play a part (Robinson and French, Pharmacol. Rev., 12:241, 1960).

4. Pharmacodynamics and Toxicity. a. Evidence for oral and sublingual absorption controversial; it may be as low as 15% (Engelberg, J.A.M.A., 169:1324, 1959).

b. In doses used to clarify lipemia, toxic effects are uncommon, but hemorrhage at the injection site, and allergic reactions, may occur.

6. Uses. a. Because prolonged hyperlipemia is associated with atherosclerotic cardiovascular disease, especially myocardial infarction, trials with heparin have been undertaken.

b. No long-term basis for judgment of effectiveness is available; therapy would seem to have to be lifetime.

c. May be tried immediately when coronary occlusion follows a large meal.

7. Preparations

HEPARIN, SODIUM

Dose: 20,000 units (about 180 mg) subcutaneously 2 times a week.

HEPARIN, POTASSIUM, SUBLINGUAL

Dose: 1,500 units (about 15 mg) held under the tongue after each meal.

GASTRIC MUCIN

Has been reported to clear plasma in the same way as heparin; suggestion that this may be a normal regulatory function (Rossi, Circulation, 18:397, 1958).

THYROXINE ANALOGUES

1. Chemistry. Some 60 analogues and derivatives of thyroxine have been studied for their effect on serum cholesterol.

2. Action and Mechanism. a. The reciprocal action between thyroid and blood cholesterol has been known for many years although its mechanism is obscure.

b. It is apparent that the effect does not lie in the metabolic stimulating property of the thyroid hormone, for derivatives with little calorigenic action effectively reduce the blood cholesterol.

c. Present hypothesis is that breakdown of cholesterol in the liver is stimulated (oxidation or hydroxylation), with subsequent excretion of the degradation products via the bile.

3. Pharmacodynamics. a. Absorbed moderately well from the gastro-intestinal tract.

b. Distributed widely in the body; excreted, partly as breakdown products in stool and urine.

4. Toxicity. a. Dextrothyroxine produces only about one-tenth the calorigenic effect of levothyroxine, but large doses may cause angina pectoris, insomnia, tremors and other signs of hypermetabolism.

b. The anticoagulant effects of coumarin anticoagulants may be increased; diabetes may be made more severe.

5. Uses. a. Used in the treatment of atherosclerosis with hypercholesterolemia, but as yet with no clear assessment of effect.

b. Used in hypercholesterolemia with xanthomas, often with reduction of the lipid deposits.

c. Reduction in blood cholesterol may be as great as 50 mg%.

6. Preparations

DEXTROTHYROXINE SODIUM (Choloxin)

Dose: 1 to 2 mg daily by mouth, increased to 4 to 8 mg.

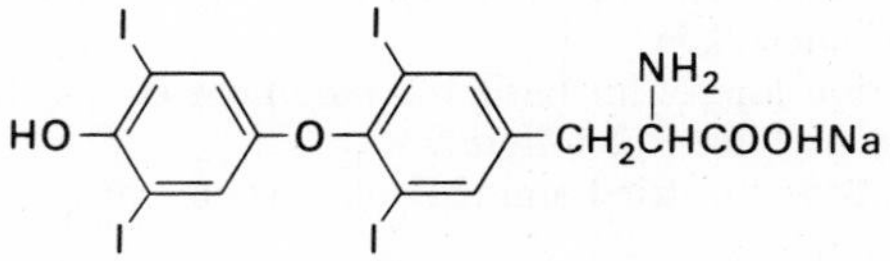

I I I I HO O NH2 $CH_2CHCOOHNa$

DETROTHYRONINE (Dextro-triiodothyronine)

Dose: 1.5 to 2 mg by mouth daily.

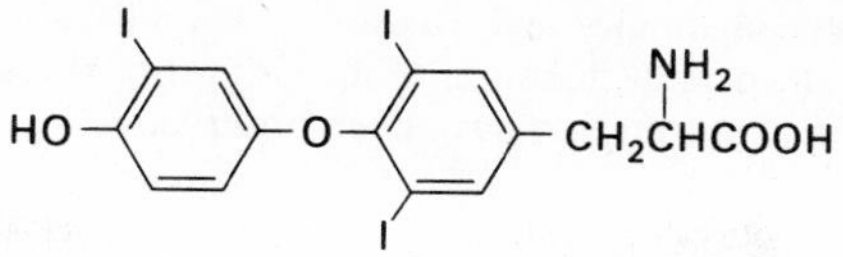

THYROPROPIC ACID (Triiodothyropropionic acid; T_3PROP; Triopron)

Dose: 1 to 3 or 4 mg daily by mouth in hypercholesterolemia, myxedema, or gout.

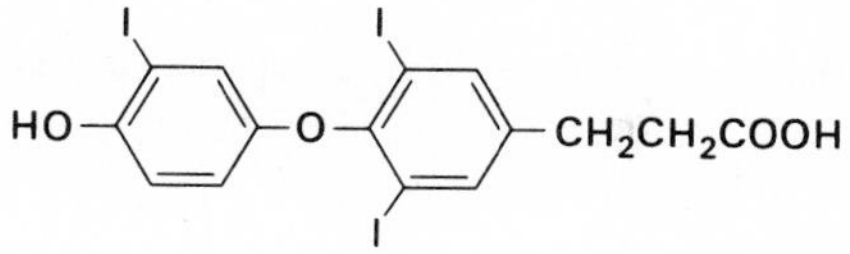

OTHERS

Thyromedan HCl; triiodothyroacetic acid (TRIAC); triiodothyroformic acid.

C. Agents Inhibiting Cholesterol Synthesis

LIPOTROPIC AGENTS

Among the earliest attempts to prevent atherosclerosis was the use of lipotropic agents. This was based on the observation that deficiency of lipotropic agents (which could contribute labile methyl groups to syntheses) produced atherosclerosis in animals, remedial by their readministration. Choline, methionine, lecithin, inositol, and whole liver were among the agents tried in human disease. The results were not encouraging, probably because of the adequate supply of substances contributing labile methyl groups in the ordinary diet. The use of lipotropic agents in atherosclerosis now appears to be obsolete.

NICOTINIC ACID

1. History. Altschul (1954) and Hoffer (1955) showed that large doses of nicotinic acid reduced serum cholesterol in man and rabbits.

2. Chemistry. (See Vitamins.)

3. Action. Serum cholesterol may be lowered over the course of several days (for instance from a serum level of 200 to 160 mg %) by large doses of nicotinic acid.

4. Mechanism. a. Cholesterol synthesis requires coenzyme A. Nicotinic acid is detoxified in the body to nicotinuric acid, which also requires coenzyme A, and thereby may reduce the amount available for cholesterol synthesis (Schön, Nature, 182:534, 1958).

b. An insulinlike action and lowered free fatty acid levels have been reported.

c. However, others believe that the effects are simply the result of dilated vessels and increased circulation.

5. Pharmacodynamics and Toxicity. Rapidly absorbed with the production of unpleasant transient flushing, but without serious toxic effects. Reversible abnormalities in liver function have been observed.

6. Uses. a. Although nicotinic acid is capable of lowering serum cholesterol, and is used to some extent for this purpose, long-term benefits have yet to be confirmed.

b. Most patients dislike it intensely because of the uncomfortable flushing and pruritus.

7. Preparations

NICOTINIC ACID (Niacin)

Dose: 1 gm 3 to 6 times a day by mouth; may be given in buffered solution to avoid the effects of the acidity.

COOH
N

ALUMINUM NICOTINATE (Nicalex)

May reduce flushing and gastric irritation.
Dose: 1 to 2 gm of nicotinic acid equivalent.

COO—Al—OOC
OH
N N

XANTHINOL NIACINATE (Complamin)

Dose: Under investigation.

CH_3
O CH_2CHCH_2—N
H_3C N OH CH_2CH_2OH
N COOH
O N N
CH_3 N

TRIPARANOL

1. Chemistry. Distant relationship to chlorotrianisene (estrogen precursor) and amotriphen (vasodilator).

2. Action and Mechanism. a. Lowers blood cholesterol by inhibiting 75% or more of endogenous synthesis. Tissue as well as blood cholesterol is reduced, including cholesterol in the bile and the adrenal.

b. Inhibition of synthesis of cholesterol in the liver at a final step before the formation of cholesterol, probably at desmosterol, which accumulates in larger than normal amounts.

3. Pharmacodynamics and Toxicity. a. Apparently well absorbed.

b. Metabolic end products excreted largely in the stool (from bile).

c. Reported to be ineffective in the presence of liver disease.

d. Nausea and vomiting with higher doses; albuminuria, but renal function said not to be impaired; rashes; euphoria with high doses; alopecia, loss of hair color, ichthyosis, cataracts.

4. Uses. a. Before withdrawal from the market because of its toxicity it had been shown that about 90% of patients slowly developed a decrease in blood cholesterol, of the order of 50 mg%.

b. A large number of compounds related to triparanol have come into investigation, but none is of general clinical use.

5. Preparation

TRIPARANOL (MER/29)

Withdrawn from market because of toxicity.

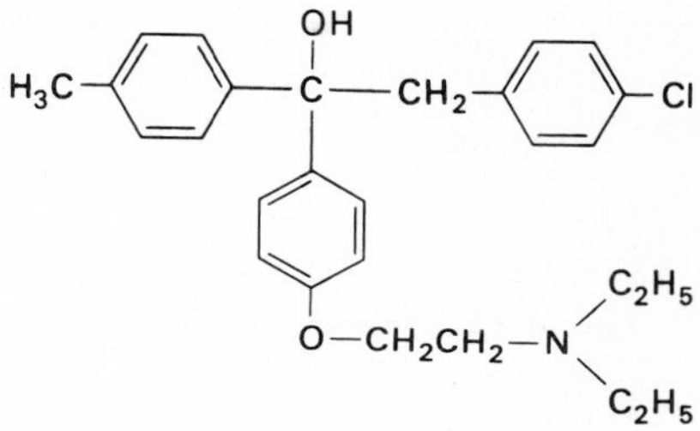

CLOFIBRATE GROUP

1. Chemistry. Aromatically substituted carboxylic acids.

2. Action and Mechanism. a. Reduce lipids in the blood, and presumably in the tissues, both cholesterol and triglycerides; also may be hypouricemic.

b. Apparently interfere with cholesterol synthesis in the liver, probably between the acetate and mevalonic acid steps.

c. Action may be by displacement of coenzymes or hormones on anionic binding sites on plasma proteins.

3. Pharmacodynamics. a. Well absorbed from the gastrointestinal tract.

b. Hydrolyzed in serum to free acid, which is highly bound to plasma proteins.

c. Largely excreted in the urine as the glucuronide.

4. Toxicity. a. May cause nausea, headache, weakness, rashes, muscle cramps; possibly stomatitis, agranulocytosis.

b. Alopecia reported but relationship uncertain.

c. No evidence of accumulation of precursors.

d. Prothrombin time may be prolonged; other evidence of effect on liver may be seen, such as increased SGOT.

5. Uses. a. Used in patients with hypercholesterolemia or hypertriglyceridemia; xanthomas generally respond poorly.

b. Under trial in atherosclerosis, especially when there is evidence of coronary disease; effect not yet evaluated, but decreases in blood cholesterol of 10% to 30% reported.

6. Preparations

PROBUCOL (Biphenabid)

Dose: 0.5 gm twice a day by mouth.

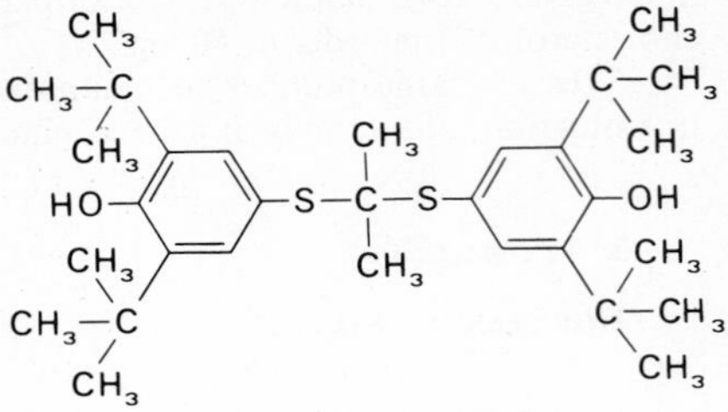

CLOFIBRATE (Atromid S)

Dose: 0.5 gm 4 times a day by mouth.

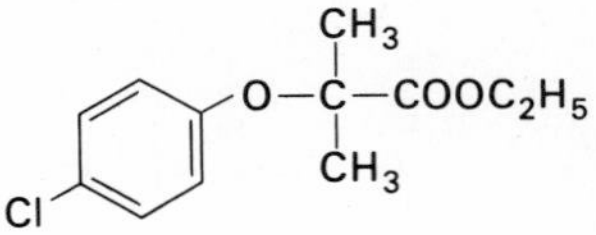

NAFENOPIN

May inhibit acetyl CoA carboxylate.
Dose: 100 to 200 mg 3 times a day by mouth.

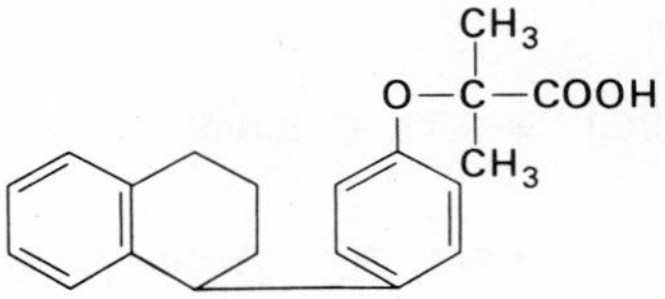

TRELOXINATE

Under investigation.

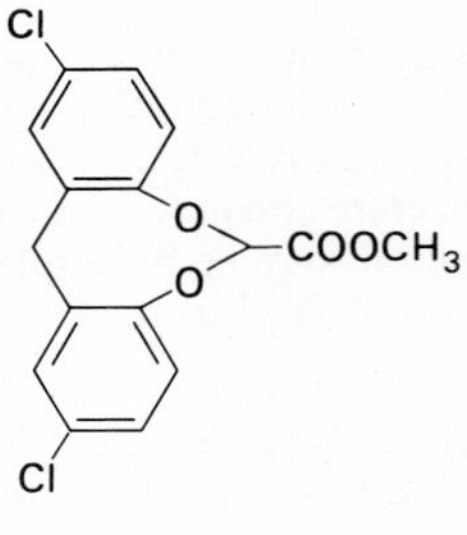

OTHER AGENTS

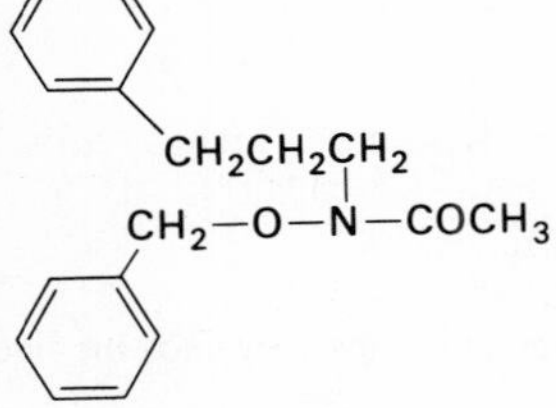

beloxamide

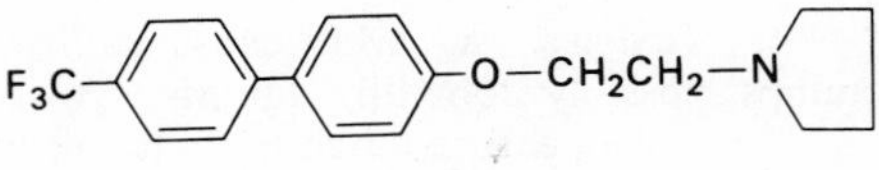

boxidine

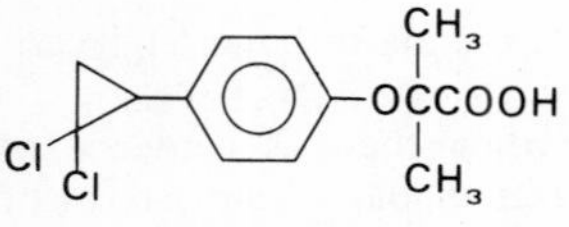

ciprofibrate

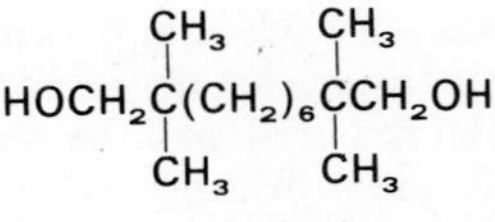

gemcadiol

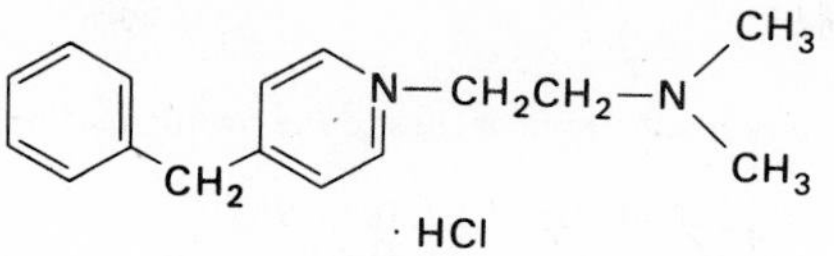

pimetine HCl

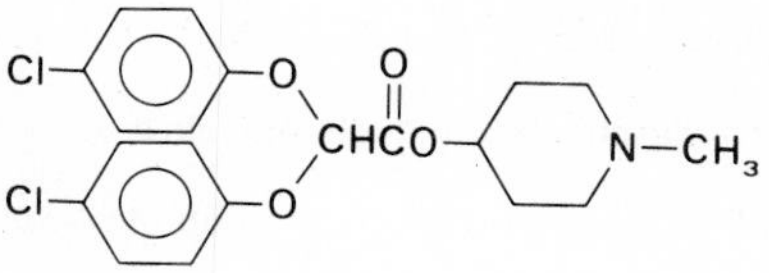

lifibrate

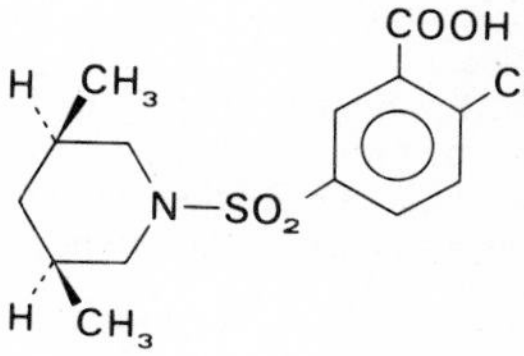

tibric acid

ESTROGENS

High doses (for example, ethinyl estradiol 1 mg daily) reduce plasma cholesterol, but feminizing effects ordinarily preclude their use in males.

SUMMARY: AGENTS IN ATHEROSCLEROSIS

TYPE	*ACTION AND MECHANISM*	*TOXICITY*	*USE*	*EXAMPLES*
Sitosterols	Compete with cholesterol absorption in intestine	Fecal impaction	Hypercholesterolemia, xanthomas	Colestipol
Unsaturated fatty acids	Uncertain	Minor	Hypercholesterolemia	Safflower oil
Heparin	Clears lipemic serum Mechanism not understood	Minor	Atherosclerosis	Heparin
Thyroxine analogues	Breakdown of cholesterol may be accelerated	Hypermetabolism	Same	Dextrothyroxine sodium
Nicotinic acid	May use up coenzyme A needed for cholesterol synthesis	Flushing	Same	Nicotinic acid
Clofibrate	Reduces synthesis of cholesterol Mechanism not clear	Minor	Hypercholesterolemia	Clofibrate

Reviews

Steinberg, D. Chemotherapeutic approaches to the problem of hyperlipidemia. Advances Pharmacol., 1:54, 1962.

Florey, H. Atherosclerosis. Endeavour, 22:107, 1963.

Dole, V., Gordis, E., and Bierman, E. Hyperlipemia and arteriosclerosis. New Eng. J. Med., 269:686, 1963.

MacMillan, D. C., Oliver, M., Simpson, J., and Tothill, P. Effects of ethylchlorophenoxyisobutyrate on weight, plasma volume, total body water and free fatty acids. Lancet, 2:924, 1965.

Pinter, K., and Van Italie, T. Drugs and atherosclerosis. Ann. Rev. Pharmacol., 6:251, 1966.

Orgain, E., Bogdonoff, M., and Cain, C. Clofibrate and androsterone effect on serum lipids. Arch. Int. Med., 119:80, 1967.

Hunninghake, D., Tucker, D., and Azarnoff, D. Long-term effects of clofibrate on serum lipids in man. Circulation, 39:675, 1969.

23. Hypotensive Agents

The clinical picture of essential hypertension is familiar, but the underlying cause remains mysterious in most instances. It is generally considered that hypertension is produced by increased peripheral resistance as a result of increased tone in the arterioles and precapillary sphincters. In general, basic therapy includes a thiazide diuretic supplemented if necessary by phenobarbital or rauwolfia in mild hypertension, by hydralazine or methyldopa in moderate disease, and by guanethidine or a ganglion blocker in severe hypertension.

Despite some lack of unanimity on the fundamental question of whether a high blood pressure should be lowered, especially in benign as contrasted to malignant hypertension, for many years therapeutic attempts to do so have been actively pursued. It is now evident that treatment is usually advisable. The traditional sedation with phenobarbital was supplemented in the 1930's by treatment with thiocyanate but in a few years the latter was abandoned as ineffective and dangerous. Modern therapy began in the 1940's with the ganglion blocking agent tetraethylammonium and now many drugs of this type, as well as others with central or peripheral action are used.

Most of the agents used in hypertension decrease sympathetic vasomotor tone, some by multiple mechanisms. Examples are shown in the following diagram:

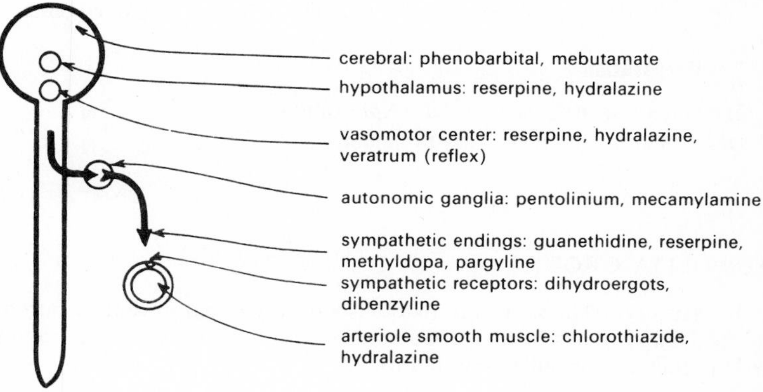

A. Centrally Acting Agents

A number of agents produce hypotension at least in part by central effects. Some, like phenobarbital and mebutamate, do not act specifically on the hypertension, but are general sedatives affecting ultimately the sensory cortex. Others exert a more specific effect, but often with accompanying peripheral actions as well.

HYDRALAZINE

1. Chemistry. A hydrazine derivative of phthalazine.

2. Action and Mechanism. a. Produces peripheral vasodilatation, possibly by acting directly on arteriolar smooth muscle.

b. In spite of the hypotension, blood flow through the kidneys and coronary arteries is not impaired.

3. Mechanism. Biochemical mechanism unknown but suggestions include chelation, inhibition of enzymatic reactions involving pyridoxal, or MAO inhibition.

4. Pharmacodynamics. a. Absorption presumably rapid, as effects are manifest in two hours.

b. Traces appear in the urine for 24 hours but fate of major portion unknown.

5. Toxicity. a. Minor side effects common: postural hypotension, angina, anxiety, headache, vomiting, tachycardia; occasional edema, urticaria, and polyneuritis.

b. Most severe toxic manifestation is acute systemic lupus erythematosus and a rheumatoid arthritis-like picture, which usually disappears when the drug is withdrawn.

6. Uses. a. To lower the blood pressure in hypertension, particularly moderately severe essential hypertension.

b. Use decreasing because of availability of less toxic newer agents.

7. Preparation

HYDRALAZINE HYDROCHLORIDE (Apresoline)
Dose: 10 to 50 mg 4 times a day by mouth.

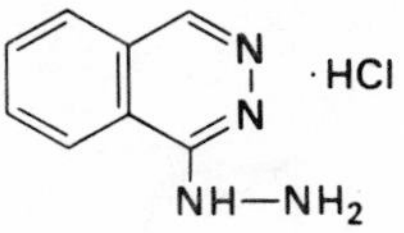

N
N
·HCl
NH—NH$_2$

RAUWOLFIA GROUP

1. History. The rauwolfia alkaloids have been used since their introduction into the United States in the 1950's as antihypertensives as well as tranquilizers (see Tranquilizers for fuller description).

2. Chemistry. Natural and semisynthetic rauwolfia alkaloids.

3. Action and Mechanism. a. Reserpine alkaloids release norepinephrine and serotonin from cellular binding sites, and prevent its reaccumulation in nerve endings, both in the brain and peripherally. The amines are then destroyed by regional enzymes, and the exhausted depots fail to respond to sympathetic stimulation.

b. Accompanying this action is sedation or tranquillity, and hypotension, the latter probably a combination of central sedation and central and peripheral depletion of pressor substances. The central effects are probably less important than the peripheral sympatholytic effects in reducing hypertension.

4. Pharmacodynamics and Toxicity. a. (See Tranquilizers.) Sedation, nightmares, parkinsonism may be troublesome side effects; less pronounced with syrosingopine than with reserpine (but also less hypotensive).

b. Sympatholytic effects: nasal stuffiness, diarrhea, and bleeding from peptic ulcers.

c. Increased incidence of breast cancer upon prolonged use.

5. Uses. The rauwolfia alkaloids alone are only moderately effective hypotensive agents, but are useful adjuncts to more potent agents and may allow reduction of dosage in the latter.

6. Preparations

RESERPINE (Reserpoid, Serpasil, and others)

Dose: 0.1 to 0.25 mg or more 2 to 3 times daily by mouth.

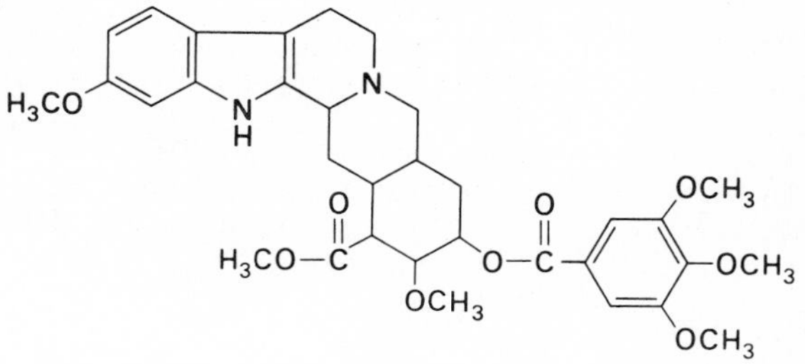

SYROSINGOPINE (Singoserp)

Dose: 0.5 to 1 mg 2 or 3 times a day by mouth.

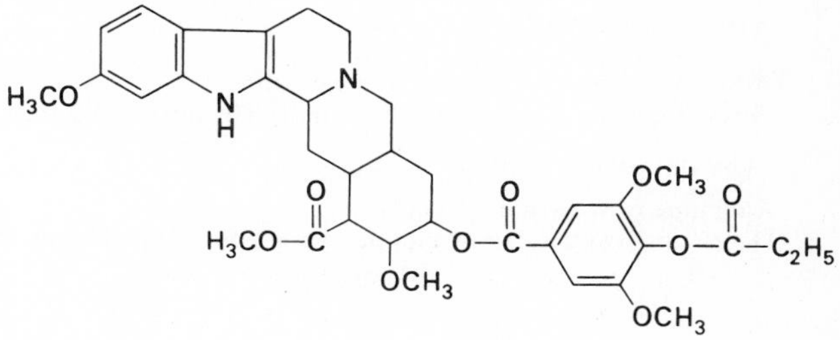

VERATRUM ALKALOIDS

1. Chemistry. *Veratrum viride* and *V. album* (green and white hellebore) are sources for a number of complex alkaloids, including protoveratrines A and B.

2. Action and Mechanism. Veratrum alkaloids stimulate vagal sensory endings in the heart and carotid sinus which reflexly diminish tonic impulses leaving the vasomotor center in the brain and thus lower blood pressure.

3. Pharmacodynamics. a. Variable absorption by mouth.

b. Slowly broken down in the body. Tachyphylaxis and tolerance have not been observed.

4. Toxicity. Flushing, salivation, nausea, relentless vomiting, and hypotensive collapse are severely limiting side effects.

5. Uses. a. Although a powerful agent, the side effects ordinarily limit use to hypertensive crises in which headache, dizziness, delirium, or blurred vision demand rapid relief.

b. Most common use has been in preeclampsia and related conditions.

6. Preparations

PROTOVERATRINES A AND B (Veralba)

Dose: 0.5 mg 4 times a day by mouth; or, more effectively, 0.05 to 0.1 mg intravenously.

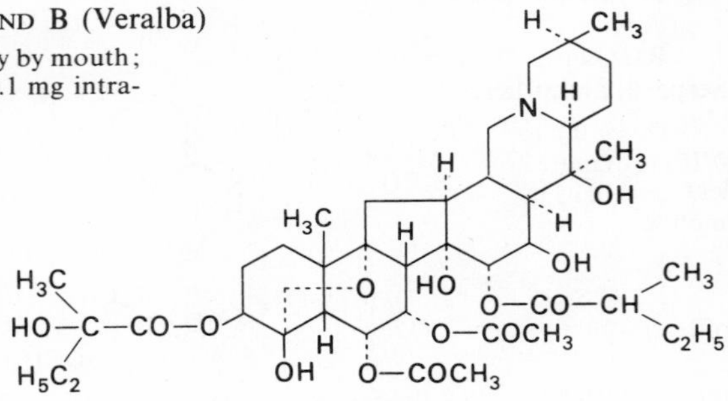

protoveratrine A

Protoveratrine A and B maleates (Provell)
Dose: 0.5 mg 4 times a day by mouth.

ALKAVERVIR (Veriloid)

A highly purified but noncrystalline mixture.
Dose: 3 to 5 mg 3 times a day by mouth; 0.05 mg intravenously.

CRYPTENAMINE (Unitensen)

A mixture of veratrum alkaloids.
Dose: 2 mg twice a day by mouth, increased as needed up to 12 mg daily; 1 mg intravenously.

DIHYDROERGOT PREPARATIONS

Hydrogenation of the components of ergotoxine produces derivatives which lower blood pressure by a central reduction of sympathetic tone together with a peripheral sympatholytic action. In Europe a mixture of these alkaloids, called Hydergine, enjoys limited use but the preparation has been largely replaced by more potent agents. (See Smooth Muscle Stimulants; also Sympathetic Depressants.)

B. Ganglion-Blocking Agents

Tonic impulses to both the parasympathetic and sympathetic peripheral nervous systems may be interrupted by removal or paralysis of the autonomic ganglia. Sympathetic block causes a loss of the impulses which maintain vascular tone, and thus results in a lowering of the blood pressure. Parasympathetic block does not contribute to the hypotension, but causes the side effects of blurred vision, dry mouth and constipation. The surgical operation of sympathectomy was formerly used to achieve sympathetic interruption. Drugs are now much more commonly used, with interruption possible at both ganglia and sympathetic nerve endings to produce hypotension or to improve the blood supply in peripheral vascular disease.

QUATERNARY AMMONIUM COMPOUNDS

1. History. a. Marshall (1914) and Dale and Burn (1915) noted the ganglion blocking properties of tetraethylammonium.

b. Acheson and Moe (1946) introduced modern interest in the agent. (See also Ganglionic Agents.)

2. Chemistry. The representatives of the group possess a structural resemblance to acetylcholine and either one, or more commonly two, quaternary nitrogens; in the latter case they are separated by five or six carbon atoms or their equivalent.

3. Action. a. Produce ganglionic blockade, with interference in the passage of both sympathetic and parasympathetic impulses.

b. The therapeutic effect desired is peripheral arteriolar relaxation from the removal of sympathetic tone. This produces hypotension, particularly when the patient is erect (postural hypotension); other effects are undesirable side actions.

4. Mechanism. The quaternary ammonium compounds presumably compete with acetylcholine for receptors at ganglial synapses.

5. Pharmacodynamics. a. Like other quaternary N compounds, absorption from the intestine is erratic, and existence in the body is primarily extracellular. For consistent therapeutic effects parenteral administration is usually desirable. Chlorisondamine, pentolinium and trimethidium may have enough regularity of absorption by mouth to allow moderately satisfactory treatment of chronic hypertension in other than acute episodes.

b. Tolerance develops gradually with use.

6. Toxicity. a. The principal side effects from sympathetic blockade include excessive postural hypotension and impaired cerebral circulation.

b. Parasympathetic interference may cause dilated pupils, dry mouth, urinary retension, and particularly constipation.

c. Other hypertensive therapy may markedly increase potency.

7. Uses. a. The members of the group have been used variously for the treatment of acute episodes of hypertension, for chronic hypertension, to produce a "bloodless field" in surgery, to increase circulation in peripheral vascular disease, and for other less certain indications such as causalgia and herpes zoster.

b. Tetraethylammonium was early superseded by hexamethonium, and the latter by pentolinium, chlorisondamine and trimethidium, for the treatment of severe essential hypertension.

c. Phenacylhomatropinium and trimethaphan produce transitory hypotension when given intravenously and have been used to control bleeding in neurosurgical and vascular operations (controlled hypotension).

8. Preparations

CHLORISONDAMINE CHLORIDE
(Ecolid)

Dose: 10 mg once daily by mouth, increased in morning and evening doses over a week or more until a daily dose of 200 mg may be reached; 2.5 mg or more every 8 hours subcutaneously or intramuscularly.

$$\text{Cl}_4\text{-isoindolinium}\ \overset{+}{N}(CH_3)-CH_2CH_2-\overset{+}{N}(CH_3)_3 \cdot 2Cl^-$$

HEXAMETHONIUM CHLORIDE
(Bistrium; Esomid; Methium)

Dose: 125 mg 4 times a day by mouth, increasing the dose as tolerance develops; or, with more consistency of effect, 50 to 100 mg intramuscularly; practically obsolete.

$$(H_3C)_3\overset{+}{N}-CH_2(CH_2)_4CH_2-\overset{+}{N}(CH_3)_3 \cdot 2Cl^-$$

PENTOLINIUM TARTRATE (Ansolysen)

Dose: 20 mg 3 times a day by mouth, increased as tolerance develops. The dose should be adjusted so that the postural hypotension produced is the maximum tolerable to the patient's activities.

$$\text{pyrrolidinium}\ \overset{+}{N}(CH_3)-CH_2CH_2CH_2CH_2CH_2-\overset{+}{N}(CH_3)\ \text{pyrrolidinium} \cdot 2C_4H_5O_6$$

PHENACYLHOMATROPINIUM (Trophenium)

Dose: 0.1% to 0.3% solution by intravenous drip.

$$C_6H_5-CH(OH)-C(=O)-O-CH \ \text{(tropane ring:}\ CH_2, CH, CH_2;\ CH_2, CH, CH_2)\ H_3C-\overset{+}{N}-CH_2-C(=O)-C_6H_5$$

TRIMETHAPHAN CAMSYLATE (Arfonad)

Dose: 0.1% solution by intravenous drip.

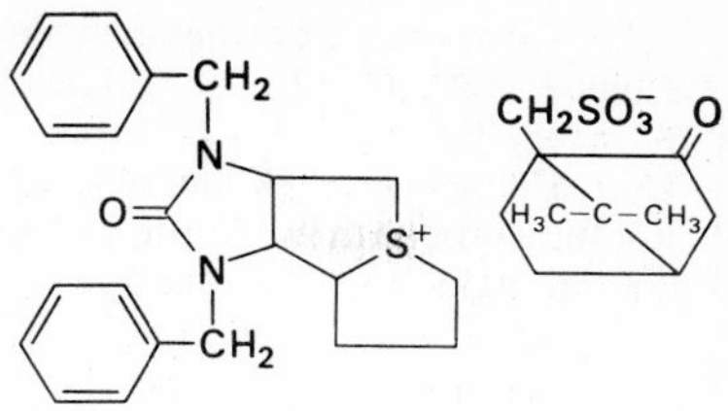

TRIMETHIDINIUM METHOSULFATE (Ostensin; Camphidonium)

Dose: 20 mg twice a day by mouth, increased as required; 1 to 3 mg intravenously.

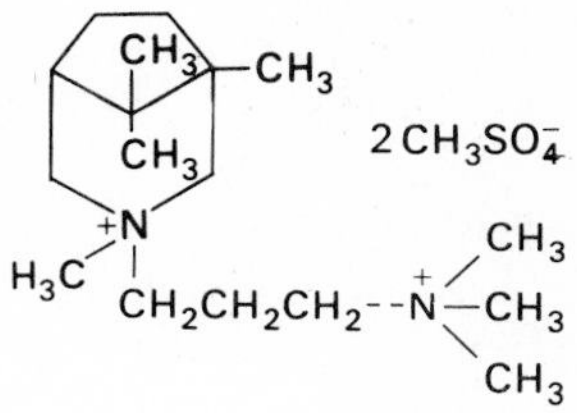

MECAMYLAMINE GROUP

1. **Chemistry.** Secondary amines; may contain a modified camphor nucleus.

2. **Action.** a. Produce ganglionic blockade and hypotension resembling that from the quaternary ammoniums, but the effect is rather more gradual and less subject to sudden hypotension.

b. In addition, a number of other effects are produced. The camphor nucleus appears to be responsible for central stimulation (choreiform movements, malaise, acute mania, seizures); spread of action to the neuromuscular junction produces a mild curare effect, with resultant weakness; smooth muscle may be depressed by a local anesthetic action, enhancing constipation.

3. **Mechanism.** Instead of competing at receptors with acetylcholine as the quaternary ammoniums do, mecamylamine is thought to enter the nerve cells of the ganglia and alter the state of their receptors so that they no longer respond normally to acetylcholine (Bennett, Lancet, 2:218, 1957).

4. **Pharmacodynamics.** a. Unlike the charged ammoniums, absorption is complete from oral administration.

b. Effects are prolonged; administration two or three times a day will give a sustained effect.

c. Tolerance develops only slowly and does not cross with the hexemethonium type.

5. **Toxicity.** a. Profound hypotension, requiring pressor amine therapy, has been observed; glomerular filtration may be impaired by reduced blood pressure.

b. Constipation and paralytic ileus may be indications for laxatives and cholinergic drugs such as bethanechol.

c. Mecamylamine may produce camphor-like central effects as noted under Actions.

6. Uses. Mecamylamine is replacing pentolinium to a considerable extent in the treatment of both moderate and severe hypertension because of the advantage of oral administration.

7. Preparations

MECAMYLAMINE (Inversine)

Dose: 2.5 mg twice daily by mouth, increasing to as much as 75 mg daily.

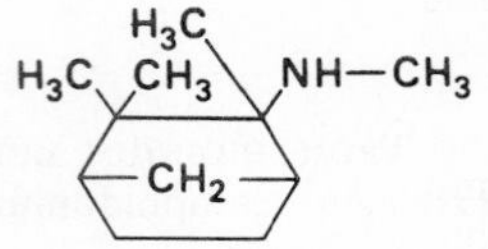

PEMPIDINE (Perolysen)

Faster and shorter acting than mecamylamine.
Dose: 1.25 to 2.5 mg twice daily by mouth.

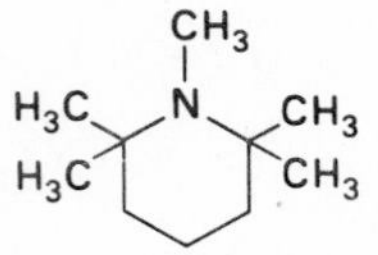

C. Sympatholytic Agents

Sympathetic transmission can be suppressed peripherally, with resultant lowering of vascular tone and hypotension, in two general areas:

a. Nerve endings: Interference in synthesis, storage, or release of norepinephrine. The more effective compounds are of this class.

b. Receptors: Interference in stimulation by norepinephrine.

AMIDINE GROUP

1. History. Guanethidine synthesized by Mull (1957).

2. Chemistry. Relatives of sympathomimetic amines, but with terminal amidine moieties.

3. Actions. a. Orthostatic hypotension, as a result of inhibition of normal pressor effects. (May be venous inhibition with hypotension from decreased cardiac output, rather than arteriolar; Page, J.A.M.A., 175:543, 1961.)

b. The orthostatic characteristics may be severe at first, but later decrease; drop in mean blood pressure about 300 mm erect and 10 mm recumbent.

c. Tolerance does not develop.

4. Mechanism. a. Interfere with the appearance of norepinephrine at sympathetic nerve endings, either by blocking synthesis or preventing release (Maxwell, J. Pharmacol. Exp. Ther., 129:24, 1960).

b. May also release amines from nerve endings (Wylie, Nature, 189:490, 1961) and increase sensitivity of receptor substance (McCubbin, J. Pharmacol. Exp. Ther., 131:340, 1961).

5. Pharmacodynamics. a. Guanethidine is relatively poorly absorbed by mouth, about one quarter of the drug passing through in the feces.

b. Effects last more than 24 hours.

6. Toxicity. a. Sympatholytic side effects noted include nasal stuffiness, drooping eyelids, bradycardia, diarrhea (may be controlled by atropine).

b. Psychotic episodes have also been described.

c. Guanoxan may cause abnormal hepatic function (Frohlich, Clin. Pharmacol. Ther., 7:599, 1966).

7. Uses. a. Valuable in hypertension (Page, J.A.M.A., 170:1255, 1959). Improvement over ganglionic blockers in treating hypertension because of lack of side effects from parasympathetic blockade.

b. May be used alone, or as a supplement to a thiazide or other hypotensive.

c. Ideal dose is that which will just bring the blood pressure to normal when the patient is standing, but without faintness. Cumulation requires careful control until maintenance is established.

8. Preparations

BETHANIDINE SULFATE

Dose: 5 mg 4 times a day, increased slowly to tolerance.

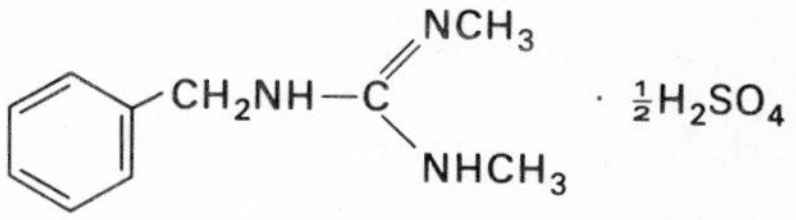

$C_6H_5CH_2NH{-}C(=NCH_3)NHCH_3 \cdot \frac{1}{2}H_2SO_4$

CLONIDINE HYDROCHLORIDE (Catapres)

Dose: 0.15 to 0.3 mg 3 times a day by mouth.

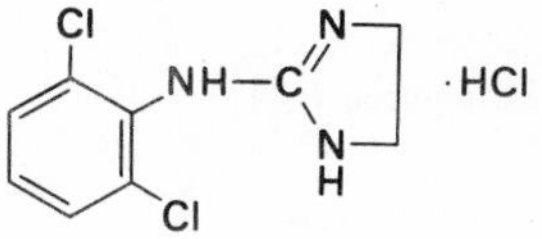

Cl, Cl, NH—C, N, N, H · HCl

DEBRISOQUIN SULFATE (Declinax)

Dose: 40 to 80 mg per day by mouth.

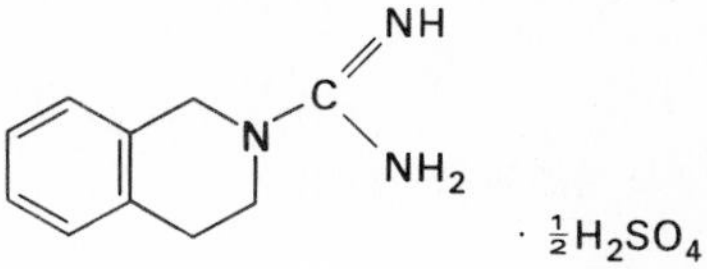

N, C, NH, NH_2 $\cdot \frac{1}{2}H_2SO_4$

GUANADREL SULFATE

Dose: 10 to 100 mg 3 to 4 times a day by mouth.

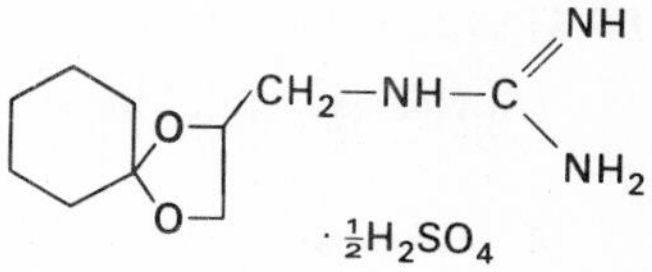

O, O, $CH_2{-}NH{-}C(=NH)NH_2$ $\cdot \frac{1}{2}H_2SO_4$

GUANETHIDINE SULFATE (Ismelin)

Dose: 10 mg twice a day by mouth, up to 50 mg 4 times a day if necessary.

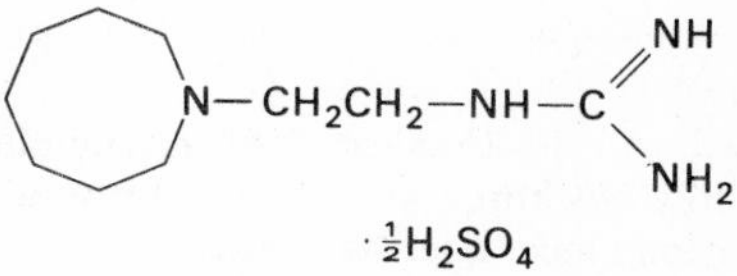

$N{-}CH_2CH_2{-}NH{-}C(=NH)NH_2$ $\cdot \frac{1}{2}H_2SO_4$

GUANOXAN SULFATE (Envacar)
Dose: 25 mg 3 times a day by mouth.

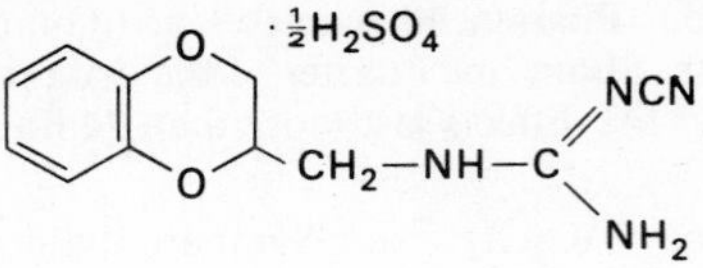

$\cdot\frac{1}{2}H_2SO_4$

NCN
CH₂—NH—C
NH₂

OTHERS

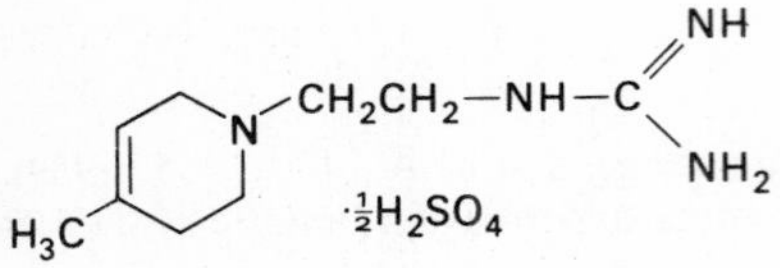

granacline sulfate

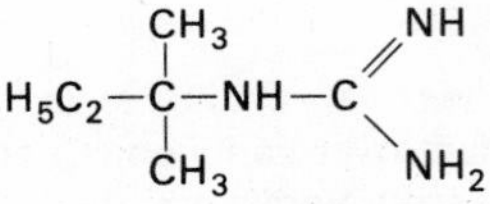

guancydine

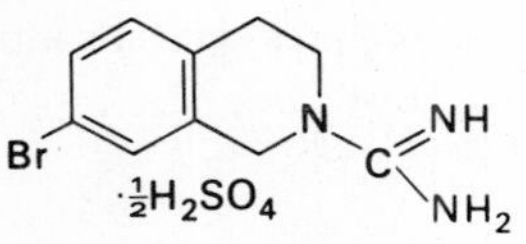

guanisoquin sulfate

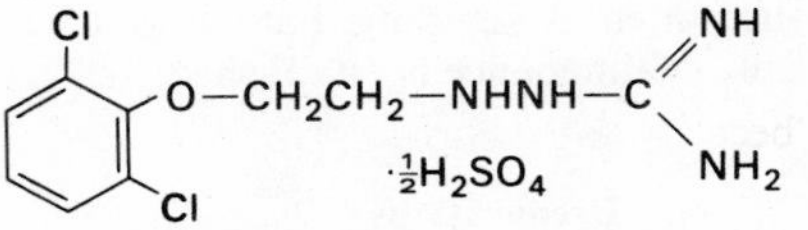

guanoclor sulfate (Vatensol)

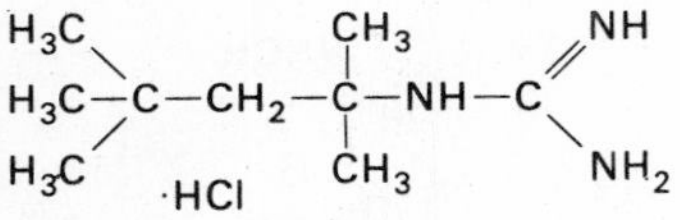

guanoctine HCl

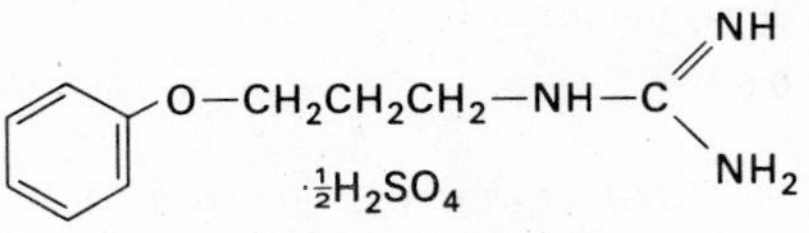

guanoxyfen sulfate

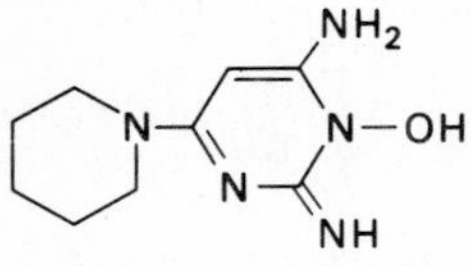

minoxidil (PDP)

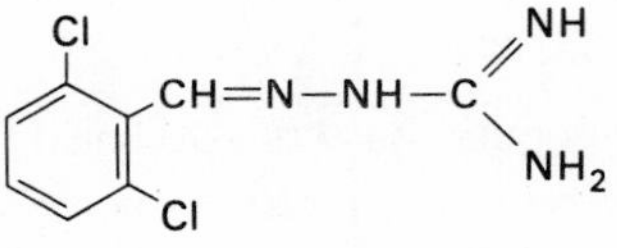

guanoxabenz

BRETYLIUM

1. **History.** Introduced by Boura (1959).

2. **Chemistry.** A quaternary N compound.

3. **Action.** Sympatholytic; producing hypotension.

4. **Mechanism.** a. Accumulates in postganglionic sympathetic fibers, probably blocking synthesis or release of norepinephrine; also impairs conduction by a strong local anesthetic effect at nerve terminals.

b. Does not block end organ receptors and therefore circulating norepinephrine and epinephrine are not interfered with. It increases the sensitivity to norepinephrine and epinephrine, like sympathectomy, and is thus potentially dangerous in pheochromocytoma.

c. There are no ganglionic effects, nor parasympathetic effects except with extratherapeutic doses.

d. Tolerance develops rapidly.

5. Pharmacodynamics. Absorption poor by mouth (quaternary), but effects begin in about 2 hours and last up to 9 hours.

6. Toxicity. a. Side effects include nasal congestion, muscular weakness, severe facial (parotid) pain, mental confusion.

b. Notably lacking are the parasympatholytic effects of ganglionic blockade: blurred vision, dry mouth, constipation.

7. Uses. Used in hypertension, but less satisfactory than guanethidine because of the earlier development of tolerance; now little used.

8. Preparation

BRETYLIUM TOSYLATE (Darenthin)

Dose: 0.1 to 0.3 gm 3 times a day by mouth initially; 0.2 to 0.6 gm 3 times a day, maintenance.

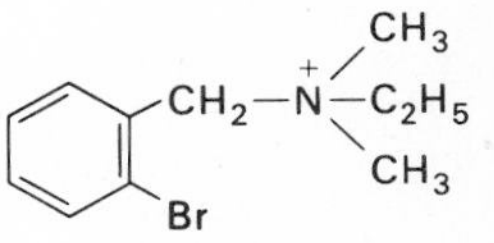

CH_3
$CH_2-\overset{+}{N}-C_2H_5$
CH_3
Br

METHYLDOPA

1. Chemistry. Methyl derivative of precursor of norepinephrine.

2. Action. a. Produces orthostatic hypotension and tranquility, possibly as a result of a reduction of brain and peripheral norepinephrine, dopamine, and serotonin.

b. Potentiated by thiazides; tolerance does not develop.

3. Mechanism.

a. Metabolized to alpha-methylnorepinephrine, a weak transmitter replacing norepinephrine, a strong transmitter.

b. The action is primarily in the central nervous system.

4. Pharmacodynamics. a. Absorption relatively poor; peak blood level by four hours.

b. Maximal lowering of blood pressure appears by second day; excretion complete in 24 hours.

5. Toxicity. Sedation frequent; occasional dry mouth, edema, weight gain, drug fever, psychic depression, aggravation of asthma, impaired liver function, elevated SGOT, hemolytic anemia, positive Coombs test. Occasional postural hypotension.

6. Uses. Useful agent in severe essential hypertension; effect may be enhanced by small doses of guanethidine or a thiazide.

7. Preparation

METHYLDOPA (alpha-methyldopa; Aldomet)

Dose: 0.25 gm 3 times a day by mouth, increased to 0.5 gm or more.

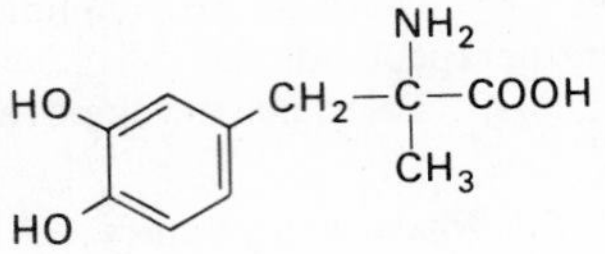

METHYLDOPATE HYDROCHLORIDE (Aldomet Ester)

Dose: 0.25 to 0.5 gm every 6 hours intravenously.

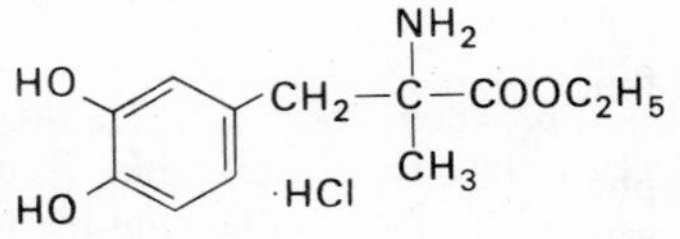

OTHERS

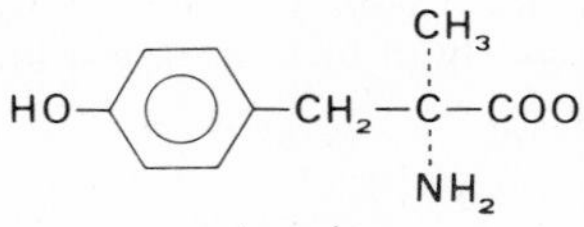

metyrosine

MAO INHIBITORS: PARGYLINE

1. Chemistry. Nonhydrazide, MAO inhibitor (see Psychic Stimulants).

2. Action and Mechanism. a. Produces long-lasting hypotension.

b. As a result of MAO inhibition, weak, "false" catecholamines are thought to collect in vascular smooth muscle, lessening its response to norepinephrine, but mechanism not established.

3. Pharmacodynamics and Toxicity. a. Oral absorption good; onset of action may be immediate or delayed several days; excreted in urine, largely unchanged.

b. Toxicity: Drowsiness or excitement, constipation, dizziness, paresthesias, hallucinations, inability to ejaculate, hypoglycemia.

c. Potentiation of other drugs with CNS or ganglionic effects: hypertensive crises when taken with sympathomimetic amines or foods containing amines (amphetamine, ephedrine, cheese, beer, wine), or other MAO inhibitors; hypotensive crises when taken with sedatives, tranquilizers, antihistamines, narcotics, alcohol.

4. Uses. Generally effective agent in moderate to severe hypertension (Maronde, J.A.M.A., 184:7, 1963).

5. Preparation

PARGYLINE (Eutonyl)

Dose: 25 to 50 mg once daily by mouth, increased to 75 or 100 mg.

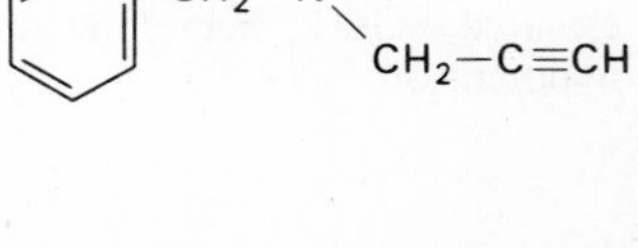

D. Thiazides

The blood pressure in essential hypertension can usually be lowered by severe restriction of dietary salt (to as little as 6 mEq daily), but the regimen need be much less strict when a thiazide diuretic is taken at the same time.

THIAZIDE DIURETICS

1. Chemistry. See Thiazide Diuretics.

2. Action and Mechanism. a. Initially, loss of Na and Cl, giving reduction of fluid volume in vessels and tissues.

b. Later, reduction of Na and water content of vessel walls decreases peripheral resistance. Some question of direct relaxation of smooth muscle in vessel walls.

c. The loss of sodium and chloride, with a resultant decrease in plasma volume may be the primary mechanism.

d. Alternatively, the walls of arterioles may contain excessive water (noted in rats), resulting in a decreased lumen, which can be restored by depletion of this water, or smooth muscle may be relaxed directly.

3. Pharmacodynamics and Toxicity. See Diuretics.

4. Uses. As adjuncts to other hypotensives and to a low sodium diet in the treatment of hypertension.

5. Preparation

HYDROCHLOROTHIAZIDE (Hydrodiuril, Esidrix)
Dose: 25 to 50 mg once or twice daily by mouth.

NONDIURETIC THIAZIDES: DIAZOXIDE

1. Action and Mechanism. a. Immediate prolonged hypotension without diuresis.

b. Result of direct, peripheral arteriolar dilatation (Rubin, J. Pharmacol. Exp. Ther., 140:46, 1963). Systolic and diastolic pressures reduced; cardiac output not impaired.

c. Cause marked salt and water retention; oxytocin inhibited.

2. Pharmacodynamics. Absorbed adequately by mouth; effective in 5 minutes after intravenous injection, with action lasting 4 to 6 hours.

3. Toxicity. Anorexia, vomiting, lacrimation, tachycardia, edema; hirsutism; increased uric acid; neutropenia, thrombopenia; orthostatic hypotension, shock; hyperglycemia.

4. Uses. a. Have been used for acute hypertensive crises, especially episodes in preeclampsia, pheochromocytoma, acute heart failure, encephalopathy, acute glomerular nephritis.

b. Use in chronic hypertension not advised because of the diabetic syndrome produced as a side effect.

c. Have been used for their hyperglycemic effects, especially in leucine-sensitive hypoglycemia, and islet cell tumours.

d. Under trial as a uterine relaxant.

5. Preparation

DIAZOXIDE (Hyperstat)

Dose: 75 to 300 mg twice daily by mouth; 300 mg intravenously (give in 30 seconds) up to 4 times a day.

Also used orally as an antihypoglemic.

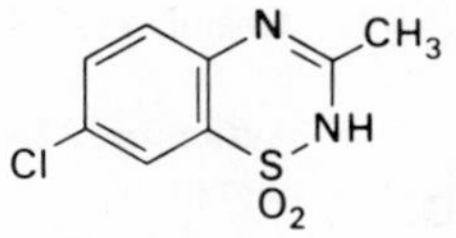

PAZOXIDE

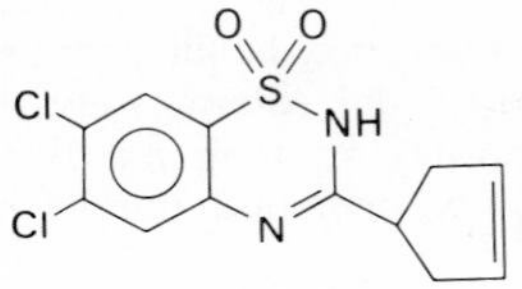

E. Antiserotonins

Serotonin stimulates vascular smooth muscle and when produced in excess by carcinoid tumors causes pulmonary stenosis, and periodic cyanosis and flushing. Despite these and other actions (see Psychotomimetic Agents) the normal role of serotonin in health is not understood. However, some antiserotonins (but not all) have been found to reduce blood pressure, presumably by counteracting an excessive amount of serotonin and thus preventing arteriolar vasoconstriction.

Although highly experimental, a number of antiserotonins have been tried clinically in hypertension. Intolerable sedation or insomnia, and even psychotic manifestations, have been limiting side effects with some of the compounds; however, they are of interest and some promise.

F. Angiotensin II. Inhibitors

Block Angiotensin receptors competitively. Lower elevated blood pressure.

SARALASIN ACETATE

Under investigation.

Sar-Arg-Val-Tyr-Val-His-Pro-Ala $\cdot$ $\chi CH_3COOH \cdot \chi H_2O$
1 2 3 4 5 6 7 8

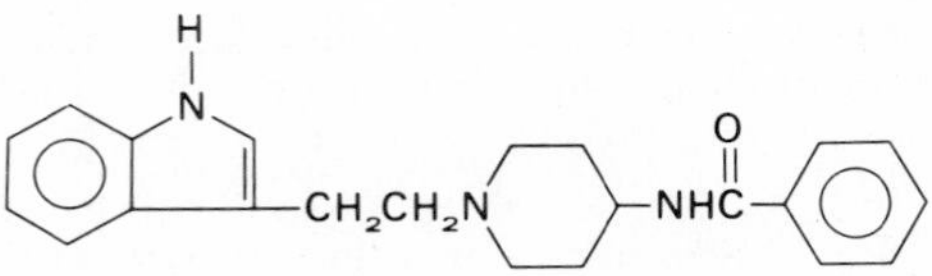

CH_2CH_2N NHC

indoramin

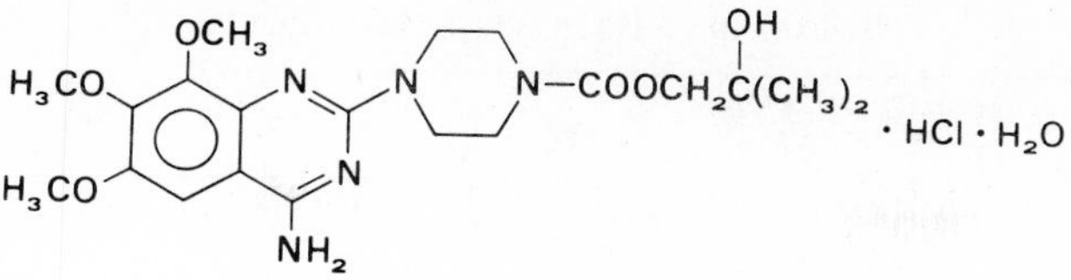

trimazosin hydrochloride

G. Quinolines and Related Compounds

HYPOTENSIVE PAPAVERINE RELATIVES

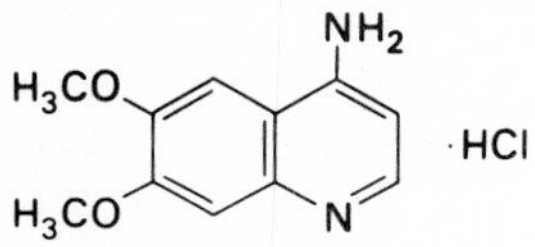

amiquinsin hydrochloride

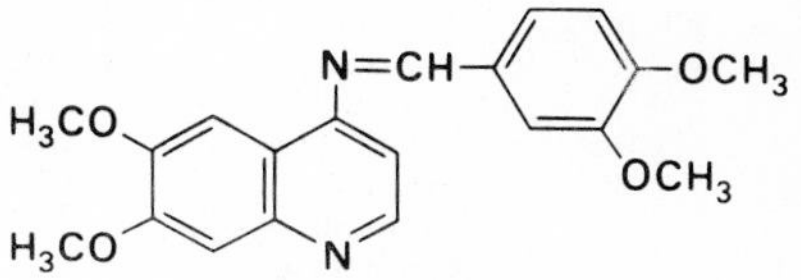

leniquinsin

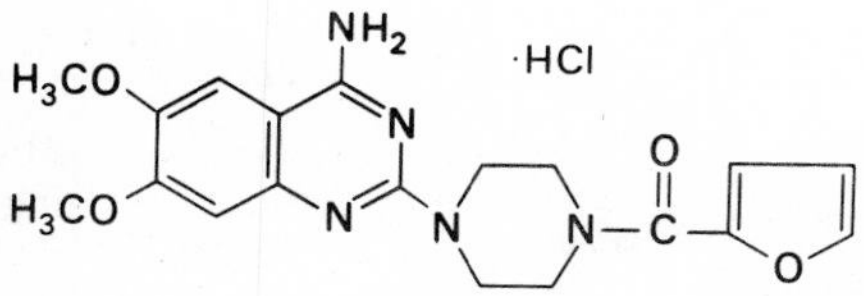

prazosin HCl

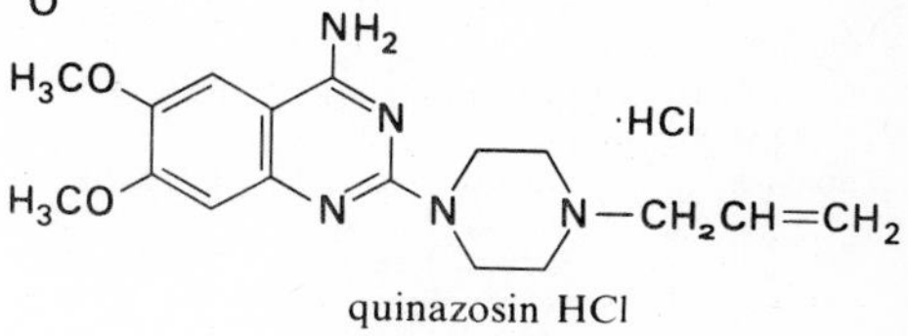

quinazosin HCl

BRONCHODILATOR PAPAVERINE RELATIVES

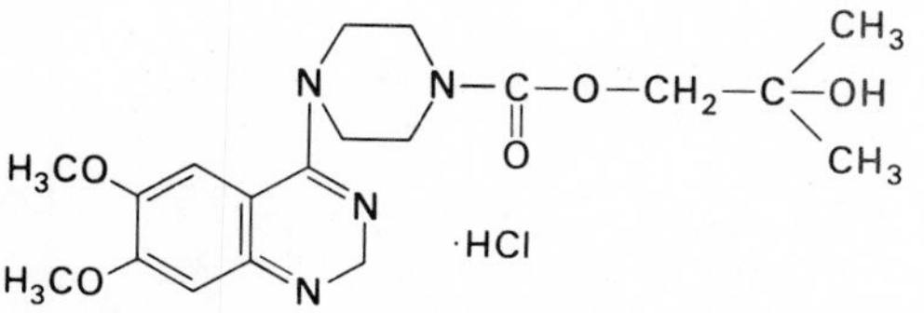

hoquizil HCl

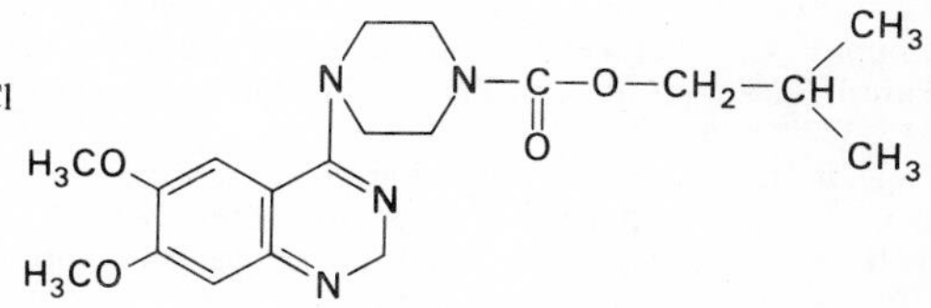

piquizil HCl

SUMMARY: HYPOTENSIVE AGENTS

TYPE	*ACTION AND MECHANISM*	*TOXICITY*	*USE*	*EXAMPLES*
Hydralazine	Sympatholytic, possibly by blocking receptors	Lupus erythematosus	Hypertension	Hydralazine
Rauwolfia group	Exhaust norepinephrine from cellular stores	Sedation, nightmares, parkinsonism	Same	Reserpine
Veratrum	Reflex through vasomotor center	Vomiting, collapse	Hypertensive crises	Protoveratrines A and B
Ganglionic blockers	Reduce sympathetic tone by ganglionic blockage, probably by competition with acetylcholine	Postural hypotension, dry mouth, urinary retention	Hypertension	Mecamylamine
Sympatholytic group	Sympathetic interference at nerve endings or receptors	Nasal stuffiness, bradycardia, diarrhea	Same	Guanethidine sulfate
MAO inhibitors	Collection of false catecholamines in vessel smooth muscle	Paresthesias, hallucinations	Same	Pargyline
Thiazides	Loss of Na reduces blood volume and later volume of blood vessels	K loss	Same	Hydrochloro-thiazide

Reviews

Green, A. F. Antihypertensive drugs. Advances Pharmacol., 1:162, 1962.
Fawaz, G. Cardiovascular pharmacology. Ann. Rev. Pharmacol., 3:57, 1963.
Copp, F. C. Adrenergic neurone blocking agents. Advances Drug Res., 1:161, 1964.
Pardo, E., Vargas, R., and Vidrio, H. Antihypertensive drug action. Ann. Rev. Pharmacol., 5:77, 1965.
Page, I. H. Drug treatment of arterial hypertension. Clin. Pharmacol. Ther., 7:567, 1966.
Bender, A. Antihypertensive agents. Topics Med. Chem., 1:177, 1967.
Tobian, L. Why do thiazide diuretics lower blood pressure in essential hypertension? Ann. Rev. Pharmacol., 7:399, 1967.
Brent, A., et al. Mechanisms of antihypertensive drug therapy. J.A.M.A., 211:480, 1970.

24. Smooth Muscle Relaxants

The smooth muscle in the walls of various types of hollow viscera may be relaxed by drugs. Thus, vasodilators may relax the smooth muscle in blood vessels, bronchodilators that in the bronchial tree, and antispasmodics that in the gastrointestinal, biliary, urinary and uterine tracts.

The smooth muscle relaxants are of two types:

a. Direct action on smooth muscle. Examples: nitrites (considered in this chapter).

b. Action primarily via the autonomic nerve supply. Examples: isoproterenol, atropine (considered in the chapters on sympathetic stimulants and parasympathetic depressants).

A. Nitrites and Nitrates

1. Chemistry. Nitrites and nitrate esters of sugars or polyols.

2. Action. a. Relaxation of the involuntary muscle of the blood vessels, both arteries and veins, and of the intestines, biliary tree, and ureter, more or less impartially.

b. All blood vessels are not equally affected, but vasodilatation is marked in the coronary arteries and in cerebral, splanchnic, and cutaneous vessels. Dilatation of small postcapillary vessels leads to venous pooling of blood. Blood flow may be increased with only minimal decrease in blood pressure. Intraocular pressure is increased. Tolerance may develop.

c. Increase in oxygenation from vasodilatation exceeds diminution from methemoglobin formation in therapeutic range.

d. In angina pectoris when plaques in large coronary vessels limit flow, relief may be the result of decreased cardiac work. This may be the result of peripheral vasodilatation induced by the nitrite.

3. Mechanism. The action is directly upon smooth muscle, without involvement of autonomic nerves or receptors, but the mechanism is not understood.

4. Pharmacodynamics. a. The rapidly acting compounds are quickly absorbed from the respiratory tract or from mucous membranes (glyceryl trinitrate) and act fleetingly within minutes; the more slowly acting compounds are absorbed from the alimentary tract and act over several hours.

b. All the compounds are broken down in the tissues.

5. Toxicity. a. Large doses may produce throbbing headache, flushing of the face, palpitation and fainting.

b. Nitrite ion may produce methemoglobinemia.

6. Uses. a. The rapidly acting compounds are widely used to relieve the pain in angina pectoris, and occasionally to relieve spasm in biliary or urinary tracts.

b. The slowly acting compounds are also widely used for assumed value in the prevention of angina and in hypertension, but the results are usually both modest and inconsistent.

7. Preparations

a. Rapidly acting

AMYL NITRITE

Dose: 0.2 ml by inhalation from a "pearl."

CH_2-NO_2
CH_2
$CH-CH_3$
CH_3

GLYCERYL TRINITRATE (nitroglycerin)

The most useful of the series.

Dose: 0.4 mg sublingually; may be taken in anticipation of anginal pain as a prophylactic.

CH_2-O-NO_2
$CH-O-NO_2$
CH_2-O-NO_2

OCTYL NITRITE

Little used.

Dose: 1% solution from an inhaler.

CH_2-NO_2
$CH-C_2H_5$
$(CH_2)_3$
CH_3

SODIUM NITRITE ($NaNO_2$)

Used to produce methemoglobinemia in cyanide poisoning.

Dose: 300 to 500 mg intravenously.

SODIUM NITROPRUSSIDE [$Na_2Fe(CN)_5NO$]

Used in hypertensive crisis.

Can cause cyanide poisoning (Medical Letter, 17:82, 1975).

b. Slowly acting

CLONITRATE (Dylate)

Dose: 0.6 mg by mouth.

H_2-C-Cl
$H-C-O-NO_2$
$H_2-C-O-NO_2$

ERYTHRITYL TETRANITRATE (Erythrol tetranitrate)

Dose: 30 mg by mouth, or 5 to 15 mg sublingually.

CH_2-O-NO_2
$CH-O-NO_2$
$CH-O-NO_2$
CH_2-O-NO_2

ISOSORBIDE DINITRATE (Isordil)

Dose: 10 to 40 mg sublingually.

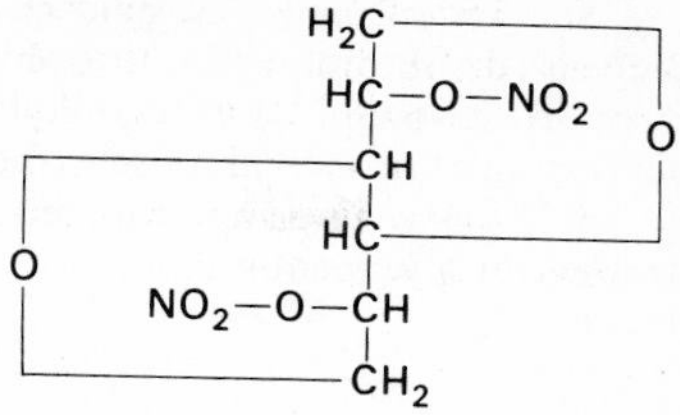

MANNITOL HEXANITRATE (Maxitate; Nitranitol)

Dose: 15 to 60 mg by mouth.

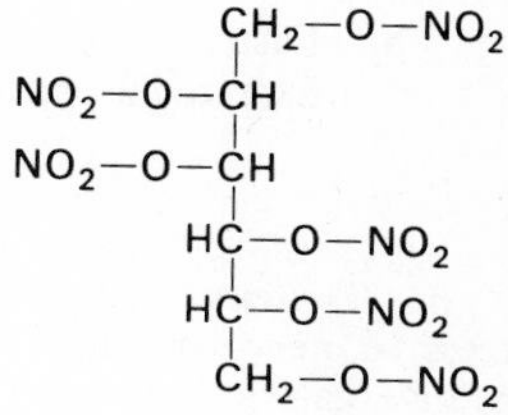

PENTAERYTHRITOL TETRANITRATE (Peritate; Pentritol)

Dose: 10 to 20 mg by mouth.

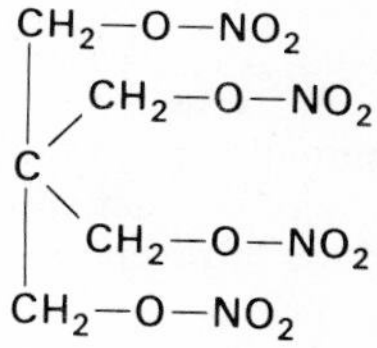

PENTRINITROL

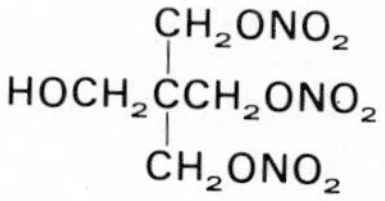

$$HOCH_2C(CH_2ONO_2)_3$$

PROPATYLNITRATE (Etrynit)

Under investigation.

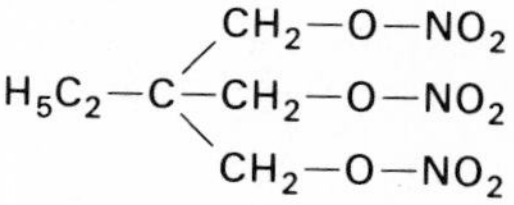

$$H_5C_2-C(CH_2-O-NO_2)_3$$

TROLNITRATE PHOSPHATE (triethanolamine trinitrate diphosphate; Metamine; Nitretamin)

Dose: 2 to 10 mg by mouth.

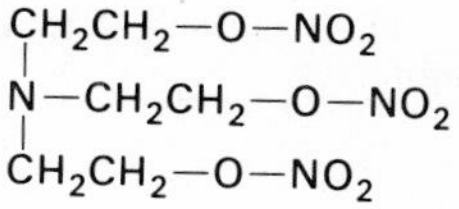

$$N(CH_2CH_2-O-NO_2)_3$$

B. Xanthines

1. History. Naturally occurring members long known in beverages (see Stimulants; Diuretics; and Psychotomimetic Agents).

2. Chemistry. Natural methylated purines, but especially theophylline, and various salts or synthetic modifications.

3. Action and Mechanism. a. Produce central stimulation (caffeine); diuresis (theobromine and theophylline preparations); myocardial stimulation and increased coronary flow (theophylline preparations); bronchial dilatation by direct depression of bronchial muscle (theophylline preparations).

b. Mechanism not understood. Increase 3′,5′-AMP in tissues which in turn accelerates glycogenolysis.

4. Pharmacodynamics. a. Well absorbed by mouth, some moderately well by rectum.

b. Distribution widespread in body, including CNS.

c. Excreted as various metabolic derivatives.

5. Toxicity. Relatively nontoxic. Caffeine may produce extrasystoles, excessive nervous stimulation and insomnia; theophylline preparations often produce gastric irritation; nausea, headache, hypotension, palpitation, and precordial pain may occur with intravenous injection; children particularly sensitive.

6. Uses. Only the theophylline preparations used as smooth muscle relaxants. Aminophylline valuable in bronchial asthma and pulmonary edema, and other theophylline derivatives similarly used. Most satisfactory relief in acute asthma follows intravenous administration.

7. Preparations

AMINOPHYLLINE (theophylline ethylenediamine)

Dose: 0.1 to 0.5 gm by mouth, intramuscularly or intravenously.

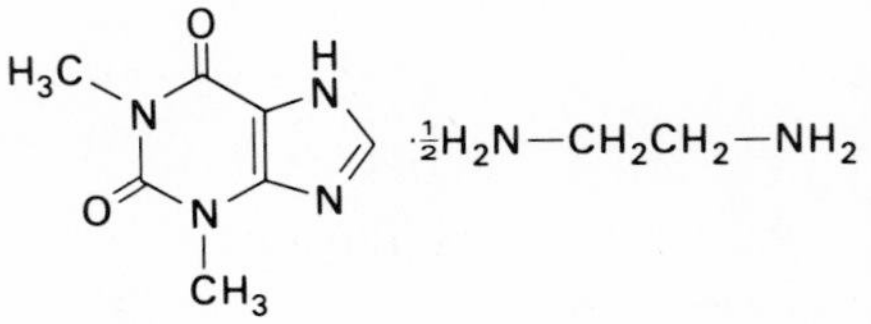

$\cdot \frac{1}{2} H_2N{-}CH_2CH_2{-}NH_2$

DIPHYLLINE

Dose: 200 mg 3 times a day by mouth.

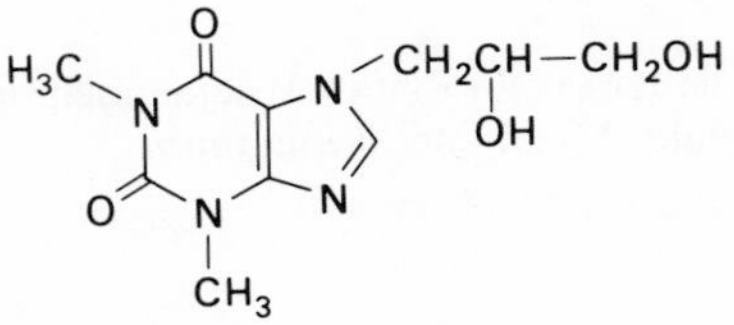

$CH_2CH(OH){-}CH_2OH$

OXTRIPHYLLINE (choline theophyllinate; Choledyl)

Dose: 0.2 gm 3 times a day by mouth.

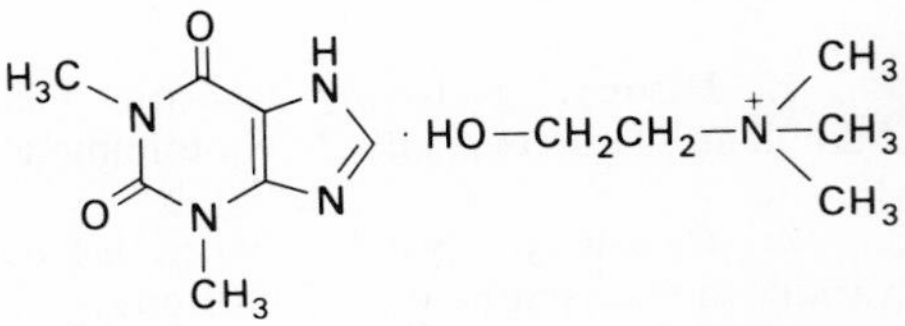

$\cdot HO{-}CH_2CH_2{-}\overset{+}{N}(CH_3)_3$

THEOPHYLLINE-METHYLGLUCAMINE (glucophylline)
Dose: 0.15 to 0.75 gm 3 times a day by mouth or rectally.

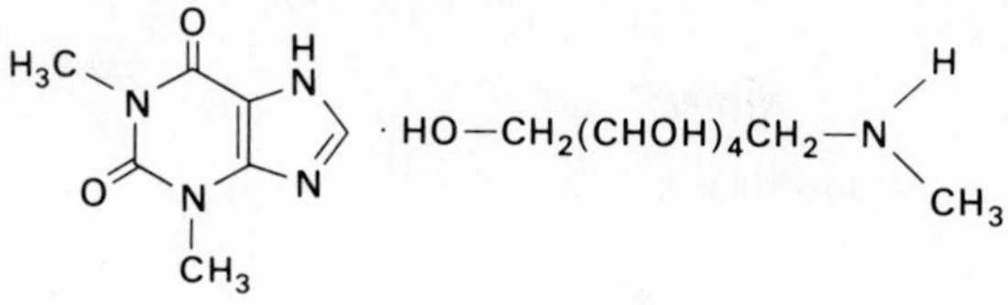

THEOPHYLLINE SODIUM GLYCINATE (Theoglycinate, and others).

Dose: 0.3 to 1 gm by mouth, rectally, or by aerosol.

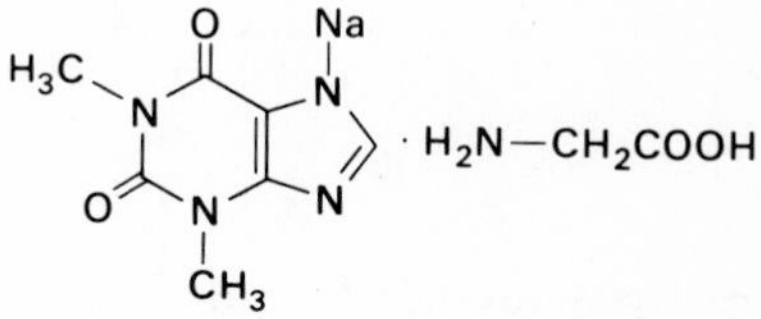

OTHERS

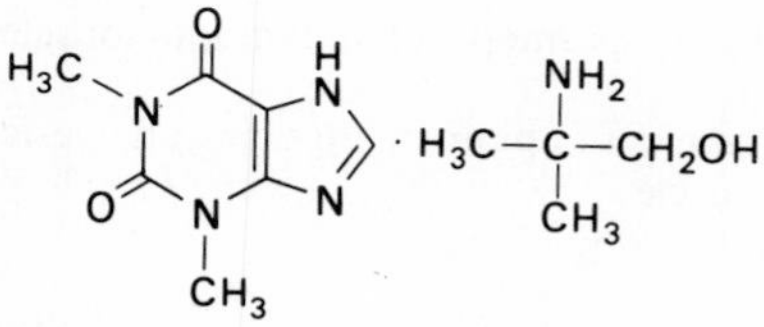

ambuphylline (in Nethaprin)

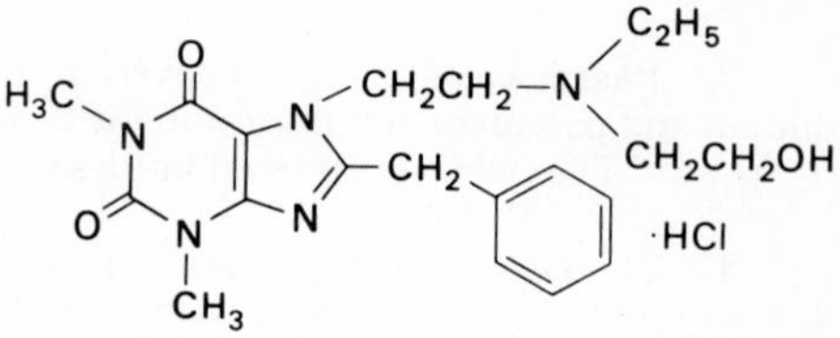

bamiphylline HCl

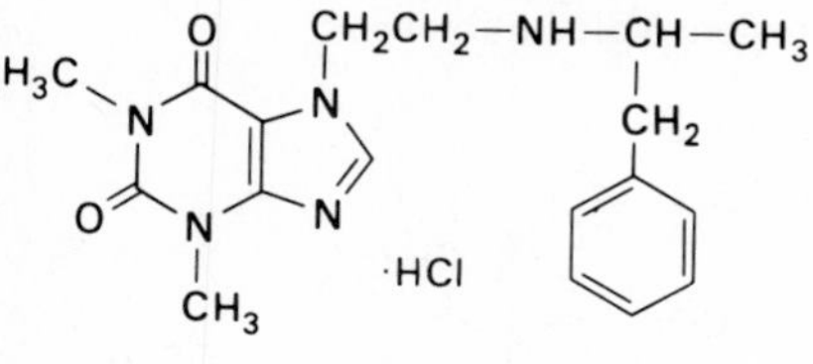

fenethylline HCl

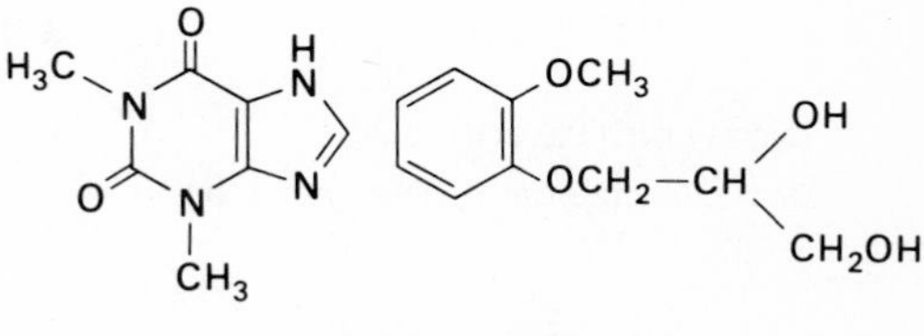

guaithylline (Eclabron)

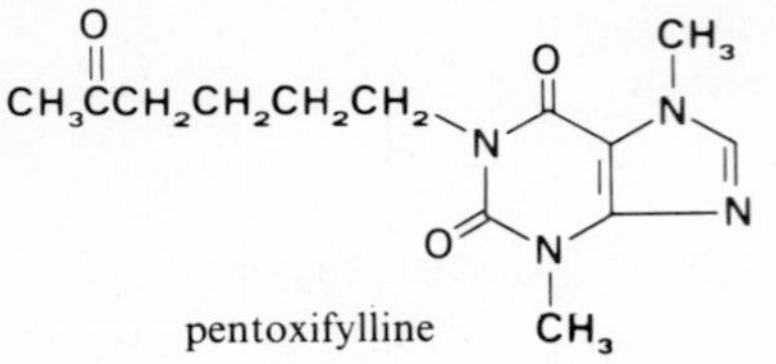

pentoxifylline

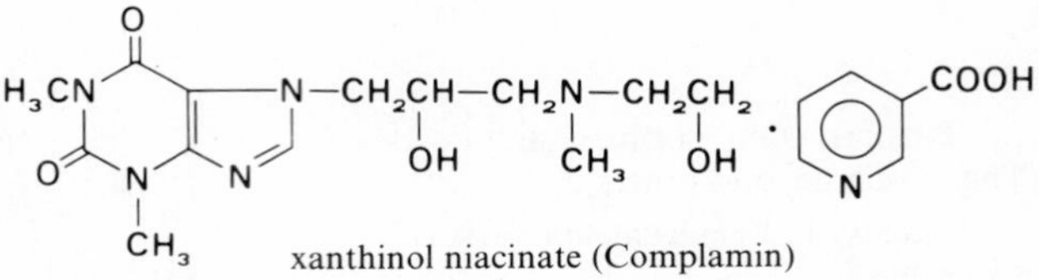

xanthinol niacinate (Complamin)

C. Papaverine Group

PAPAVERINE GROUP

1. Chemistry. Isoquinoline opium alkaloids and synthetic analogues.

2. Action and Mechanism. a. Strongly antispasmodic on the smooth muscle of blood vessels and the abdominal viscera.

b. Differ from the phenanthrene derivatives of opium in not being analgesic or habituating, or causing spasm of smooth muscle.

c. The mechanism of action is not understood.

3. Pharmacology. a. Papaverine is destroyed fairly rapidly when given by mouth and parenteral administration is therefore preferable.

b. Dioxyline is absorbed more satisfactorily.

4. Toxicity. Although relatively safe, cardiac arrhythmias from depressed conduction have been reported with large doses; also reversible liver damage.

5. Uses. To produce vasodilatation in coronary and peripheral vascular disease, particularly in acute vascular occlusion. Value dubious.

6. Preparations

PAPAVERINE HYDROCHLORIDE

Dose: 60 mg orally, subcutaneously, or intravenously.

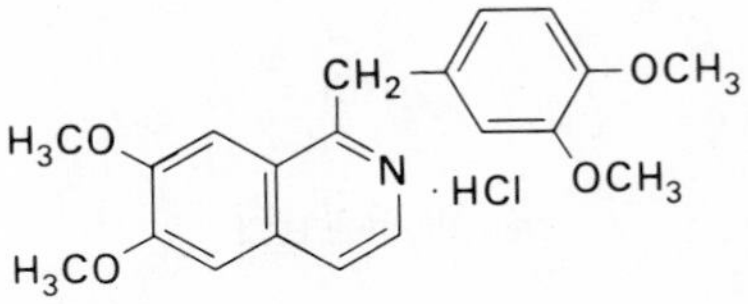

DIOXYLINE (Paveril)

Dose: 200 mg 3 times a day by mouth.

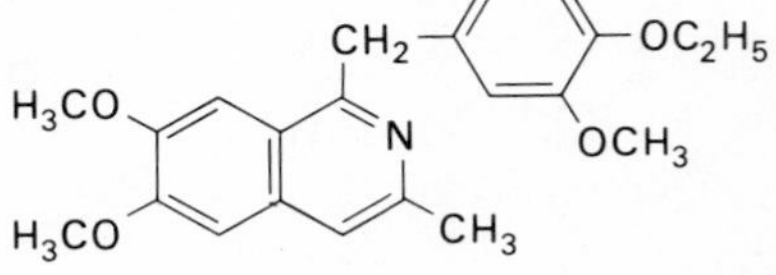

ETHAVERINE

Dose: 60 to 200 mg orally; 15 to 100 mg intravenously.

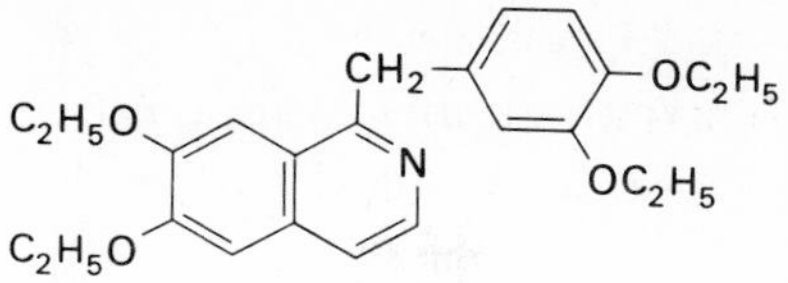

OTHERS

(See also Quinolines and Related Compounds under Hypotensive Agents.)

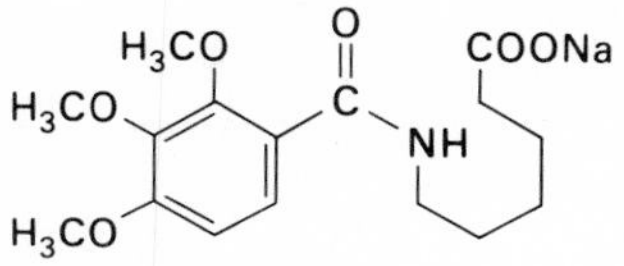

capobenate sodium

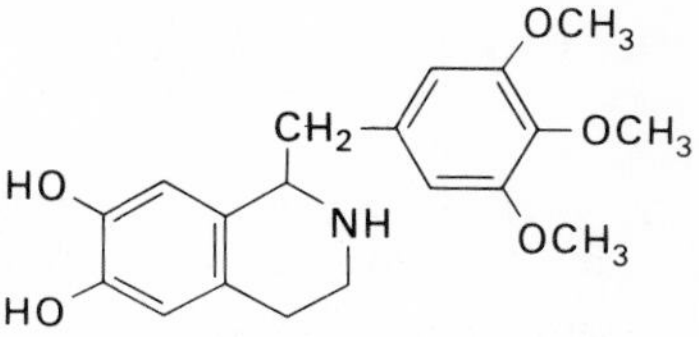

droverine

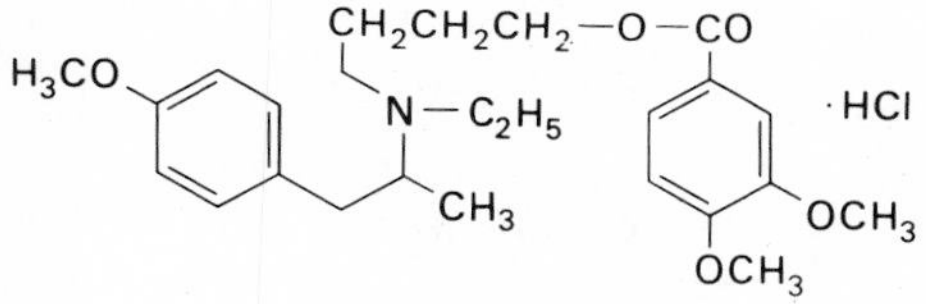

mebeverine HCl

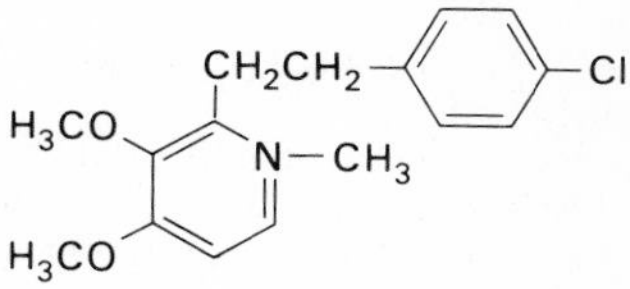

methoquoline

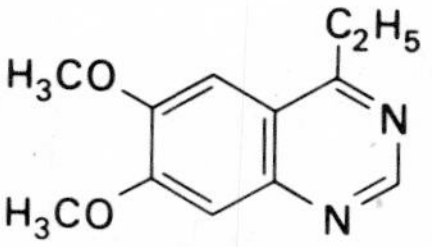

quazodine

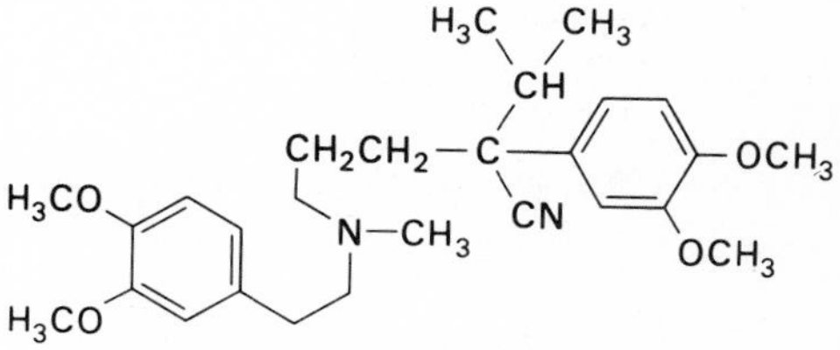

verapamil (Isoptin)

CYCLANDELATE

1. Action and Mechanism. Antispasmodic closely resembling papaverine in action. Mechanism unknown.

2. Pharmacodynamics and Toxicity. Active after oral administration. May produce flushing, tingling, headache, and dizziness.

3. Uses. Although it has been used in peripheral vascular disease, both spastic and obliterative, experience has not shown advantages over other vasodilators.

4. Preparation

CYCLANDELATE (Cyclospasmol)

Dose: 200 mg 4 times a day by mouth.

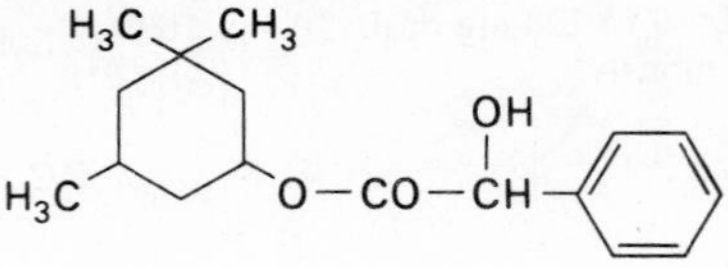

D. Amotriphene Group

1. Chemistry. General resemblance to antihistamines; some contain stilbene nucleus.

2. Action and Use. a. Coronary dilators; resemble nitroglycerin in effect.
b. Used in angina; as a group seem relatively ineffective.

3. Preparations

ALVERINE CITRATE (Spascolin)

Dose: 120 mg 1 to 3 times a day by mouth.

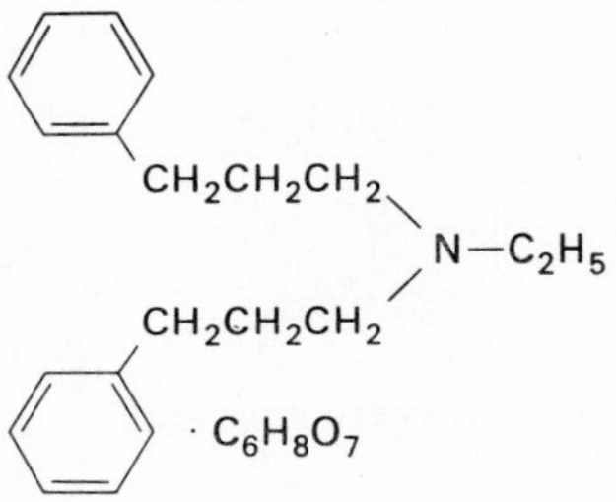

PERHEXILINE MALEATE

Under trial in angina pectoris.
Dose: 300 to 400 mg 3 to 4 times a day by mouth.

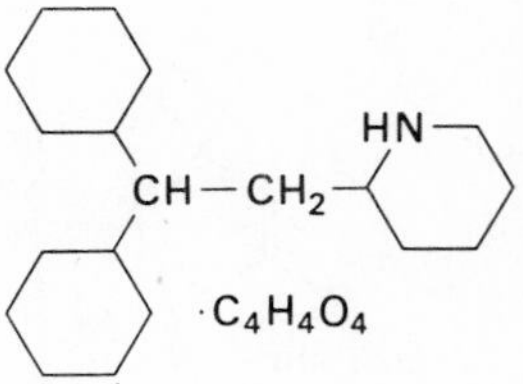

OTHERS

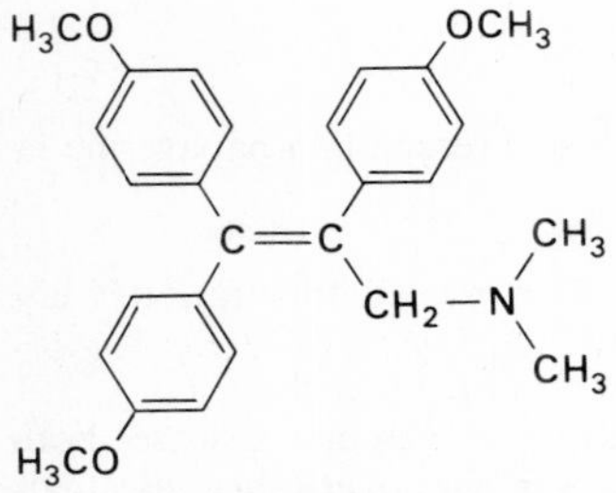

amotriphene

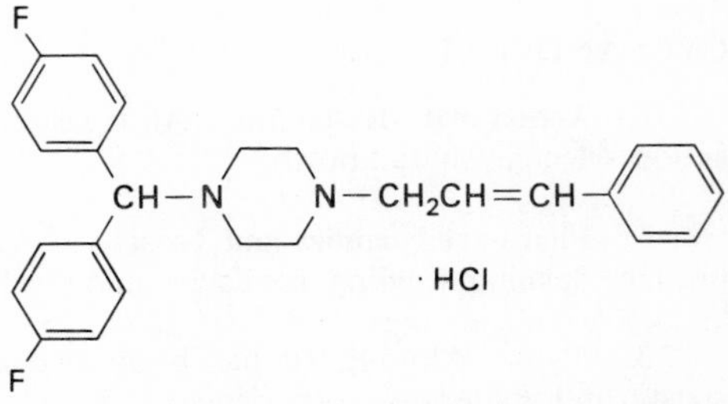

flunarizine

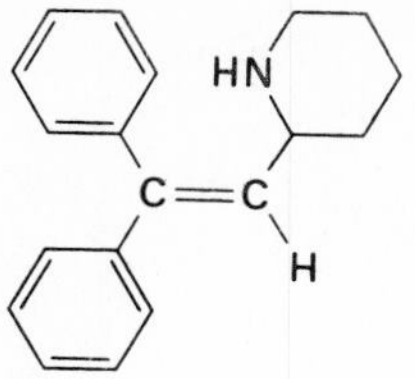

hexadiline

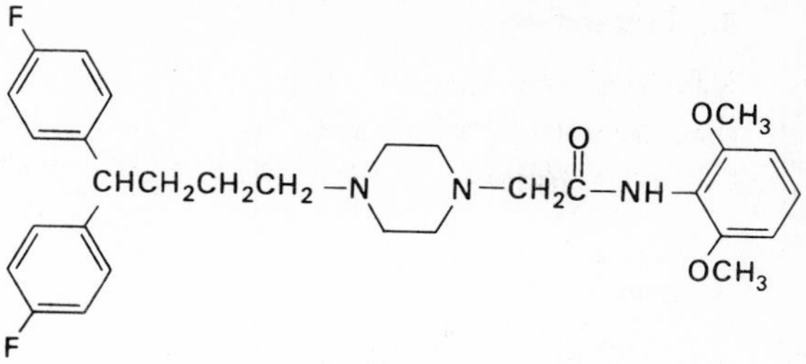

lidoflazine

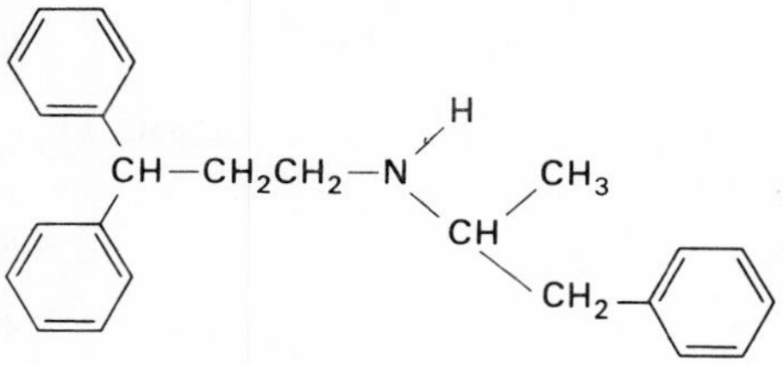

prenylamine

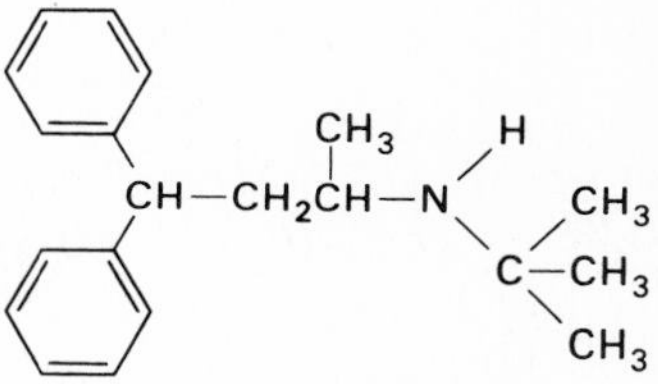

terodiline

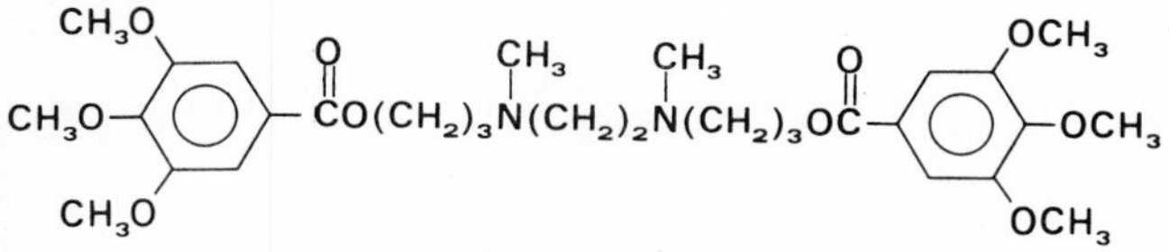

hexobendine

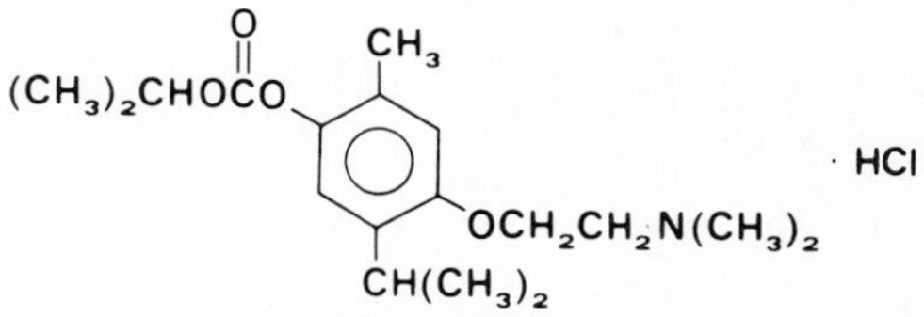

iproxamine hydrochloride

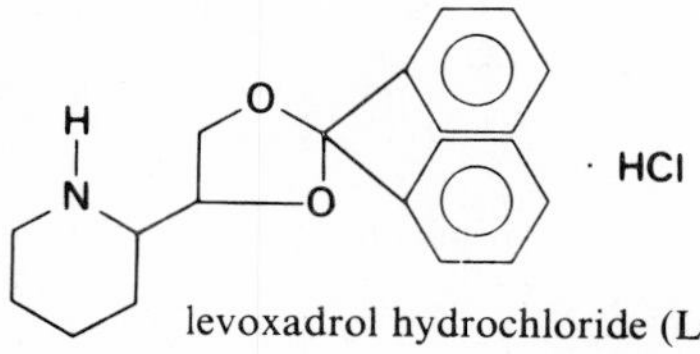

levoxadrol hydrochloride (Levoxan)

E. Nicotinic Acid Derivatives

NICOTINIC ACID

1. Action. Vitamin of the B group (see Vitamins; also Atherosclerosis). Also vasodilator, causing transient, generalized peripheral vasodilatation.

2. Uses. Occasionally used in peripheral vascular disease in an attempt to relieve intermittent claudication.

3. Preparations

NICOTINIC ACID (niacin)

Dose: 50 to 100 mg 3 or 4 times a day.

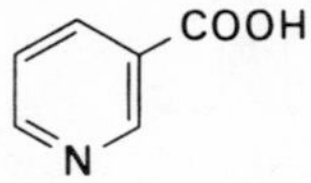

OTHERS

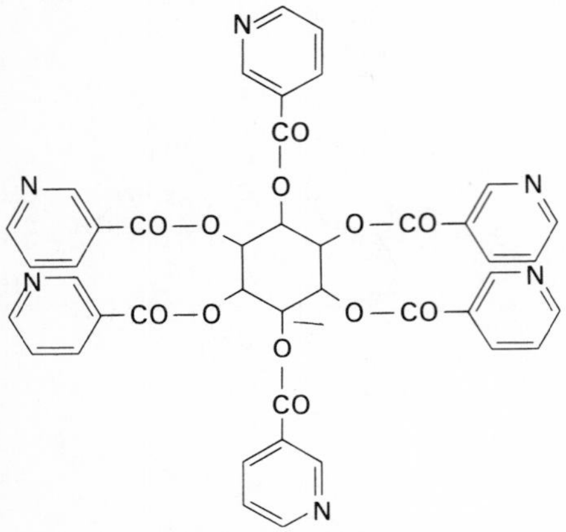

inositol niacinate (Palohex)

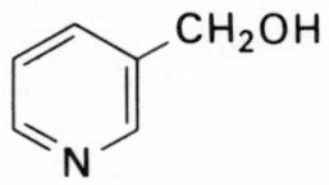

nicotinyl alcohol (Roniacol)

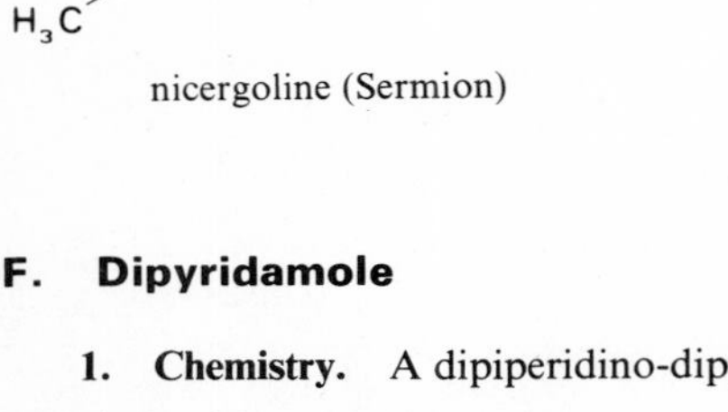

nicergoline (Sermion)

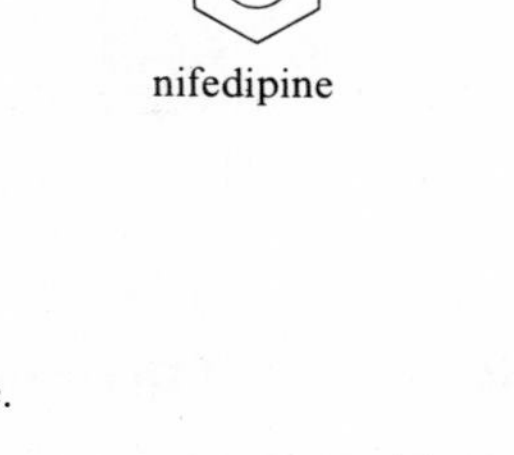

nifedipine

F. Dipyridamole

1. Chemistry. A dipiperidino-dipyrimidine.

2. Action and Mechanism. a. In general similar to papaverine. Increases coronary blood flow without significant change in blood pressure or peripheral flow in therapeutic doses.

b. Improves efficiency of utilization of oxygen in heart muscle by accelerating restitution of ATP in sarcosomes; may act as an electron acceptor in oxidations leading to ATP and nucleotide formation.

3. Pharmacodynamics and Toxicity. Absorbed by mouth. Excreted via the bile in the feces.

4. Toxicity. Headache, dizziness, nausea, weakness, large doses may give peripheral vasodilatation.

5. Uses. a. Reported to be effective in angina pectoris and for coronary vasodilatation after the acute phase of myocardial infarction; other reports do not confirm this effect. Not rapid enough for acute angina.

b. Increases exercise tolerance; may aid nocturnal dyspnea. May decrease blood coagulability.

6. Preparation

DIPYRIDAMOLE (Persantin)

Dose: 25 to 50 mg 2 or 3 times a day by mouth before meals.

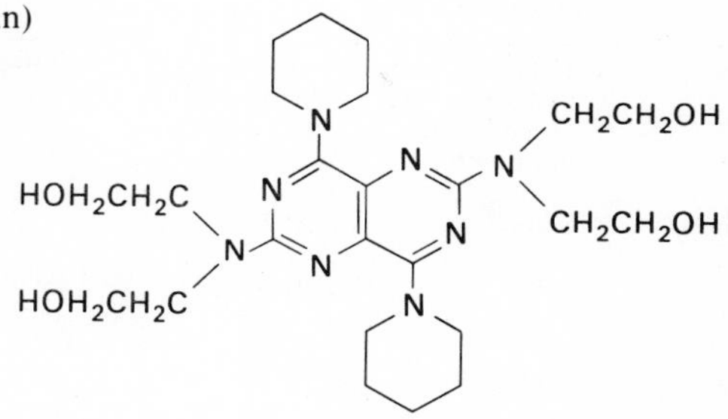

HOH_2CH_2C HOH_2CH_2C N N N N N N N CH_2CH_2OH CH_2CH_2OH

G. Other Agents, of Uncertain Value

ADENOSINE PHOSPHATE (My-B-Den)

Natural constituent of muscle essential for formation of ATP. Claimed to be vasodilating and anti-inflammatory. Used in varicose veins, thrombophlebitis, bursitis.

Toxicity: flushing, dizziness, anaphylaxis.

Dose: 20 to 200 mg daily intramuscularly; reduced to 3 times.

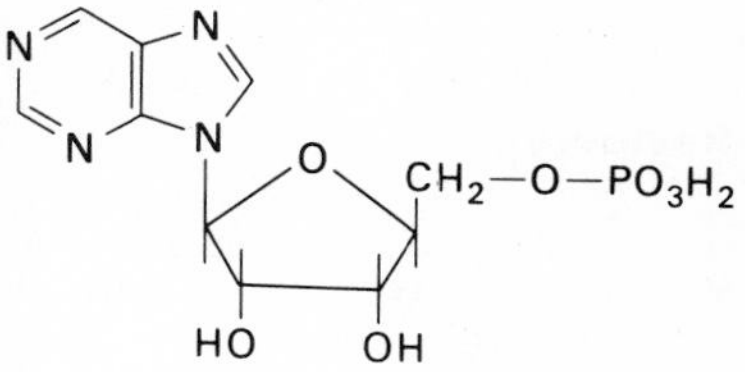

N N N N O $CH_2—O—PO_3H_2$ HO OH

CHROMONAR HYDROCHLORIDE (Intensain)

Dose: 225 mg 3 times a day by mouth.

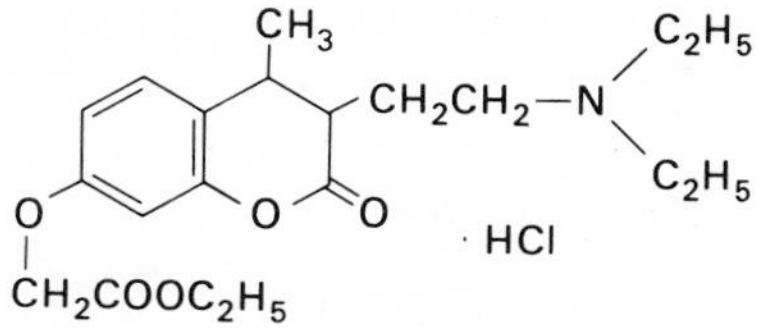

CH_3 $CH_2CH_2—N$ C_2H_5 C_2H_5 O O O $CH_2COOC_2H_5$ · HCl

CROMOLYN SODIUM (Intal)

Pulmonary antispasmodic.

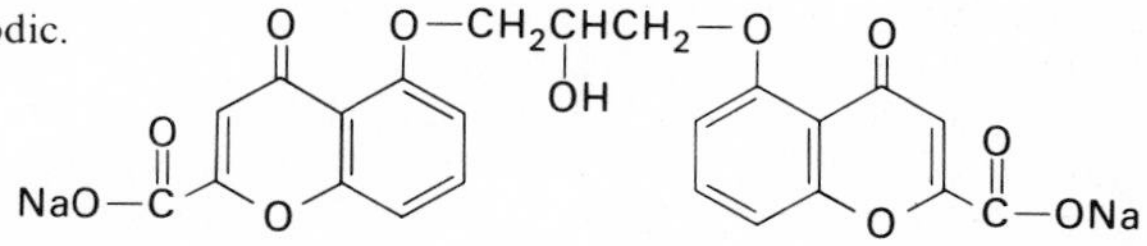

O O—CH_2CHCH_2—O O OH O NaO—C O O C—ONa

FLAVOXATE HYDROCHLORIDE
Urinary antispasmodic.

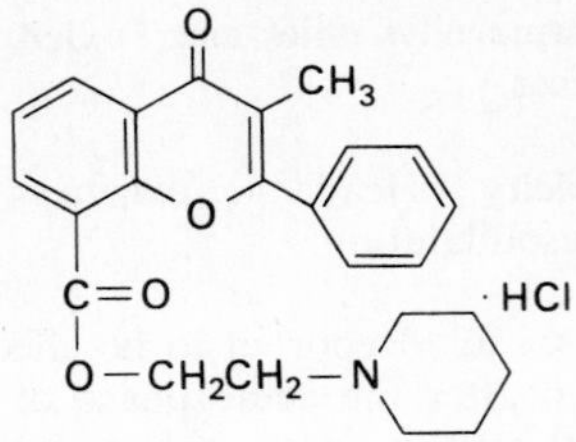

SUMMARY: SMOOTH MUSCLE RELAXANTS

TYPE	*ACTION AND MECHANISM*	*TOXICITY*	*USE*	*EXAMPLES*
Nitrites	Relax smooth muscle directly Mechanism unknown	Headache, palpitation, fainting	Angina pectoris	Glyceryl trinitrate
Xanthines	Same	Minor	Asthma	Aminophylline
Papaverine group	Same	Minor	Acute vascular occlusion	Papaverine HCl
Amothiphene group	Same	Minor	Angina pectoris	Perhexiline maleate
Dipyridamole	May improve utilization of oxygen in heart	Headache, weakness, peripheral vasodilatation	Same	Dipyridamole

Reviews

Charlier, R. Coronary Dilators. London, Pergamon, 1961.

Winsor, T., and Hyman, C. Clinical pharmacology of vasodilating drugs. Clin. Pharmacol. Ther., 2:636, 1961.

Rowe, G. Pharmacology of the coronary circulation. Ann. Rev. Pharmacol., 8:95, 1968.

Miller, J., and Lewis, J. Drugs affecting smooth muscle. Ann. Rev. Pharmacol., 9:147, 1969.

25. Smooth Muscle Stimulants

Drugs may stimulate, or induce spasm in, smooth muscle by two means:

a. Direct stimulation of the muscle, as by ergot or posterior pituitary (considered in this chapter).

b. Stimulation via the autonomic mechanism, as by neostigmine or bethanecol (considered under Parasympathetic Stimulants).

The direct stimulants are useful agents to cause constriction of scalp or cerebral vessels in migraine and to cause contraction of the uterus during or after labor. Most are polypeptides.

A. Ergot Alkaloids

1. History.

a. Epidemics of ergotism in the Middle Ages from eating bread made from contaminated flour (as in 994 and 1129 in France) exhibited two clinical pictures:

a′. Gangrenous ergotism (Holy Fire; St. Anthony's Fire), characterized by hot extremities, becoming numb, then vesiculation and black coloration, finally mummification and loss of extremities at joints without bleeding.

b′. Convulsive ergotism, characterized by twitching, numbness in fingers and toes progressing to terrible pain with shrieking and vomiting.

b. The first description of ergot for contracting the uterus was by Stearns (1808) who described it as "a Remedy for quickening Child-birth."

2. Chemistry. a. Ergot is a fungus, *Claviceps purpura*, that grows on rye.

b. It contains a number of pharmacologically active agents: ergosterol, tyramine, histamine, acetylcholine, ergot alkaloids.

c. The identification of the ergot alkaloids as lysergic acid derivatives, mostly polypeptides, has been largely the work of Stoll in Switzerland. Each alkaloid occurs as an isomeric pair, of which the levo form, derived from lysergic acid, is pharmacologically active, while the dextro form, from isolysergic acid, is inactive.

d. Three groups of alkaloids have been separated: the ergotamine group, ergotoxine group, and ergonovine group.

ERGOTAMINE GROUP

1. History. Ergotamine was isolated by Stoll (1918); ergosine by Smith and Timmis (1936); dihydroergotamine synthesized by Stoll (1943).

2. Chemistry. a. The two pairs of naturally occurring alkaloids, i.e., ergotamine and ergotaminine, and ergosine and ergosinine, consist of a lysergic acid amide moiety combined with a condensed polypeptide.

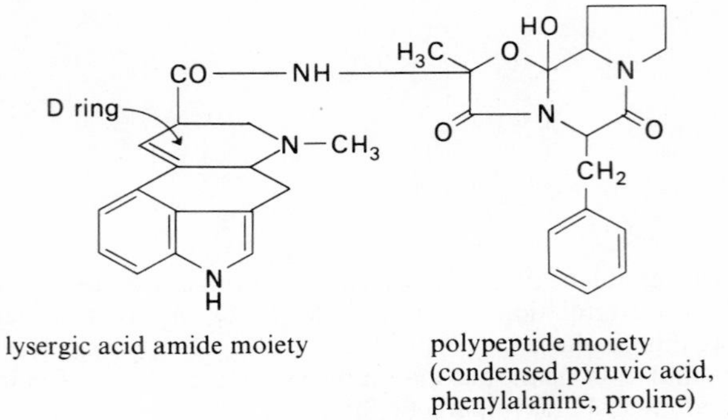

lysergic acid amide moiety

polypeptide moiety (condensed pyruvic acid, phenylalanine, proline)

ergotamine

b. Hydrogenation of the double bond in the D ring of ergotamine gives the semisynthetic product, dihydroergotamine.

c. The ergosine pair has no therapeutic significance.

3. Action. a. Ergotamine is a potent vasoconstrictor and uterine stimulant; large doses stimulate gastrointestinal smooth muscle and the pupil.

b. In laboratory preparations, sympatholytic effects and epinephrine reversal may be demonstrated (see Sympathetic Depressants); but in man, side effects preclude the use of blocking doses.

c. Dihydroergotamine is generally similar but with greater sympatholysis and a relaxing effect on nonpregnant uterine muscle; oxytocic on pregnant uterus at term.

4. Mechanism. a. Muscle stimulant mechanism not fully explained but probably drugs stimulate cellular receptors directly; may be related to structurally similar serotonin, which also stimulates smooth muscle.

b. Sympatholytic action could be related to competition with sympathomimetic amines.

5. Pharmacodynamics. a. Oral absorption incomplete and delayed; fate unknown but effects last for several hours.

b. Biological test: after injection into rooster, comb and wattles turn purple from vasoconstriction.

6. Toxicity. a. Nausea and vomiting.

b. Possibility of damage to capillary endothelium and tissues from peripheral vascular spasm. Circulatory changes prominent in chronic poisoning.

7. Uses. a. Both ergotamine and dihydroergotamine are useful in migraine, presumably by constricting the dilated vessels in or around the scalp or brain.

b. Ergotamine is inferior to ergonovine as uterine stimulant because its actions are more diffuse, oral administration is less satisfactory, and there is a latent period after intravenous administration.

8. Preparations

ERGOTAMINE TARTRATE (Gynergen)

Dose: 0.5 to 1 mg by mouth repeated every hour for 8 hours if needed (migraine); 0.25 to 0.5 mg subcutaneously (more effective).

DIHYDROERGOTAMINE MESYLATE (DHE-45)

Dose: 1 to 2 mg subcutaneously.

ERGOTOXINE GROUP

1. History. a. Tanret (1875) isolated an early crystalline preparation from ergot (ergotinine); Barger and Carr (1906) separated an amorphous mixture (ergotoxine) thought for many years to be an entity.

b. Stoll and Burckhardt (1937) separated ergotoxine into three crystalline alkaloids: ergocristine, ergokryptine and ergocornine; Stoll (1943) hydrogenated the three to make dihydroergocristine, dihydrokryptine, and dihydrocornine.

2. Chemistry. a. Three pairs of naturally occurring isomers differing in polypeptide moieties: ergocristine and ergocristinine, ergokryptine and ergokryptinine, and ergocornine and ergocorninine.

b. In the dihydro forms the double bond in the D ring has been hydrogenated.

lysergic acid amide moiety

polypeptide moiety (condensed isovaleric, phenylalanine, and proline)

ergocristine

3. Action. a. In general the actions of the three natural alkaloids are similar to those of ergotamine, with blood vessel and uterine stimulation.

b. Sympatholytic effects are greater than with ergotamine.

c. The hydrogenated forms show little or no direct effects on blood vessels and do not stimulate the nonpregnant uterus, but have an increased adrenolytic action and a moderately strong central action inhibiting the vasomotor center.

4. Mechanism. Unknown; possibilities same as for ergotamine.

5. Pharmacodynamics and Toxicity. a. The natural mixture, ergotoxine, is primarily a laboratory tool, traditionally used to demonstrate epinephrine reversal (sympatholysis).

b. The hydrogenated mixture is not absorbed reliably and is therefore given by injection; its action may last many hours. It is relatively nontoxic. With it, central vasomotor inhibition overcomes peripheral vasoconstriction.

6. Uses. The hydrogenated mixture (Hydergine) has been used in peripheral vascular spasm and in chronic hypertension, but uncommonly in the United States, where it is generally considered to be ineffective.

7. Preparation

METHANESULFONATE DERIVATIVES OF DIHYDROERGOTOXINE ALKALOIDS (Hydergine)

Dose: 0.3 mg parenterally.

BROMOCRIPTINE (Parlodel)

Stimulates CNS dopamine-receptors. Inhibits secretion of growth hormone and prolactin. Under investigation in treatment of Parkinson's disease, galactorrhea, and acromegaly.

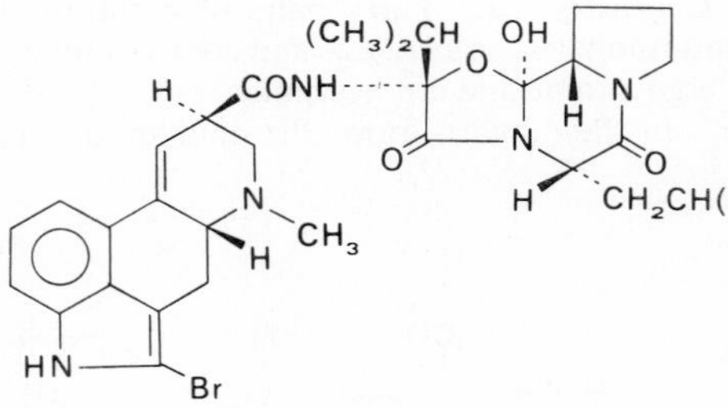

BROMOCRIPTINE (Parlodel)

ERGONOVINE GROUP

1. History. Nearly simultaneous isolation of ergonovine in 1935 by Dudley and Moir, Stoll and Burckhardt, Karasch and Legault, and by Thompson.

2. Chemistry. Ergonovine and the related partial synthetic, methyl ergonovine, differ from the preceding alkaloids in having an isopropyl instead of a polypeptide substitution and in being easily soluble.

3. Action and Mechanism. a. Almost exclusively oxytocic by direct action on uterine muscle.

b. Practically no action on blood vessels, and no sympatholytic or central effects.

c. Mechanism unknown but probably similar to that of ergotamine.

4. Pharmacodynamics. a. Unlike the preceding alkaloids, these smaller, nonpolypeptide molecules are quickly absorbed by mouth.

b. Effects begin in 5 minutes after oral administration; in 1 minute after intravenous injection. The effects last for about 4 hours.

5. Toxicity. The only likely deleterious possibility is rupture of the uterus from excessive or premature administration.

6. Uses. Almost routinely given to women at the end of the second stage of labor to cause uterine contraction and reduce bleeding.

7. Preparations

ERGONOVINE MALEATE (Ergotrate)

Dose: 0.5 mg by mouth, or 0.2 mg subcutaneously.

CH_3 / CO—NH—CH / CH_2OH; N—CH_3; N; $\cdot C_4H_4O_4$

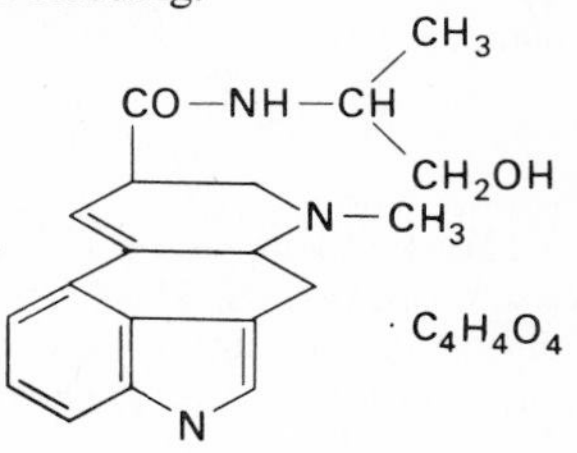

METHYL ERGONOVINE TARTRATE (Methergine)

Dose: 0.5 mg by mouth, or 0.2 mg subcutaneously.

METHYSERGIDE MALEATE (Deseril; Sansert)

Antiserotonin; used in prevention of migraine (see Antiserotonins).

Dose: 2 mg 2 to 4 times a day.

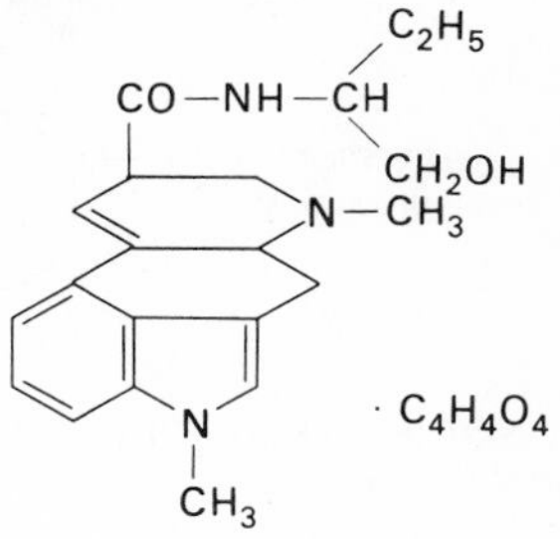

C_2H_5 / CO—NH—CH / CH_2OH; N—CH_3; N—CH_3; $\cdot C_4H_4O_4$

B. Prostaglandins

(See Autacoids and Hormones.)

C. Posterior Pituitary Hormones

1. History. a. Physiology: Oliver and Schäfer (1895) showed that whole pituitary was pressor; Howell (1898) showed that the pressor action came from the posterior lobe; Dale (1906) showed that it also increased uterine activity.

b. Chemistry: Abel (1908) isolated histamine and later oxytocic principle from posterior lobe; Kamm (1927) recognized two factors, oxytocic and pressor; Du Vigneaud (1953) synthesized separate factors.

2. Chemistry. a. Closely related octapeptides.

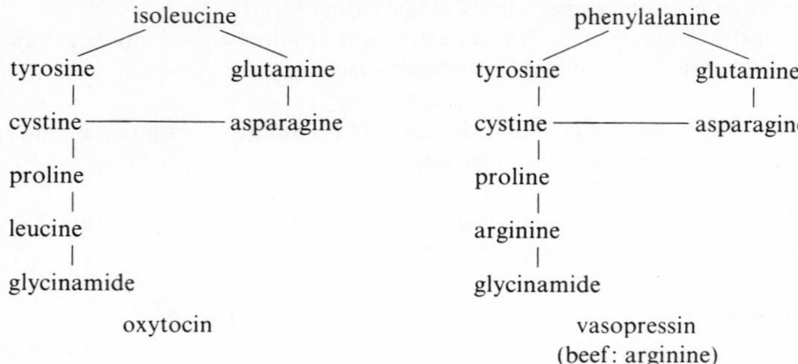

b. The oxytocic factor is the same in all species, but there are species differences in vasopressins. Thus, hog vasopressin is lysine vasopressin, fowls have arginyl-oxytocin (vasotocin) in place of vasopressin, and felypressin is synthetic.

c. The posterior pituitary hormones are formed in the hypothalamic nuclei, from which they migrate as granules down axones to the posterior lobe where they are stored.

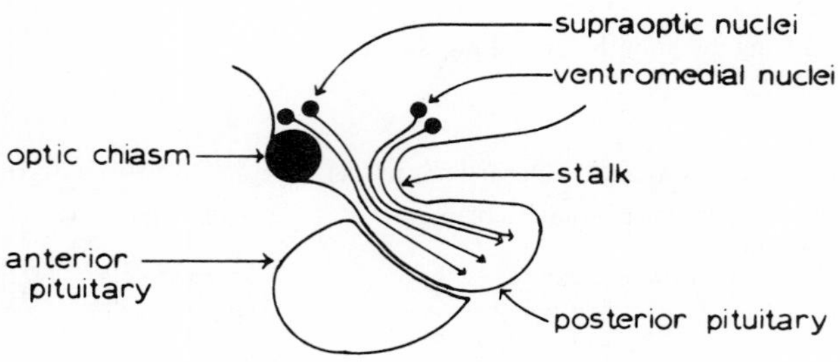

3. Action and Uses. Composite action of individual components as described in the next sections.

4. Preparation

POSTERIOR PITUITARY INJECTION

Dose: 0.3 to 0.5 ml subcutaneously or intramuscularly.

OXYTOCIN

1. Action. a. Oxytocin causes strong contractions of the uterus when given at term; whether it plays any part in the normal induction of labor is uncertain.

b. Also the "letdown" factor in lactation, causing smooth muscle in the breast to contract in response to sucking.

c. Little action on vascular smooth muscle or on the intestine; the antidiuretic effect of vasopressin is augmented, probably by a similar action on the renal tubules.

2. Mechanism. No satisfactory explanation has been given for the means by which oxytocin stimulates smooth muscle directly.

3. Pharmacodynamics. a. Ineffective orally, but acts within 5 minutes of intramuscular injection; the duration is 2 to 3 hours.

b. Natural oxytocin contains up to 0.5 u of pressor activity per ml; synthetic oxytocin is free of vasopressor.

4. Toxicity. The danger of rupture of the uterus from overly vigorous contractions before the cervix effaced is present when oxytocin is used to induce labor.

5. Uses. To hasten the third stage of labor. To induce labor (caution).

6. Preparations

OXYTOCIN INJECTION (Pitocin)

Dose: 0.1 to 0.5 ml intramuscularly, or on pledgets of cotton inserted into the nose; 0.5 to 2 ml of intravenous drip (1 ml = 10 units).

OXYTOCIN (Syntocinon, synthetic)

Dose: 0.1 to 0.5 ml intramuscularly.

OXYTOCIN CITRATE (Pitocin citrate)

Dose: 200 u as buccal tablet.

VASOPRESSIN

1. Action. a. Antidiuretic, increasing reabsorption of water in the distal tubules.

b. Constriction of blood vessels and gastrointestinal smooth muscle by direct musculotropic action.

c. It is possibly a factor in stress as direct perfusion of the adrenal with vasopressin (dog) increases the output of hydrocortisone.

2. Mechanism. a. The mechanism of the direct stimulation of smooth muscles has not been explained.

b. Mechanism of antidiuresis is controversial. The vasopressins may act by increasing 3′,5′-cyclic AMP. It has also been suggested that vasopressin releases hyaluronidase in the kidney tubules and so lets water be reabsorbed more easily, or that the effect is on Na^+ and may be through activation of carbonic anhydrase (Nature, 184:991, 1959).

3. Pharmacodynamics. a. Vasopressin is inactive orally.

b. Effects last 3 to 4 hours after intramuscular injection.

4. Toxicity. a. Side effects include pallor, nausea, abdominal cramps.

b. More serious effects of overdosage may be cerebral or coronary arterial spasm; water intoxication.

5. Uses. a. Most useful agent in diabetes insipidus, in which a lesion in the pituitary stalk may interfere with the transfer of the hormone to the posterior lobe.

b. Also used as a stimulant of intestinal motility in paralytic ileus and abdominal distension.

c. Should be used with care in patients with coronary disease.

6. Preparations

VASOPRESSIN INJECTION (antidiuretic hormone; ADH; Pitressin)

Dose: 0.3 to 1 ml subcutaneously or intramuscularly.

VASOPRESSIN TANNATE (Pitressin tannate):

Longer acting form, also available as a suspension in oil.
Dose: 0.3 to 1 ml intramuscularly.

OTHERS

Felypressin (2-phenylalanine-8-lysine vasopressin; PLV-2); lypressin (8-lysine vasopressin; Diapid).

D. Serotonin and Related Compounds

(See Autacoids and Hormones.)

E. Other Polypeptides of Mammalian Origin

(See Autacoids and Hormones.)

F. Other Agents

BARIUM

Soluble salts of barium are potent stimulants of smooth, cardiac, and skeletal muscle, and much used in pharmacological experiments. In the intact animal barium is a CNS depressant. Death from respiratory depression or cardiac arrest is usual.

HISTAMINE

Histamine stimulates the smooth muscle of bronchioles strongly, intestine weakly and uterus irregularly, while dilating capillaries. (See Autacoids and Hormones.)

SPARTEINE SULFATE (Tocosamine)

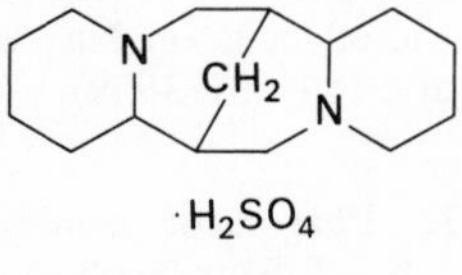

Quinidine-like stimulant for the induction of labor; also has quinidine-like cardiac actions.

Dose: 150 mg intramuscularly, repeated up to 3 times at intervals of 1 to 2 hours.

N CH$_2$ N $\cdot H_2SO_4$

QUIPAZINE MALEATE

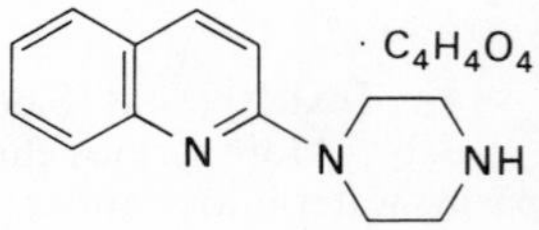

Oxytocic.
Under investigation.

$\cdot C_4H_4O_4$ N N NH

SUMMARY: SMOOTH MUSCLE STIMULANTS

TYPE	*ACTION AND MECHANISM*	*TOXICITY*	*USE*	*EXAMPLES*
Ergot alkaloids	Vasoconstrictors uterine stimulants Mechanism uncertain	Nausea, vomiting, vessel damage, uterine rupture	Migraine after labor	Ergotamine tartrate
Oxytocin	Uterine contraction Mechanism uncertain	Uterine rupture	To induce or conclude labor	Oxytocin
Vasopressin	Vasoconstrictor, antidiuretic Mechanism uncertain	Abdominal cramps, vascular spasm, water intoxication	Diabetes insipidus, paralytic ileus	Vasopressin
Antiserotonins	Inhibit action of serotonin	Confusion, retroperitoneal fibrosis	Migraine	Methysergide
Angiotensin	Increase in BP, aldosterone secretion	Hypertension	Shock	Angiotensin amide
Bradykinin	Vasodilator, stimulates other smooth muscle May be involved in pain mechanism	Not known	None	Bradykinin
Prostaglandins	Vasodilation or vasoconstriction, smooth muscle stimulation or depression	Not known	None	Prostaglandin PGE_1

Reviews

Erspamer, V. Pharmacologically active substances of mammalian origin. Ann. Rev. Pharmacol., 1:175, 1961.

Euler, U. S. Bradykinin and vasodilating polypeptides. Biochem. Pharmacol., 10:1, 1962.

Erdös, E. G. Structure and function of biologically active peptides. Bull. N.Y. Acad. Sci., 104:1, 1963.

Schachter, M. Kinins—A group of active peptides. Ann. Rev. Pharmacol., 4:281, 1964.

Collier, H. O. J. Bradykinin and its allies. Endeavor, 27:14, 1968.

Von Euler, U. S. Prostaglandins. Clin. Pharmacol. Therap., 9:228, 1968.

Bergström, S., Carlson, L., and Weeks, J. The Prostaglandins. Pharmacol. Rev., 20:1, 1968.

Kellermeyer, R., and Graham, R. Kinins. Possible physiologic and pathologic roles in man. New Eng. J. Med., 279:754, 1968.

Du Vignaud, V., and Graham, R. Hormones of the mammalian posterior gland and their naturally occurring analogues. Johns Hopkin's Med. J., 127:53, 1969.
Pickles, V. Prostaglandins. Nature, 224:221, 1969.

26.
Agents in Anemia

1. AGENTS IN IRON DEFICIENCY ANEMIA

A. Iron

1. History. Blaud, in 1831, used ferrous carbonate pills for anemia.

2. Chemistry. a. Iron is active in the body in hemoglobin and other large molecules consisting of an iron-containing porphyrin unit combined with a protein.

b. The total amount of iron is about 5 grams, distributed as follows:

Hemoglobin	60% to 70%
Myohemoglobin	3% to 5%
Cytochrome, etc.	0.1%
Transferrin	0.1%
Ferritin	15%
"Tissue" or unaccounted	10± %

c. Heme, the iron-containing porphyrin of hemoglobin, shows the general structure of iron compounds in the body.

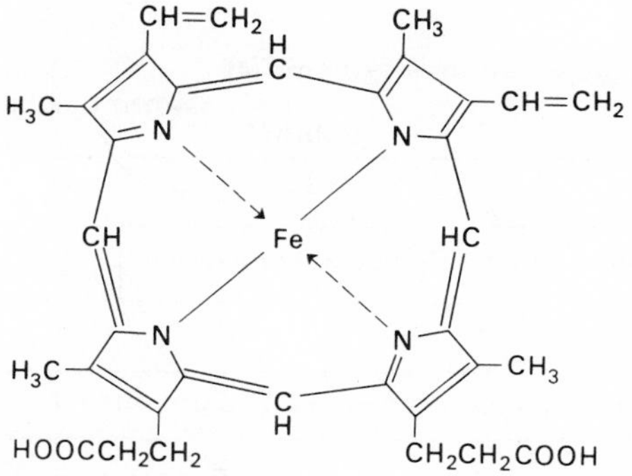

CH=CH₂ CH₃ H C H₃C— —CH=CH₂ N N CH Fe HC N N H₃C— —CH₃ C H HOOCCH₂CH₂ CH₂CH₂COOH

heme

3. Action and Mechanism. a. Iron enters into the body metabolism as a necessary component of hemoglobin and the other substances mentioned.

b. Physiological needs of iron normally vary as follows:

Normal adult	1 to 3 mg per day
During growth	2 to 3 mg per day
Menstrual period	2 to 3 mg per day
Pregnancy	3 to 4 mg per day

c. The metabolic pathway of iron is complicated, as shown in the following diagram:

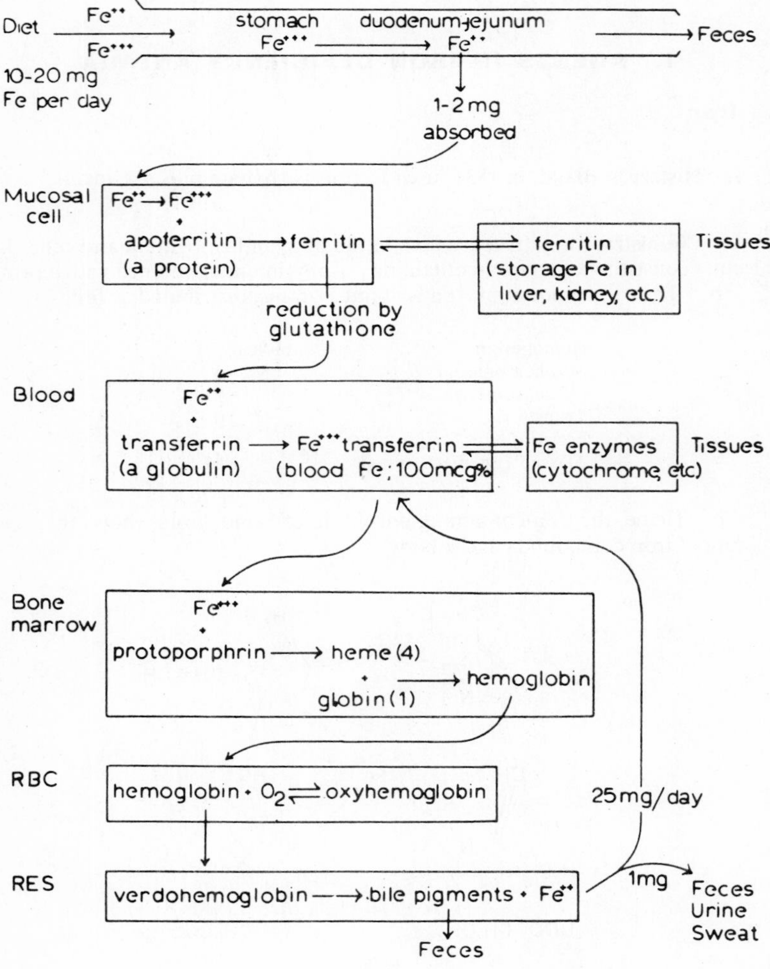

4. Pharmacodynamics. a. Absorption from gastrointestinal tract poor, usually about 10% of dietary iron.

b. Absorption may be increased by perhaps another 10% by increasing the iron intake, through complete saturation of all the available apoferritin or possibly by the formation of more apoferritin; however, when all the apoferritin is saturated and no more can be formed, absorption of iron stops. Maximum oral absorption obtained from about 200 mg of Fe^{++} daily; larger intake may inhibit absorption.

c. Excretion of iron in feces, urine and sweat amounts to 1 mg daily, about the amount absorbed, while 25 mg is returned to the cycle for re-use.

5. Toxicity. a. Most iron salts are astringent in the alimentary tract and thus may produce indigestion, or even fatal mucosal necrosis in children when large doses are accidentally taken.

b. Parenteral administration may produce "nitritoid" reactions.

c. Excessive parenteral iron may produce a condition resembling hemochromatosis, with the deposition of ferritin and hemosiderin in the tissues.

d. Hemochromatosis is an inborn disease in which iron is stored excessively in the tissues, both as ferritin, and as the abnormal pigment, hemosiderin. Hemofuscin and melanin are also deposited in excess. The disease probably is the result of increased iron absorption, possibly in turn related to an increased ability of cells to reduce ferritin to Fe^{++}. The total amount of iron in the body may be increased from a normal of about 5 gm to as much as 30 gm.

e. Ferritin has been thought to enter the circulation in shock ("vasodepressor factor") prolonging the hypotension.

6. Uses. a. Iron is specifically remedial in iron deficiency anemia.

b. It is not particularly beneficial in other microcytic anemias such as may be present in chronic infections or malignancy.

c. Iron is ordinarily given by mouth, parenteral administration being reserved for patients who do not tolerate oral therapy because of gastrointestinal irritation (McCurdy, J.A.M.A., 191:859, 1965). Some physicians, however, commonly give the total calculated iron needed in a few injections to hasten therapy (600 mg to replace storage Fe, plus 150 mg for each 1 gm deficit of Hb, expressed as gm% in the blood).

7. Preparations

a. Oral forms

FERROCHOLINATE (Chel-Iron, Ferrolip)

Somewhat better tolerated than ferrous sulfate.
Dose: 0.3 to 0.7 gm 3 times a day by mouth.

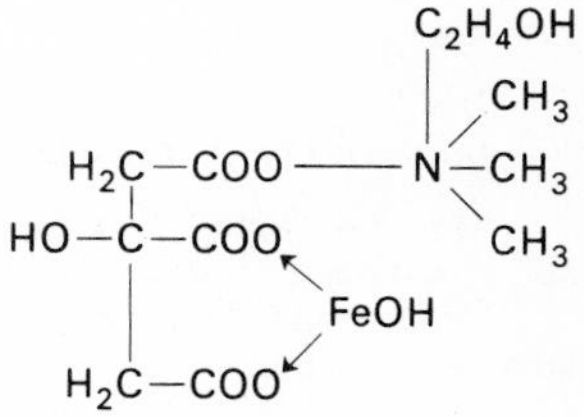

C_2H_4OH
$H_2C{-}COO$ — $N{-}(CH_3)_3$
$HO{-}C{-}COO$
FeOH
$H_2C{-}COO$

FERROUS FUMARATE (Toleron, Firon, and others)

Also may be better tolerated.
Dose: 0.5 gm 3 times a day by mouth.

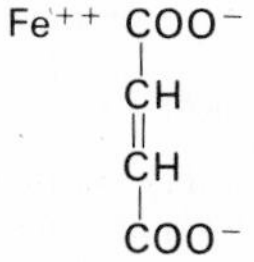

Fe^{++} COO^-
CH
‖
CH
COO^-

FERROUS GLUCONATE (Fergon, and others)

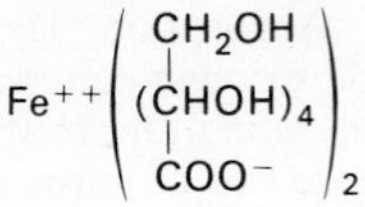

Somewhat less irritating than ferrous sulfate.
Dose: 0.5 gm 3 times a day after meals by mouth.

$$Fe^{++}\left(\begin{array}{c} CH_2OH \\ | \\ (CHOH)_4 \\ | \\ COO^- \end{array}\right)_2$$

FERROUS SULFATE (Feosol, and others): $FeSO_4$

Probably the most commonly used iron salt.
Dose: 0.25 gm 4 times a day after meals by mouth.

OTHERS

FERRIC AMMONIUM CITRATE

Dose: 1 gm 3 times a day in a syrup.

IRON-POLYSACCHARIDE COMPLEX (Niferex, Nu-Iron)

Nonionizable preparation.
Dose: 150 mg 2 times a day.

POLYFEROSE (Jefron)

Iron chelated in a polymerized carbohydrate.

b. Parenteral forms

DEXTRIFERRON (Astrafer)

Dose: 1.5 ml (30 mg Fe) intravenously on first day; then 2 to 5 ml daily.

FERRIC FRUCTOSE (Ferritose)

Under investigation.

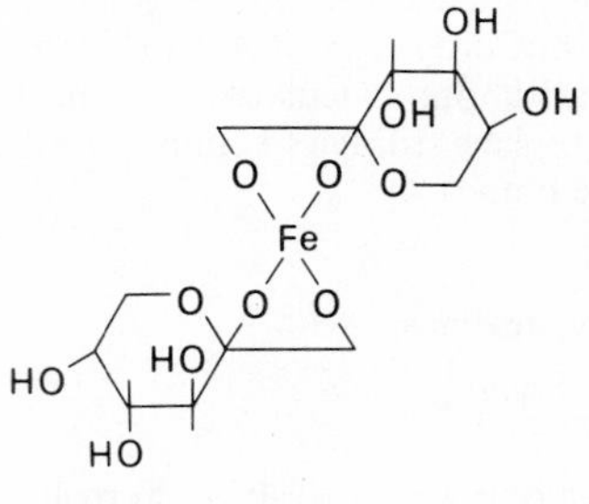

IRON DEXTRAN COMPLEX (Imferon)

More satisfactory than saccharated iron oxide, but protracted administration questionably carcinogenic in rats. Fatalities have been reported from anaphylactic shock.

Dose: 1 ml (50 mg Fe) intramuscularly on first day; then 2 to 4 ml daily to total calculated requirement.

IRON OXIDE, SACCHARATED (Proferrin, Feojectin, and others)

Dose: 5 ml (100 mg Fe) intravenously, slowly.

IRON SORBITEX (Jectofer)

Dose: 1.5 mg per kg body weight up to a total dose of 100 mg (2 ml) daily until the total calculated requirement is reached, intramuscularly.

II. AGENTS IN PERNICIOUS ANEMIA AND OTHER MEGALOBLASTIC ANEMIAS

Megaloblastic (hyperchromic; primary) anemias are characterized by the presence of megaloblasts, large abnormal cells from a maturation arrest in the development of RBC. Examples are pernicious anemia and the megaloblastic anemias of nutritional deficiency, infancy, pregnancy and puerperium, and sprue. Therapy for the group became effective with the advent of liver preparations in the 1920's.

A. Liver and Stomach

1. History. a. Whipple and Robscheit-Robbins (1920–25) found that the administration of liver remedied the anemia produced in dogs by bleeding.

b. Minot and Murphy (1926) used liver in pernicious anemia.

c. Castle (1929) recognized the extrinsic and intrinsic factors in pernicious anemia.

2. Chemistry. The original extracts of liver and stomach were crude, but liver extracts were gradually purified (Cohn) until they were potent preparations of vitamin B_{12}, even though the latter had not yet been recognized.

3. Action. a. Liver, and liver extracts, contain both folic acid and vitamin B_{12} and were effective by mouth in pernicious anemia and megaloblastic anemias in restoring the normal blood picture. Response in pernicious anemia, where absorption of vitamin B_{12} is greatly impaired, was the result of the very large amounts (100 to 300 mcg) ingested daily.

b. Pernicious anemia is the result of deficiency of vitamin B_{12} (extrinsic factor), the absorption of which is promoted by intrinsic factor. Stomach preparations contained intrinsic factor and presumably acted by enabling dietary B_{12} to be absorbed.

4. Mechanism. Considered in the special sections that follow.

5. Pharmacodynamics and Toxicity. Require parenteral injection; early solutions produced local soreness.

6. Uses. a. Oral preparations have long been obsolete.

b. Injectable preparations are seldom used, having been largely replaced by vitamin B_{12} in the treatment of pernicious anemia.

7. Preparation

Liver injection

Dose: 1 ml daily subcutaneously, decreasing in frequency (each ml contains 10 or 20 mcg of cyanocobalamin).

B. Vitamin B_{12}

1. History. a. Shorb (1947) showed that a growth factor for *Lactobacillus lactis* was present in liver extracts.

b. Rickes and others (1948) used this criterion for the isolation of the anti-pernicious anemia factor, vitamin B_{12} in place of the previous laborious testing on patients; at the same time Smith, using chromatography, isolated the factor.

2. Chemistry. a. Vitamin B_{12} (cyanocobalamin) is a member of a family of active cobalamins (hydroxy, nitro, etc.) which contain cobalt.

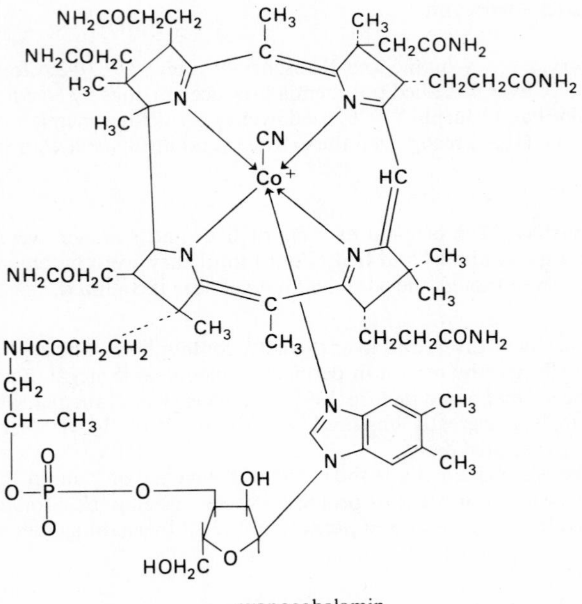

cyanocobalamin

b. Vitamin B_{12} enriches most animal products in the human diet; although made by intestinal bacteria it is not absorbed from the lower intestine of man, whose supply must therefore be exogenous.

c. In drug manufacture it is made by cultures of various *Streptomyces* and *Propionibacteria*.

3. Action. a. Vitamin B_{12} is necessary for normal growth, normal hematopoiesis, and for the proper maintenance of epithelium and probably myelin; requirement 1 microgram per day.

b. The animal protein factor (APF) is identical with vitamin B_{12} and is necessary for growth in lower animals and fowls but its absence in them does not produce pernicious anemia.

4. Mechanism. a. Present view is that vitamin B_{12} is necessary for the synthesis of DNA.

b. May be the result of failure of reduction of ribose nucleotides to deoxyribose nucleotides (Castle, Clin. Pharmacol. Ther., 7:147, 1966).

5. Pharmacodynamics and Toxicity. a. Soluble, but not well absorbed from the diet by man in the absence of intrinsic factor.

b. Elderly persons may have low blood levels (200 ng) but even this is above the level of pernicious anemia (100 ng). Dietary deficiency possible only if no animal or spoiled (bacteria) food eaten.

c. Nontoxic.

6. Uses. The parenteral administration of vitamin B_{12} (or the oral administration with suitable intrinsic factor) controls pernicious anemia: blood, neural, and epithelial abnormalities.

7. Preparations

CYANOCOBALAMIN (vitamin B_{12})

Dose: 20 mcg daily intramuscularly until remission; then 50 mcg intramuscularly monthly (maintenance).

HYDROXOCOBALAMIN (alpha-Redisol)

Similar to cyanocobalamin but may give a longer, higher serum level.
Dose: 50 mcg 2 or 3 times a week intramuscularly until remission; then 100 mcg monthly.

CYANOCOBALAMIN Co 60

Used as a diagnostic test of intrinsic factor activity by measuring the amount of radioactivity lost in the urine. After a 1 mg dose by mouth, normals excrete 10% or more; pernicious anemics excrete 2.5% or less.

MECOBALAMIN

Similar to cyanocobalamin, the CN group replaced by CH_3.

C. Intrinsic Factor

1. Chemistry. a. Intrinsic factor is formed in the gastric mucosa and consists of mucoproteins, three of which have been isolated from pigs or human gastric mucosa, with molecular weights of 5,000, 15,000, and 40,000.

b. Other compounds (sorbitol and polyols) are also said to enhance the absorption of vitamin B_{12} to some extent.

2. Action. Pernicious anemia results from a deficiency of intrinsic factor, which is necessary for the proper absorption of the cobalamins from the diet.

3. Uses. A satisfactory preparation of intrinsic factor would allow pernicious anemia to be treated orally, but no completely satisfactory preparations are available.

4. Preparation

CYANOCOBALAMIN WITH INTRINSIC FACTOR CONCENTRATE
Under investigation; tolerance may develop.

D. Folic Acid and Folinic Acid

1. History. a. Wills (1931) noted that the anemia of pregnancy responded to yeast; Snell and Peterson (1940) showed that a liver factor was essential for the growth of *Lactobacillus casei;* Mitchell (1941) showed that a spinach factor would also support the growth of *L. casei.*

b. Angier (1946) synthesized folic acid and it was shown to be the common factor in the preceding observations.

c. Nichol (1950) showed the function of folinic acid.

2. Chemistry. a. Molecule contains glutamic acid, PABA, and pteridine components.

b. Present in yeast, green vegetables, liver and many other foods.

3. Action. a. Deficiency of folic acid causes inadequate nucleic acid synthesis with early megaloblastic anemia, failure in growth, and inadequate maintenance of the intestinal epithelium.

b. The normal human requirement is 0.1 to 0.2 mg daily.

4. Mechanism. a. Folic acid is the precursor of folinic acid, which is formed from it by partial hydrogenation to tetrahydrofolic acid (requiring ascorbic acid) and the addition of a formyl group.

b. Folinic acid then transfers the formyl units in various methylations (such as ethanolamine to choline), and contributes them to the synthesis of purines and pyrimidines required for nucleic acid synthesis.

HCOO (formate) ← formate, glycine, serine, methionine, choline, betaine
+
folic acid
folinic acid
5-aminoimidazole carboxamide
hypoxanthine
uracil
thymine

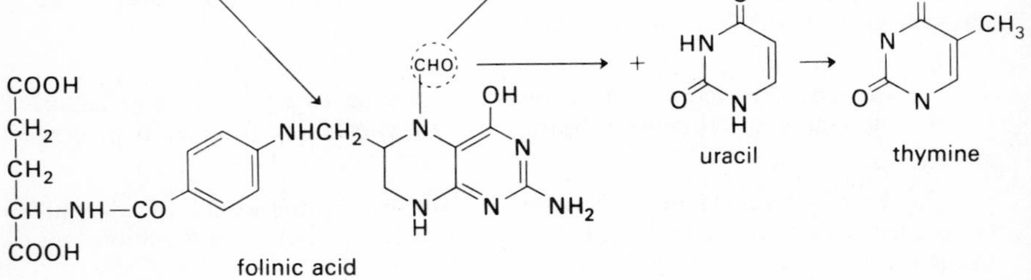

5. Pharmacodynamics and Toxicity. Both folic acid and folinic acid are well absorbed by mouth; nontoxic.

6. Uses. a. Folic acid remedies the megaloblastic anemias and is used in these anemias and the anemias of sprue. However, it will not correct the underlying metabolic effect allowing gliadin toxicity in nontropical sprue.

b. It also will induce an initial hematological response in pernicious anemia, but does not affect the other manifestations, and the response fails as soon as available cobalamin is exhausted. This is highly dangerous because the CNS changes will continue to advance.

c. Folinic acid has no advantage over folic acid except as an antidote for poisoning with folic acid antagonists (aminopterin, methotrexate).

7. Preparations

FOLIC ACID (pteroylglutamic acid; PGA)

Dose: 5 to 10 mg daily by mouth.

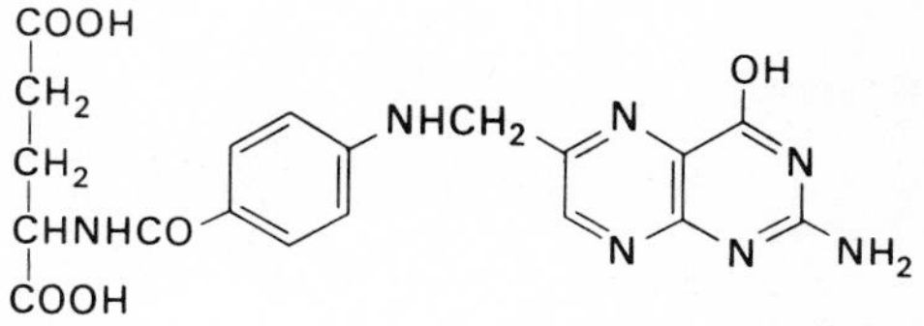

FOLINIC ACID (citrovorum factor)

Administered as: CALCIUM FOLINATE (Leucovorin).

Dose: 3 mg daily by mouth.

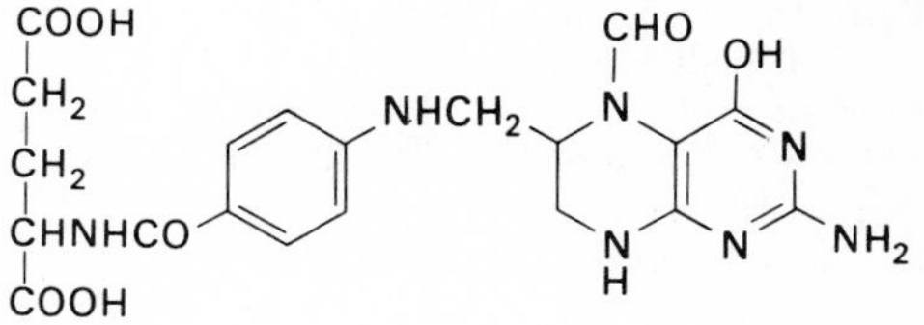

E. Other Factors

ERYTHROPOIETIN

1. Chemistry. a. A glycoprotein, 28,000 mol. wt., containing sialic acid and hexosamine. Not completely isolated.

b. In the presence of renal hypoxia, a renal factor (REF) is produced which acts enzymatically on an alpha-2-globulin in the plasma to generate an active protein, erythropoietin.

2. Action and Mechanism. a. Increases rate of production and release of RBC from marrow.

b. May be deficient in renal damage, causing anemia; however, may be excessively produced in kidney tumor and other conditions.

c. May be blocked by specific antibodies and cause aplastic anemia.

3. Uses. Not available commercially.

SUMMARY: AGENTS IN ANEMIA

TYPE	*ACTION AND MECHANISM*	*TOXICITY*	*USE*	*EXAMPLES*
Iron salts	Hemoglobin defective when iron insufficient	Astringent, deposition of iron pigments	Iron deficiency anemia	Ferrous sulfate
Liver and derivatives	Vitamin B_{12} necessary for hematopoiesis Involved in synthesis of DNA	Minor	Pernicious anemia	Cyanocobalamin
Folic acid and derivatives	Inadequate nucleic acid synthesis	Minor	Megaloblastic anemias	Folic acid

Reviews

Wallerstein, R. O., and Mettier, S. R. Iron in clinical medicine. Berkeley, Univ. Calif. Press, 1958.
Beutler, E. Iron Metabolism. Ann. Rev. Med., 12:195, 1961.
Bothwell, T., and Finch, C. Iron Metabolism. Boston, Little, Brown, 1962.
Friend, D. Iron therapy. Clin. Pharmacol. Ther., 4:419, 1963.
Castle, W. B. Treatment of pernicious anemia: Historical aspects. Clin. Pharmacol. Ther., 7:147, 1966.
Fisher, J. Erythropoietin. N.Y. Acad. Sci., 149:1, 1968.
Finch, C. Erythropoietin. Triangle, 9:127, 1969.

27. Anticoagulants and Coagulants

Coagulation of the Blood. In simplest outline the coagulation of the blood may be expressed as follows: Tissue damage releases thromboplastin, which changes prothrombin to thrombin, which changes fibrinogen to fibrin, the clot. The latter is then slowly dissolved by fibrinolysin.

tissue damage → thromboplastin
prothrombin → thrombin
fibrinogen → fibrin (clot)
profibrinolysin → fibrinolysin
polypeptides

In detail the process is extremely complicated, involving a dozen or more blood and tissue factors, largely a series of enzymes and their activators, several requiring calcium.

1. SYSTEMIC ANTICOAGULANTS

A. Heparin and Related Compounds

HEPARIN

1. History. a. McLean (1916) found an anticoagulant in liver (hence heparin); Howell (1925), Best (1933), Jorpes (1935) purified.

b. Murray and Best (1937) and Crafoord (1937) introduced clinical use.

2. Chemistry. a. Disaccharide polymer mixtures containing two to three sulfuric acid groups (45%); or corresponding tetrasaccharides; mol. wt. about 20,000. Is highly acidic and negatively charged; sulfamic linkage unique.

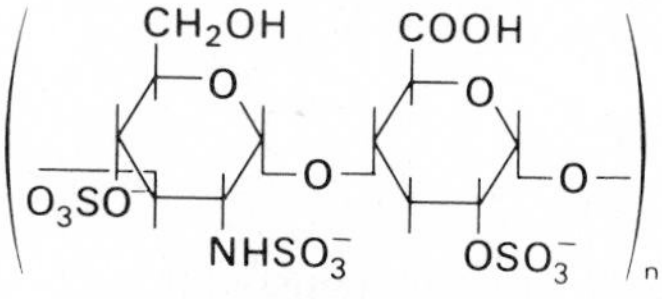

CH_2OH $COOH$ O_3SO $NHSO_3^-$ OSO_3^- n

heparin (polymeric unit)

b. Chemically similar to chondroitin sulfuric acid, and mucoitin sulfuric acid.

c. Heparin is formed normally in the mast cells, whose granules are a heparin-lipoprotein complex, and is released readily from these cells; commercial sources: lungs or liver.

3. Action and Mechanism. a. Heparin is probably the most important natural anticoagulant of the body. Its principal action is as an antithromboplastin. It prevents activation of clotting factor IX (Christmas) and, with a cofactor, inhibits the action of thrombin.

b. It is released in allergic shock and may be responsible for disturbed coagulation in such reactions.

c. In subanticoagulant amounts heparin reduces hyperlipemia by activating a lipoprotein lipase in the blood which hydrolyses the tryglycerides to fatty acids and glycerol. This action has led to its trial in atherosclerosis (see Agents in Atherosclerosis).

d. Action is related to strong acidity.

4. Pharmacodynamics and Toxicity. a. Not well absorbed by mouth.

b. Intravenous administration gives a peak in the blood in 10 minutes which may last 3 hours; subcutaneous administration gives a peak in 1 hour which lasts 4 to 6 hours.

c. Disappears from blood, partly by combination with plasma protein, partly by inactivation by heparinase; 25% in urine as uroheparin.

d. Nontoxic except for danger of bleeding from excessive dosage.

5. Uses. a. May be used as the initial anticoagulant agent in thrombophlebitis and coronary thrombosis; gives quick effects and may be continued until simultaneously administered coumarin derivative begins to act.

b. Therapy must be controlled by observations on the clotting time, not on the prothrombin time, as the latter is not affected by heparin.

c. Used to prevent thrombosis in cardiac vascular surgery.

6. Preparations

HEPARIN SODIUM

Dose: 5,000 units (about 45 mg) every 2 to 4 hours intravenously; (1 mg = about 100 units).

HEPARIN REPOSITORY INJECTION (Depo-heparin; and others)

Heparin in a gelatin-dextrose menstruum.
Dose: 40,000 units (about 360 mg) every 2 to 3 days intramuscularly.

OTHERS

LYAPOLATE SODIUM (Peson)

$$\left[-CH_2\underset{\displaystyle SO_3Na}{\underset{|}{C}H}-\right]_n$$

B. Heparin Antagonists

1. Chemistry. Highly basic compounds; protamine, a protein, has replaced tolonium chloride and hexadimethrine bromide.

2. Action and Mechanism. Heparin antagonists act by neutralizing the acid heparin in the body.

3. Pharmacodynamics and Toxicity. a. Protamine is not absorbed by mouth.

b. It may give shock with overdosage.

4. Uses. Indicated whenever heparin is to be neutralized, as after overdosage, after cardiac surgery in which extracorporeal circulation has been used, or when surgery is necessary for a patient on heparin therapy.

5. Preparations

PROTAMINE SULFATE

Dose: 1 to 1.5 mg for each mg of heparin, intravenously, slowly (not more than 50 mg in 10 minutes).

C. Coumarin and Indandione Derivatives

COUMARIN DERIVATIVES

1. History. a. Schofield (1922) described "sweet clover disease" of cattle as a clotting defect; Roderick (1931) showed the cause to be a prothrombin deficiency. Quick (1935) accelerated the investigation by developing a method of prothrombin estimation.

b. Link (1934–40) isolated bishydroxycoumarin as the prototype toxic agent; Butt and Allen (1949) used it in thrombosis.

2. Chemistry. Derivatives of coumarin; resemblance to vitamin K.

3. Action and Mechanism. a. Cause hypoprothrombinemia; also inhibit proconvertin.

b. Active only in vivo.

c. Interfere with synthesis of prothrombin in the liver, probably by competition with vitamin K.

4. Pharmacodynamics. a. Absorbed readily but not effective for about 24 hours (time to use up prothrombin already present).

b. Bound to plasma proteins; then released to the liver and slowly metabolized over a week; little excreted as such.

5. Toxicity. a. Vomiting, diarrhea, urticaria.

b. More serious danger is widespread hemorrhages, often first manifested as hematuria.

c. Toxicity may be increased by large doses of salicylates or chloral hydrate; decreased by phenobarbital, which induces coumarin-destroying enzymes.

d. Treat poisoning with fresh whole blood and phytonadione (see Vitamin K).

7. Uses. a. Used in thrombophlebitic and thromboembolic states, including postoperative thrombophlebitis, pulmonary embolism, and especially coronary thrombosis.

b. May initiate therapy with heparin to achieve rapid anticoagulant effect.

c. Contraindicated in bleeding syndromes, severe hypertension, or hepatic or renal insufficiency.

d. Therapy should be closely controlled by prothrombin levels (clotting time of recalcified blood in excess of thromboplastin). Maintain 15% to 30% of normal activity; below 15% dangerous. Coagulation or bleeding times inadequate as they are still normal at dangerous levels of prothrombin. Vitamin K should be carried; 5 to 20 mg taken at once if bleeding occurs.

8. Preparations

ACENOCOUMAROL (Sintrom)

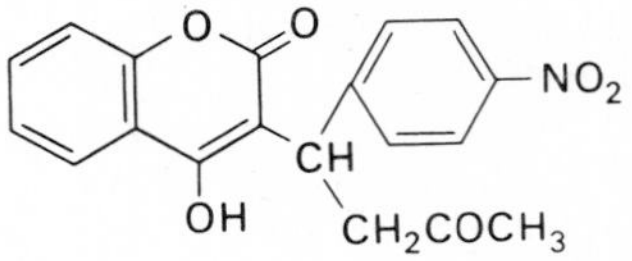

Moderately rapid effect (24 to 48 hours); rapid exit (48 hours).

Dose: 15 to 25 mg by mouth initially, then 2 to 10 mg any day prothrombin activity is over 20%.

O, O, NO_2, CH, OH, CH_2COCH_3

DICUMAROL (Bishydroxycoumarin; dicoumarin)

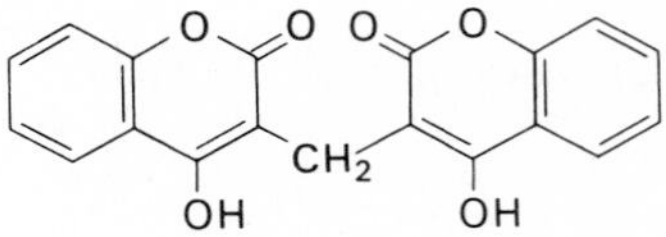

Dose: 300 mg by mouth, then 100 to 200 mg maintenance as above.

O, O, O, O, CH_2, OH, OH

ETHYLBISCOUMACETATE (Tromexan)

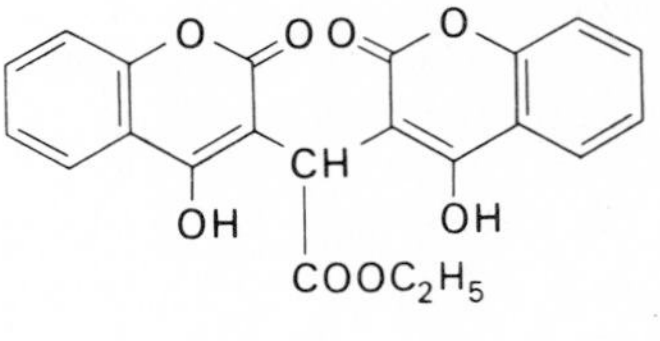

More rapid in transit than bishydroxycoumarin, but more variable.

Dose: 1 gm by mouth initially, then 0.5 to 1 gm maintenance as above.

O, O, O, O, CH, OH, OH, $COOC_2H_5$

PHENPROCOUMON (Liquamar)

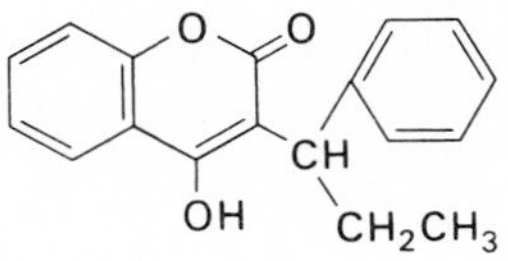

Slow effect (36 to 48 hours); slow recovery (7 to 14 days).

Dose: 20 to 30 mg by mouth initially, then 0.75 to 6 mg maintenance as above.

O, O, CH, OH, CH_2CH_3

WARFARIN SODIUM (Coumadin; Athrombin)

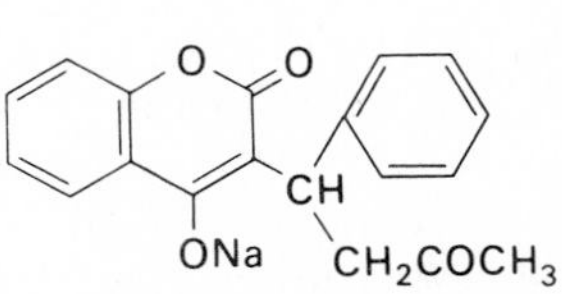

Said to be the easiest coumarin to control. Also used as rodent poison.

Dose: 30 to 40 mg by mouth, or subcutaneously or intravenously initially; then 10 mg maintenance as above.

O, O, CH, ONa, CH_2COCH_3

WARFARIN POTASSIUM (Athrombin-K)

INDANDIONE DERIVATIVES

1. **Chemistry.** Indandione derivatives resembling the coumarins.

2. **Action and Mechanism.** Essentially similar to the coumarins.

3. **Pharmacodynamics.** Absorbed by mouth. Diphenadione slower in onset than phenindione or most coumarins (48 to 72 hours), and most protracted in action (up to 20 days).

4. **Toxicity.** a. Same hemorrhagic dangers as exhibited by the coumarins.
   b. May also cause allergic sensitivity and agranulocytosis.

5. **Uses.** a. Satisfactory agents except for toxicity.
   b. Probably should be reserved for patients sensitive to the coumarins.
   c. Require the same controls and precautions as with the coumarins.

6. **Preparations**

ANISINDIONE (Miradon)

Similar to phenindione.
Dose: 300 mg (initial); then 25 to 300 mg daily, according to prothrombin time.

O O OCH_3

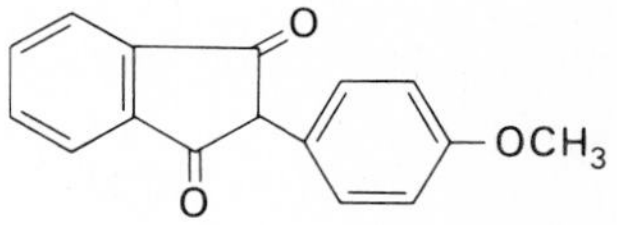

BROMINDIONE (Halinone)

Long-acting derivative of phenidione.
Dose: 10 to 15 mg by mouth on the first day, then 2 to 3 mg daily, or 6 mg every 3 days.

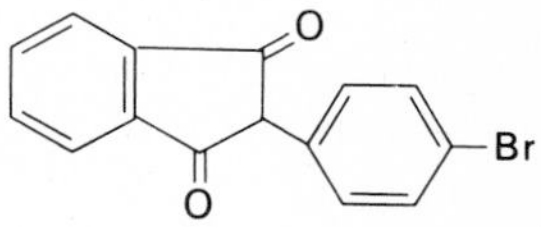

O O Br

DIPHENADIONE (Dipaxin)

Less toxic than phenindione.
Dose: 20 to 30 mg orally on the first day, then 0 to 15 mg daily, according to prothrombin time.

O O CO—CH

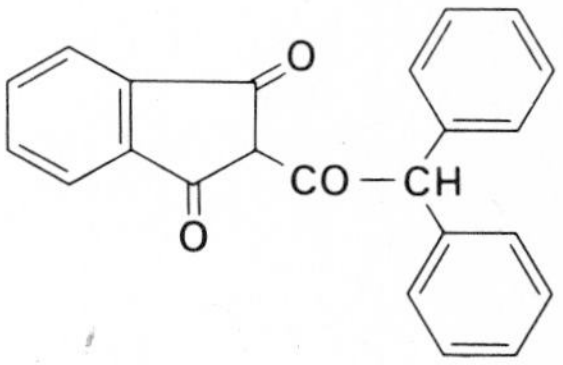

PHENINDIONE (Danilone; Hedulin; Indon)

Dose: 100 to 150 mg twice daily by mouth the first day, then 25 to 50 mg twice daily on any day that prothrombin activity is over 20%.

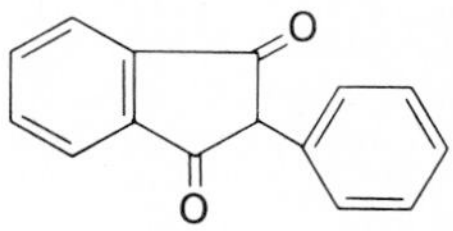

O O

II. LOCAL AND SPECIAL ANTICOAGULANTS

A. Proteolytic and Dornase Enzymes

A number of enzyme preparations are in use to liquefy clotted blood and pus and to reduce inflammation. They are principally proteolytic, but some also contain dornase (DNAase); they are derived from man, lower animals, and plants.

FIBRINOLYSIN (PLASMIN)

1. Chemistry. Human fibrinolysin (plasmin) is an enzyme prepared by the action of streptokinase on profibrinolysin (plasminogen) isolated from human plasma.

2. Action. a. Whenever tissues are damaged, thromboplastin is liberated, setting the clotting mechanism in action.

b. At the same time, fibrinolysis is liberated, setting a corresponding lytic chain in action to dissolve the fibrin deposits in blood vessels; hence to increase tissue permeability and hasten resorption of exudate.

3. Mechanism. a. Fibrinolysin exists in the blood in the form of a precursor, profibrinolysin, which is activated by plasminogen activators; it then breaks down fibrin into large, soluble polypeptides. Circulating antifibrinolysin neutralizes any excess fibrinolysin.

b. Fibrinolysin can be activated in vitro by a number of substances including streptokinase and trypsin; it can break down other proteins as well as fibrin: fibrinogen, casein, gelatin.

c. In shock, the fibrinolysin-antifibrinolysin balance may be disturbed, resulting in excessive fibrinolysis; this may be rectified by adrenal corticoids.

4. Pharmacodynamics and Toxicity. a. Fibrinolysin must be injected intravenously.

b. Febrile reactions are common, and allergic reactions, including rashes, urticaria and edema, have been observed. Excess streptokinase probably partly responsible, as may activate endogenous profibrinolysin.

5. Uses. a. Advised to limit or dissolve clots in thrombophlebitis, phlebothrombosis, and pulmonary embolism; subsidence of pain, edema, and inflammation are claimed.

b. Despite considerable use no reliable assessment is possible; probably somewhat effective in preventing spread of thrombus but ineffective in removing it.

6. Preparation

FIBRINOLYSIN (Human) (Thrombolysin; Actase)

Dose: 50,000 to 500,000 units per day intravenously, given over periods of 1 to 6 hours; repeat on 1 to 3 subsequent days. Smaller doses for thrombophlebitis; larger for arterial emboli.

The powder is dissolved in a small volume (10 ml) of water and then added to an intravenous infusion of 5% dextrose.

STREPTOKINASE

1. Chemistry. Metabolic product of beta-hemolytic streptococci.

2. Action and Mechanism. Activates plasminogen to form plasmin (fibrinolysin) causing a breakdown of fibrin.

3. Pharmacodynamics and Toxicity. a. The highly purified preparations are well tolerated.

b. Therapeutic plasma levels can be rapidly achieved and be maintained for several days.

c. Antigenic in man, no retreatment for 3–4 months.

d. Bleeding from sites of injury.

4. Uses. To treat acute major pulmonary embolism, deep vein thrombosis, and arterial occlusion.

5. Preparations

STREPTOKINASE (Streptase)

Dose: Initial: 250,000 to 600,000 units intravenously by slow infusion (10–30 min.). Maintenance: 100,000 units hourly by slow intravenous infusion.

UROKINASE

1. Chemistry. Plasminogen activator purified from human urine.

2. Action. Helps breakdown of fibrin.

3. Pharmacodynamics and Toxicity. a. Nonantigenic, nonpyrogenic.

b. Causes bleeding from sites of injury.

4. Uses. Similar to Streptokinase.

5. Preparations

UROKINASE (Win-Kinase, Abbokinase)

Dose: Initial: 3,500–7,000 units per kg by slow (10 min.) intravenous injection. Maintenance: same dose per kg hourly.

TRYPSIN AND CHYMOTRYPSIN

1. Chemistry. Crystalline enzymes obtained from pancreas.

2. Action and Mechanism. a. Minute quantities activate prothrombin to thrombin causing coagulation.

b. Large quantities have the opposite action and liquefy blood clots and debride surfaces by proteolytic action.

3. Pharmacodynamics and Toxicity. a. Inactive pharmacologically.

b. Rapidly inactivated by blood and viable tissue.

c. Toxicity minor when applied locally but may give histaminelike flushing when injected or used as an irrigation.

4. Uses. a. Trypsin used chiefly for the liquefaction of coagulated blood and exudate in the debridement of wounds, ulcers, and empyemas; parenteral use investigative.

b. Chymotrypsin advised for use intramuscularly in various inflammations: dermatitis, trauma, strains, sprains, hematoma, and many others. Further clinical experience needed before value can be assessed.

5. Preparations

TRYPSIN, CRYSTALLINE (Parenzyme; Tryptar)

Dose: Applied locally on dry or wet dressings, or in irrigations; 0.25 to 0.5 mg 1 to 4 times a day intramuscularly.

CHYMOTRYPSIN (Chymar)

Dose: 0.5 to 1.0 ml 3 times a day intramuscularly (prepared solution in water or oil).

ALPHA-CHYMOTRYPSIN

Said to be useful in cataract operations to loosen the lens after incision of the cornea.

OTHER PROTEOLYTIC AND ANTICOAGULANT AGENTS

ASPERKINASE (Megazyme)

Proteolytic and diastatic enzymes from *Aspergillus oryzae*. Tried in tissue swelling after trauma or dental surgery.

BRINOLASE

Fibrinolytic enzyme produced by *Aspergillus oryzae*.

PANCREATIC DORNASE (Dornavac)

A dornase (deoxyribonuclease) derived from pancreas; employed to reduce the tenacity of pulmonary secretions.

Dose: 50,000 to 100,000 units 3 times a day by aerosol inhalation for 2 to 6 days.

PAPAIN (Caroid)

Proteolytic enzyme concentrate from *Carica papaya*. Used for edema of trauma, hematoma, inflammation. Urticaria, pruritis, diarrhea, reported as side effects, but evidence of absorption inadequate.

Dose: 10,000 u by mouth, or buccally, every 2 hours.

PLANT PROTEASE CONCENTRATE (Bromelains; Ananase)

Proteolytic enzymes from pineapple plant. May act as depolymerizers and permeability modifiers. Used in injuries, sprains, contusions. Evidence for absorption inadequate.

Dose: 100,000 u 4 times a day by mouth.

PROTEOLYTIC ENZYME, DENATURED (Protamide)

An enzyme from hog stomach claimed to relieve pain from neuritis and to suppress inflammation of nerve roots and radicular pain, as in herpes zoster.

Dose: 1.3 ml intramuscularly daily for 3 to 5 days.

SNAKE VENOMS

Proteolytic snake venoms, such as Russel's viper venom (Stypven), resemble trypsin in action (see Sherry and Fletcher, Clin. Pharm. Therap., 1:202, 1960).

SUTILAINS (Travase)

Proteolytic enzyme from *Bacillus subtilis*.

B. Antiproteolytic Agents

APROTININ (Trasylol)

Purified polypeptide from bovine lung and liver. Inhibits proteolytic enzymes including plasmin and kallikrein. Anticoagulant and vasodilator.

Used in endotoxin, traumatic and anaphylactic shock. Effect doubtful in acute pancreatitis (Skinner, J.A.M.A., 204: 945, 1968).

Dose: Continuous infusion in excess of 100,000 units per hour.

C. Other Enzymes

HYALURONIDASE

1. Chemistry. Enzyme prepared from testis.

2. Action and Mechanism. a. Hydrolyzes mucopolysaccharides of the hyaluronic acid type, which are components of the ground substance of tissues.

b. This dissolution allows spreading of extracellular material.

3. Pharmacodynamics and Toxicity. a. Relatively nontoxic, but rarely may spread infectious processes.

b. Sensitivity infrequent.

4. Uses. a. To promote the spread and absorption of hypodermoclysis solutions.

b. To increase the diffusion of blood and transudates after injuries.

5. Preparation

HYALURONIDASE (Alidase, Diffusin, and others)

Dose: 150 units added extemporaneously to hypodermoclysis and other solutions.

ALPHA AMYLASE (Buclamase)

Amylase from *Bacillus subtilis*; splits starches and polysaccharides into simple sugars. Claimed to hasten resolution of exudates; used in cellulitis, thrombophlebitis, edema. Evidence of absorption inadequate.

Dose: 20 mg 3 times a day buccally.

D. In Vitro Anticoagulants

ANTICOAGULANT SODIUM CITRATE SOLUTION

Contains 2.5% sodium citrate.

Sodium citrate prevents blood from clotting by rendering the calcium insoluble as calcium citrate and is the most commonly used anticoagulant in blood transfusions. It cannot be used safely for systemic anticoagulant effects.

III. SYSTEMIC COAGULANTS

A. Vitamin K and Related Compounds

1. History. a. Dam (1929) described chick hemorrhagic disease.

b. Dam (1935) and Almquist (1935) isolated vitamin K from alfalfa and fish meal. Thayer (1938) determined its structure; Butt (1938) used it clinically.

2. Chemistry. a. A large series (vitamin K_1, K_2, etc.) of substituted naphthoquinones; lipid-soluble.

b. Present in green vegetables and animal sources; menadione synthetic.

3. Action and Mechanism. Promote the formation of prothrombin in the liver, probably by inducing RNA formation for the synthesis (derepresses operator by combining with the repressor; Olson, Science, 145:926, 1964).

4. Pharmacodynamics and Toxicity. a. Inactive pharmacologically; not stored in the body.

b. In premature infants large doses have caused jaundice and fatal kernicterus, presumably because of competition between vitamin K and bilirubin for an inadequate glucuronide transferase system.

5. Uses. Effective in hypoprothrombinemia due to biliary obstruction or fistula (use parenteral route or give with bile salts), malabsorption, or poisoning with coumarin type drugs. Useful in hypoprothrombinemia of the newborn, but should not be given to mothers prophylactically.

6. Preparations

MENADIONE

Dose: 1 mg orally.

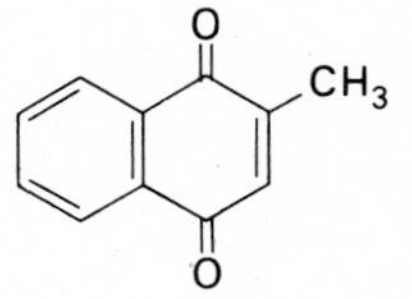

O
CH3
O

MENADIONE SODIUM BISULFATE (Hykinone)

Water-soluble salt.

Dose: 1 to 2 mg subcutaneously or intravenously.

O
CH3
SO3Na
O

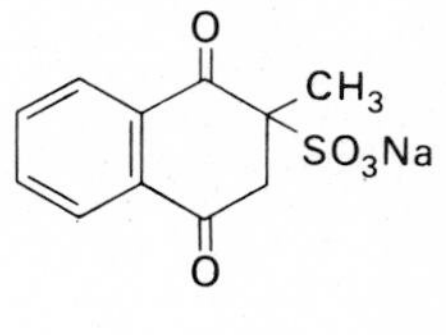

MENADIONE SODIUM DIPHOSPHATE (Synkavite)

Also a water-soluble salt.

Dose: 3 to 6 mg orally, subcutaneously or intravenously.

NaO ONa
O—P=O
CH3
O—P=O
NaO ONa

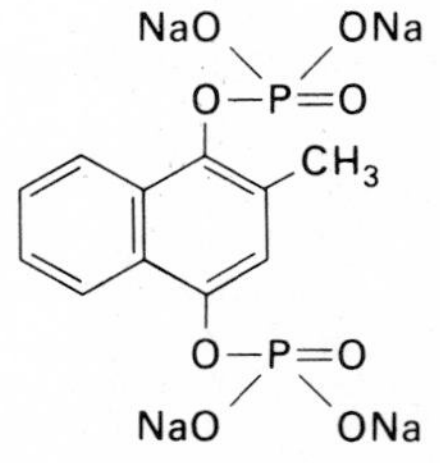

PHYTONADIONE (vitamin K_1, Mephyton)

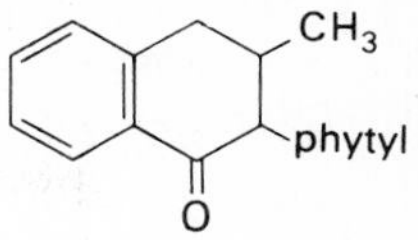

Emulsion used in coumarin poisoning.
Dose: 5 to 50 mg intramuscularly or intravenously; infants 1 to 2 mg.

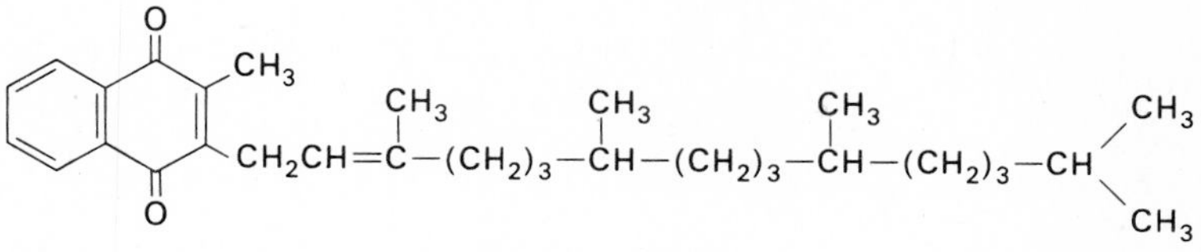

phytyl group

PHYTONADIOL SODIUM DIPHOSPHATE (dihydro-vitamin K_1)

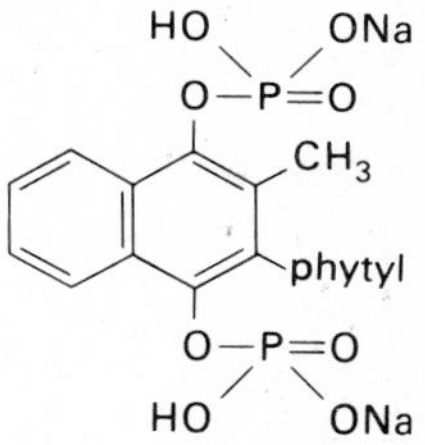

Preferred agent in coumarin poisoning; water-soluble.
Dose: 100 to 200 mg intravenously.

VITAMIN K_1 OXIDE

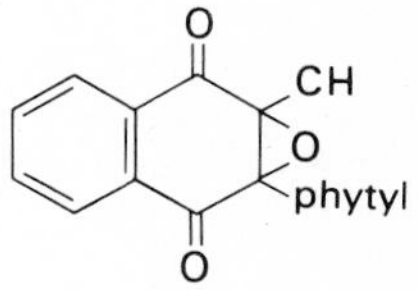

Slower acting; probably changed to vitamin K_1.

OTHERS

Oxamarin.

B. Agents Derived from Blood

ANTIHEMOPHILIC GLOBULIN

1. Chemistry. A globulin, factor VIII, prepared from human plasma.

2. Action. Required in the formation of thromboplastin. Deficient in hemophilia.

3. Uses. Given intravenously to stop bleeding in hemophiliacs; usually supplemented with fresh blood.

4. Preparation

ANTIHEMOPHILIC GLOBULIN
Dose: 200 mg intravenously.

FIBRINOGEN, HUMAN

1. Chemistry. Prepared from human plasma. Irradiated to inactivate hepatitis virus.

2. Action. Supplements natural fibrogen.

3. Uses. In fibrinogenemia or hypofibrinogenemia (congenital, excess of fibrinolysin, abruptio placentae) when fibrinogen level is 50 mg per 100 ml of blood or lower.

4. Preparation

FIBRINOGEN, HUMAN
Dose: 2 to 6 gm intravenously.

C. Other Coagulants

AMINOCAPROIC ACID (EACA: Amicar)

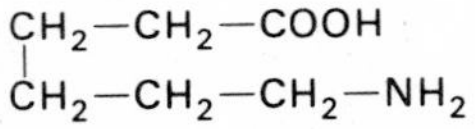

CH_2-CH_2-COOH
$CH_2-CH_2-CH_2-NH_2$

Antifibrinolytic agent discovered by Okamoto; acts by specific inhibition of plasminogen activation. Effective immediately; rapidly excreted.

Toxic effects include renal cortical necrosis (Ratnoff, New. Eng. J. Med., 280:1124, 1970).

Used to prevent bleeding in hemophilia, and after heart and prostate operations in which plasminogen or urokinase may be activated.

Dose: 10 gm per day by mouth; or 6 gm intravenously initially, plus 6 gm slowly over next 24 hours up to a total of 0.2 gm per kg.

TRANEXAMIC ACID (Transamin)

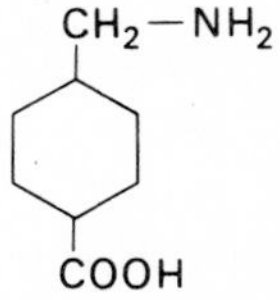

CH_2-NH_2
COOH

Cyclic aminocaproic acid. Potent plasmin inhibitor; hence antifibrinolytic.

About 10 times more potent than EACA.

CARBAZOCHROME SALICYLATE (Adrenosem; Adrestat; Adona)

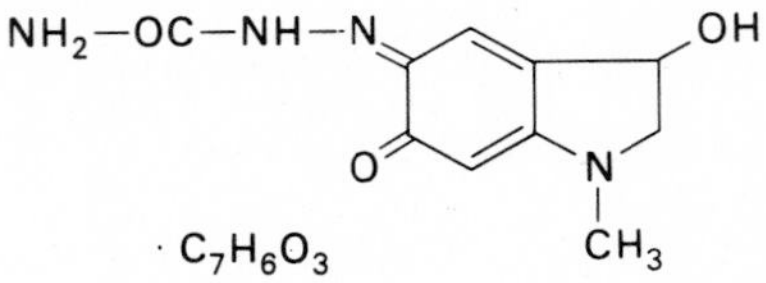

$NH_2-OC-NH-N$ OH O N CH_3 $\cdot C_7H_6O_3$

Claimed to decrease capillary permeability; clinical value doubtful.

Dose: 1 to 5 mg 4 times a day by mouth or intramuscularly.

IV. LOCAL COAGULANTS

OCCLUSIVES

STERILE WAX
Occlusive preparation for stopping oozing from bone surfaces.

OXIDIZED CELLULOSE (Hemopak; Oxycel)

Gauze or cotton treated with NO_2; absorbed in 2 days to 6 weeks; forms an artificial clot.

ABSORBABLE GELATIN SPONGE (Gelfoam)

Porous gelatin material, often applied with thrombin; absorbed in 3 to 5 weeks.

FIBRIN FOAM

Acts as a mechanical network to enmesh oozing blood; often saturated with thrombin.

COAGULANTS

THROMBOPLASTIN

Coagulant; extract of cattle brain; little used.

THROMBIN

Mixture of bovine prothrombin, thromboplastin, and calcium; used on oozing surfaces, often with one of the foregoing occlusive preparations.

ETHAMSYLATE

Hemostatic.

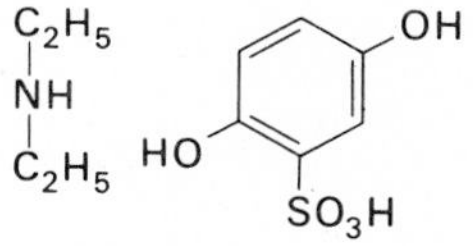

C_2H_5–NH–C_2H_5 · HO–C_6H_3(OH)–SO_3H

SUMMARY: ANTICOAGULANTS AND COAGULANTS

TYPE	*ACTION AND MECHANISM*	*TOXICITY*	*USE*	*EXAMPLES*
Heparin group	Principally an antithrombin Action related to strong acidity	Bleeding	Thrombosis	Heparin sodium
Heparin antagonist	Neutralizes by its alkalinity	Shock	Heparin overdosage	Protamine sulfate
Coumarin derivatives	Interfere with synthesis of prothrombin	Bleeding	Thrombosis	Bishydroxy-coumarin
Proteolytic enzymes	Lyse clots by enzymatic action directly or by activating fibrinolysin	Fever, allergic reactions	To liquefy clotted blood or exudate thrombosis?	Streptokinase-streptodornase
Hyaluronidase group	Hydrolyzes muco-saccharides in tissues allowing spreading of injected material	Minor	To promote diffusion of injected solutions	Hyaluronidase

(cont.)

SUMMARY: ANTICOAGULANTS AND COAGULANTS (cont.)

TYPE	*ACTION AND MECHANISM*	*TOXICITY*	*USE*	*EXAMPLES*
Vitamin K group	Coagulant by promoting formation of prothrombin	Generally minor	Hypoprothrombinemia, as from coumarin drug excess	Phytonadione

Reviews

Moser, R. H. II. Cardiac and vascular diseases. Clin. Pharmacol. Ther., 2:456, 1961.
Weiner, M. Pharmacological considerations of antithrombic therapy. Advances Pharmacol., 1:277, 1962.
Sherry, S. Symposium on thrombosis and anticoagulation. Amer. J. Med., 33:619, 1962.
Potter, L. Theory and Practice of Anticoagulant Therapy. Baltimore, Williams and Wilkins, 1962.
Pechet, L. Fibrinolysis. New Eng. J. Med., 273:966, 1965.
Jacques, L. B. Anticoagulant Theory. Springfield, Ill., Charles C Thomas, 1965.
Russell, F. E. Pharmacology of animal venoms. Clin. Pharmacol. Ther., 8:849, 1967.
Coon, W., and Willis, P. Some aspects of the pharmacology of oral anticoagulants. Clin. Pharmacol. Ther., 11:312, 1970.

28. Drugs Used in the Alimentary Tract

A. Agents Used in the Mouth

MOUTHWASHES

1. Chemistry. Mouthwashes are aqueous or alcoholic solutions, flavored with volatile oils, and often containing bicarbonates or borates.

2. Action and Uses. a. Mouthwashes are useful to flush out debris after eating.

b. Any disinfecting quality is relatively useless.

c. Similar preparations may be used for gargling; throat irrigations are usually simply warm water or saline solution.

3. Preparation

ANTISEPTIC SOLUTION

Contains boric acid, essential oils, water, and alcohol.

DENTIFRICES

1. Chemistry. Contain the following types of ingredients:

a. Detergent: soap or synthetic detergent, e.g., sulfocolaurate.
b. Abrasive: calcium salts, aluminum silicate, bentonite.
c. Emollient and vehicle: glycerin, propylene glycol.
d. Flavoring: essential oils.
e. Sweetening: saccharin.
f. Medicaments: urea, penicillin, chlorophyll, all of dubious utility in toothpastes; fluoride, efficacy compared to inclusion in drinking water under investigation.

2. Action and Uses. a. Primarily to promote the use of a toothbrush for oral cleanliness and presumptive inhibition of caries.

b. Etiological factors in caries include sugars, phosphoric acid, acid-producing bacteria, fluoride deficiency, molybdenum deficiency (?).

ANTICARIES AGENTS

SODIUM FLUORIDE (NaF); STANNOUS FLUORIDE (SnF_2)

Fluorides may be incorporated during tooth development into the apatite structure of tooth enamel; fluoroapatite has decreased solubility in acid media, resulting in resistance to caries.

Fluoride may be supplied as fluoridated drinking water (1 ppm of fluoride ion). Concentrations over 2 ppm may cause dental fluorosis. Where fluoridated water is not available, topical application of NaF (2% solution) or SnF_2 (8% solution) may be applied to the teeth by a dentist periodically throughout childhood. Dentifrices containing SnF_2 also appear to be effective.

OTHERS

Dectaflur, hetaflur, olaflur, sodium monofluorophosphate.

B. Digestives

STOMACHICS

1. Action and Uses. a. Bitter substances, popularly thought to improve gastric function and hence appetite.

b. Presumed to act by local or reflex action, but the effects are probably largely functional.

c. Widely used in appetizers, tonics, cocktails, bitters and patent medicines.

2. Preparations

ELIXIR OF IRON, QUININE, AND STRYCHNINE

Bitter "tonic." Ingredients inadequate to exert any specific therapeutic effect.

COMPOUND TINCTURE OF GENTIAN

Similarly used bitter.

DIGESTIVES

1. Action and Use. Agents alleged to aid digestion.

2. Preparations

GLUTAMIC ACID HYDROCHLORIDE

Used as a replacement for HCl.

HYDROCHLORIDE ACID

Sometimes prescribed in anacidity, but seldom in quantity adequate to represent replacement therapy.

PANCREATIN

Plausible use in pancreatic deficiency with steatorrhea, but seldom beneficial.

PEPSIN

No real utility.

CARMINATIVES

1. Action and Uses.

a. Mild irritants and volatile oils which are assumed to increase peristalsis and therefore to relieve the distension of overeating.

b. Effects largely psychic.
c. Widely used as after-dinner mints, chewing gum, liqueurs, cordials.

C. Antacids

ALKALINE SALTS

1. Chemistry. Inorganic salts with alkaline reaction.

2. Action. a. To neutralize, or partially neutralize, gastric acidity.
b. This relieves pain and discomfort in peptic ulcer and functional indigestion either by removing the direct (painful?) digestion of the ulcer by acid, or by removing painful spasm by readjustment of muscle tone.

3. Pharmacodynamics and Toxicity. Systemic alkalosis possible from excessive dosage (of soluble salts only).

4. Use. For quick, often transient, relief of indigestion.

5. Preparations

SODIUM BICARBONATE ($NaHCO_3$)

Quickest and most effective, but produces the greatest rebound of acidity after its action passes and the greatest chance of alkalosis with overuse.
Dose: 2 gm repeated as needed.

CALCIUM CARBONATE ($CaCO_3$)

Less effective, and constipating, but with longer action and less rebound; insoluble, hence little likelihood of alkalosis.
Dose: 2 gm repeated as needed.

MAGNESIUM OXIDE (MgO)

Produces loose stools; insoluble.
Dose: 0.25 gm, repeated as needed, and often mixed with one of the preceding drugs.

COLLOIDAL ANTACIDS

1. Chemistry. Insoluble salts with buffering properties.

2. Action. a. Buffer gastric acidity at about pH 4.
b. Action much less brisk than with sodium bicarbonate and relief probably on the basis of decreased acidity rather than on any sudden shift of muscle tone.
c. May protect the surface of an ulcer by mechanical coating.

3. Pharmacodynamics and Toxicity. a. Constipation; occasional impaction (Al salts); diarrhea (Mg salts).
b. No danger of alkalosis; little rebound.

4. Uses. Often preferred to alkaline salts, even though less rapidly effective, because of lack of rebound and more prolonged effect.

5. Preparations

ALGELDRATE
Aluminum hydroxide

ALMADRATE SULFATE
Aluminum magnesium hydroxide oxide sulfate.

ALUMINUM HYDROXIDE GEL [$Al(OH)_3$] (Amphogel; Creamalin)

Contains aluminum hydroxide and oxide in a suspension.
Dose: 0.6 gm (or 8 ml of the liquid preparation) by mouth every 2 to 4 hours as needed.

ALUMINUM HYDROXIDE GEL WITH MAGNESIUM HYDROXIDE (Maalox; Aludrox)

Mixture of aluminum and magnesium hydroxides.
Dose: 8 ml every 2 to 4 hours by mouth as needed.

ALUMINUM PHOSPHATE ($AlPO_4$) (Phosphajel)

Dose: 8 ml every 2 to 4 hours as needed.

BASIC ALUMINUM CARBONATE (Basaljel)

An aluminum carbonate-aluminum hydroxide gel.
Dose: 8 ml every 2 to 4 hours as needed. Also used in larger doses (30 ml 4 times a day) to diminish phosphate absorption in urinary calculi through combination with phosphate in the intestine.

DIHYDROXYALUMINUM AMINOACETATE (Alglyn): $C_2H_6AlNO_4$

Dose: 0.5 to 1 gm every 4 hours as needed.

DIHYDROXYALUMINUM SODIUM CARBONATE (Rolaids)

GLUCALDRATE, POTASSIUM (Aciquel)

Dose: Under investigation.

$$\left(\begin{array}{c} H_2O \quad O \\ HO \quad O- \\ Al \\ HO \quad O- \\ H_2O \quad C_4H_9O_4 \end{array} \right)^- K^+$$

MAGALDRATE (Riopan): $[Mg(OH)]_4 \cdot [(OH)_4Al(OH)(OH)Al(OH)_4]$

Dose: 0.8 gm 4 times a day by mouth.

MAGNESIA AND ALUMINA (Maalox)

MAGNESIUM TRISILICATE: $2\ MgO \cdot 3\ SiO_2$

Dose: 1 gm every 4 hours by mouth as needed.

SILODRATE: $2\ MgO \cdot Al_2O_3 \cdot 3\ SiO_2 \cdot xH_2O$

OTHERS

Gastric mucin

Protective and emollient; usually combined with other antacids. Mucotin contains mucin, aluminum hydroxide, and magnesium silicate.

Polignate sodium

A sodium salt of lignosulfonic acid. Described as a pepsin inhibitor.

Polyamine-methylene resin (Exorbin; Resinat)

Polyethylene-polyamine substituted resins which adsorb acid and pepsin in the stomach, with release in the alkaline intestine. Bulky, somewhat distasteful and irritating; no rebound. Little used.

Dose: 0.5 to 1 gm every 2 hours by mouth as needed.

Polyethadene

Polymer of polyethyleneimine and diepoxybutane.

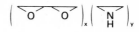

D. Gastric Acid Production Inhibitors

H_2 histamine antagonists (see Autacoids and Hormones).
Prostaglandins (see Autacoids and Hormones).

E. Emetics

LOCALLY ACTING

1. Chemistry. Various substances with irritative properties, such as inorganic salts.

2. Action. Empty the stomach by vomiting, induced by direct irritation.

3. Toxicity. Possibilities of erosion, systemic absorption, aspiration pneumonia, and accidents from increased intravascular pressure.

4. Uses. a. To empty the stomach in poisoning; possibly also to relieve cough reflexly.

b. Alternatives to mechanical irritation, as by tickling the throat or gastric tube, which, however, are often safer and more convenient.

5. Preparations

Salt water, or Mustard in water

Household remedies.

Syrup of ipecac

Contains emetine. Used in emergencies, particularly in children; produces vomiting in 15 to 30 minutes.

Dose: 15 ml.

ZINC SULFATE

Dose: 50 ml of 1% solution. (Copper sulfate in phosphorus poisoning only.)

CENTRALLY ACTING

APOMORPHINE HYDROCHLORIDE

A morphine derivative prepared by treatment with concentrated HCl; direct stimulant of vomiting center and strong central depressant.

Dose: 5 to 10 mg subcutaneously.

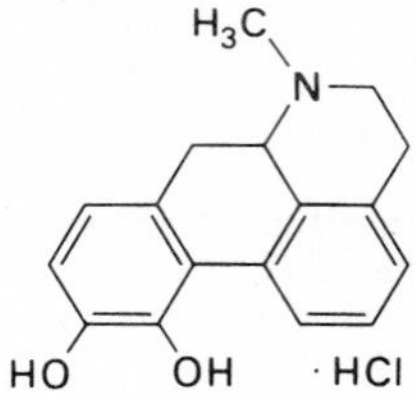

H_3C N HO OH · HCl

F. Antiemetics

See Antiemetics under Tranquilizers.

G. Choleretics

1. Chemistry. Steroids or analogues related to cholic acid, normal component of bile.

2. Action and Mechanism. a. Bile salts emulsify fat in the intestine and thereby enhance its absorption.

b. Choleretics increase bile production; hydrocholeretics increase the volume of the bile.

c. Bile salts, which contain cholic acid, are assumed to be choleretic; dehydrocholic acid is preponderantly hydrocholeretic.

3. Pharmacodynamics and Toxicity. Nontoxic except for occasional diarrhea.

4. Uses. a. Bile salts have been used by mouth to improve the absorption of vitamin K in patients with biliary obstruction.

b. Dehydrocholic acid has been used to wash out fragments of gallstones and, vaguely, to drain the biliary tree.

5. Preparations

BILE SALTS; BILE ACIDS; OX BILE EXTRACT

Preparations containing cholic acid or related compounds.

Dose: 0.5 gm.

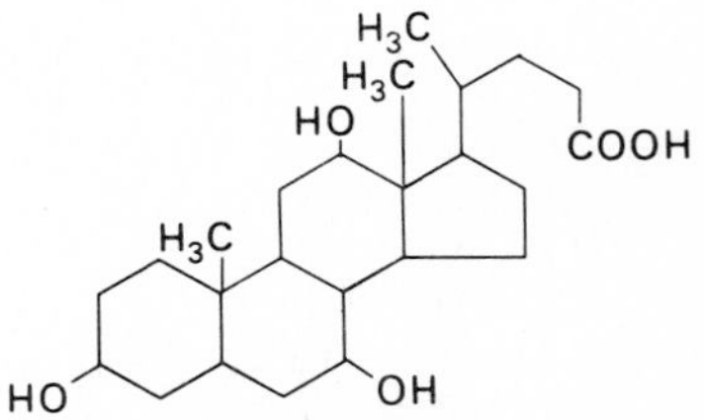

H_3C H_3C HO COOH H_3C HO OH

cholic acid

DEHYDROCHOLIC ACID (Decholin)

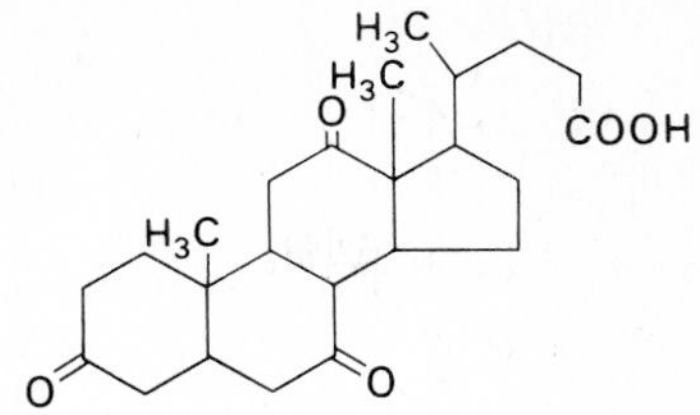

Oxidized derivative of cholic acid.

Dose: 0.25 to 0.5 gm 2 to 3 times a day by mouth after meals.

Sodium dehydrocholate injection

Dose: 5 to 10 ml daily intravenously for 3 days. Single dose for circulation time.

FLORANTYRONE (Zanchol)

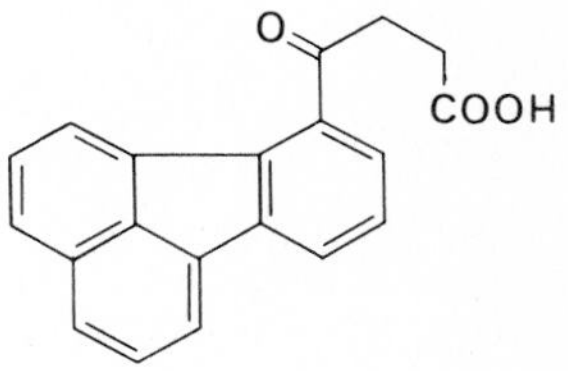

Synthetic relative similar in effect to dehydrocholic acid.

Dose: 1 gm by mouth daily.

PIPROZOLIN

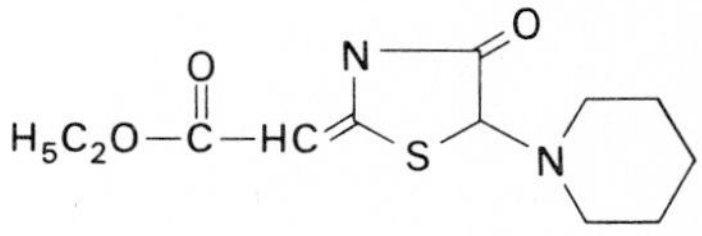

Under investigation.

SINCALIDE (Kinevac) Asp-Tyr(SO_3H)-Met-Gly-Trp-Met-Asp-Phe—NH_2 (1 2 3 4 5 6 7 8)

C-terminal octapeptide of cholecystokinin. Produces rapid contraction of the gall bladder.

Dose: 20 pg (picogram, 10^{-12} gm).

TOCAMPHYL (Gallogen; Syncuma)

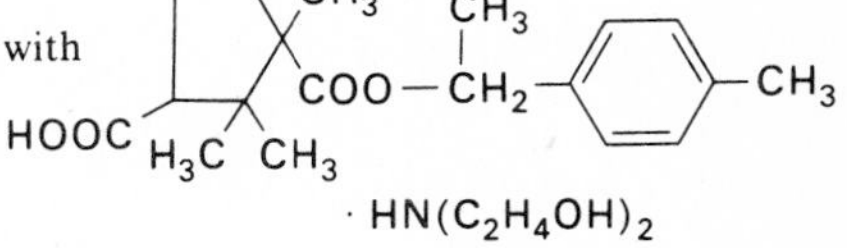

Dose: 75 mg 3 times a day by mouth with meals.

$\cdot HN(C_2H_4OH)_2$

H. Cathartics

Cathartics once constituted a major part of a physician's drugs. He distinguished between laxatives (mild) and cathartics, purges, purgatives, physics and drastics (more and more severe). Attention to the bowels is now much simpler, but still may contribute much to a patient's comfort. In the hospital constipation may result from the inactivity of illness, but often is a carryover of chronic constipation. The latter is often basically dissatisfaction with bowel movements rather than inadequate bowel movements, but is a common complaint, and one in which excessive use of drugs often plays a part. In its treatment reeducation and the mildest of drugs are to be preferred.

LUBRICANTS

1. Action. Lubricants are simple oils and emulsions which soften and lubricate the bowel contents.

2. Pharmacodynamics and Toxicity. a. Absorption of lubricants is minimal, but deposition in the liver may occur.

b. More important are possible loss of fat-soluble vitamins, and inhalation, with lipoid pneumonia, in infants or the infirm.

3. Uses. Widely used in chronic constipation, especially during attempts to eliminate the use of more potent agents.

4. Preparations

MINERAL OIL (liquid petrolatum)

Dose: 15 ml by mouth at bedtime.

EMULSION OF LIQUID PETROLATUM (Petrogalar, and others)

More expensive, but anal leakage less likely.
Dose: 15 ml by mouth once or twice daily.

SOFTENERS

1. Chemistry. Wetting agents (anionic surface-acting agents).

2. Action. Soften feces by surface action of the wetting agent. Effect develops slowly, over several days.

3. Pharmacodynamics and Toxicity. Inert, tasteless.

4. Uses. a. Alternative to lubricants in chronic constipation.

b. In megacolon, fissure, and other conditions where soft stools are desired. Often appreciated by the elderly.

5. Preparations

DIOCTYL CALCIUM SULFOSUCCINATE (Surfak)

Dose: 250 mg by mouth daily.

DIOCTYL SODIUM SULFOSUCCINATE (Colace; Doxinate)

Dose: 10 to 60 mg by mouth daily.

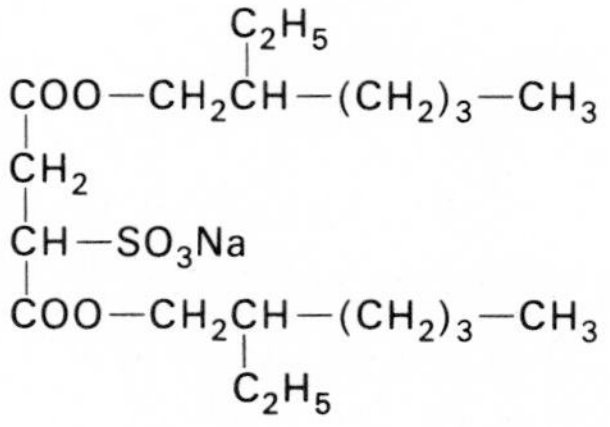

$$
\begin{array}{l}
\qquad\qquad\quad C_2H_5 \\
\qquad\qquad\quad | \\
COO-CH_2CH-(CH_2)_3-CH_3 \\
| \\
CH_2 \\
| \\
CH-SO_3Na \\
| \\
COO-CH_2CH-(CH_2)_3-CH_3 \\
\qquad\qquad\quad | \\
\qquad\qquad\quad C_2H_5
\end{array}
$$

POLOXAMER 182LF (Pluronic L-62LF)

POLOXAMER 188 (Pluronic F-68, Polykol, Magcyl)

POLOXAMER 331 (Pluronic L-101)
Dose: 100 to 200 mg by mouth daily.

BULKY SUBSTANCES

1. Chemistry. Vegetable polysaccharides.

2. Action and Mechanism. a. The polysaccharide gums swell when wet, producing a bulky, bland mass.

b. This distends the intestine and induces increased peristalsis which aids bowel movement as well as furnishing satisfying bulk.

3. Pharmacodynamics and Toxicity. a. Pharmacology inert.

b. Inadequate fluid intake may result in inspissation of the fecal mass and impaction.

4. Uses. a. Often the most desirable agents in the treatment of chronic constipation.

b. In the treatment of chronic constipation, patients should be instructed as to proper bowel habits, fluid intake, exercise, and interpretation of their mental concern.

c. Bulky substances should substitute entirely for cathartics if possible, and in turn be reduced in amount as improvement allows.

5. Preparations

METHYCELLULOSE (Cellothyl; Methocel; and others)
Dose: 1 to 1.5 gm 2 to 4 times a day.

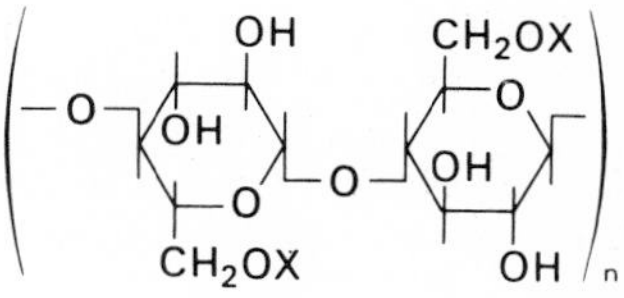

$X = H, CH_3$

PSYLLIUM HYDROPHILIC MUCILLOID (Metamucil, Konsyl)
Dose: 4 to 7 gm 1 to 3 times a day.

SODIUM CARBOXYMETHYLCELLULOSE (Carmethose)
Dose: 1.5 gm 3 times a day.

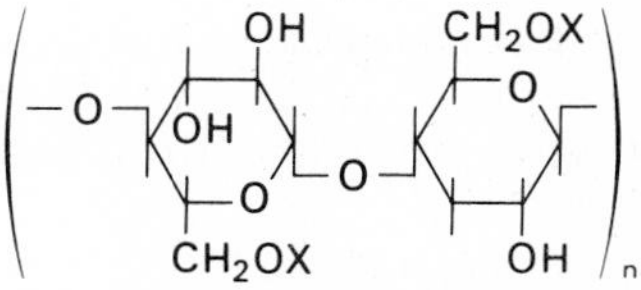

$X = H, CH_2COONa$

Other preparations contain agar (relatively ineffective), karaya or bassora gums (highly satisfactory plant gums), and bran (inadvisable because of irritating qualities).

SALINE CATHARTICS

1. Chemistry. Soluble inorganic salts.

2. Action and Mechanism. a. Although soluble, the salts are not absorbable, and therefore retain water in the intestine through osmotic effect.

b. The retained water distends the intestine and thus stimulates peristalsis, which results in a brisk bowel movement, usually liquid, within a few hours.

3. Pharmacodynamics and Toxicity. Inert; toxicity from absorption rare.

4. Uses. Most satisfactory cathartics where quick action is desired, as in poisoning, in connection with vermifuges, and in acute illness.

5. Preparations

MAGNESIUM SULFATE (epsom salts) ($MgSO_4$)

The most useful saline cathartic.
Dose: 15 gm by mouth.

MILK OF MAGNESIA (magnesia magma)

Dose: 15 ml by mouth.

SOLUTION OF MAGNESIUM CITRATE

Dose: 200 ml by mouth.

SODIUM PHOSPHATE and SODIUM SULFATE (NaH_2PO_4; Na_2SO_4)

Less commonly used.
Dose: 4 gm and 15 gm, respectively, by mouth.

EMODIN CATHARTICS

1. History. a. Cascara sagrada introduced by Bundy in 1877.

b. Others include rhubarb (Chinese), aloe, and senna.

2. Chemistry. Contain anthracene glycosides that release emodin and other polyhydroxyanthroquinones from bacterial action in the large bowel.

3. Action and Mechanism. a. Emodin and related compounds are irritating to the bowel, inducing increased peristalsis and a bowel movement 6 to 8 hours later.

b. May also inhibit Na^+ ion transport from lumen to cells, with retention of water in lumen and resultant stimulation of peristalsis.

4. Pharmacodynamics and Toxicity. Excessive purgation may be produced.

5. Use. The milder preparations are commonly used in chronic constipation.

6. Preparations

AROMATIC FLUIDEXTRACT OF CASCARA SAGRADA

Dose: 4 to 8 ml by mouth, usually in the evening.

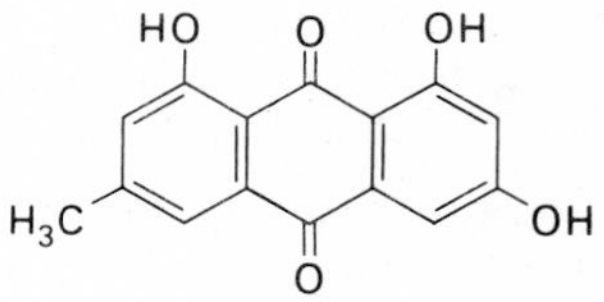

HO O OH
H_3C OH
O

emodin

DANTHRON (Chrysazin)

Dose: 50 to 150 mg by mouth at bedtime.

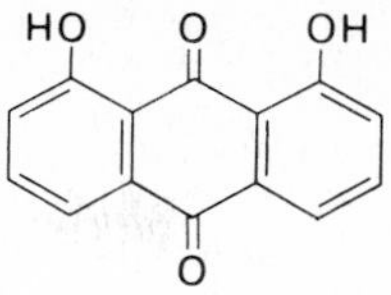

OTHERS

Senna, Casanthranol, Peri-Colace.

RESIN GROUP

Contain resins which are irritating all through the digestive tract; no modern use. Examples include elaterin, jalap, podophyllum (but used on warts), colocynth.

IRRITANT OILS

1. Chemistry. Contain irritating fatty acids; thus castor oil on hydrolysis liberates ricinoleates which act on the small bowel, and croton oil contains "croton resin" which is reputed to be the most potent cathartic. Examples: castor oil, croton oil.

2. Use. Castor oil may be used to prepare the large bowel for x-ray examination.

3. Preparation

CASTOR OIL

Dose: 15 ml by mouth.

PHENOLPHTHALEIN AND ISATIN DERIVATIVES

1. Chemistry. a. Phthalic anhydride and isatin derivatives.
b. Some of the latter natural agents in prunes.

2. Action and Mechanism. Inhibit sodium and water absorption from the large bowel.

3. Pharmacodynamics and Toxicity. a. Mild cramping or, with larger doses, excessive purgation.

b. Sensitization with rashes has been reported from phenolphthalein. Oxyphenisatin has been reported to cause hepatitis.

4. Use. Much used in chronic constipation, especially in proprietary medicines.

5. Preparations

BISACODYL (Dulcolax)

Acts in 6 hours.

Dose: 10 to 15 mg by mouth or 10 mg in suppositories.

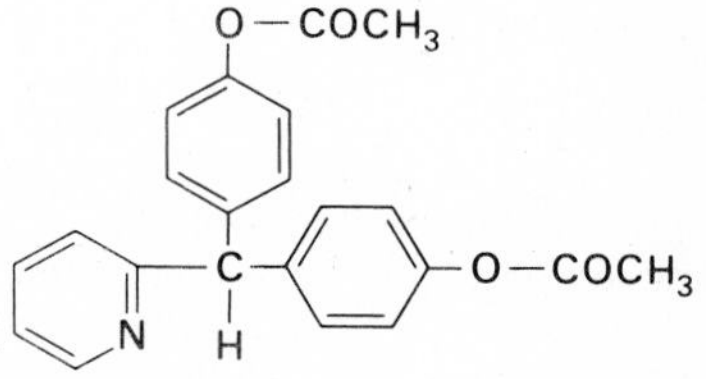

BISACODYL TANNEX
(Clysodrast)

OXYPHENISATIN (Lavema)
Acts directly on the colon.
Dose: 10 to 20 mg in an enema.

Oxyphenisatin acetate (Isocrin and others)
Dose: 5 mg by mouth.

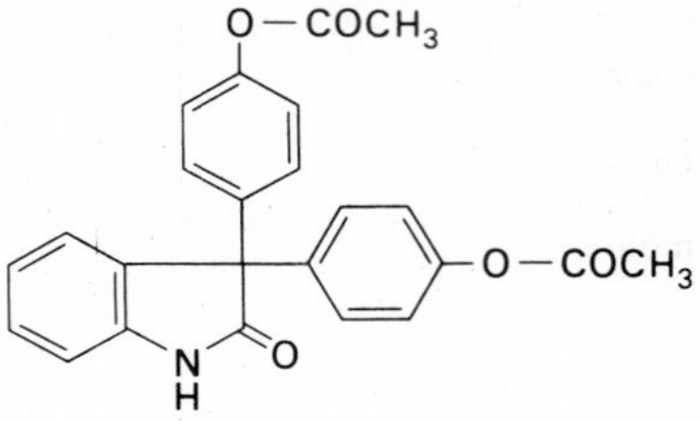

O—COCH3
O—COCH3
N
H
O

PHENOLPHTHALEIN
Effective in about 6 hours.
Dose: 60 mg by mouth.

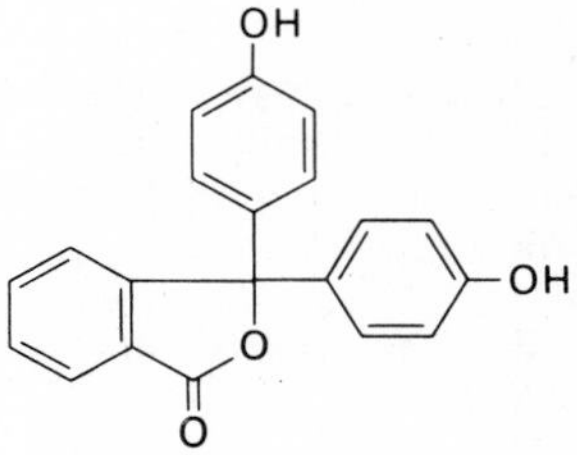

OH
OH
O
O

OTHERS
Bisoxatin acetate (Tolsis).

OTHER CATHARTICS

CALOMEL (mild mercurous chloride): $HgCl_2$
Weak, irritant; long obsolete.

LACTULOSE
Neutralizes intestinal ammonia. Used in hepatic encephalopathy.

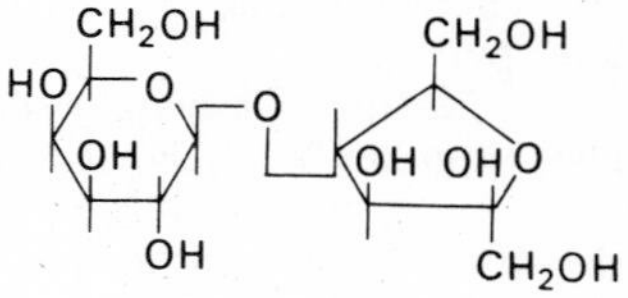

CH_2OH CH_2OH
HO O O
OH OH OH O
OH CH_2OH

ENEMAS

Acute distension of the rectum by various fluids results in evacuation in 20 or 30 minutes. For quick, uncomplicated effects in acute illnesses enemas are often the preferred method for obtaining a bowel movement. The fluid may be tap water, saline, or soapsuds. Retention enemas, sometimes containing oil, may be used to soften impacted feces. Nutritive enemas are relatively unsatisfactory as absorption is poor. Prepared enemas in disposable containers have the advantage of simplicity.

DEFOAMING AGENTS

SIMETHICONE (Antifoam A; Mylicon; Silain)

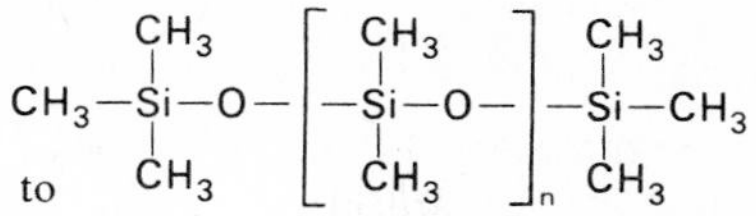

$$CH_3-\underset{CH_3}{\overset{CH_3}{Si}}-O-\left[-\underset{CH_3}{\overset{CH_3}{Si}}-O-\right]_n-\underset{CH_3}{\overset{CH_3}{Si}}-CH_3$$

Defoaming agent; enables pockets of gas to coalesce.

Uses: Antiflatulant; in aerophagia; in pulmonary edema.

Dose: 40 mg after meals and at bedtime by mouth.

POLOXALENE (Therabloat; Bloat Guard)

See Surface-Acting Compounds under Local Antiinfectives.

I. Agents Used to Control Diarrhea

A number of nonspecific agents are useful for the symptomatic control of diarrhea. Examples include:

BISMUTH SUBCARBONATE [$(BiO)_2CO_3$]

A bland protective and astringent.
Dose: 1 gm by mouth, repeated as needed.

CHARCOAL, ACTIVATED

In combination with magnesium oxide and tannic acid used as universal antidote in poisonings.
Dose: 1 to 8 gm by mouth, repeated as needed.

DIPHENOXYLATE HYDROCHLORIDE (in Lomotil)

Analgesic related to meperidine (see Narcotic Analgesics). Used to diminish diarrhea by inhibiting smooth muscle of bowel.

KAOLIN (in Kaopectate); CLAYSORB (in Polymagma); ATTAPULGITE, activated (Attasorb)

Adsorbent clays for the symptomatic control of diarrhea; often mixed with pectin.

LOPERAMIDE HYDROCHLORIDE (Imodium)

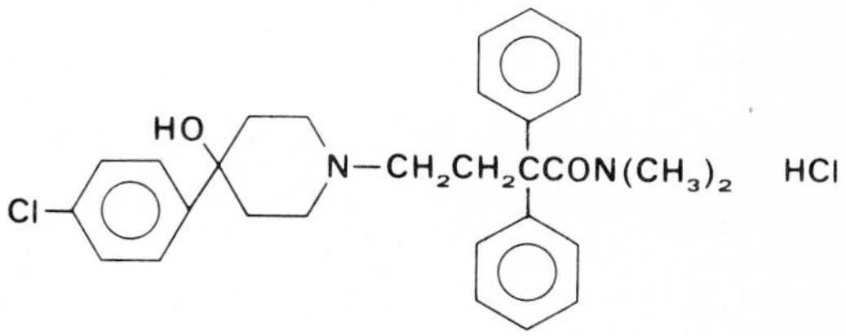

HO, Cl, $N-CH_2CH_2CCON(CH_3)_2$ HCl

PAREGORIC (camphorated tincture of opium)

Widely used; after initial stimulation, intestine is paralyzed, especially lower bowel.
Dose: 4 ml by mouth, repeated as needed.

PECTIN

Dose: 0.5 gm; usually in combinations.

POLYCARBOPHIL (in Sorboquel); CALCIUM POLYCARBOPHIL (in Carbophil); MALETHAMER

Adsorptive polymers for the symptomatic relief of diarrhea.

TINCTURE OF OPIUM (laudanum)

Dose: 0.6 ml by mouth.

J. Enzymes

CELLULASE (Dorase)

Enzyme claimed to aid in digestion of cellulose.

PANCRELIPASE (Cotazym, Lipan)

Pancreatic lipase reported to control lipase deficiency. Used in pancreatitis and viscidosis.

Dose: 300 mg before meals, 100 mg at intermeal feedings.

SODIUM AMYLOSULFATE (Depepsen)

Enzyme inhibitor under investigation for treatment of peptic ulcer.

SUMMARY: DRUGS USED IN THE ALIMENTARY TRACT

TYPE	*ACTION AND MECHANISM*	*TOXICITY*	*USE*	*EXAMPLES*
Agents used in the mouth	Cleansing, anticaries	Minor	Dentifrices, prevent caries	Sodium fluoride
Digestives	No important actions	Minor	Aid digestion	Hydrochloride acid
Antacids	Lower gastric acidity	Alkalosis	Indigestion	Aluminum hydroxide gel
Emetics	Induce vomiting by direct irritation or reflexly	Gastric irritation	Poisoning	Syrup of ipecac
Choleretics	Increase bile flow	Minor	Improve absorption of vitamin K	Dehydrocholic acid
Lubricant cathartics	Soften stool	Minor	Chronic constipation	Mineral oil
Bulky substance cathartics	Increase volume of stool	Minor	Chronic constipation	Methylcellulose

SUMMARY: DRUGS USED IN THE ALIMENTARY TRACT (cont.)

TYPE	*ACTION AND MECHANISM*	*TOXICITY*	*USE*	*EXAMPLES*
Saline cathartics	Increase volume of stool by retaining water in bowel osmotically	Minor	To produce acute bowel movement	Magnesium sulfate
Emodin cathartics and other irritant types	Irritate bowel wall and induce forward peristalsis	Excessive bowel activity	Constipation	Cascara sagrada
Antidiarrheal	Decrease intestinal activity	Minor	Diarrhea	Paregoric

Reviews

Law, D. H., Smith, F. W., and others. Drug therapy of gastrointestinal disease. Amer. J. Med. Sci., 238:160, 1959.

Kirsner, J. D., Dooley, J., Scott, G., and Kraft, S. Gastroenterology. Ann. Rev. Med., 10:21, 1959.

Kirsner, J. Facts and fallacies of current medical therapy for uncomplicated duodenal ulcer. J.A.M.A., 187:423, 1964.

Phillips, R., Love, A., and others. Cathartics and the sodium pump. Nature, 206:1367, 1965.

Holtz, S. Drug action on the digestive system. Ann. Rev. Pharmacol., 8:171, 1969.

29.
Diagnostic Agents

Many agents of pharmacological nature are used as diagnostic aids. Like drugs, they must be effective yet without excessive toxicity.

A. Plasma and Blood Volume

1. **Chemistry.** Dyes and radioactive isotopes.

2. **Preparations**

CHROMIC CHLORIDE $Cr^{51}(Cr^{51}Cl_3)$

SODIUM CHROMATE Cr^{51} (Chromitope Sodium) $Na_2Cr^{51}O_4$

Both used in estimating whole blood volume.

EVANS BLUE

An azo dye which combines firmly with plasma albumin; measurable color depends on volume of blood in which dye is diluted.
Dose: 25 mg in 6 ml of dilute saline intravenously.

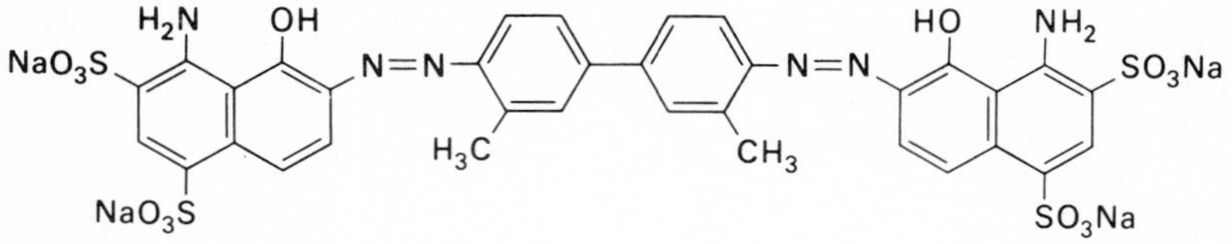

H_2N OH HO NH_2 NaO_3S N=N N=N SO_3Na H_3C CH_3 NaO_3S SO_3Na

IODINATED I^{131} SERUM ALBUMIN

After intravenous injection leaves the blood slowly; radioactivity of plasma proportional to dilution of agent. Used to study blood volume, circulation time, and cardiac output; also for localization of brain tumors.

SODIUM ANAZOLENE (Coomassie blue); HO N=N SO_3Na NaO_3S SO_3Na NH

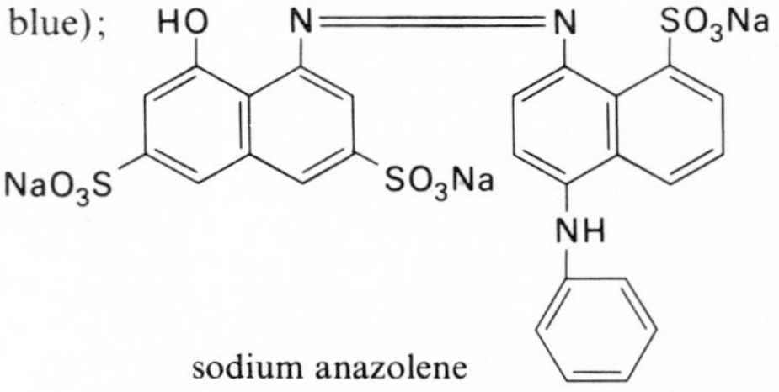

sodium anazolene

INDOCYANINE GREEN (Cardio green)

For measuring cardiac output by the indicator dilution technique.

SODIUM CHROMATE $Cr^{51}(Na_2Cr^{51}O_4)$

Diffuses into RBC and is then fixed to the globulin. Used to study red cell volume and survival.

B. Gastric Acidity

1. Preparations

AZURESIN (Diagnex blue)

A blue dye resin (azure A carbacrylic resin) from which the dye may be displaced by H^+ ions in the stomach; the dye is then absorbed and excreted in the urine where it may be estimated by colorimetric means. Used to estimate gastric acidity.

Dose: 2 mg (fasting), usually 1 hour after a stimulant of gastric secretion, such as betazole.

BETAHISTINE HYDROCHLORIDE (Serc)

Histamine potentiator.
Has been used for vertigo of Ménière's disease.
Dose: 4 mg 2 to 4 times a day by mouth.

(pyridine ring, N) $CH_2CH_2-N(H)(CH_3)$ · HCl

BETAZOLE HYDROCHLORIDE (Histalog)

Histamine substitute with fewer side effects.
Dose: 50 mg subcutaneously, or 100 mg by mouth.

(pyrazole ring, N, NH) $CH_2CH_2-NH_2$ · HCl

HISTAMINE PHOSPHATE (or dihydrochloride)

Stimulates maximum gastric acidity; side effects include flushing and fall in blood pressure.

Dose: 1 mg subcutaneously.

(imidazole ring, HN, N) $CH_2CH_2-NH_2$ · H_3PO_4

PENTAGASTRIN

Potent stimulator of gastric secretion.
Under investigation.
Dose: 6 μg/kg subcutaneously.

β-ala—C(=O)—O—C(CH₃)₃
|
tryp
|
meth
|
asp
|
phen—NH_2

C. Hypertension

Sympatholytic drugs, such as phentolamine or piperoxan, cause a diagnostic fall of blood pressure in patients with an excess of circulating norepinephrine in pheocromocytoma (see Sympathetic Depressants).

D. Kidney Function

1. Preparations

INULIN [$(C_6H_{10}O_5)_3$]

A starchlike carbohydrate from dahlia bulbs. Inulin clearance measures glomerular filtration rate.

MANNITOL

A hexahydric alcohol. Filtered by the glomeruli (10% reabsorbed by tubules; none secreted) and used to measure glomerular filtration rate.

$HO{-}CH_2CH(OH)CH(OH)CH(OH)CH(OH)CH_2{-}OH$

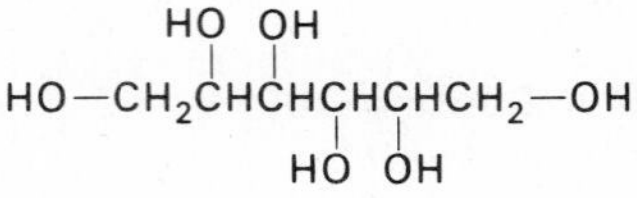

PHENOLSULFONPHTHALEIN (phenol red)

Acts similarly to *p*-aminohippurate but indicates about two thirds of effective renal plasma flow.

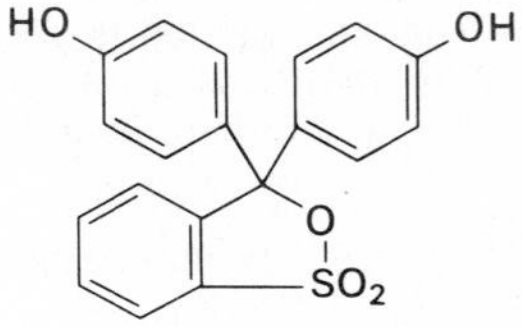

SODIUM *p*-AMINOHIPPURATE

Filtered by glomeruli and excreted by tubules. Used to measure renal plasma flow, and tubular excretion.

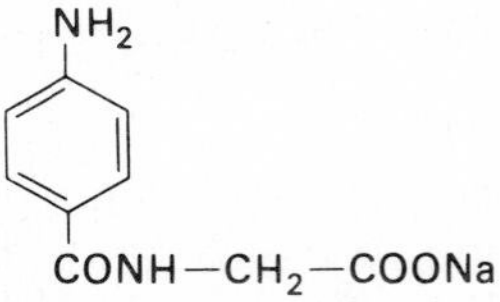

SODIUM INDIGOTIN DISULFONATE (indigo carmine)

Colored dye used to indicate and measure kidney function.

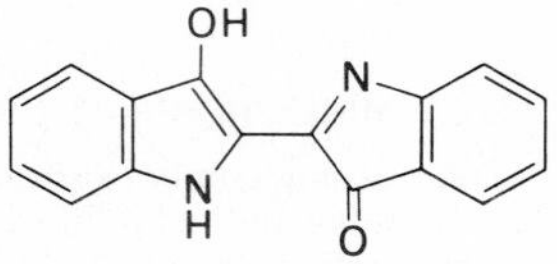

indigotin

SODIUM THIOSULFATE

Also used to measure glomerular filtration, but less accurately, as there is some tubular excretion and reabsorption.

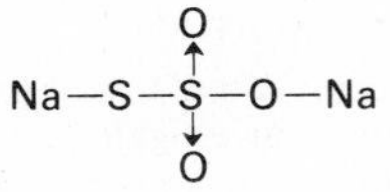

$Na{-}S{-}S(\rightarrow O)_2{-}O{-}Na$

E. Circulation Time

SODIUM DEHYDROCHOLATE (Decholin)

See Choleretics.

Dose: 5 mg in 20% solution gives average time of 12 sec.

SODIUM SUCCINATE

Dose: 1.5 mg in 30% solution gives average of 17 sec.

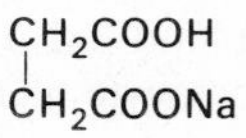

CH_2COOH
CH_2COONa

F. Hypoalbuminemia

TOLPOVIDONE I 131 (Raovin)

To measure excretion of albumin in stool.
Dose: 4 to 25 microcuries intravenously.

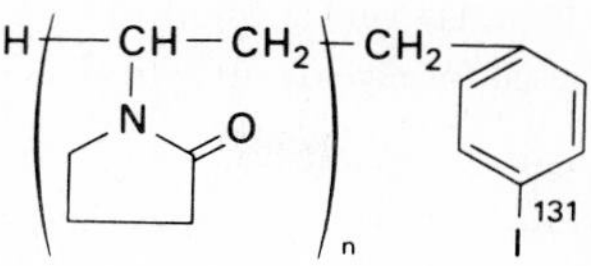

G. Liver Function

1. Preparations

GALACTOSE TOLERANCE TEST

Liver normally converts galactose to glycogen; in liver disease galactose is excreted in urine.

Dose: 40 gm galactose by mouth (measure galactose in urine), or 0.5 gm intravenously (measure galactose in blood).

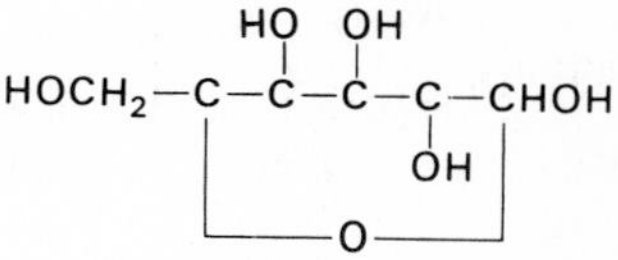

HIPPURIC ACID TEST

Benzoic acid normally conjugated with glycine in the liver forming hippuric acid. Deficient excretion of hippuric acid (measured after hydrolysis to benzoic acid) in urine in liver disease.

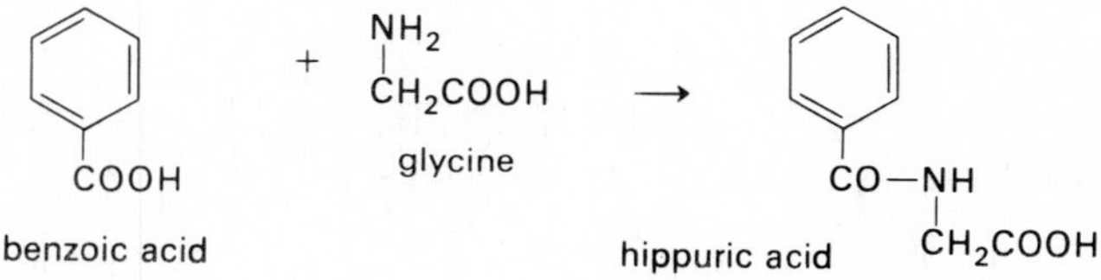

benzoic acid + glycine → hippuric acid

SULFOBROMPHTHALEIN SODIUM (Bromthalein)

Dye which liver normally removes from blood after intravenous injection. Retention in blood indicates degree of liver damage.

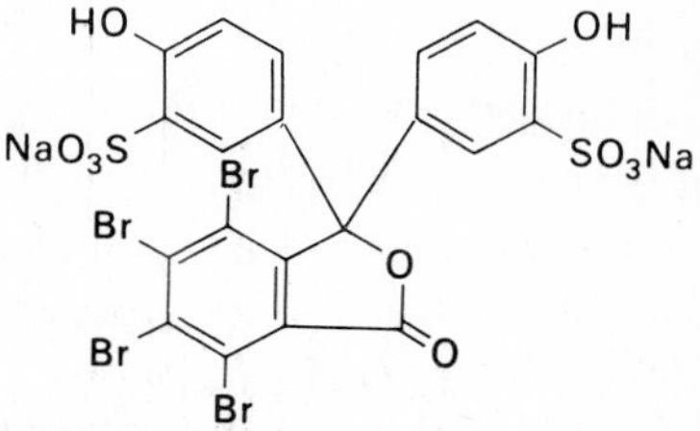

H. Radiopaque Media

IODIZED OILS

1. **Chemistry.** Oils or fatty acids containing iodine (radiopaque).

2. **Toxicity.** May produce local irritation.

3. **Uses.** Injected into cavities for the visualization of the bronchial tree, spinal canal, uterine tubes, bile ducts, fistulas, etc.

4. Preparations

IODIZED OIL (Lipiodol), and IODIZED POPPY SEED OIL
Used for myelography (danger of arachnoiditis).

CHLORIODIZED OIL (Iodochlorol), and IODOBRASSID (Lipoiodine)
Used for bronchography, hysterosalpingography, to outline fistulas, etc.

ORGANIC IODINE COMPOUNDS

1. Chemistry. Principally iodinated benzene or pyridone derivatives.

2. Toxicity. a. Insoluble, oral preparations may cause minor nausea or vomiting.
b. Soluble, oral or intravenous preparations may cause cardiovascular collapse; also anaphylactic reactions in persons sensitive to iodine.

3. Uses. a. Insoluble preparations used largely for cholecystography; well absorbed and subsequently concentrated in the bile.
b. Soluble preparations given orally or intravenously for visualization of the gallbladder, urinary tract, bronchial tree, blood vessels and other structures.

4. Preparations

a. Benzene derivatives

ETHYL CARTRIZOATE
Bronchographic agent.

IOCETAMIC ACID (Cholebrine)
For oral cholecystography.

IODAMIDE (Uromiro)

IODOALPHIONIC ACID (Priodax)
For oral cholecystography.

IOGLYCAMIC ACID (Biligram); IOGLYCAMATE MEGLUMINE (Biligram)
For intravenous cholangiography and cholecystography.

IOPANOIC ACID (Telepaque)
Similar use.

IOPHENDYLATE (Pantopaque)
For myelography or injection into biliary tree.

IOPHENOXIC ACID (Teridax)
Similar use. Repeated, large doses (over 4 or 5 gm) may produce renal tubule necrosis.

IOSEFAMIC ACID
For intravenous cholangiography and cholecystography.

PROPYLIODONE

SODIUM ACETRIZOATE (Urokon)

For intravenous or retrograde urography; angiocardiography. No longer marketed.

SODIUM BUNAMIODYL (Orabilex)

For oral cholecystography. Renal tubular necrosis may follow large doses. Withdrawn from market.

SODIUM DIATRIZOATE (Hypaque)

For intravenous urography; meglumine salt for angiography or oral use.

SODIUM DIPROTRIZOATE (Miokon)

For intravenous urography.

SODIUM IODIPAMIDE; IODIPAMIDE MEGLUMINE (Chlorografin)

For cholangiography.

SODIUM IODOHIPPURATE (Hippuran)

For intravenous or retrograde pyelography.

SODIUM IODOPHTHALEIN (Tetraiodophthalein, Iodeikon)

Orally or intravenously for gallbladder visualization.

SODIUM IPODATE (Oragrafin)

For oral cholecystography and cholangiography.

SODIUM IOTHALAMATE (Angio-Conray; Conray-400)

For intravascular use; maglumine salt for urography and angiography.

SODIUM METHIODAL (Skiodan)

For urography.

SODIUM METRIZOATE (Isopaque)

SODIUM PHENTETIOTHALEIN (Iso-Iodeikon)

Similar but better tolerated.

SODIUM TYROPANOATE (Bilopaque)

Oral cholecystographic agent.

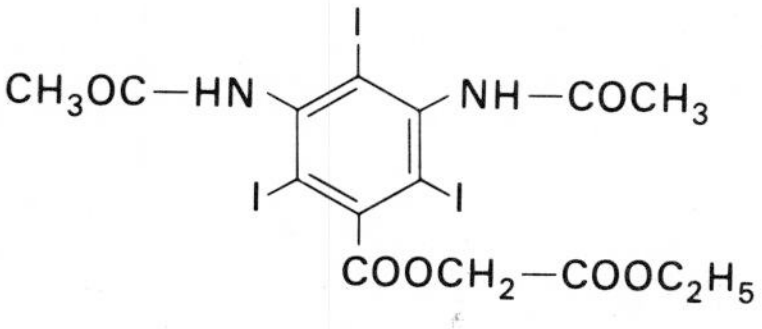

I

$CH_3OC—HN$ $NH—COCH_3$

I I

$COOCH_2—COOC_2H_5$

ethyl cartrizoate

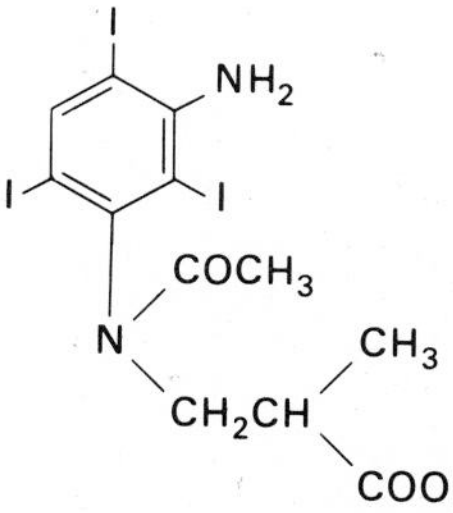

I

NH_2

I I

$COCH_3$

N CH_3

CH_2CH

COOH

iocetamic acid (Cholebrine)

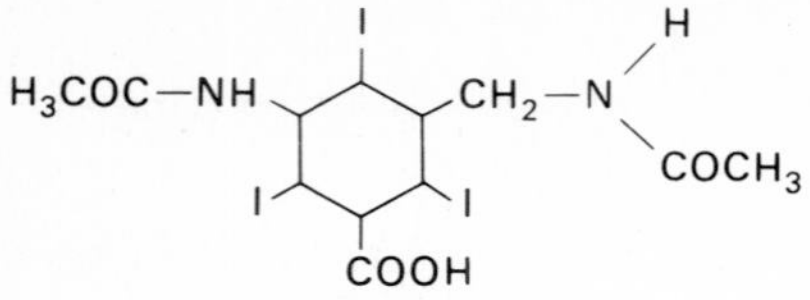

I
$H_3COC-NH$ $CH_2-N(H)(COCH_3)$
I I
COOH

iodamide

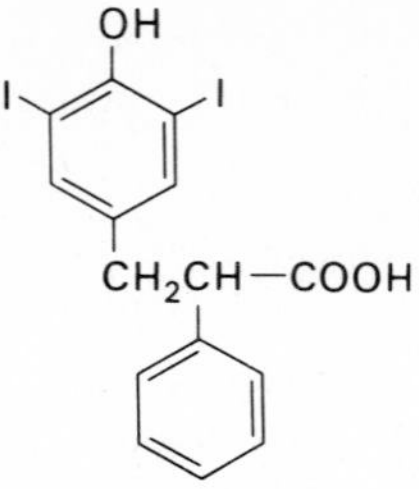

OH
I I
$CH_2CH-COOH$
(phenyl)

iodoalphionic acid

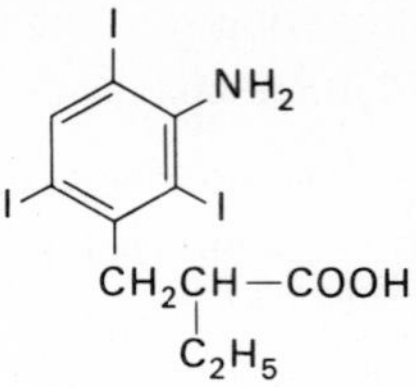

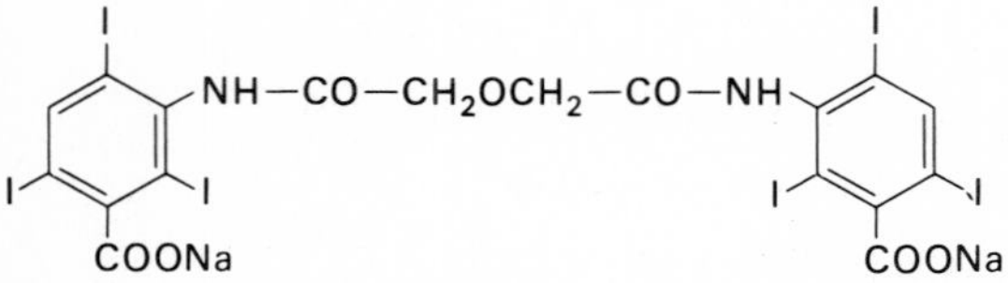

I
NH_2
I I
$CH_2CH-COOH$
C_2H_5

I
$NH-CO-CH_2OCH_2-CO-NH$
I I
COONa

I
I I
COONa

ioglycamic acid

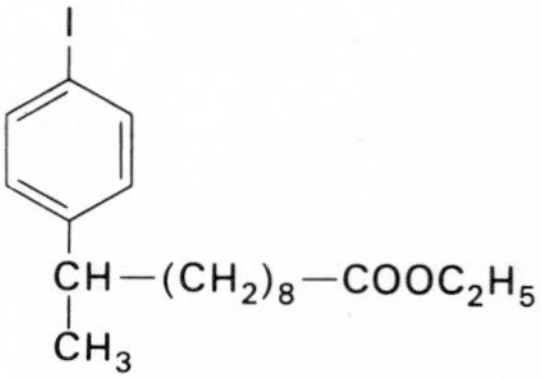

I
$CH-(CH_2)_8-COOC_2H_5$
CH_3

iophendylate

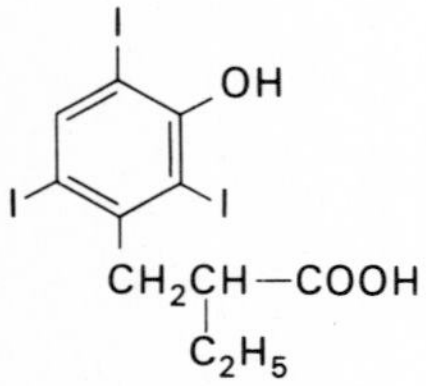

I
OH
I I
$CH_2CH-COOH$
C_2H_5

iophenoxic acid

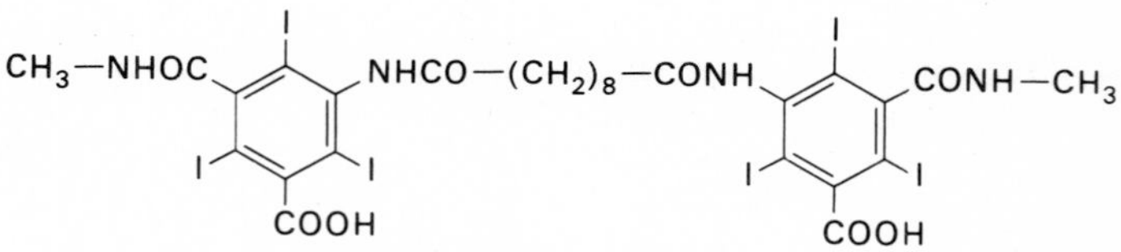

I
CH_3-NHOC $NHCO-(CH_2)_8-CONH$ I $CONH-CH_3$
I I I I
COOH COOH

iosefamic acid

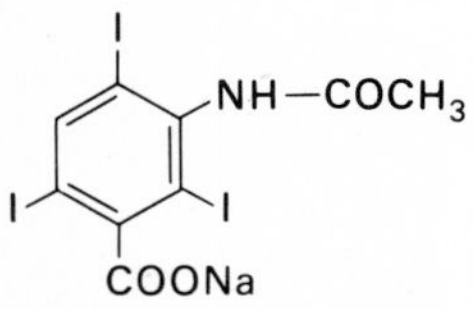

I
$NH-COCH_3$
I I
COONa

sodium acetrizoate

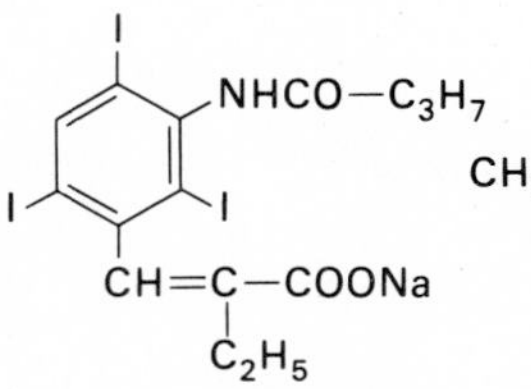

I
$NHCO-C_3H_7$
I I
$CH=C-COONa$
C_2H_5

sodium bunamiodyl

I
CH_3OC-HN $NH-COCH_3$
I I
COONa

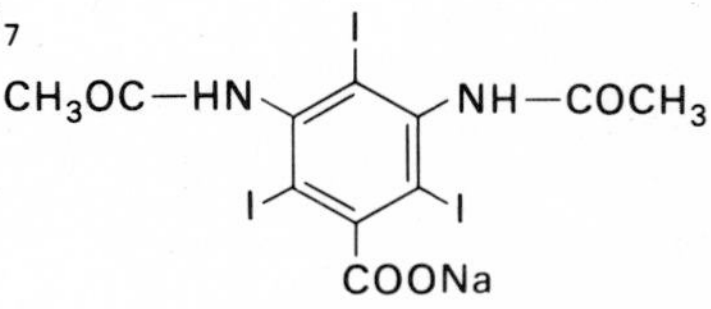

sodium diatrizoate

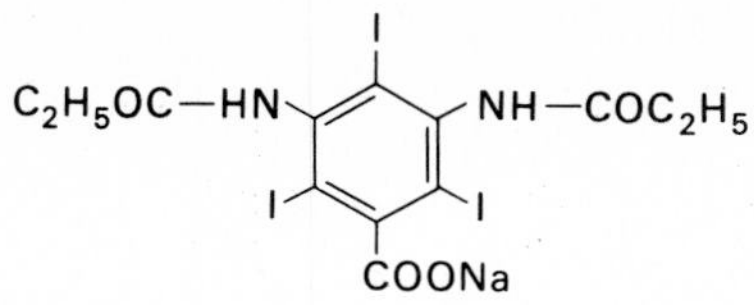

C_2H_5OC-HN $NH-COC_2H_5$ I I I $COONa$

sodium diprotrizoate

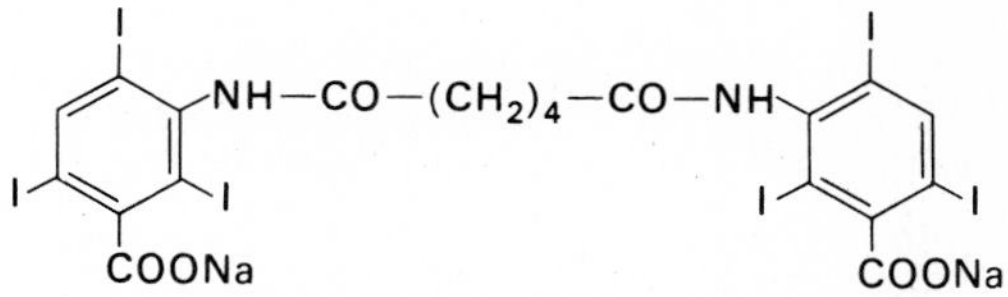

I $NH-CO-(CH_2)_4-CO-NH$ I I I I I $COONa$ $COONa$

sodium iodipamide; iodipamide meglumine

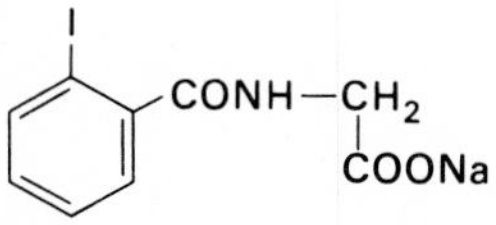

I $CONH-CH_2$ $COONa$

sodium iodohippurate

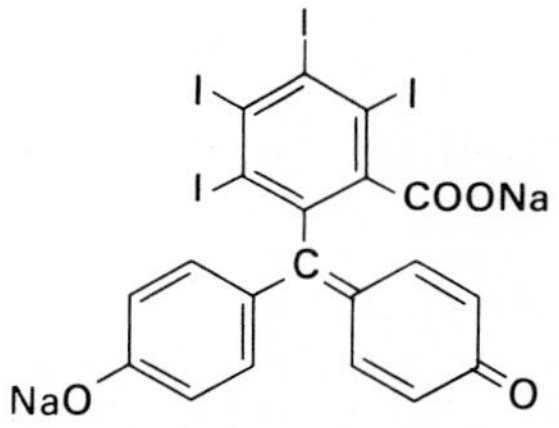

I I I I $COONa$ C NaO O

sodium iodophthalein

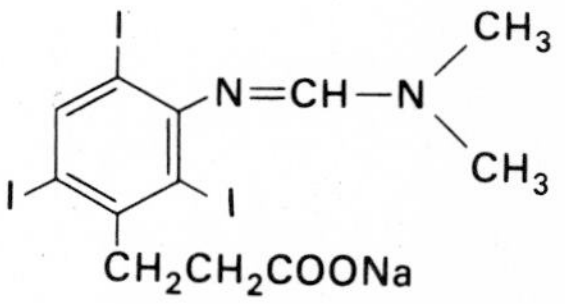

I $N=CH-N$ CH_3 CH_3 I I CH_2CH_2COONa

sodium ipodate

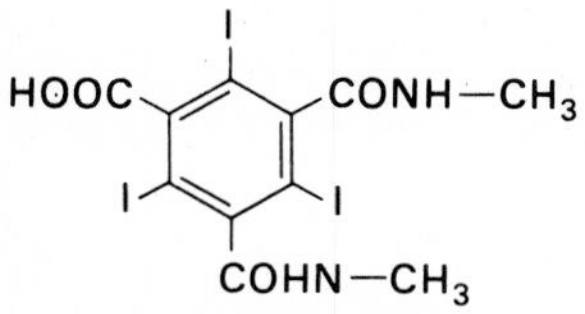

I HOOC $CONH-CH_3$ I I $COHN-CH_3$

sodium iothalamate

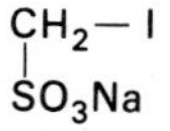

CH_2-I SO_3Na

sodium methiodal

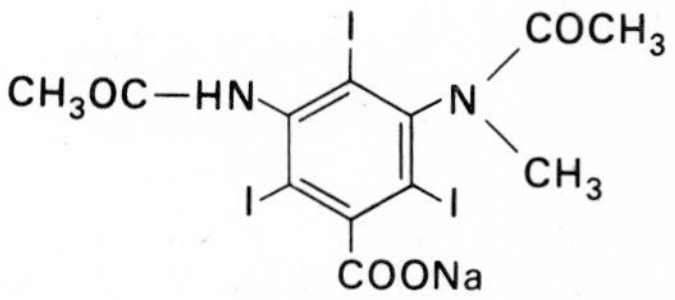

I CH_3OC-HN N $COCH_3$ CH_3 I I $COONa$

sodium metrizoate

$COONa$ C I I NaO O I I

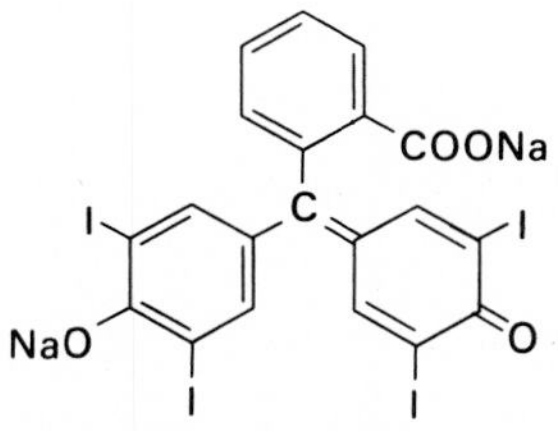

sodium phentetiothalein

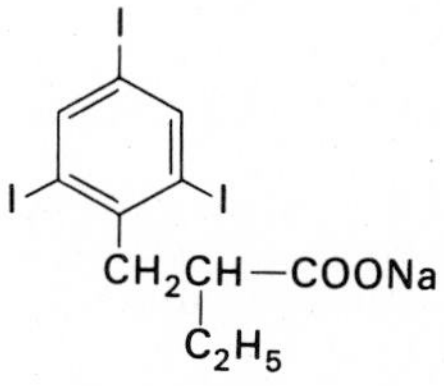

I I I $CH_2CH-COONa$ C_2H_5

sodium tyropanoate

b. Pyridone derivatives

IODOPYDOL (in Hytrast)
Bronchographic medium.

IODOPYDONE (in Hytrast)
Bronchographic medium.

IODOPYRACET COMPOUND (Diodrast)
For intravenous or retrograde pyelography. Concentrated solution for intravenous visualization of heart and vessels; cholangiography.

PROPYLIODONE (Dionosil)
For intratracheal bronchography; may be used in patients sensitive to iodine.

SODIUM IODOMETHAMATE (Neo-Iopax)
For intravenous urography.

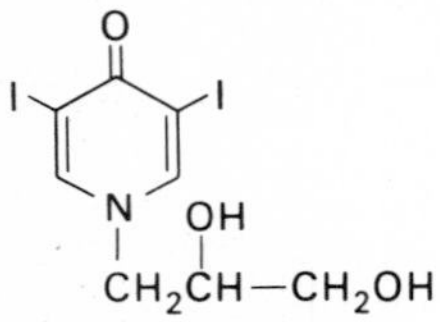

iopydol

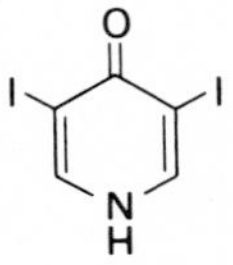

iopydone

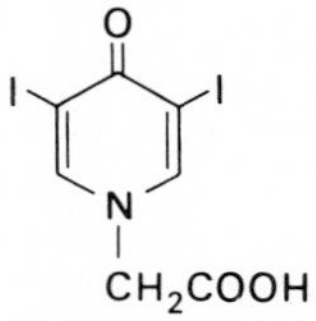

iodopyracet compound

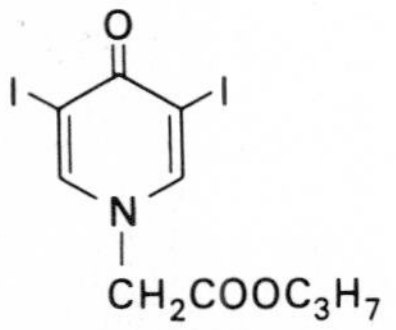

propyliodone

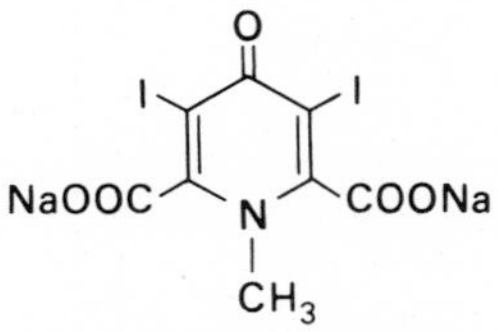

sodium iodomethamate

INSOLUBLE RADIOPAQUES

1. Preparation

BARIUM SULFATE ($BaSO_4$)
Many different suspensions used orally or rectally for gastrointestinal visualization.

I. Radiopharmaceuticals

Arsenic	SODIUM ARSENATE As 74
Bromine	POTASSIUM BROMIDE Br 82
Calcium	CALCIUM CHLORIDE Ca 45, Ca 47
Cesium	CESIUM CHLORIDE Cs 131 (Cescan 131)

Chromium	SODIUM CHROMATE Cr 51 (Rachromate 51, Chromitope sod. Cr 51)
	CHROMATED Cr 51 SERUM ALBUMIN (Chromalbumin)
	CHROMIC CHLORIDE Cr 51 (Chromitope chloride Cr 51)
Cobalt	COBALTOUS CHLORIDE Co 57, Co 60 (Cobatope Co 57, Co 60)
	CYANOCOBALAMIN Co 57, Co 60 (Racobalamin Co 57, Co 60, Rubratope Co 57, Co 60)
Copper	CUPRIC ACETATE Cu 64
Deuterium	DEUTERIUM OXIDE (stable isotope)
Gold	GOLD Au 198 (Aurcoloid 198, Aureotope Au 198)
Iodine	SODIUM DIATRIZOATE I 131 (Hypaque 131 sod., Radio-Renografin I 131)
	DIOHIPPURIC ACID I 125, I 131
	DIOTYROSINE I 125, I 131
	ETHIODIZED OIL I 131
	INSULIN I 125, I 131
	SODIUM IODIDE I 125, I 131 (Iodotope I 125, I 131; Theriodide I 131)
	IODINATED I 125, I 131, SERUM ALBUMIN (Risa 125, 131; Albumotope I 125, I 131)
	IODINATED I 125, I 131, SERUM ALBUMIN AGGREGATED (Albumotope LS)
	SODIUM IODIPAMIDE I 131 (Radio-Cholografin I 131)
	IODOANTIPYRINE I 131
	SODIUM IODOHIPPURATE I 125, I 131 (Hippuran 131; Hipputope I 125, I 131)
	IODOPYRACET I 131 (Diodrast 131)
	IOMETHIN I 125, I 131
	SODIUM IOTHALAMATE I 131 (Glofil 131)
	IOTYROSINE I 131
	LIOTHYRONINE I 131 (Triomet 131, Tri-thyrotope I 131)
	OLEIC ACID I 131, I 125 (Raoleic 131, Oleotope I 131, I 125)
	POVIDONE I 125, I 131
	SODIUM ROSE BENGAL I 125, I 131 (Robengatrope I 125, I 131)
	THYROXINE I 125, I 131
	TOLPOVIDONE I 131 (Raovin 131)
	TRIOLEIN I 125, I 131 (Raolein 131, Trioleotope I 131)
Iridium	IRIDIUM Ir 192 (Iriditope)
Iron	FERRIC CHLORIDE Fe 59
	FERROUS CITRATE Fe 59 (Ferrutope Fe 59)
	FERROUS SULFATE Fe 59
	KRYPTON CLATHERATE Kr 85
Mercury	CHLOROMERODRIN Hg 197, Hg 203 (Neohydrin 197, 203)
	MERISOPROL Hg 197 (Merprane)
	MERISOPROL ACETATE Hg 197, Hg 203 (MPH Acetate Hg 197, Hg 203)
Phosphorus	CHROMIC PHOSPHATE P 32 (Chromophosphotope P 32)
	POLYMETAPHOSPHATE P 32
	SODIUM PHOSPHATE P 32 (Phosphotope P 32)
Potassium	POTASSIUM CHLORIDE K 42
Rubidium	RUBIDIUM CHLORIDE Rb 86
Selenium	SELENOMETHIONINE Se 75 (Sethotope)
Sodium	SODIUM CHLORIDE Na 22 (Natritope chloride)
Sulfur	SODIUM SULFATE S 35
Strontium	STRONTIUM CHLORIDE Sr 85
	STRONTIUM NITRATE Sr 85 (Strotope)
Technitium	SODIUM PERTECHNETATE Tc 99m
	TECHNETIUM Tc 99m (Technetope)
Tritium	TRITIATED WATER (Tritiotope)
Ytterbium	PENTETATE TRISODIUM CALCIUM Yb 169
Zinc	ZINC CHLORIDE Zn 65

SUMMARY: DIAGNOSTIC AGENTS

TYPE	*ACTION AND MECHANISM*	*TOXICITY*	*USE*	*EXAMPLES*
Blood volume	Plasma dilution	Minor	To measure blood volume	Evans blue
Gastric acidity	Evoke maximum secretion	Flushing	Gastric acidity	Histamine phosphate
Kidney function	Renal clearance	Minor	To measure kidney function	Inulin
Circulation time	Time for transmission to sensing area	Minor	To measure circulation time	Sodium dehydrocholate
Liver function	Dye retention	Minor	To measure liver function	Sulfobromphthalein sodium
Iodized oil	Opaque medium	Local irritation	To visualize cavities	Iodized oil
Organic iodine compounds	Opaque medium	Anaphylactic reactions	To visualize gallbladder and other organs	Sodium diatrizoate
Inorganic iodine compound	Opaque medium	Minor	To visualize gastrointestinal tract	Barium sulfate
Radiopharmaceuticals	Localization measurable	Radioactivity	For diagnosis or therapy	Sodium iodide I 125

Reviews

Crocker, D., and Vandam, L. Untoward reactions to radiodiagnostic media. Clin. Pharmacol. Ther., 4:654, 1963.

Knoefel, P. Radiopaque diagnostic agents. Ann. Rev. Pharmacol., 5:321, 1965.

Rabinowitz, J., and Bruns, G. Radioactive drugs. Topics Med. Chem., 1:357, 1967.

Shockman, A. Radiologic diagnostic agents. Topics Med. Chem., 1:381, 1967.

30. Agents for Immunity and Immunologic Disease

A. Agents for Immunity

AGENTS FOR ACTIVE IMMUNITY

Active immunity is produced by the administration of various antigens, especially as microorganisms or their products. An increase in the host's antibody follows, which lasts briefly or longer, more or less according to that produced by the corresponding natural disease. In general, however, such artificially induced immunity is less profound than from the natural disease; and that produced by killed microorganisms is less effective than that from living vaccines. Nevertheless, ideal preparations, at least as regards viruses, would consist only of the protein and other substances of an organism toward which the antibodies are directed, and would not contain the nucleic acids of the organism, upon which actual infection depends.

a. Toxins and Toxoids

Toxins are antigenic and harmful proteins elaborated by microorganisms. When the harmfulness is disguised by combination with antibody (toxin-antitoxin combinations) or, better, by treatment with formaldehyde or like agents (toxoids), the preparations are useful in the production of immunity.

1. Preparations

DIPHTHERIA TOXOID; DIPHTHERIA TOXOID, ALUM PRECIPITATED, ALUMINUM HYDROXIDE ADSORBED, or ALUMINUM PHOSPHATE ADSORBED

For the prevention of diphtheria.
Dose: 0.5 or 1 ml (as specified on the label) subcutaneously, repeated in 4 to 6 weeks.

TETANUS TOXOID; TETANUS TOXOID, ALUM PRECIPITATED, OR ALUMINUM HYDROXIDE ADSORBED

For the prevention of tetanus.
Dose: 0.5 or 1 ml (as specified on the label) subcutaneously, repeated in 3 to 4 weeks; 1 ml booster at time of injury or yearly.
(And various combinations of the above, with or without pertussis vaccine or poliomyelitis vaccine.)

b. Vaccines

Vaccines are preparations of bacteria, viruses or other microbes suitably altered so that they have lost their ability to produce harmful disease, but have retained their antigenicity. The alteration may consist of killing, as with heat or formaldehyde. Or, attenuated, or antigenically related, strains may be used.

1. Preparations

CHOLERA VACCINE

Killed bacteria; of doubtful value.
Dose: 0.5 ml subcutaneously, then 1 ml at 10 and 20 days.

INFLUENZA VIRUS VACCINE, POLYVALENT; or MONOVALENT, TYPE A

Killed virus.
Dose: 1 ml subcutaneously.

MEASLES VIRUS VACCINE, INACTIVATED, ADSORBED (Pfizer-Vax Measles-K)

Dose: 0.5 to 1 ml subcutaneously monthly for 3 months.

MEASLES VIRUS VACCINE, LIVE ATTENUATED (Rubeovax)

Dose: 0.5 ml of reconstituted vaccine subcutaneously; often followed by 0.02 ml per kg weight Immune Serum Globulin (human) intramuscularly.

MENINGOCOCCAL MENINGITIS VACCINE

Killed Group A bacteria.

MUMPS VIRUS VACCINE, INACTIVATED

Killed virus.
Dose: 1 ml subcutaneously, repeated in 1 to 4 weeks.

MUMPS VIRUS VACCINE, LIVE, ATTENUATED

Dose: 0.5 ml of reconstituted vaccine.

PERTUSSIS VACCINE; PERTUSSIS VACCINE, ALUM PRECIPITATED, or ALUMINUM HYDROXIDE ADSORBED

Killed bacterial vaccine.
Dose: 0.5 ml subcutaneously, repeated in 4 and 8 weeks.

PLAGUE VACCINE

Killed bacteria; of doubtful value.
Dose: 0.5 ml subcutaneously, followed by 1 ml in 7 to 10 days.

POLIOMYELITIS VIRUS VACCINE

Killed or attenuated virus.
Dose: 1 ml subcutaneously or intramuscularly, repeated in 1, 6, and 12 months.

POLIOMYELITIS VACCINE, LIVE, ORAL. TYPES I, II, III

Dose: orally, according to directions.

POLYVALENT PNEUMOCOCCAL PNEUMONIA VACCINE

Immune polysaccharides from the bacterial capsule.

RABIES VACCINE

Killed or attenuated virus.
Dose: 1 ml subcutaneously daily for 14 days.

ROCKY MOUNTAIN SPOTTED FEVER VACCINE
Active immunizing agent.

RUBELLA VIRUS VACCINE, LIVE (Cendevax and other)
For active immunization.

SMALLPOX VACCINE
Related living vaccinia virus.
Dose: By multiple pressure into the skin.

TUBERCULOSIS VACCINE (BCG)
Attenuated strain of bacteria.
Dose: according to label.

TYPHOID VACCINE, and TYPHOID and PARATYPHOID VACCINE
Killed bacteria.
Dose: 0.5 ml subcutaneously, repeated at 2 and 4 weeks.

TYPHUS VACCINE (epidemic typhus vaccine)
Killed rickettsiae.
Dose: according to label.

YELLOW FEVER VACCINE
Attenuated 17D strain.
Dose: 0.5 ml subcutaneously.

AGENTS FOR PASSIVE IMMUNITY

Passive immunity differs from active immunity in that antibodies, premade in another individual, are simply injected into the person to be protected. His own immune mechanism plays no part in the process. Protection lasts only as long as the foreign antibody continues to circulate in the new host, usually about three weeks. When the antibody has been made in a different species, sensitivity may be present, or may be induced, with resultant anaphylaxis, or other allergic manifestations, or subsequent serum sickness.

a. Serums prepared in man

Protective antibodies may be obtained from other human beings, usually from a pool of adult serums which will contain many antibodies; or, they may be obtained from individuals convalescent from the disease in question, or from donors who have recently been vaccinated. Preparations may consist of whole serum, or fractions of it which contain gamma globulin.

1. Preparations

ANTI-RHO (D) IMMUNE GLOBULIN
To prevent Rh immunization of a mother after labor.
Dose: 1 to 1.5 ml intramuscularly.

HYPERIMMUNIZED GAMMA GLOBULIN
Dose: 1.5 to 4.5 ml intramuscularly (mumps, pertussis, rabies).

IMMUNE SERUM GLOBULIN (Human)

Contains antibodies against poliomyelitis, measles, infectious hepatitis.
Dose: 2 to 10 ml intramuscularly.

PERTUSSIS IMMUNE SERUM (Human)

Dose: 20 ml every 2 days for 3 or 4 doses intramuscularly or intravenously.

POLIOMYELITIS IMMUNE GLOBULIN (Human)

Dose: 0.044 ml per kg body weight (measles or infectious hepatitis) intramuscularly to 0.31 ml per kg (poliomyelitis).

SCARLET FEVER IMMUNE SERUM (Human)

Dose: 20 ml intramuscularly.

TETANUS IMMUNE GLOBULIN (Human)

Preferred to tetanus antitoxin as not antigenic for man.

Dose: 250 u (adults), 4 u per kg (children), intramuscularly (prophylactic); 6,000 u (therapeutic).

VACCINIA IMMUNE GLOBULIN (Human)

Dose: 0.3 ml/kg.

b. Serums prepared in animals

Horses and rabbits are the most commonly used animals for the preparation of antiserums. Testing the intended recipient for sensitivity must precede the use of such agents.

1. Preparations

ANTIVENIN (Crotalidae) POLYVALENT

Dose: 10 to 50 ml subcutaneously, intramuscularly, or intravenously.

ANTIVENIN (Latrodectus mactans)

Dose: 2.5 ml intramuscularly.

GAS GANGRENE ANTITOXIN, BIVALENT, TRIVALENT, or PENTAVALENT and MIXTURES WITH TETANUS ANTITOXIN

Dose: 10,000 units of each constituent subcutaneously or by local infiltration.

DIPHTHERIA ANTITOXIN

Dose: 20,000 to 150,000 units of which 20,000 to 40,000 units may be given intravenously, the balance intramuscularly.

TETANUS ANTITOXIN

Dose: 10,000 to 20,000 units subcutaneously (prophylactic); 20,000 to 80,000 units intravenously or intramuscularly (therapeutic).

Human tetanus immune globulin is now replacing that from animal sources.

ALLERGENIC PREPARATIONS

Allergenic preparations contain small amounts of the antigenic substances responsible for atopic hypersensitivity. They have been prepared from a great variety of inhalants and ingestants (e.g., danders and foods), and from contact agents (e.g., plant leaves). The mechanism by which such preparations reduce hypersensitivity is not clear, though this may be by increased production of blocking antibodies, or possibly by exhaustion of the antibody-producing cells, promoted by the frequent small injections of the allergens. The subcutaneous route of injection is apparently important.

AGENTS FOR SKIN TESTING

Susceptibility to disease, or the presence of disease, may be indicated by the type of reaction which follows the intradermal injection of a small amount of the relevant antigen into the skin. Toxins (diphtheria; streptococcus) produce a red area in the absence of antibodies, thus indicating susceptibility; other (delayed) antigens (tuberculosis, mumps) produce a red area in the presence of tissue hypersensitivity, indicating past or present infection.

1. Preparations

BLASTOMYCIN

Dose: 0.1 ml (of 1:100 dilution of commercial material) intradermally.

COCCIDIOIDIN

Dose: 0.1 ml (of 1:100 dilution of commercial material) intradermally.

DIPHTHERIA TOXIN (Schick test)

Dose: 0.1 ml intradermally.

MUMPS SKIN TEST ANTIGEN

Dose: 0.1 ml intradermally.

OLD TUBERCULIN

Dose: 0.01 cu mm diluted to 0.1 ml, intradermally, increased to 0.1 to 1.0 on subsequent tests in negative reactors.

PURIFIED PROTEIN DERIVATIVE OF TUBERCULIN (PPD)

Dose: 0.02 mcg (first dose), 0.2 (second dose), and 5.0 (third dose) intradermally.

STREPTOCOCCUS TOXIN (Dick test)

Dose: 0.2 ml intradermally.

B. Agents in Hypersensitivity

The immunologic diseases most amenable to treatment are those of the immediate hypersensitivity group, specifically asthma, hay fever, urticaria, angioneurotic edema, and allergic dermatitis. Avoidance of the responsible antigen, or desensitization to it, may be helpful, but treatment must often be nonspecific. The principal agents employed, in addition to sedation and appropriate antibiotic therapy if bacteria are involved, include the following:

a. Sympathomimetic amines: To constrict vessels (hives) and dilate bronchi (asthma) (see Sympathetic Stimulants).

b. Xanthines: To dilate bronchi (asthma) (see Smooth Muscle Relaxants).

c. Adrenal corticoids and ACTH: To restrain inflammatory and allergic mechanisms (all forms) (see The Adrenal).

d. Iodides and detergents: To thin mucus (asthma).

e. Antihistamines: Considered in the next section.

C. Immunosupressors

1. Uses. To prevent rejection of transplanted organs and in treatment of severe immunological disorders (disseminated lupus erythematosus, nephrosis, collagen vascular disease, rheumatoid arthritis, etc).

2. Agents used for immunosuppression

a. Adrenocorticosteroids: cortison, prednison, and others.

b. Cancer chemotherapeutics:

a′. Alkylating agents (cyclophosphamide and others).

b′. Antimetabolites (mercaptopurine, thioguanine, and others).

c′. Natural products (dectinomycin and others).

D. Immunostimulation

1. Uses. To enhance the body's defense mechanism in infections and in malignancy.

2. Agents used

a. Stimulants of the reticuloendothelial system (RES): bacterial antigens (BCG and others), polynucleotide.

b. Enhance humoral immune body production: amantadine, tilorone.

c. Enhance cellular immunity.

a′. Transfer factor (TF). Small molecular weight, unknown structure; supposedly capable of transferring to the lymphocyte of nonsensitive individuals the immunologic "memory" of the sensitive donor. Species specific, experimental, not yet available for therapeutic use.

b′. Tetromisole, levanisole, lentinan.

d. Enhance cellular resistance: interferon and its inducers.

F. Drug Sensitivity

Drug toxicity is of two general types, the expected and the unexpected. Expected toxicity is that from overdosage and the manifestations are those of the regular pharmacological action of the drug. Thus, one expects nausea if too much digitalis is given, and sleepiness if too much barbiturate. Unexpected toxicity, or drug sensitivity in the specific sense, is not a manifestation of overdosage, but of an unusual constitution on the part of the patient. Thus, agranulocytosis from aminopyrine or aplastic anemia from chloramphenicol are uncommon and totally unrelated to the usual action of the drugs. At least two explanations for this type of drug sensitivity are known, one on the basis of immunologic disease and the other on genetic abnormality.

a. Immunologic disease: Drugs attached to an individual's cells may act as antigens; the individual's antibodies may then harm his own cells. Why the drugs are able to act as antigens in some persons but not in most is certainly not clear; very possibly genetic abnormalities may be influential.

The following are examples of pathological states and drugs that appear to be responsible. The examples could be expanded to include a large percentage of drugs but, as with most of those mentioned, the guilt is by association, for actual immunologic demonstrations have not been made, nor has the factor of genetic defect been assessed.

Agranulocytosis: aminopyrine, gold salts, phenylbutazone, thiouracil.
Thrombocytopenic purpura: barbiturates, diphenhydramine, gold salts, arsenicals, Sedormid.
Hemolytic anemia: sulfanilamide, tetracyclines, mephenesin.
Aplastic anemia: chloramphenicol, nitrofurantoin, trimethadione.

b. Genetic abnormality: Drug sensitivity on the basis of genetic abnormality is usually the result of the absence of an enzyme normally present in most persons. In the absence of this enzyme the drug is not handled normally by the body. The drug, or an intermediate in its metabolism, may accumulate, a necessary end product may not be made, or an unusual enzyme may take over with the production of different end products. Examples include:

Apnea: succinylcholine (deficiency of pseudocholinesterase).
Hemolytic anemia: primaquine, sulfanilamide, nitrofurans, naphthalene, acetanilid, acetophenetidin (deficiency of glucose-6-phosphate dehydrogenase which causes an altered glutathione metabolism in RBC with resultant instability).

SUMMARY: AGENTS FOR IMMUNITY AND IMMUNOLOGIC DISEASE

TYPE	*ACTION AND MECHANISM*	*TOXICITY*	*USE*	*EXAMPLES*
Active immunity	Induce antibody formation	Local inflammation, systemic malaise and fever	Prevent infection	Smallpox vaccine
Passive immunity	Provide antibodies	Hypersensitivity phenomena	Treat infection	Tetanus antitoxin
Histamine	Stimulates (bronchial) or relaxes (vascular) smooth muscle	Flushing, hypotension	Diagnostic, gastric juice	Histamine phosphate
Antihistamines	Competitive interference with histamine at receptors	Drowsiness, dizziness, dry mouth, nausea	Hay fever, urticaria	Tripelennamine
Anti-motion sickness	Vestibular depression	Same	Motion sickness	Dimenhydrinate

Reviews

Raffel, S. Immunity, 2nd ed. New York, Appleton-Century-Crofts, 1961.
Samter, M., and Berryman, G. Drug allergy. Ann. Rev. Pharmacol., 4:265, 1964.
Haurowitz, F. Antibody formation and the coding problem. Nature, 205:847, 1965.
Carr, E. A. Allergic responses to allergic agents. Fed. Proc., 24:39, 1965.
Kahlson, G., and Rosengren, E. Histamine. Ann. Rev. Pharmacol., 5:305, 1965.
Wood, C., and Graybill, A. A theory of motion sickness based on pharmacological reactions. Clin. Pharmacol. Ther., 11:621, 1970.

31. Histamine, Serotonin, Peptides, Prostaglandins, and Antagonists

A. Histamine and Antihistamines

HISTAMINE

1. History. a. Windaus and Vogt (1907) synthesized histamine.

b. Barger and Dale (1910) isolated from ergot; recognizing the similarity of various allergic phenomena, including smooth muscle stimulation and capillary dilatation, they proposed histamine as the mediating agent.

c. Dragstedt (1945–48) demonstrated that the blood level of "histamine" rose after passage of antigen through sensitized guinea pig lungs, but also that histamine failed to explain coagulation abnormalities, leucopenia, eosinophilia, delayed death.

2. Chemistry. a. Histamine is an amine, found in many tissues, and synthesized by intestinal bacteria.

b. Made in the body by decarboxylation of histidine, and excreted as histamine, acetylhistamine, methylhistamine and other products.

$CH_2CH(COOH)-NH_2$ (imidazole ring: N, NH)	→	$CH_2CH_2-NH_2$ (imidazole ring: N, NH)	→	CH_2COOH (imidazole ring: N, NH)
histidine (precursor)	decarboxylase	histamine	diamineoxidase (histaminase)	imidazole acetic acid (and other excretion products)

c. Marked species and organ differences exist (Dale and Best, 1911–27). Man: low in blood, high in skin; rabbit: high in blood; guinea pig: medium in blood, low in liver; dog: high in liver.

3. Action and Mechanism. a. Histamine is a potent dilator of capillaries, giving a flare reaction in the skin, and hypotension.

b. It is a strong stimulant of bronchial muscle and uterus, less of bowel and arterial smooth muscle.

c. It stimulates the secretion of gastric acid and causes the release of epinephrine from the adrenal medulla.

4. Pharmacodynamics. a. Not effective orally.

b. Released from tissues by many diverse agents (Paton, Pharmacol. Rev., 9:269, 1957): venoms and toxins, trypsin and other enzymes, surface active agents, and a number of alkylamines, including the interesting Compound 48/80, a condensation product of *p*-methoxyphenethylmethylamine with formaldehyde. The mechanism by which compound 48/80 releases histamine from mast cells is thought to be by replacing it on heparin, which acts as a cationic exchanger:

histamine: heparin + 48/80 → heparin: 48/80 + histamine

5. Toxicity. a. Excessive dosage causes flushing, throbbing headache, hypotension.

b. Presumably released from tissues in allergic reactions.

6. Uses. The only important use for histamine is as a diagnostic stimulant of gastric secretion (see Diagnostic Agents).

ANTIHISTAMINES

1. History. a. Early trials with desensitization to histamine and histaminase.

b. Fourneau and Bovet (1933), Halpern (1942), Mayer (1945) developed and introduced ethylenediamine series of antihistamines; Loewi (1945) the aminoalkyl ether series.

c. Black et al. (Nature 236: 385, 1972) introduced burinamide as an antagonist to the gastric acid secretion stimulating effect of histamine and defined the H_2 histamine receptor.

H_1 ANTAGONISTS

1. Chemistry. The antihistamines can be classified somewhat arbitrarily into three groups, on the basis of their relationship to the aminoethyl side chain of histamine; thus:

a. Ethylenediamine series: Relationships can also be pointed out between some members of this large group and sympatholytic agents (i.e., antazoline with phentolamine) (Bovet, Science, 129:1255, 1959).

b. Aminoalkylether series: The members of this series are closely related to the spasmolytics, e.g., adiphenine (see Parasympathetic Depressants).

c. Alkylamine series.

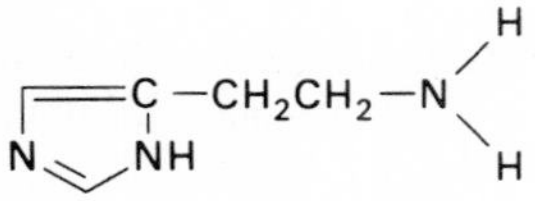

histamine

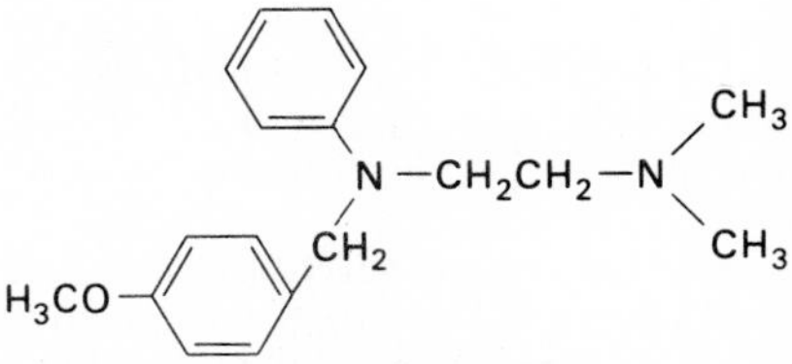

pyrilamine (maleate)
(ethylenediamine
series)

$$\mathrm{(C_6H_5)_2HC{-}O{-}CH_2CH_2{-}N(CH_3)_2}$$

diphenhydramine (HCl)
(aminoalkylether series)

$$\mathrm{(C_6H_5)(C_5H_4N)HC{-}CH_2CH_2{-}N(CH_3)_2}$$

pheniramine (maleate)
(alkylamine series)

2. Action. a. Strongly oppose the action of histamine on capillaries, less strongly on bronchioles and intestine, weakly on uterus, without effect on glandular secretion.

b. Also show local anesthetic action, antispasmodic effects, sedation (except phenindamine), antihyaluronidase activity, and variously, antiparkinsonian, antimotion, antiemetic and antipururitic effects.

3. Mechanism. a. The antihistamine effect is primarily the result of competitive interference with histamine at the H_1 receptors.

b. It may also be partly inhibition of mast cell damage and consequent histamine release (Mota, Brit. J. Pharmacol., 15:396, 1960).

c. It appears not to be due to chemical or physical neutralization, or interference with production.

d. The effect is more pronounced when histamine is presumed to be circulating (hives) than when it is released in proximity to the receptor (asthma).

4. Pharmacodynamics. Well absorbed by mouth; effects appear within 30 minutes. Distributed widely; excreted satisfactorily.

5. Toxicity. a. Side effects vary considerably but may include some degree of drowsiness, dizziness, dry mouth, headaches, nausea, muscular twitching, and rarely hyperpyrexia.

b. Allergic hypersensitivity is uncommon with oral administration, but not uncommon with topical application.

6. Uses. a. The H_1 antihistamines are highly useful in urticaria, but less so in hay fever, most dermatoses, or asthma. Relative effectiveness is as follows:

Urticaria, angioneurotic edema, anaphylaxis	80%
Hay fever, vasomotor rhinitis	50%
Allergic dermatitis	20%
Asthma	1%

b. Topical preparations, although widely used, are of little value.

c. Parenteral administration may occasionally be useful to hasten effects, but should not replace epinephrine in anaphylaxis.

d. Because of individual patient variation, it is usual to select agents in turn from the different chemical groups when the first to be tried is ineffective.

8. Preparations

a. Ethylenediamine group

ANTAZOLINE PHOSPHATE (Antistine)

Dose: 100 to 200 mg 4 times a day; 0.5% solution for instillation in the eye.

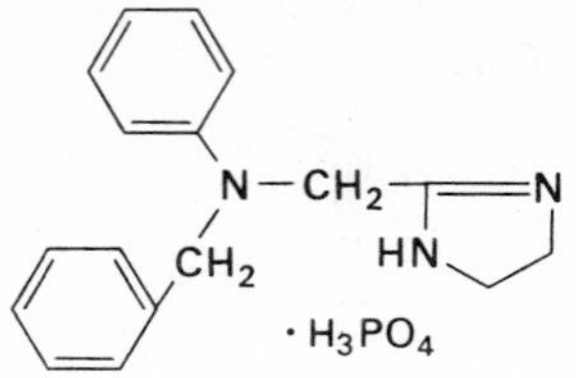

N—CH₂ HN N CH₂ · H_3PO_4

CLEMIZOLE HYDROCHLORIDE (Allercur)

Dose: 25 mg 2 to 3 times a day by mouth.

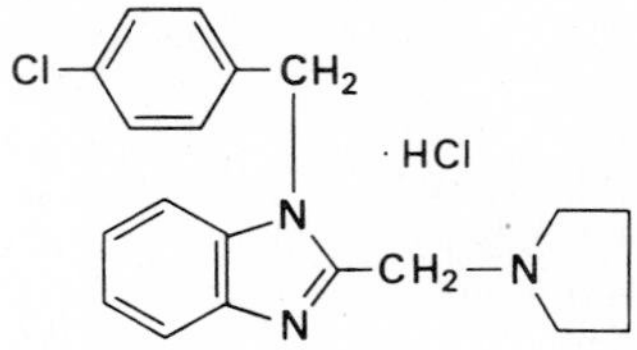

Cl CH₂ · HCl N CH₂—N N

CHLORCYCLIZINE HYDROCHLORIDE (DiParalene; Perazil)

Long acting.
Dose: 50 mg 2 or 3 times a day.

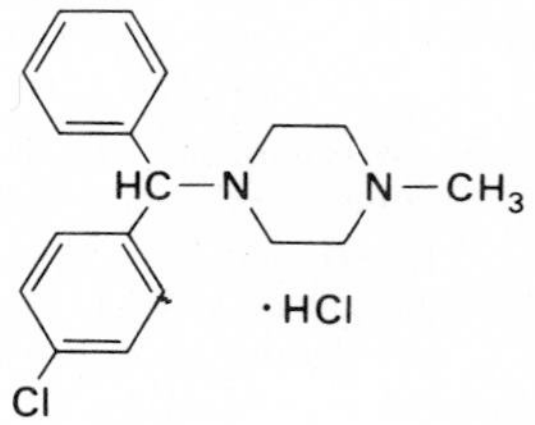

HC—N N—CH₃ · HCl Cl

CHLOROTHEN

Chlorothen citrate (Tagathen)
Dose: 25 mg 3 or 4 times a day by mouth.

N CH₃ N—CH₂CH₂—N Cl S CH₂ CH₃ $C_6H_8O_7$

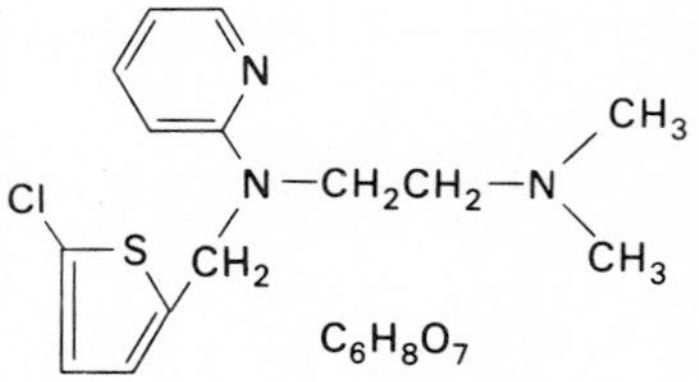

METHAPHENILINE HYDROCHLORIDE (Diatrine)

Dose: 50 mg 4 times a day by mouth.

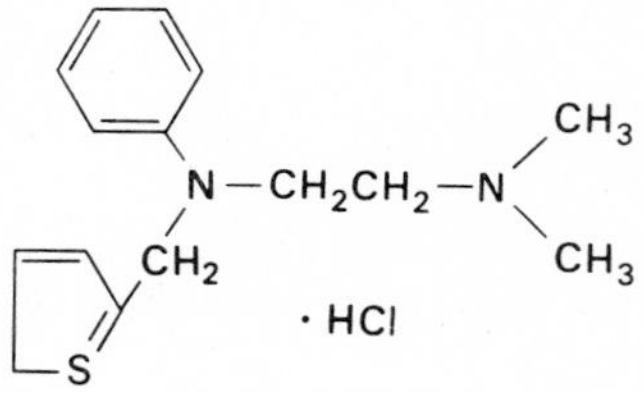

CH₃ N—CH₂CH₂—N CH₂ CH₃ · HCl S

METHAPYRILENE HYDROCHLORIDE (Histadyl; Thenylene; and others)

Dose: 50 to 100 mg 3 or 4 times a day by mouth; also intravenously.

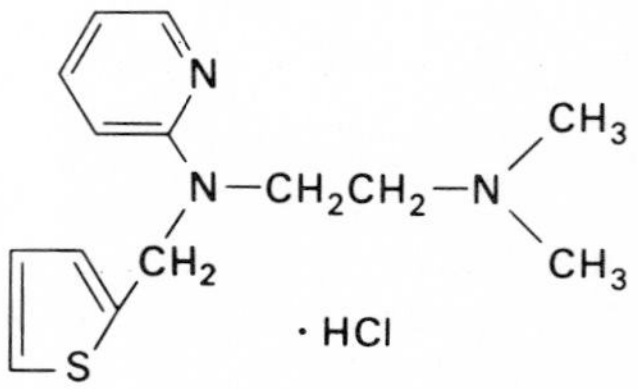

N CH₃ N—CH₂CH₂—N CH₂ CH₃ · HCl S

METHDILAZINE HYDROCHLORIDE (Tacaryl)

Dose: 8 mg twice a day by mouth.

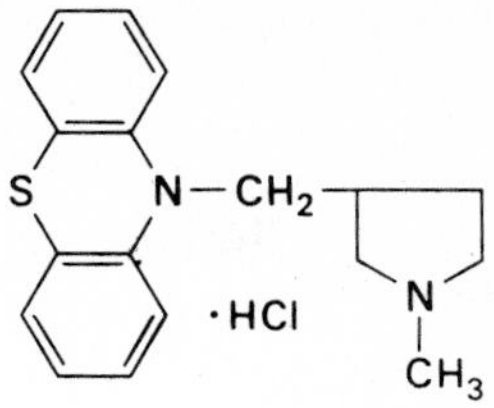

PROMETHAZINE HYDROCHLORIDE (Phenergan)

More potent and longer lasting than most antihistamines (similarity to promazine, tranquilizer), and used considerably as a sedative and potentiator of analgesics.

Dose: 25 mg once daily at bedtime.

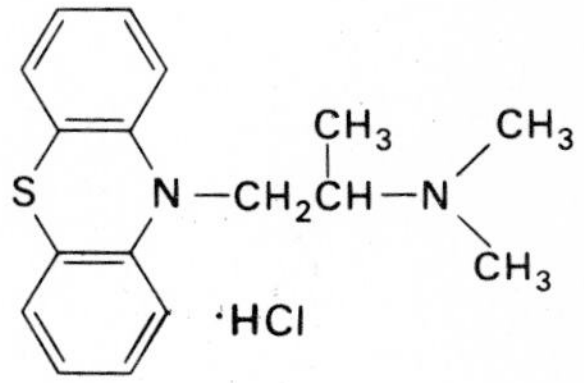

PYRATHIAZINE HYDROCHLORIDE (Pyrrolazote)

Dose: 25 to 50 mg 3 or 4 times a day by mouth.

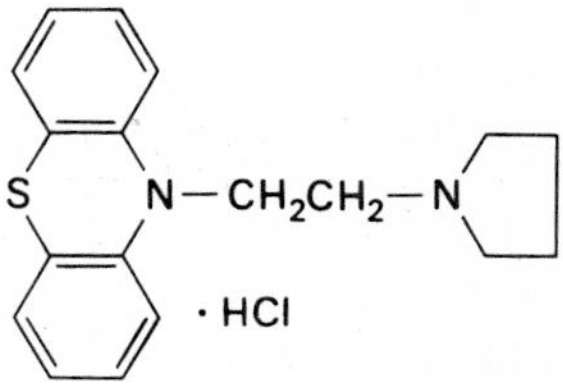

PYRILAMINE MALEATE (Neoantergan)

Dose: 25 to 50 mg 3 or 4 times a day by mouth.

Pyrabrom (pyrilamine bromotheophyllinate; Glybrom)

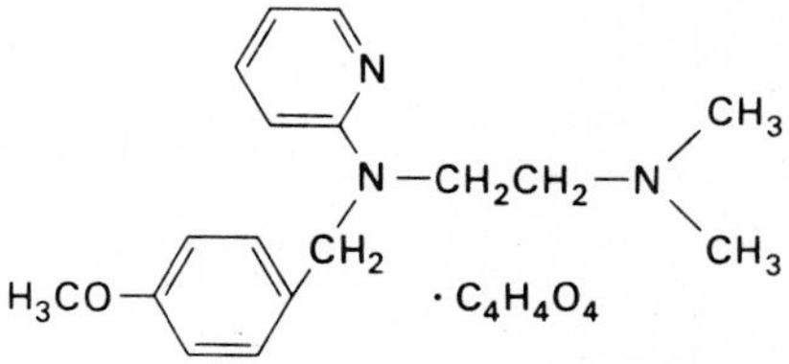

QUINETOLATE (aureoquin diamate; Ventaire)

Bronchodilator; antihistamine.
Under investigation.

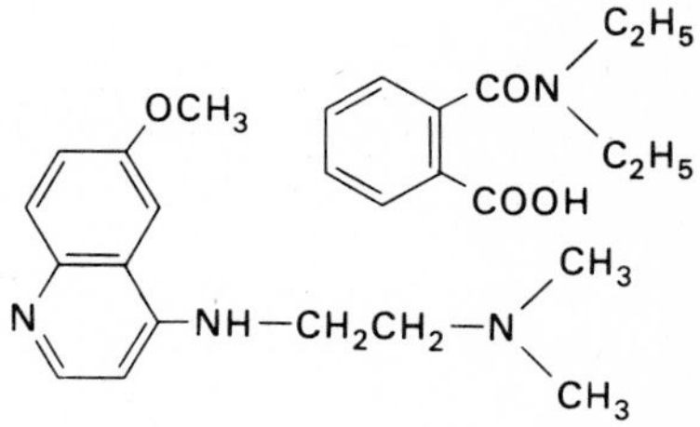

THENALIDINE (Sandostene)

Under investigation.

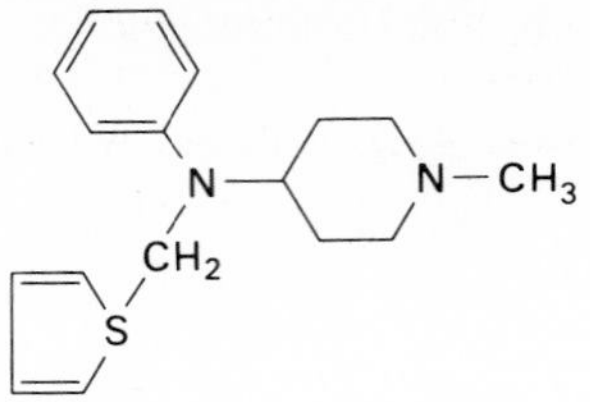

THENYLDIAMINE HYDROCHLORIDE (Thenfadil)

Dose: 15 to 30 mg 3 or 4 times daily by mouth.

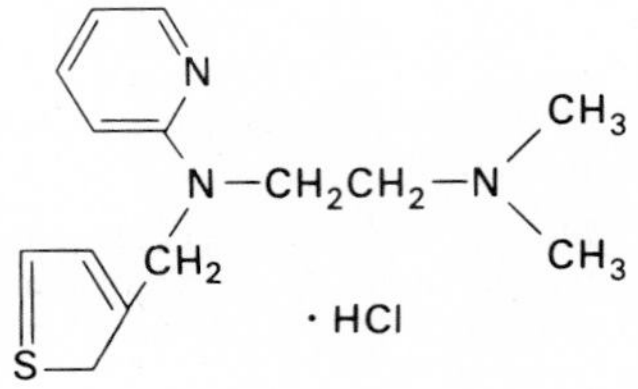

THONZYLAMINE HYDROCHLORIDE (Anahist; Neohetramine)

Dose: 50 to 100 mg 4 times a day by mouth.

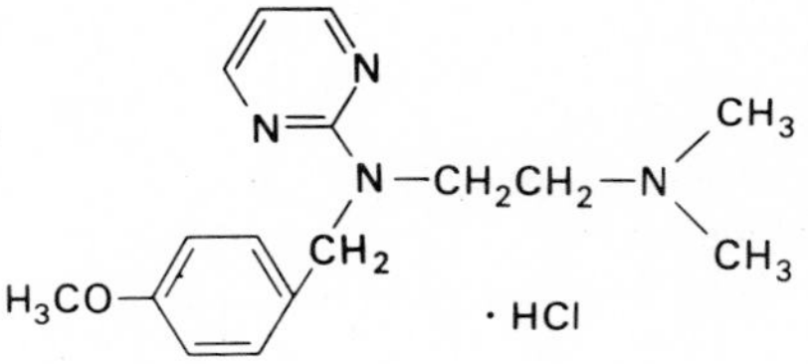

TRIPELENNAMINE (Pyribenzamine)

Widely used example; strong sedative.

Dose: 25 to 50 mg 3 times a day by mouth. Also topically, 2% in creams and ointments; and in injectable forms.

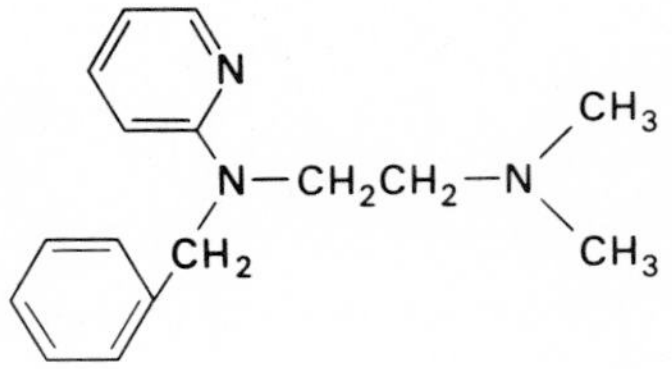

ZOLAMINE HYDROCHLORIDE (in Otodyne)

Dose: 1% solution locally.

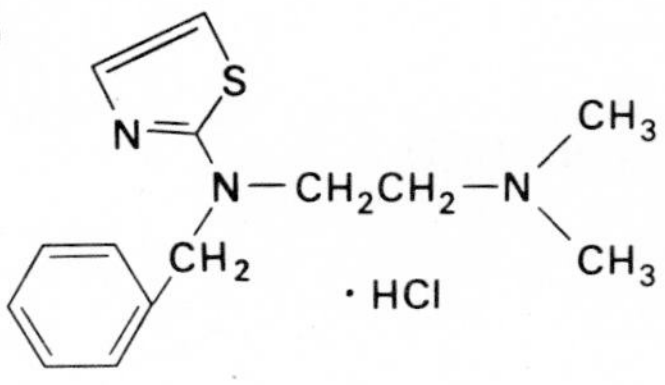

b. Aminoalkylether group

CHLORPHENOXAMINE HYDROCHLORIDE (Systral)

Under investigation.

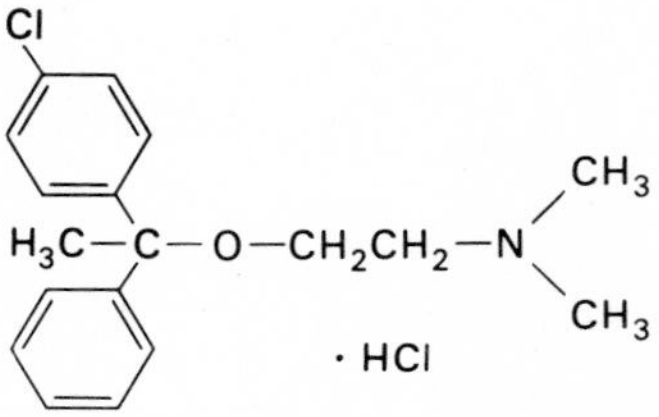

CARBINOXAMINE MALEATE (Clistin)

Dose: 4 mg 3 or 4 times a day by mouth.

Rotoxamine tartrate (Twiston)
More potent levo isomer.
Dose: 2 mg 3 or 4 times a day by mouth.

Cl
HC—O—CH_2CH_2—N
N
CH_3
CH_3
· $C_4H_4O_4$

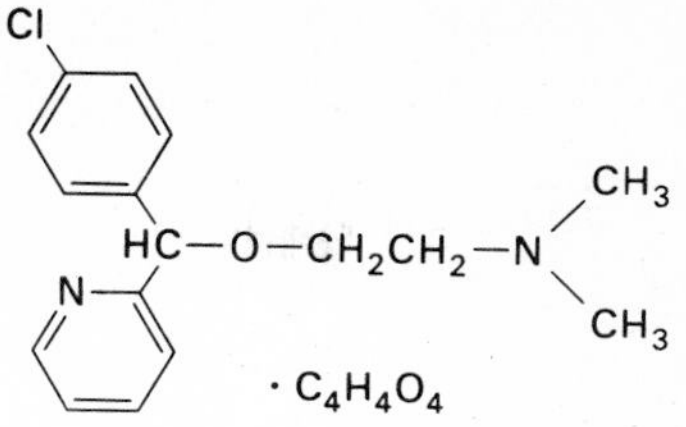

CLEMASTINE (Tavist)

Dose: 1 mg twice a day by mouth.

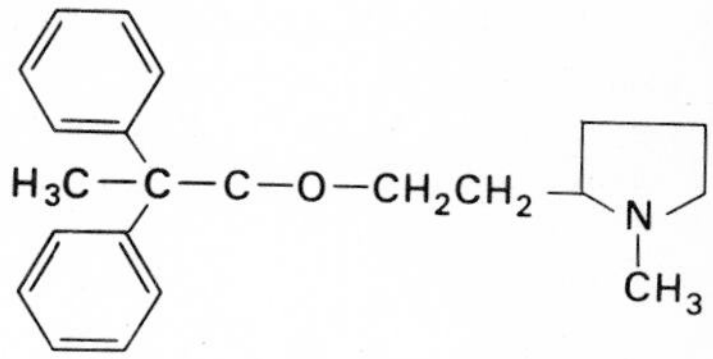

H_3C—C—C—O—CH_2CH_2
N
CH_3

DIPHENHYDRAMINE HYDROCHLORIDE (Benadryl)

Earliest member of this group; widely used; strongly sedative.

Dose: 50 mg 3 or 4 times a day; 2% topically; also intravenously.

Dimenhydrinate (Dramamine)
See Anti-Motion Sickness Agents.

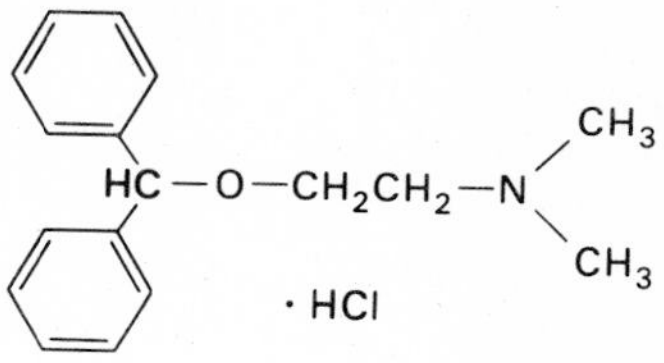

HC—O—CH_2CH_2—N
CH_3
CH_3
· HCl

DIPHENYLPYRALINE HYDROCHLORIDE (Diafen, Hispril)

Potent; may produce drowsiness, headache, dizziness, flushing, dry mouth and nose.

Dose: 2 mg 3 or 4 times a day by mouth.

HC—O—
N—CH_3
· HCl

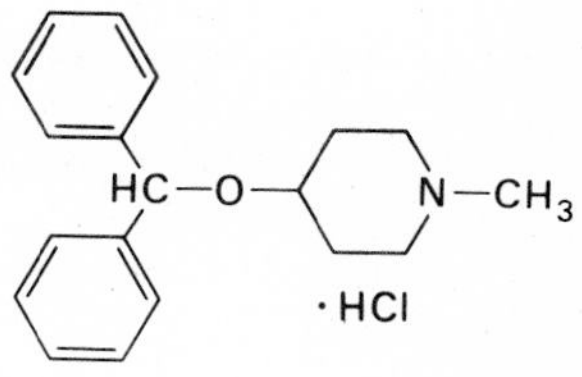

DOXYLAMINE SUCCINATE (Decapryn)

Also strongly sedative.

Dose: 12.5 to 25 mg 2 or 3 times a day by mouth.

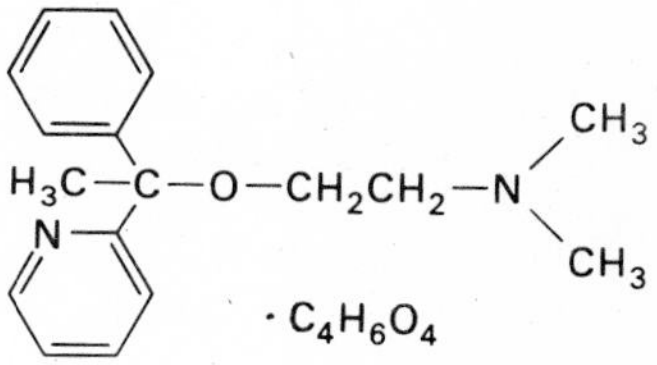

H_3C—C—O—CH_2CH_2—N
N
CH_3
CH_3
· $C_4H_6O_4$

PYROXAMINE MALEATE

May produce drowsiness.

Dose: 40 to 60 mg daily by mouth.

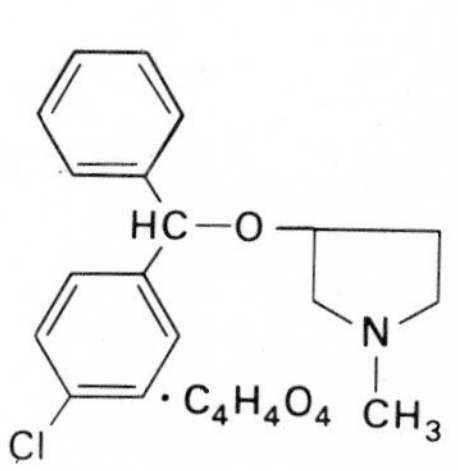

HC—O
N
Cl
· $C_4H_4O_4$
CH_3

c. Alkylamine group

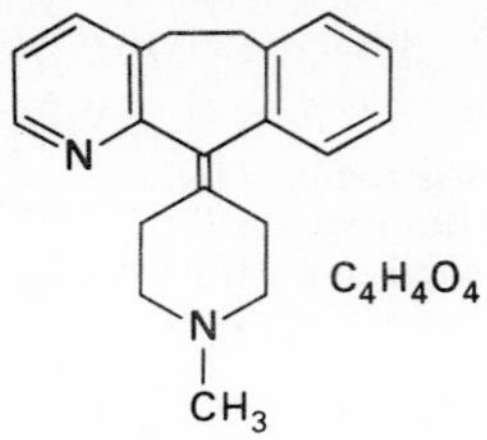

AZATADINE MALEATE (Optimine)

Recommended only for adults.
Dose: 2 mg twice daily.

$C_4H_4O_4$

BROMODIPHENHYDRAMINE HYDROCHLORIDE (Ambodryl hydrochloride)

Dose: 25 mg 3 times daily.

CYPROHEPTADINE HYDROCHLORIDE (Periactin)

Does not cause stimulation; antihistamine and antiserotonin. Used against itching.
Dose: 2 to 20 mg daily.

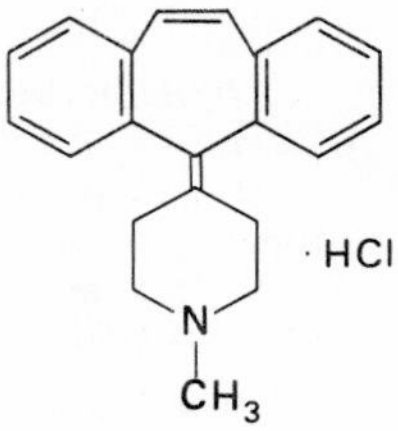

$\cdot HCl$

DIMETHINDENE MALEATE (Forhistal)

Also used as an antipruritic.
Dose: 1 to 2 mg 3 times a day by mouth.

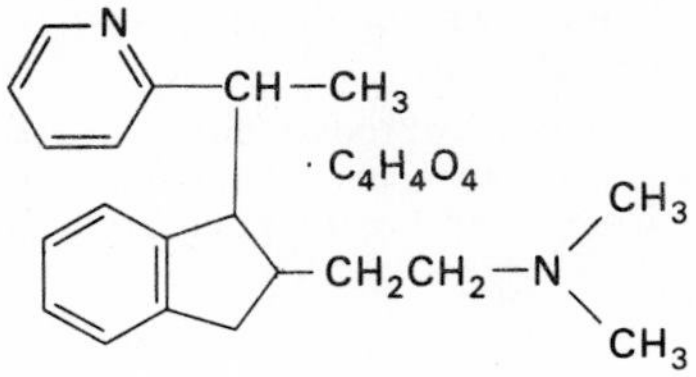

$\cdot C_4H_4O_4$

PHENINDAMINE TARTRATE (Thephorin)

Less likely to produce sedation and may cause stimulation.
Dose: 25 mg 4 times a day by mouth.

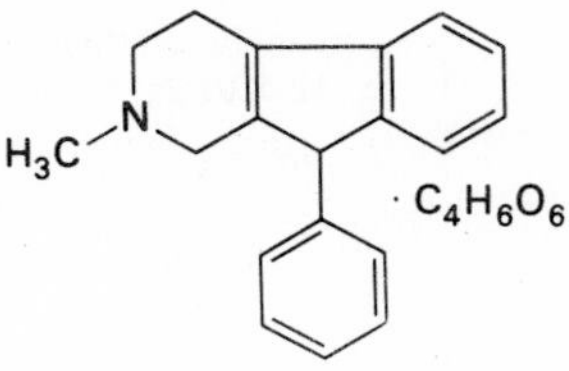

$\cdot C_4H_6O_6$

PHENIRAMINE MALEATE (Trimeton)

Dose: 25 mg 3 times a day by mouth.

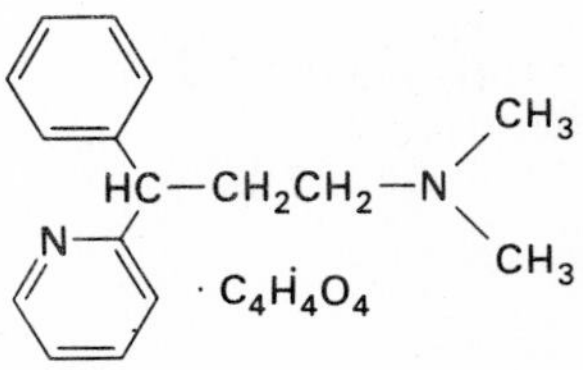

$\cdot C_4H_4O_4$

BROMPHENIRAMINE MALEATE (Dimetane)
Dose: 4 to 8 mg 1 to 4 times daily by mouth.

DEXBROMPHENIRAMINE MALEATE (Disomer)
Dose: 2 mg 3 times daily.

CHLORPHENIRAMINE MALEATE (Chlor-Trimeton)

Dose: 2 to 4 mg 3 times a day by mouth; 5 to 20 mg subcutaneously, intramuscularly, or intravenously.

Dextrochlorpheniramine (Polaramine)
Dose: 2 mg 3 to 4 times a day by mouth.

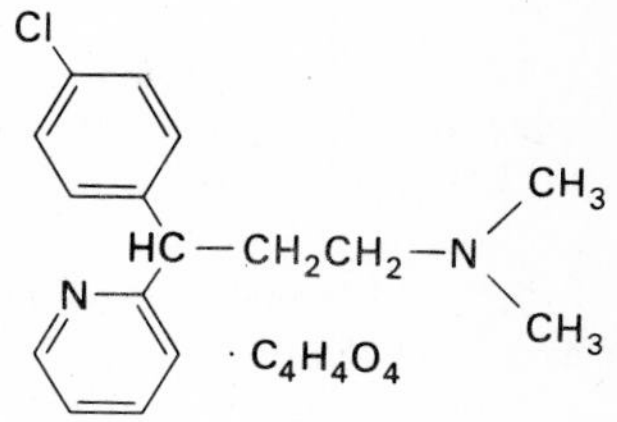

Cl, HC—CH_2CH_2—N, CH_3, CH_3, N, $\cdot\ C_4H_4O_4$

MIANSERIN HYDROCHLORIDE

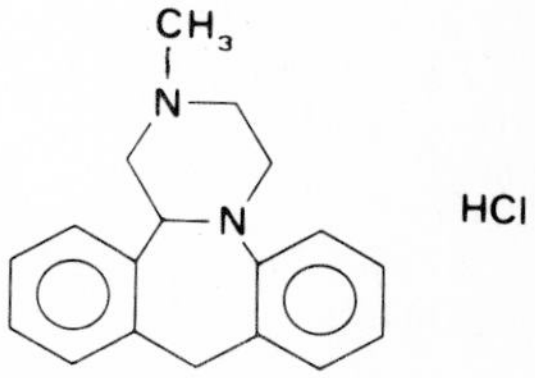

CH_3, N, N, HCl

PYRROBUTAMINE PHOSPHATE (Pyronil)
Long acting.
Dose: 15 mg 3 or 4 times a day by mouth.

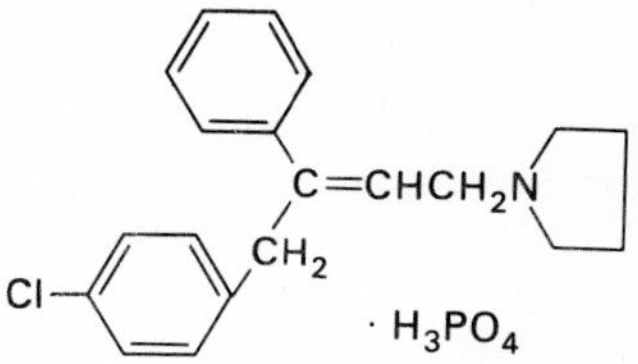

C=$CHCH_2N$, CH_2, Cl, $\cdot\ H_3PO_4$

TERFENADINE

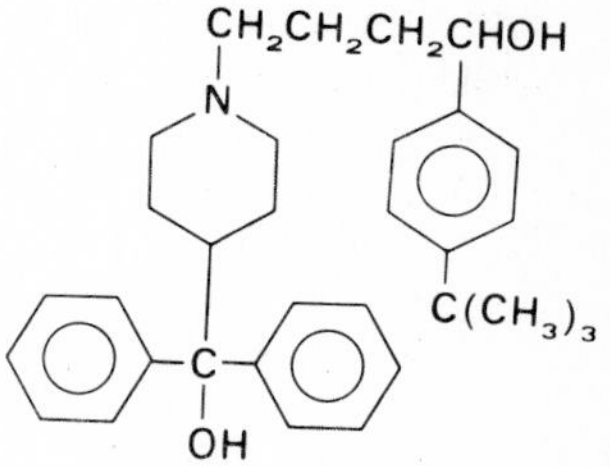

$CH_2CH_2CH_2CHOH$, N, $C(CH_3)_3$, C, OH

TRIPROLIDINE HYDROCHLORIDE (Actidil)
Long acting.
Dose: 2.5 mg 2 or 3 times a day by mouth.

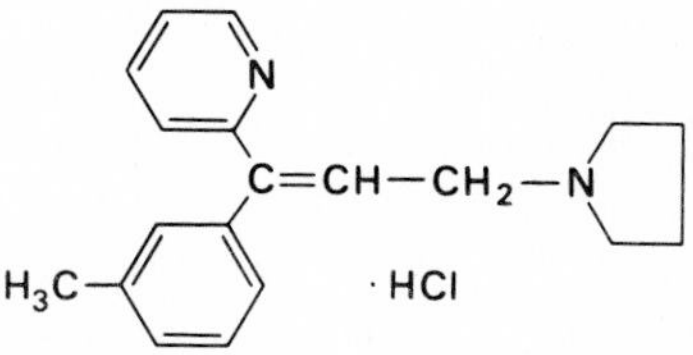

N, C=CH—CH_2—N, H_3C, $\cdot$ HCl

ANTI-MOTION SICKNESS AGENTS

Motion sickness originates in the vestibular apparatus. Although it bears no relationship to allergy, certain of the antihistamines are surprisingly effective in prevention and control, and have largely replaced scopolamine, the most effective of the older agents.

1. Chemistry. Largely antihistamines (diphenhydramine, dimenhydrinate, promethazine, pheniramine, pyrathiazine) or related compounds (see Trumbull, Clin. Pharmacol. Ther., 1:280, 1960).

2. Action and Mechanism. a. Stop motion sickness by vestibular and labyrinthine depression, but the mechanism for this action is not clear.

b. It is uncertain whether receptors or afferent nerves may be involved; the vomiting center may be depressed.

c. The action is not solely antihistaminic, as many antihistamines are ineffective; nor is it purely antiemetic, as chlorpromazine, a good antiemetic, is not a good anti-motion sickness agent; most of the active compounds antagonize acetylcholine.

3. Pharmacodynamics and Toxicity. a. Similar to that of the antihistamines generally.

b. Cyclizine and meclizine have produced teratogenic effects in animals.

4. Uses. a. To decrease or prevent motion sickness.

b. To control Ménière's disease.

c. Also used against vomiting from other causes but certain tranquilizers usually are more effective (see Antiemetics).

d. Should not be used in pregnancy.

5. Preparations

BUCLIZINE HYDROCHLORIDE (Softran)

Mild sedative; used in motion sickness and vertigo; should not be used in nausea of pregnancy.

Dose: 50 mg 1 to 3 times a day by mouth.

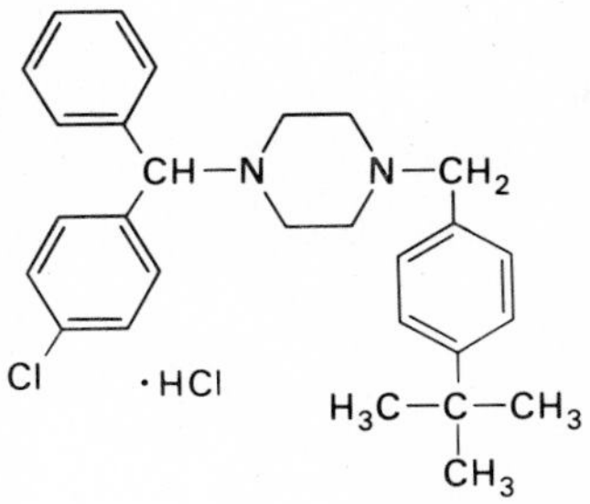

CINNARIZINE HYDROCHLORIDE (Mitronal)

Under investigation.

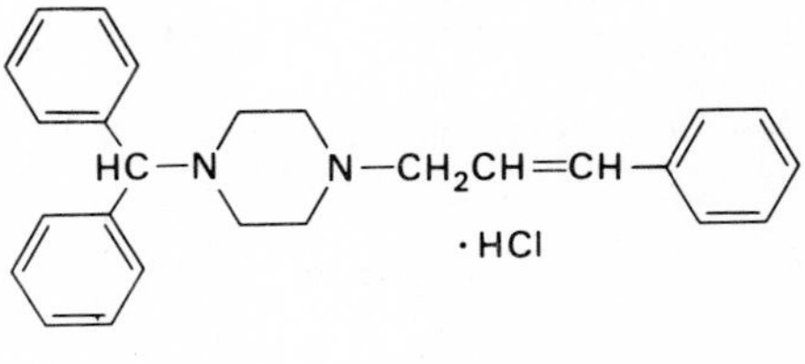

CYCLIZINE HYDROCHLORIDE (Marezine)

Dose: 50 mg 3 times a day by mouth.

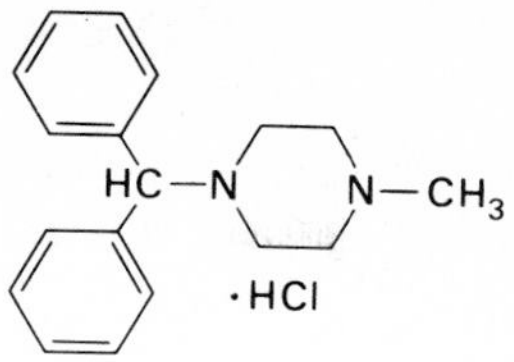

DIMENHYDRINATE (Dramamine)

(8-chlorotheophylline derivative of diphenhydramine)

Dose: 50 mg 3 times a day by mouth.

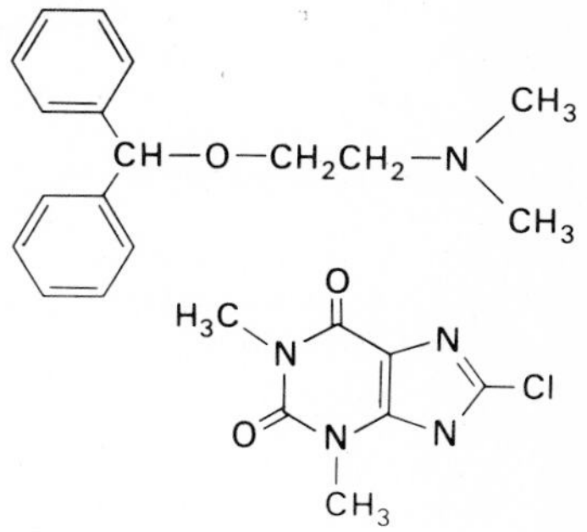

DIPHENIDOL (Vontrol)

Antiemetic; depresses labyrinthine excitability. May cause hallucinations. Used in motion sickness and Ménière's disease.

Dose: 25 mg every 4 hours by mouth; 20 to 40 mg intramuscularly or by intravenous drip.

Diphenidol hydrochloride, pamoate.

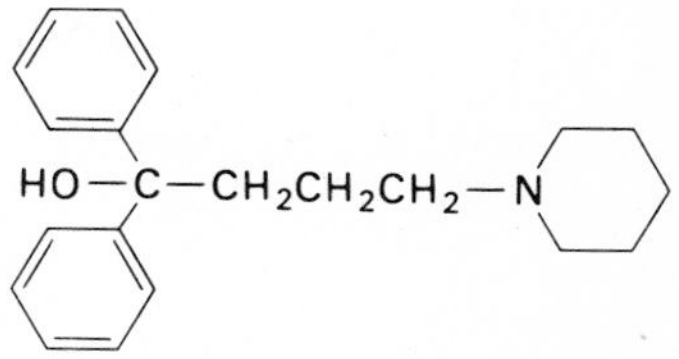

MECLIZINE HYDROCHLORIDE (Bonine)

Long acting; up to 24 hours.

Dose: 25 to 50 mg once daily by mouth.

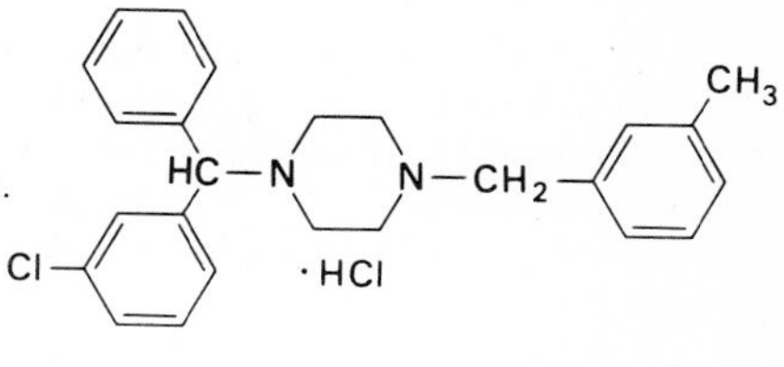

METOCLOPRAMIDE HYDROCHLORIDE (Reglan)

Antiemetic.

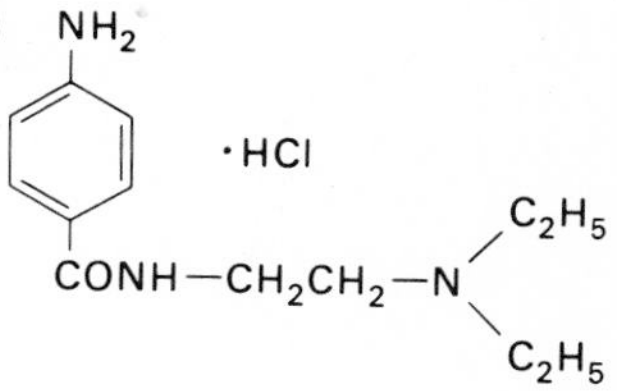

PHENGLUTARAMIDE (Aturban)

Dose: 2.5 mg by mouth.

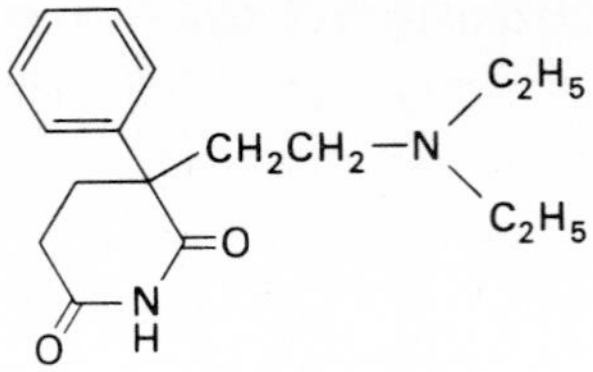

SCOPOLAMINE

(See Parasympathetic Depressants)

OTHER COMPOUNDS

BROCRESINE PHOSPHATE

Inhibitor of histidine decarboxylase.
Under investigation.

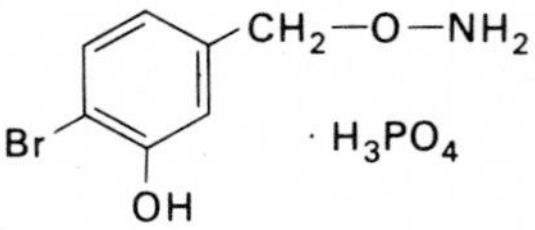

H_2 ANTAGONISTS

1. Chemistry. Possess the imidazole ring of histamine.

2. Action. Antagonize the effect of histamine on gastric acid secretion.

3. Mechanism. Competitive inhibition of the action of histamine on the H_2 receptor.

4. Pharmacodynamics. Burimamide is poorly absorbed, metiamide and cimetidine are well absorbed. Cimetidine is excreted in the urine, half-life approximately 2 hours.

5. Toxicity

a. Well tolerated. Dizziness, diarrhea, muscular pain, occasional rash.

b. No anticholinergic side effects (no dry mouth, urinary retention or blurred vision). No sedation, no local anesthetic action.

6. Uses. In the treatment of peptic ulcer.

7. Preparations

BURIMAMIDE

First drug introduced in the group. Only of historical interest.

METIAMIDE

Good clinical effect but occasional bone marrow depression.

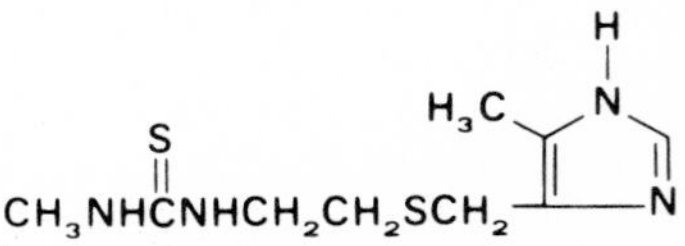

CIMETIDINE (Tagamet)

Dose: 300 mg 4 times a day by mouth.

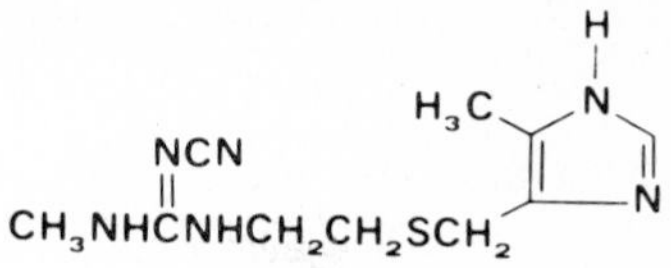

$$CH_3NHC(=NCN)NHCH_2CH_2SCH_2\text{-(4-methylimidazol-5-yl)}$$

B. Serotonin and Related Compounds

SEROTONIN

1. History. a. Erspamer (1937) isolated serotonin (enteramine) from intestine and showed that it was a smooth muscle stimulant.

b. Page (1947) showed it to be a pressor substance in clotted blood, and (1953) to be present in the brain.

2. Chemistry. Serotonin is 5-hydroxytryptamine (5HT).

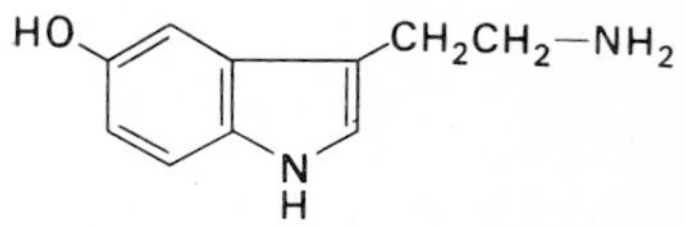

$$HO\text{-}C_8H_5N\text{-}CH_2CH_2\text{—}NH_2$$

3. Action and Mechanism

a. In the body, excluding the brain:

a′. Pharmacology: Found in argentaffin and other cells; present in bound state in platelets, mast cells (with histamine and heparin), and epidermis (with histamine). When liberated from bound state rapidly deaminated by MAO, especially in the lungs, and excreted as 5-hydroxyindole acetic acid (portions also acetylated, oxidized, and conjugated). Does not penetrate into the brain.

b′. Function: Uncertain; inhibits gastric secretion; stimulates vascular and smooth muscle. Neurohormonal transmitter in *Mercenaria mercenaria* (clam).

c′. Carcinoid tumors (argentaffinomas): Liberate excessive amounts of serotonin producing episodic flushing, tachycardia, and hypertension followed by cyanosis and diarrhea; asthma; pulmonary and tricuspid stenosis; acute symptoms may be induced by injected epinephrine (Peart, Lancet, 1: 577, 1961).

b. In the brain:

a′. Pharmacology: "Separate" occurrence in brain; concentration parallels norepinephrine and monoamineoxidase (MAO), high in hypothalamus.

b′. Function: Uncertain; presumed to be a chemical transmitter; theories:

a″. Excess serotonin may cause CNS stimulation. Evidence: Transient mental stimulation occurs after the release of serotonin by reserpine; precursor, 5-hydroxytryptophan, also produces stimulation; stimulation follows block of MAO by iproniazid. However, direct injection into the ventricles produces CNS depression.

b″. Deficient serotonin may cause CNS depression. Evidence: Mental depression follows release and exhaustion of serotonin by reserpine because free serotonin quickly inactivated by MAO. Or, conversely, by preventing storage of serotonin (and other amines), reserpine may provide continuing levels of free serotonin (Brodie).

4. Uses. No clinical applications at present.

ANTISEROTONINS

1. Chemistry. A large number of antiserotonins have been synthesized, most being indole derivatives:

2. Action. a. Variously counteract the effects of serotonin.

b. Some (not all) are hypotensive; some inhibit immediate toxicity of serotonin or prevent experimental inflammation or fibroplasia (methysergide).

3. Pharmacodynamics and Toxicity. a. Generally absorbed adequately by mouth.

b. Methysergide may produce weakness, nausea, diarrhea; angina, claudication, edema; tingling, drowsiness, dizziness, confusion, nightmares, anxiety, psychoses, and retroperitoneal fibrosis.

c. Cyproheptadine may produce drowsiness, dry mouth, nausea, dizziness, skin rashes.

4. Uses. a. Methysergide may be administered for the prevention (not treatment) of migraine; its value is not yet adequately documented and is hampered by its potential severe chronic toxicity (retroperitonial fibrosis).

b. Benanserin is under trial as a sedative and hypotensive.

c. Cyproheptadine, although more commonly used as an antihistaminic and antipruritic, has been used to control symptoms in carcinoid tumor (Brown, Clin. Res., 8:61, 1960).

5. Preparations

CYPROHEPTADINE HYDROCHLORIDE (Periactin)

Dose: 2 to 4 mg 4 times a day by mouth.

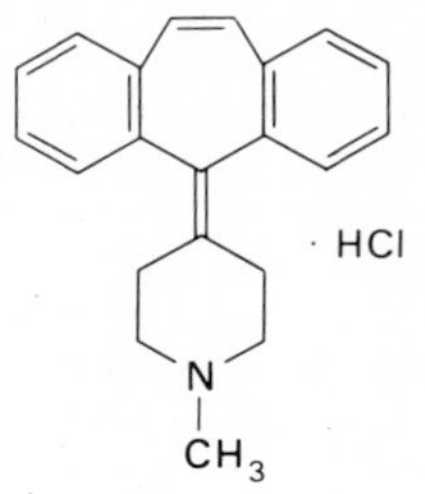

· HCl

N

CH_3

FENCLONINE

Inhibits synthesis of serotonin; has been tried in carcinoid tumor.

Dose: 4 gm daily by mouth.

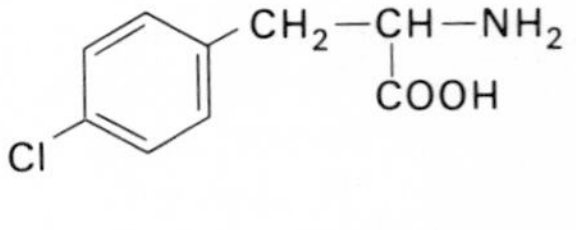

$CH_2-CH-NH_2$

COOH

Cl

METHYSERGIDE MALEATE
(Deseril; Sansert)

Dose: 2 mg 2 to 4 times a day by mouth.

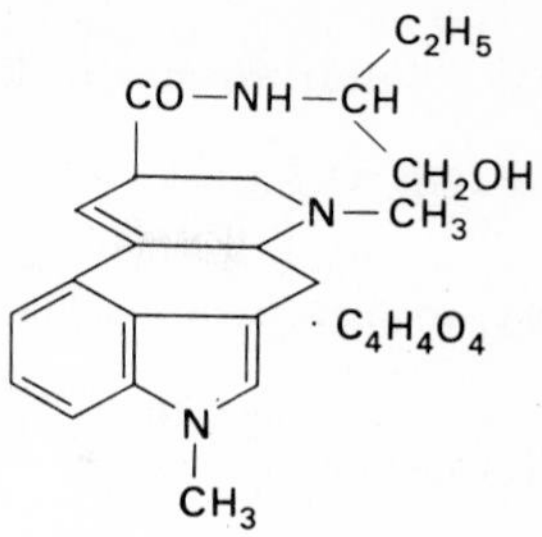

C_2H_5 CO—NH—CH CH_2OH N—CH_3 · $C_4H_4O_4$ N CH_3

OTHERS

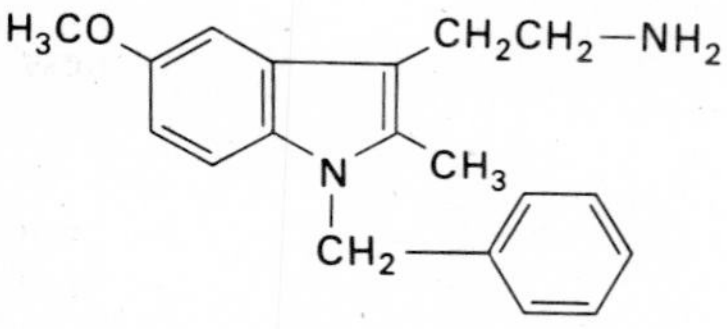

H_3CO CH_2CH_2—NH_2 N CH_3 CH_2

benaserin HCl

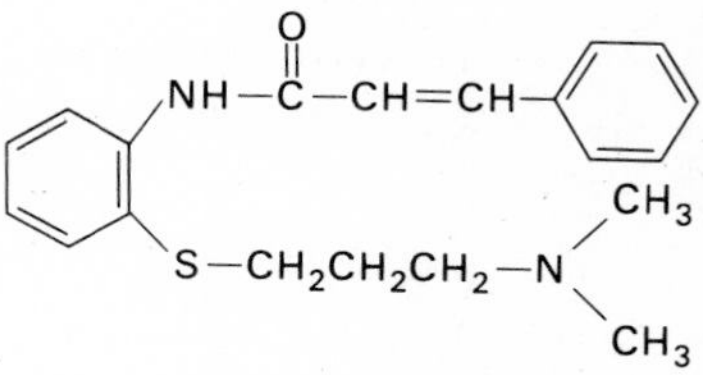

O NH—C—CH=CH— S—$CH_2CH_2CH_2$—N CH_3 CH_3

cinanserin

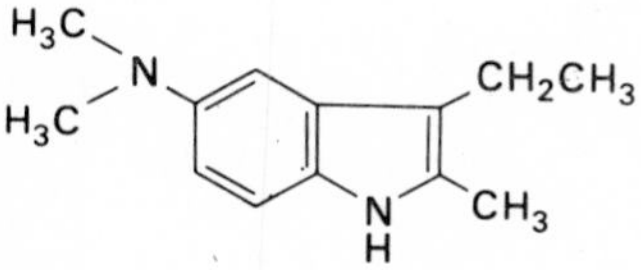

H_3C N H_3C CH_2CH_3 N H CH_3

medmain

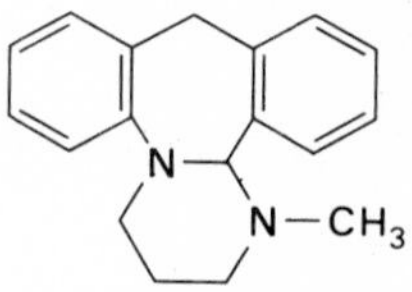

N N—CH_3

mianserin HCl

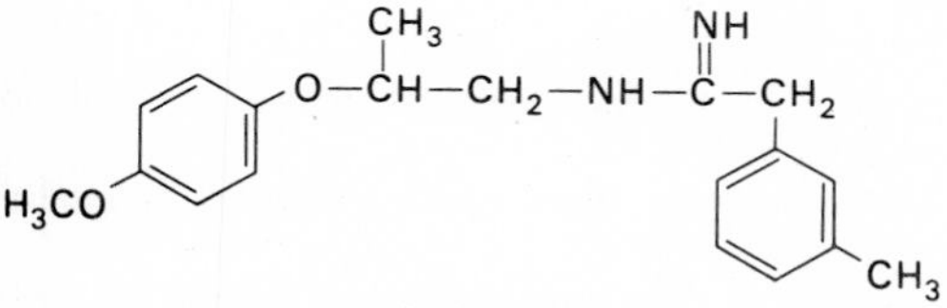

CH_3 NH O—CH—CH_2—NH—C—CH_2 H_3CO CH_3

xylamidine

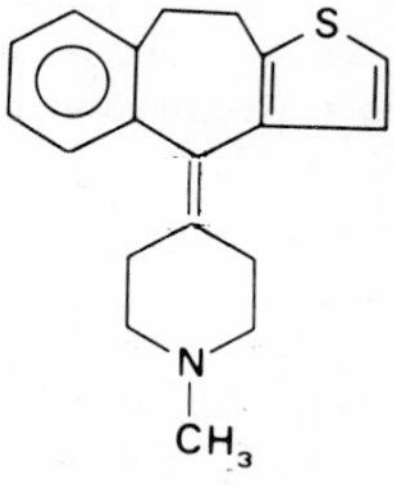

S N CH_3

pizotyline

D. Other Polypeptides of Mammalian Origin

ANGIOTENSIN

1. History. a. Volhard in 1928 suggested that the kidney might secrete a hypertensive agent, and unilateral removal of a diseased kidney has occasionally been curative.

b. Page, Braun-Menendez, Peart and others (see Science, 127:242, 1958) isolated and synthesized angiotensin.

2. Chemistry. a. The angiotensins are polypeptides; several active analogues have been made.

b. The following steps are involved in the formation of angiotensin II, the pressor substance:

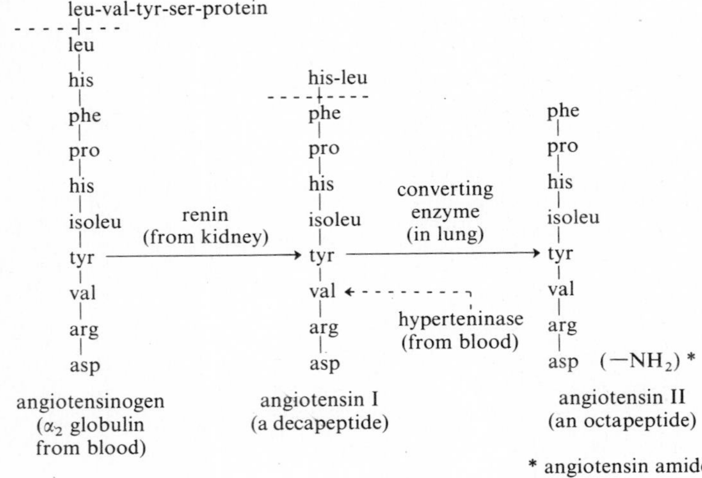

3. Action. a. Powerful pressor substance giving increase of blood pressure; constricts renal and splanchnic arteriolar beds, not venous; little change in heart rate or output; not followed by reflex hypertension or resistance, but response lessens as clinical condition deteriorates; decreased urine flow.

b. Stimulates aldosterone secretion, causing sodium retention.

c. Association with hypertensive disease uncertain, but reported to be increased in some patients with malignant hypertension.

4. Mechanism. a. Baroreceptor in kidney responds to reduced blood pressure, releasing renin from juxtaglomerular cells.

b. Renin reacts in blood with angiotensinogen, which is changed to angiotensin I and then II.

c. Angiotensin II stimulates smooth muscle of arteriolar wall directly and may increase effectiveness of endogenous norepinephine; also stimulates secretion of aldosterone from zona glomerulosa of adrenal, which in turn produces sodium retention.

5. Pharmacodynamics and Toxicity. a. Rapidly destroyed in body; does not cause sloughing or arrhythmia.

b. Rapid infusion may elevate blood pressure excessively.

6. Uses. Potent agent in acute shock, but superiority to pressor amines questioned (Udhoji, New Eng. J. Med., 270:501, 1964).

7. Preparation

ANGIOTENSIN AMIDE (Hypertensin)

Dose: 2.5 mg in 500 ml of saline by *slow* intravenous drip; exact rate determined by titration of increasing doses against blood pressure (Council on Drugs, J.A.M.A., 186:1158, 1963).

BRADYKININ

1. History. Rocha e Silva (1948) discovered; Boissonnas and others (1960) synthesized.

2. Chemistry. a. Kininogen, an α_2 globulin, is present in plasma as the bradykinin precursor.

b. Kallikrein, an enzyme in plasma, may be activated by low pH (inflammation), damaged surfaces (burns with activated Hageman factor), snake venom, or other stimuli; it then releases a polypeptide, lysylbradykinin, from the precursor.

c. Another enzyme, converting factor, shortens the polypeptide to the active substance, bradykinin.

d. Other enzymes, kininases, then rapidly break down bradykinin to inactive fragments.

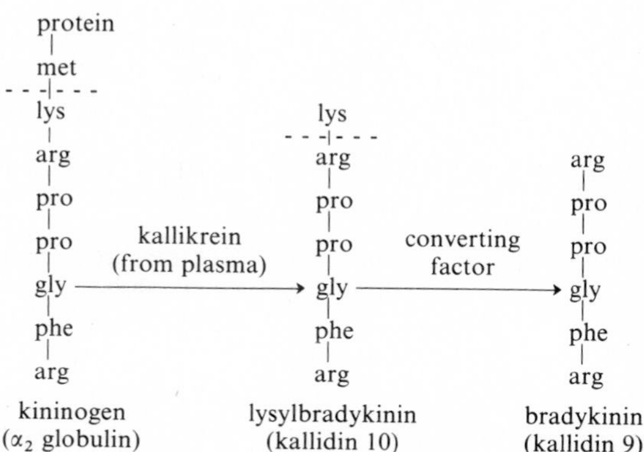

3. Action and Mechanism. a. Potent vasodilator, especially of skin, head, coronaries.

b. Smooth muscle stimulant, especially bronchi, gastrointestinal tract, uterus.

c. May be responsible for some elements of local pain; may be released in carcinoid syndrome; may be mediator of inflammation and of parts of the allergic reaction.

d. Function may be as a local hormone that mediates defense reactions.

4. Uses. No present use: brief action would make use difficult.

PROSTAGLANDINS

1. History. a. Actions recognized by Kurzrok and Lieb (1930) and von Euler (1935).

b. Isolated by Bergstrom (1956); synthesized by Pike and Beal (1966).

2. Chemistry. a. Derivatives of prostanoic acid, a 20-C lipid acid with a 5-membered ring; 16 different derivatives known.

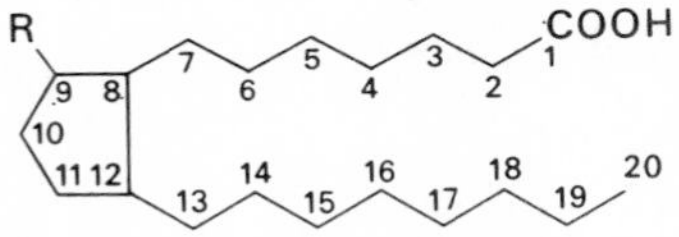

b. Classified as PGA, PGB, PGE, PGF, with subscripts 1, 2, etc. E derivatives have =O at R; F derivatives —OH; the 1 and 2 series have 1 and 2 double bonds, respectively, in the side chains.

c. Probably synthesized in most cells of most animal species, though first recognized in semen.

3. Action and Mechanism. a. Many actions, varying with the derivative and the species used in testing. Include smooth muscle stimulation or depression, vasoconstriction or dilatation, inhibition of platelet aggregation, inhibition of gastric secretion, inhibition of lipolysis, depression of corpus luteum, induction of sodium excretion.

b. The E series (PGE_1, PGE_2, etc.) tend to be vasodilators and smooth muscle depressors; the F series (PGF_{1a}, etc.) tend to be pressor in some species (dogs, rats) and depressor in other (cats, rabbits).

c. The primary action appears to be on cell membranes; receptors may be involved. Tentatively, the prostaglandins modify or inhibit the action of adenyl cyclase, which alters the formation of cyclic AMP, the mediator of most hormone actions.

4. Pharmacodynamics and Toxicity. a. Salicylates, indomethacin, and other antirheumatic drugs inhibit synthesis.

b. Absorption and excretion inadequately studied; most derivatives are inactivated in the lungs.

c. Toxicity inadequately studied.

5. Uses. No presently accepted uses, but proposed for peptic ulcer, abortion, contraception, sterility, induction of labor, thrombosis, hypertension, asthma, nasal congestion, and probably others.

6. Preparations

DOXAPROST

Smooth muscle relaxant, bronchodilator.

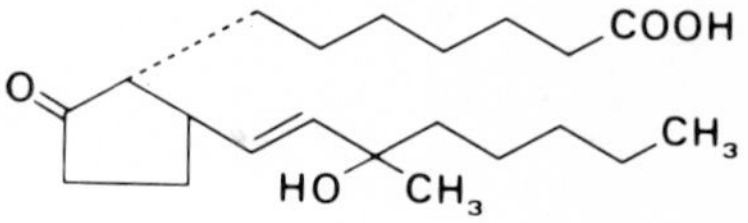

DINOPROSTONE (Brostin E_2)
PGE_2. Oxytocic.

For abortion from the 12th week through the second trimester.

Dose: 20 mg in vaginal suppository, repeat after 3 to 5 hours.

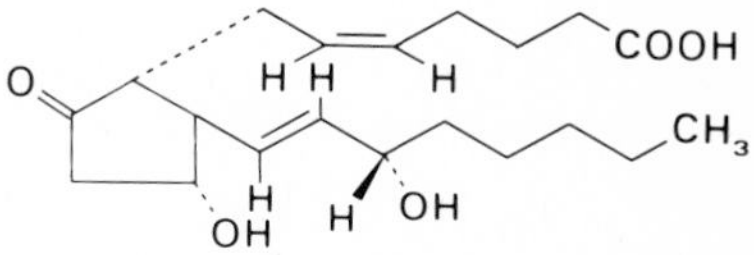

CARBOPROST ($PGF_{2\alpha}$)
Oxytocic.

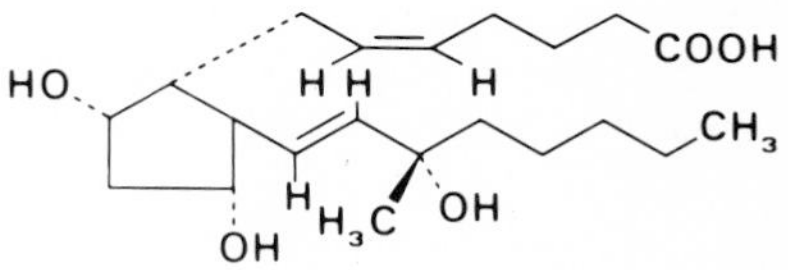

DINOPROST (Prostin F_2 Alpha)
Oxytocic.

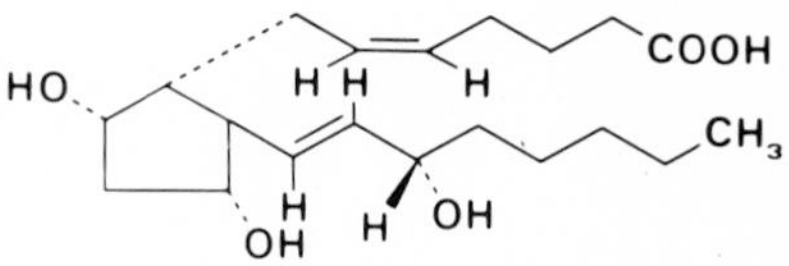

DINOPROST TROMETHAMINE

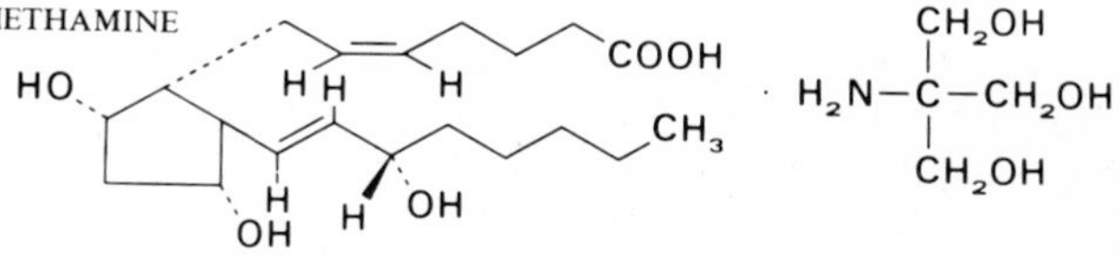

OTHER AGENTS

SUBSTANCE P

A polypeptide found in the intestine and brain that causes contraction of the intestine, but dilatation of blood vessels. May be a transmitter of pain impulses.

ELEDOISIN

An 11-polypeptide from octopus salivary gland. Potent pressor; unrelated to angiotensin.

32. Anterior Pituitary Hormones and Related Agents

A. Corticotropin (ACTH)

1. History. a. Evans (1932) and Li prepared adrenocorticotropic extracts from the anterior pituitary.

b. Shephard (1956) determined structure; Hoffmann (1960) and Schwyzer (1963) synthesized active molecules.

2. Chemistry. ACTH is a single chain polypeptide of 39 amino acids and a molecular weight of 4,566.

ser-tyr-ser-met-glu-his-phe-arg-try-gly-lys-pro-val-gly-lys-lys
1 2 3 4 5 6 7 8 9 10 11 12 13 14 15 16

NH_2

ala-leu-glu-asp-glu-ala-gly-asp-pro-tyr-val-lys-val-pro-arg-arg
32 31 30 29 28 27 26 25 24 23 22 21 20 19 18 17

glu-ala-phe-pro-leu-glu-phe
33 34 35 36 37 38 39

3. Action. a. Corticotropin is one member of the chain of substances and events that result in the production of adrenal cortical hormones. The sequence is diagrammed on p. 341.

a′. Corticotropin releasing factor (CRF): the hypothalamus contains a polypeptide (10 amino acids; similar to FSH) called CRF. This substance can release ACTH from the anterior pituitary.

b′. Corticotropin (ACTH): ACTH stimulates the adrenal cortex to produce cortical hormones (mostly glycosteroids) from cholesterol, in the presence of vitamin C.

c′. Cortical steroids: Carry on peripheral actions in the tissues, but also inhibit further ACTH liberation.

d′. Other factors: A number of other agencies can also cause ACTH release by stimulating CRF production (or release). These include trauma (stress) which influences CRF via neural pathways, drugs, such as barbiturates and anesthetics, which act via the reticular activating center, and influences from other parts of the brain, transmitted through the hypothalamus (Sayers, Ann. Rev. Physiol., 20:243, 1958).

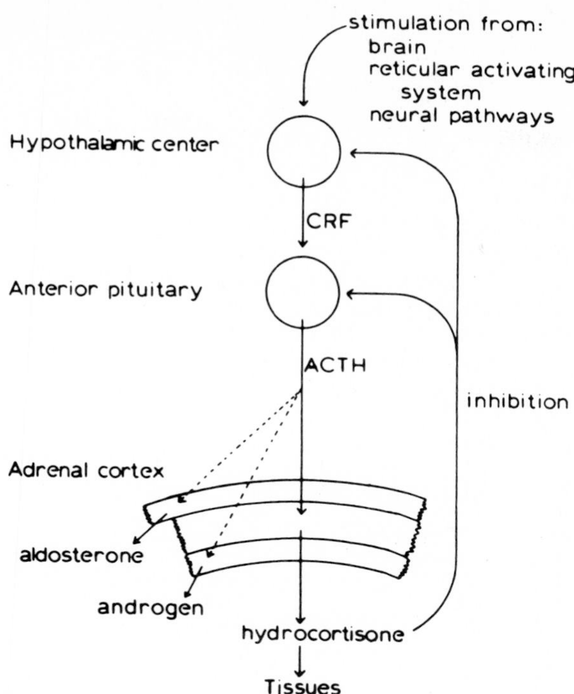

b. The effects of ACTH are in general those of the administration of cortisone; however, the actions also include moderate salt and water retention and androgenic effects. The asthenia upon withdrawal is shorter and less severe than after cortisone.

4. Mechanism. ACTH stimulates adenyl cyclase in the adrenal cell wall to synthesize cyclic AMP. This then stimulates conversion of cholesterol to pregnenolone by forcing accumulation of cholesterol by the adrenal.

5. Pharmacodynamics. Parenteral administration is necessary. The injected hormone rapidly disappears from the circulation (half-life approximately 15 min.). Does not appear in the urine.

6. Toxicity. Aside from the effects of increased cortical hormones there is little toxicity, although allergic sensitivity may occur. The pigmentation in Addison's disease may be due to ACTH, as it appears in adrenalectomized Cushing's disease patients; (see Melanocyte Stimulating Hormones).

7. Uses. In inflammatory states as an alternative to glycosteroids; rheumatoid arthritis, ulcerative colitis, exfoliative dermatitis.

8. Preparations

Cosyntropin (Cortrosyn)

Synthetic corticotropin, consisting of the first 24 amino acids.

For diagnostic purposes.

Dose: 0.25 mg intravenously or intramuscularly.

Corticotropin (ACTH; Acthar; Cortrophin)

Dose: 10 to 20 units 4 times a day intramuscularly or intravenously.

Corticotropin, purified (ACTH, purified; Depo-ACTH; and others)
Suspended in a gel which gives prolonged effects.
Dose: 40 to 80 units once daily subcutaneously or intramuscularly.

Corticotropin-zinc hydroxide (Cortrophin-Zinc)
Dose: 40 to 80 units once daily intramuscularly (long acting).

B. Melanocyte Hormones

MELANOCYTE STIMULATING HORMONES (MSH)

1. Chemistry. a. Derived from the pituitary.
b. α-MSH is identical with the first 13 amino acid sequence of ACTH; β-MSH, with 18 amino acids, is similar but varies with the species.

CH_3CO-ser-tyr-ser-met-glu-his-phe-arg-try-gly-lys-pro-val-NH_2

α-MSH

2. Action. a. α-MSH causes dispersion of melanin granules and darkening of darked-skinned persons within 24 hours (Lerner, Nature, 189:176, 1961); β-MSH effective in some persons.
b. Both are natriuretic in rats.

MELATONIN

1. Chemistry. a. Present in pineal and peripheral nerves of man.
b. N-acetyl - 1 serotonin.

2. Action. Most effective melanophore contractor; lightens color (Lerner, J. Amer. Chem. Soc., 81:6084, 1959). Secretion is stimulated by light, via sympathetics, and slows estrus cycle in rats (Wurtman, Sci. Amer., 213:50 [July], 1965).

3. Use. No therapeutic use.

C. Thyrotropic Hormone (TSH)

1. History. a. Smith (1922) demonstrated thyroid stimulating property of anterior pituitary.
b. Evans (1934) prepared potent extracts.

2. Chemistry. Thyrotropic hormone (TSH) is a glycoprotein produced by basophil cells of the anterior pituitary; mol. wt. 28,000.

3. Action and Mechanism. a. TSH is the normal regulator of thyroid function. It acts to produce hypertrophy of the thyroid and increased formation of thyroid hormones.

b. The stimulating effect appears to be on many of the steps involved in the synthesis of thyroxin, but is more quantitative than qualitative.

c. The production of TSH by the anterior pituitary is controlled by the thyroid releasing factor (TRF) from the hypothalamus, which is released in response to a lowered level of thyroid hormone in the blood.

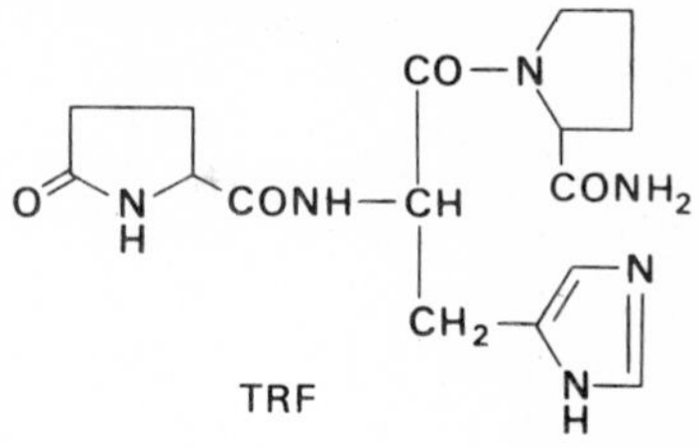

CO—N
O N H CONH—CH CONH$_2$
N
CH$_2$
TRF N H

4. Role in Disease. a. Although administration of TSH will produce hyperthyroidism with exophthalmos, natural hyperthyroidism appears to be the effect of a long-acting thyroid stimulator (LATS). This substance, found in the blood of patients with hyperthyroidism, acts more slowly than TSH, but similarly increases I_2 uptake and the production of calorigenic hormone. It is associated with gamma globulin and may be a manifestation of immunological disease.

b. The associated exophthalmus appears not to be due to intact TSH, but to an allied agent, probably a break-down product; the orbital muscles are swollen and infiltrated with lymphocytes, eosinophils, and mast cells; water is bound by mucopolysaccharides.

5. Uses. a. Available preparations induce refractoriness to the thyroid stimulating effect in three or four weeks, an effect probably the result of the formation of antibodies to the species of the source of the preparation. These antibodies have been called antihormones, but do not appear to be different from ordinary antibodies.

b. Used diagnostically in conjunction with radioactive iodine to test functional capacity of the thyroid as TSH normally increases the amount of radioactivity leaving the thyroid.

6. Preparation

THYROTROPIN (Thytropar)

Dose: 10 u daily for 3 to 5 days.

D. Pituitary Gonadotropins

FOLLICLE STIMULATING HORMONE (FSH)

1. History. a. Smith and Engle (1927) produced sexual precocity in rats by anterior pituitary implantation.

b. Evans and Li (1949) purified; Steelman (1956) isolated.

2. Chemistry. a. Glycoprotein (containing glucosamines).
b. Probably produced by the basophil cells of the anterior pituitary.

3. Action and Mechanism. a. Induces development of ovarian follicles (female), and maintains spermatogenesis (male).
b. Production controlled by FSH releasing factor (FRF), a small polypeptide from the hypothalamus.

4. Role in Disease. Deficiency gives sterility (and, in the female, menstrual abnormalities); excess gives premature maturity.

5. Uses. Not available, but see Menotropins under Nonpituitary Gonadotropins.

E. Luteinizing Hormone

LUTEINIZING HORMONE (LH, INTERSTITIAL CELL STIMULATING HORMONE, ICSH) AND LUTEINIZING HORMONE RELEASING FACTOR (LHRF)

1. History. Li and Evans (1940) isolated the hormone.

2. Chemistry. a. Glycoprotein.
b. Probably produced by the acidophils of the anterior pituitary.

3. Action and Mechanism. a. Induces continued follicular development with maturation, ovulation, and corpus luteum formation (female), and maintains production of androgens by interstitial cells (male).

LUTEINIZING HORMONE RELEASING FACTOR (LHRF)

1. Chemistry. Decapeptide.

2. Action. It is elaborated by the hypothalamus and reaches the anterior pituitary by the hypophyseal portal circulation and there stimulates production and release of LH.

3. Uses. Increases female fertility.

4. Preparations.

GONADORELIN ACETATE

$$\underset{1}{\text{5-oxoPro}}\text{-}\underset{2}{\text{His}}\text{-}\underset{3}{\text{Trp}}\text{-}\underset{4}{\text{Ser}}\text{-}\underset{5}{\text{Tyr}}\text{-}\underset{6}{\text{Gly}}\text{-}\underset{7}{\text{Leu}}\text{-}\underset{8}{\text{Arg}}\text{-}\underset{9}{\text{Pro}}\text{-Gly-}NH_2 \cdot 2C_2H_4O_2 \cdot 4H_2O$$

GONADORELIN HYDROCHLORIDE

PROLACTIN (LUTEOTROPIC HORMONE, LTH)

1. History. a. Riddle (1939) identified action on crop sac of the pigeon.

b. White (1949) isolated the hormone.

2. Chemistry. Similar to growth hormone. One hundred and ninety-one amino acids; mol. wt. 22,000.

3. Action and Mechanism

a. Stimulates the growth of the female breast, with the assistance of estrogen and progestin, and initiates lactation.

b. Prolongs function in the corpus luteum in mice and rats.

c. Bromocriptine (see Ergot Alkaloids) inhibits prolactine secretion.

4. Role in disease. May be involved in pathogenesis of gynecomastia and galactorrhea.

5. Uses. No therapeutic preparations are available.

F. Nonpituitary Gonadotropins

HUMAN CHORIONIC GONADOTROPIN (HCG)

1. History. Gey (1938) showed the placental origin of certain gonadotropins.

2. Chemistry. a. Glycoprotein: mol. wt. about 20,000.

b. Produced by the Langhans cells of the trophoblast; obtained from human pregnancy urine.

3. Action and Mechanism. In general resembles ICSH; luteinizing in rats but not in humans. Normal function probably to maintain corpus luteum of early pregnancy.

4. Uses. In cryptorchidism or hypogonadism in the male.

5. Preparation

GONADOTROPIN, CHORIONIC (Antuitrin, S., APL, Follutein and others)

Dose: 1,000 to 4,000 units 2 or 3 times a week intramuscularly.

MENOTROPINS (Human Follicle Stimulating Hormone; Humegon; Pergonal)

From human postmenopausal urine; mostly FSH and LH. May induce ovulation in ovarian failure. Under trial in infertility; has been responsible for multiple births.

Dose: 75–150 units daily intramuscularly for 9 to 12 days followed by 10,000 i.u. gonadotropin.

PREGNANT MARE SERUM GONADOTROPIN (PMSG)

1. History. Cole and Hart (1930) and Zondek (1930) described preparations.

2. Chemistry. a. Possibly a mixture of glycoproteins.

b. Produced by the endometrium of pregnancy in the horse (formerly thought placental).

3. Action. Shows both FSH and ICSH actions.

4. Uses. No clearly established therapeutic use.

G. Growth Hormone

GROWTH HORMONE (STH)

The anterior pituitary forms at least one further hormone, the growth hormone, in addition to the adrenocorticotropic, thyrotropic, and gonadotropic hormones previously described (Matsuzaki, Ann. Rev. Pharmacol., 5:137, 1965).

1. History. Evans and Long (1921) produced gigantism in animals by anterior pituitary injections; Li (1945) isolated growth hormone, (1970) synthesized human growth hormone (HGH) with Yamashiro.

2. Chemistry. a. Bovine hormone a polypeptide chain, mol. wt. about 46,000; human, mol. wt. 21,500 with 190 amino acids.

b. Produced by the eosinophils of the anterior pituitary. Release stimulated by the hypothalmic Growth Hormone Releasing Factor (GHRF, GRF) and inhibited by the tetradecapeptide, somatostatin, also produced in the hypothalamus. Release also inhibited by the synthetic ergot-alkaloid Bromocriptine (see Bromocriptine).

3. Action. a. Stimulates growth, probably in all body cells.

b. Causes nitrogen retention.

c. Produces an increase in glucose turnover ("diabetogenic hormone," Evans, 1935).

d. Increases oxidation of fat ("pancreatotrophic" or "ketogenic" hormone, Hoffmann and Anselmino, 1931).

e. Maintains lactation; maintains renal function.

4. Mechanism. a. Enhances transport of some or all amino acids through cell membrane to interior of the cell.

b. May control mRNA synthesis and hence protein synthesis and growth (Komer, Recent Progr. Hormone Res., 21:205, 1965).

c. Some of the effects may be mediated through cyclic AMP (cyclic adenosine 3′5′-monophosphate).

5. Role in Disease. a. Deficiency in childhood produces pituitary dwarfism.

b. Excess in childhood produces gigantism; in adults acromegaly.

c. Chronic administration in animals may produce diabetes, and tumors (rats).

6. Uses. a. The hormone has been promising experimentally in pituitary dwarfism and cachexia and recently a modified growth hormone from cattle has been tried for the promotion of growth, muscle development, and wound healing

(Forsham, Med. Sci., 5:359, 1959).

b. No commercial preparations are available.

SUMMARY: ANTERIOR PITUITARY HORMONES AND RELATED AGENTS

TYPE	*ACTION AND MECHANISM*	*TOXICITY*	*USE*	*EXAMPLES*
Corticotropin	Stimulates production of adrenal cortical hormones Increases cyclic AMP: cholesterol converted to pregnenolone	Minor	Alternative to glycosteroids	Corticotropin (ACTH)
Thyrotropic hormone	Stimulates production of thyroid hormone	Hyperthyroidism	To test function of thyroid	Thyrotropin
Pituitary gonadotropins (FSH)	Induces follicular development and maintains spermatogenesis	Minor	Not in use	None
(LH)	Continues preceding and induces ovulation and corpus luteum	Minor	Not in use	None
Nonpituitary gonadotropins	Induce ovulation	Multiple births	Infertility	Menotropins
Growth hormone	Stimulates growth in all cells	Minor	Pituitary dwarfism	Experimental

Reviews

Li, C. The ACTH molecule. Sci. Amer., 209:46, 1963.

Fridhandler, L., and Pincus, G. Pharmacology of reproduction and fertility. Ann. Rev. Pharmacol., 4:177, 1964.

Friesen, H., and Astwood, E. Hormones of the anterior pituitary body. New Eng. J. Med., 272:1216, 1965.

Daughaday, W., and Parker, M. Human pituitary growth hormone. Ann. Rev. Med., 16:47, 1965.

33. Adrenal Cortical Hormones

A. The Adrenal Cortex

1. History. a. Addison (1855) described disease of the adrenal capsules.

b. Pfiffner and Swingle (1929), Hartman (1930) made potent adrenal cortical extracts; Kendall, Pfiffner, Reichstein, Wintersteiner (1934+) independently isolated crystalline steroids; Reichstein (1937) synthesized desoxycorticosterone.

c. Sarett (1948) synthesized cortisone; Hench (1949) showed clinical use; Wendler (1950) synthesized hydrocortisone; Luetscher (1952) and Tait and the Simpsons (1952) isolated aldosterone from urine and the adrenals respectively.

2. Chemistry. a. The adrenal cortex elaborates three types of corticosteroids from acetate via cholesterol and pregnenolone, as in the following examples:

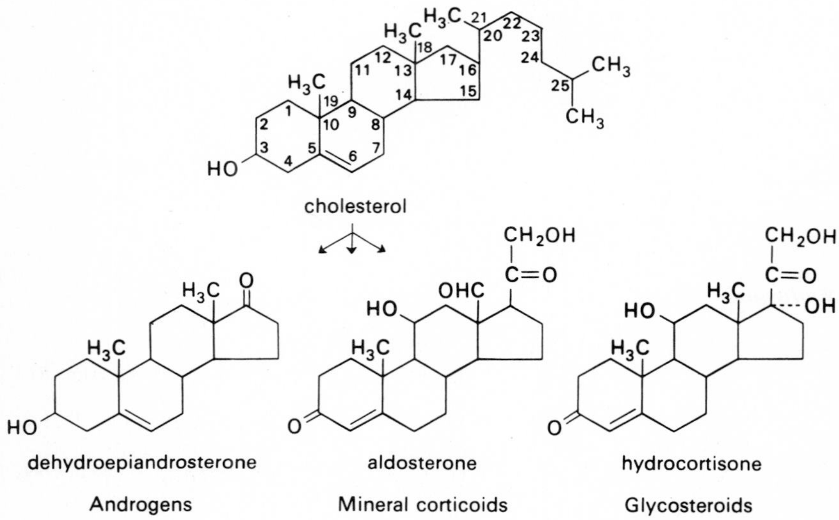

b. Mineral corticoids are formed in the glomerular (outer) layer of the cortex; glycosteroids in the fascicular (middle) layer; and androgenic steroids in the reticular (inner) layer.

3. Physiological Production. a. Normal production in man: hydrocortisone, 25 mg per day; aldosterone, 0.125 mg.

b. The glycosteroids and mineral corticoids show some overlapping in physiological effect, as may be seen from the following table of approximate physiological activities.

STEROID	RELATIVE ACTIVITY MINERAL CORTICOID	GLYCOSTEROID
Aldosterone	10,000	50
Desoxycorticosterone	100	1
Cortisone	5	100
Hydrocortisone	10	150

c. Corticosteroid production is under the general control of ACTH, which acts on the cell membrane to activate adenyl cyclase, which in turn increases production of cyclic AMP. The latter appears to promote corticosteroid synthesis between cholesterol and pregnenolone.

4. Preparation

ADRENAL CORTICAL EXTRACT
Obsolete.

B. Mineral Corticoids

ALDOSTERONE

1. History. Demonstrated by Luetscher (1952) as salt-retaining factor in urine (SRF) and isolated from the adrenals by Tait and the Simpsons (1952).

2. Chemistry. a. Has O at 11. Type mineral corticoid is C-21 hydroxysteroid, with O at 11, at 17, or neither.

b. Exists largely as the hemiacetal.

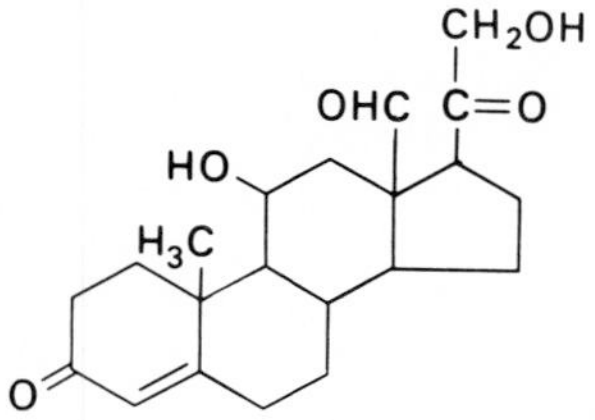

CH_2OH, OHC C=O, HO, H_3C, O

aldosterone

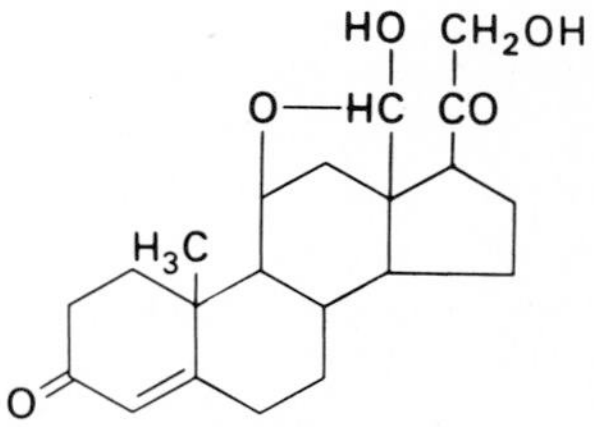

HO CH_2OH, O—HC CO, H_3C, O

hemiacetal form

3. Action and Mechanism. a. Aldosterone is the natural salt-retaining factor of the body. It acts to increase reabsorption of Na in the distal renal tubules by influencing active transport (probably also to restrict Na loss by sweat, salivary, and gastrointestinal glands), and to increase the excretion of K. Aldosterone and hydrocortisone appear to share in the control of electrolytes, but homeostasis is maintained almost entirely by aldosterone.

b. It also has considerable glycosteroid effect (half that of cortisone) but is present in such small amounts in the blood that quantitatively this is inconsequential.

c. The secretion of aldosterone is governed mainly by the level of angiotensin, which is increased when the blood pressure falls (see Angiotensin); synthesis is facilitated between cholesterol and pregnenolone. A receptor in the diencephalon near the pineal body appears to be a secondary means of regulation; this elaborates a lipid hormonal substance when the fluid volume or Na concentration of the body falls. The hypophysis (ACTH) may also be necessary for full aldolsterone secretion (hypophysectomy decreases production by 60% or more, but temporarily), but this appears not to be a factor in the ordinary fluctuations of aldosterone which are controlled by the diencephalic factor (Farrell, Endocrinology, 65:239, 1959).

d. Aldosterone, and many other hormones, may act by "exposing" specific DNA templates, which then proceed to direct the synthesis of messenger RNA; the RNA, in turn, directs the synthesis of enzyme or other protein which provides the specific action (Castles, Proc. Soc. Exp. Biol. Med., 119:308, 1965).

4. Role in Disease. a. In the edema of heart failure, the nephrotic syndrome, cirrhosis, and the toxemia of pregnancy, the production and excretion of aldosterone is increased, and aldosterone is instrumental in the production of the edema.

b. In primary aldosteronism, caused by an adrenal cortical tumor which produces excessive aldosterone, however, edema is not present; characteristically there are hypernatremia, hypokalemia, and increased urinary aldosterone, with weakness, hypertension, polyuria, polydypsia, and hyperchloremic, hypokalemic alkalosis.

5. Uses. Aldosterone is not available as a therapeutic agent.

DESOXYCORTICOSTERONE

1. History. Synthesis by Reichstein (1937).

2. Chemistry. Source synthetic, but has been demonstrated in adrenal glands.

3. Action and Mechanism. Causes retention of Na and water, and loss of K, by acting on the renal tubules similarly to aldosterone; does not produce glycosteroid effects.

4. Pharmacodynamics and Toxicity. a. Poorly absorbed by mouth but parenteral routes satisfactory.

b. Excreted in part as pregnanediol.

c. Excessive retention of Na may cause edema and hypertension.

d. Excessive depletion of K may cause weakness, and myocardial and skeletal muscle necrosis.

5. Uses. a. Used to control the electrolyte defect in adrenal insufficiency, particularly before the advent of cortisone; now may be used as a supplement.

b. Has been given in many forms: crystalline suspension intramuscularly, pellets implanted subcutaneously, aerosol droplets.

6. Preparation

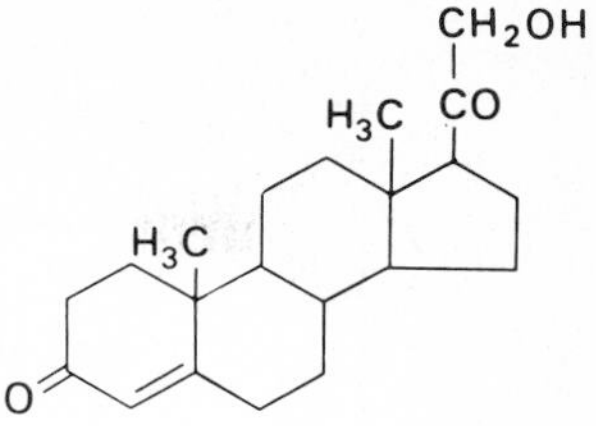

DESOXYCORTICOSTERONE
(11-desoxycorticosterone)

Desoxycorticosterone acetate (DOCA; Percorten)
Solution in sesame oil.
Dose: 1 to 3 mg daily intramuscularly; 10 to 20 mg in emergency.

CH_2OH | H_3C CO | H_3C | O

C. Glucocorticoids

NATURAL GLUCOCORTICOIDS

1. Chemistry. a. Source: adrenal cortex; also synthetic.
b. Cortisone and hydrocortisone have an O at C-11, and an OH at C-17.
c. Production takes place under the stimulation and control of ACTH.

2. Action. It is difficult to propose a single, unifying action for cortisone. The most fundamental action is apparently an alteration of protein metabolism, with the production of a negative protein balance. However, whether this is the result of the inhibition of protein synthesis, or of increased breakdown, and whether in all cells or only in certain cells, is not clear. On a descriptive basis, actions may be observed affecting the following functions:

a. Protein metabolism: Increased protein breakdown, osteoporosis, negative N balance, cessation of growth; also increased excretion of amino acids and uric acid.

b. Carbohydrate metabolism: Increased gluconeogenesis (manufacture of sugar from protein), increased blood sugar.

c. Fat metabolism: Abnormal mobilization and deposition of fat.

d. Electrolytes: Increased Na and water retention; increased K excretion.

e. Endocrines: Inhibited ACTH secretion.

f. Glandular secretions: Increased saliva, sweat, gastric acid, sebaceous secretions.

g. Blood: Increased clotting, increased neutrophils (but poor quality); decreased lymphocytes and eosinophils.

h. Central nervous system: Stimulation and euphoria.

3. Mechanism. a. The underlying mechanism of action is unknown.
b. Several theories suggest an effect on enzyme or protein synthesis:

a′ Interaction with genetic apparatus resulting in stimulation of DNA-dependent RNA production, with subsequent increase (or decrease) in enzyme and protein manufacture (Samuels, New Eng. J. Med., 271:1252, 1964).

b′ Stimulation of cytoplasmic enzymes to increased protein manufacture (in liver) (Litwack, Topics Med. Chem., 1:3, 1967).

c′. Interference in the phosphogluconate shunt between glucose-6-phosphate and pentose. This could then result in decreased nucleic acid production, and subsequently in decreased protein synthesis.

c. Effect on membranes or intercellular material:

a′. Stabilization of organelle membranes, preventing rupture of lysosomes with consequent release of contained lytic enzymes.

b′. Possible inhibition of sulfation of polysaccharides in synthesis of mucopolysaccharides of connective tissue (Whitehouse, Nature, 189:37, 1961); antiinflammatory activity may be related to chelation of copper (Wiesel, Amer. Coll. Clin. Pharm., Chicago, 1965).

c′. Prevention of formation of vasoactive kinins (Cline, Science, 153:1135, 1966).

4. Actions in Extraphysiological Dosage. a. Inflammation: General suppression. Inhibition of exudation; inhibition of cell proliferation; inhibition of capillary dilatation (may exclude locally irritating substances, like histamine, from cells; see Wool, Nature, 186:728, 1960). Effects may be local actions; perhaps by stabilization of lysosome membranes preventing release of damaging enzymes.

b. Muscle work: Increased performance.

c. Allergy: Suppressed allergic phenomena. Possible explanations include decreased antibody formation (but not in man?) from decreased protein metabolism, or from decreased lymphocytes and plasma cells; decreased eosinophils; inhibition of histidine decarboxylase which would reduce the production of histamine; other inhibition of formation or storage of histamine; direct smooth muscle relaxation (Aviado, J. Clin. Pharmacol., 10:3, 1970); however, the effects may be primarily from the antiinflammatory action.

d. Endocrine: Adrenal cortical atrophy.

5. Pharmacodynamics

a. Preparations variably soluble and variably absorbed.

b. Metabolically transformed in liver into tetrahydrocortisone and a large number of other derivatives before excretion.

c. Hydrocortisone more potent than cortisone, gives more salt retention but less CNS stimulation; may be in equilibrium with cortisone in the body.

6. Toxicity. a. Serious toxic potentialities in extraphysiological dosage include particularly the production of Cushing's disease with the following manifestations: moon face, striae, hirsutism, acne, hypothyroidism, amenorrhea, adrenal atrophy, negative N balance, osteoporosis, muscle wasting, sodium and water retention with edema, K, Ca, and P loss, hypertension, transformation of rheumatoid vasculitis into necrotizing arteritis.

b. Other hazards include the spread of infections from lack of restraint of inflammation and interference with immune mechanisms, especially dissemination of tuberculosis; aggravation of diabetes; aggravation of herpetic keratitis; induction of glaucoma; aggravation of peptic ulcer without symptoms until hemorrhage or perforation; masking of myocardial infarction; prolongation of wound healing; insomnia, psychosis.

7. Uses. a. For physiological replacement in adrenal insufficiency (Addison's disease); may be combined with small amounts of desoxycorticosterone acetate, and adequate salt and sugar intake. Also occasionally for suppression of adrenal cortical hyperactivity.

b. In immunologic diseases: Rheumatoid arthritis, rheumatic fever, disseminated lupus erythematosus, hypersensitivity reactions (asthma, serum sickness), hemolytic anemia, drug reactions, agranulocytosis, and others.

c. In inflammation: Ulcerative colitis, exfoliative dermatitis, pemphigus, gout, and others.

d. In acute shock; in overwhelming infection.

e. In neoplasm.

f. In nephrosis: May produce diuresis, when given with Na restriction (0.5 gm), but supplemental K (3 gm KCl).

8. Preparations

CORTISONE ACETATE (Cortone; Cortogen)

Dose: 5 to 20 mg daily by mouth (adrenal insufficiency) to 10 to 500 mg daily by mouth, intramuscularly, intravenously or topically, in tablets, microcrystalline suspensions or ointments (for extraphysiological effect in various diseases).

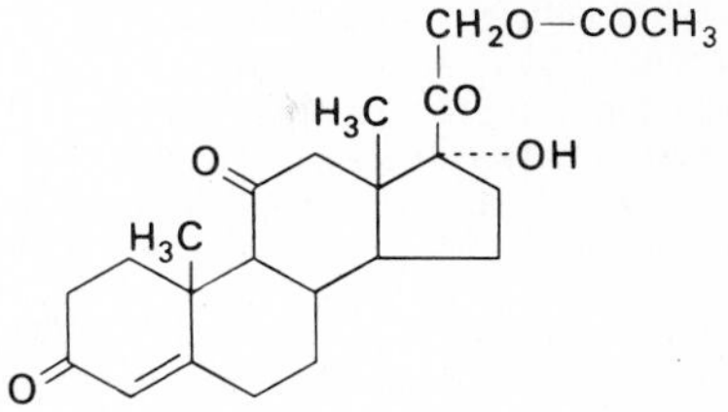

HYDROCORTISONE (cortisol; Cortef; Cortril; and others).

Dose: 10 to 20 mg 4 times a day by mouth initially, then adjusted as needed; also locally in several forms in 0.5% to 2.5% concentrations; not parenterally owing to poor solubility and absorption.

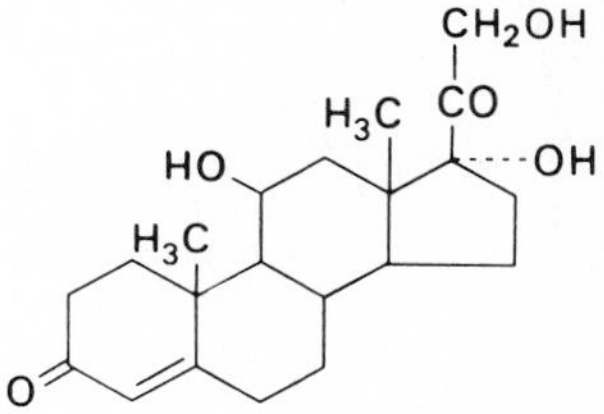

Hydrocortisone acetate (Cortef acetate, etc.)

Dose: 0.5% to 2.5% in topical or ophthalmic preparations; 10 to 25 mg or more of crystalline suspension into joints and bursae.

Hydrocortisone cyclopentylpropionate: Suspension of an ester for oral administration in the same doses as hydrocortisone.

Hydrocortamate hydrochloride (Magnacort): An ester salt for topical application in 0.5% preparations.

Hydrocortisone sodium succinate (Solu-Cortef): A soluble ester salt allowing intravenous administration.

Dose: 50 mg or more intramuscularly or intravenously.

CARBENOXOLONE SODIUM

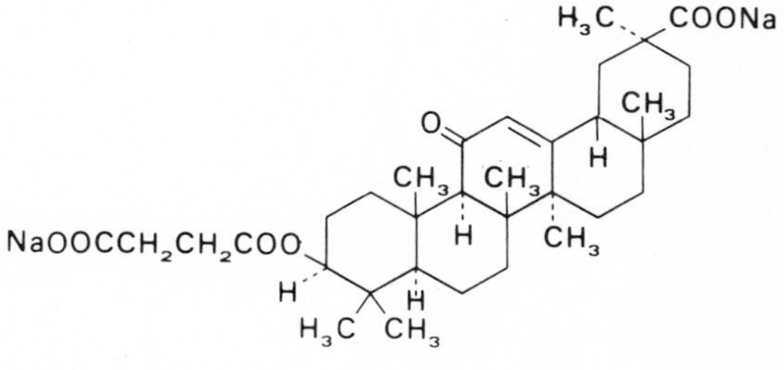

Prepared from liquorice. Glucocorticoid with some mineral corticoid effect.
Primary use in treatment of peptic ulcer.
Dose: First week: 100 mg 3 times a day, thereafter 50 mg 3 times a day by mouth.
(Baron and Sullivan, eds. Carbonoxolone Sodium. Butterworth, London, 1970.)

SYNTHETIC DERIVATIVES

1. Chemistry. a. A large number of derivatives of the glycosteroids have been made in an effort to produce compounds with greater glycosteroid effect (and hence greater antiinflammatory effect), but with fewer side effects, especially Na retention. The first has been accomplished much more easily than the second.

b. Some generalization as to the relationship of chemical structure to activity can be made. Introduction of a double bond at 1-2, as in prednisone and prednisolone, increases glycosteroid activity more than mineral corticoid activity. Halogenation (F) usually increases both. Methylation at 2 increases electrolyte activity; at 16 it increases glycosteroid activity and decreases electrolyte activity.

c. Topical absorption is enhanced in the acetate or acetonide derivatives.

2. Action. Qualitatively similar to cortisone, but with quantitative differences in potency of glycosteroid and electrolyte effect. Glycosteroid potency is illustrated by the following list of dosages which produce equivalent effects:

EQUIVALENT DOSAGES

Cortisone	25 mg
Hydrocortisone	20
Prednisone	5
Prednisolone	5
Triamcinolone	4
Paramethasone	2
Dexamethasone	0.75

3. Pharmacology and Toxicity. The full side effects of cortisone, except for salt retention in some cases, may be produced, and clinical toxicity is frequent and may be severe.

4. Uses. Similar to those for cortisone and hydrocortisone.

5. Preparations

a. Cortisone and hydrocortisone derivatives

CORTODOXONE (cortexolone)

Under investigation.

FLUCETONIDE

Under investigation.

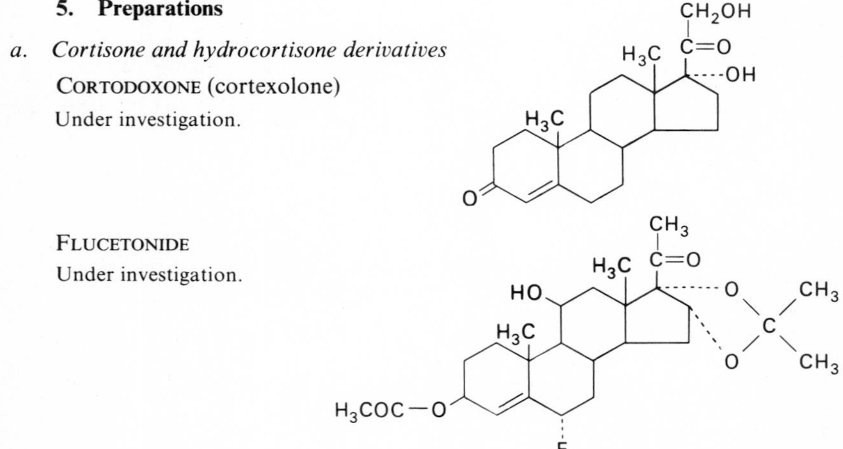

FLUDROCORTISONE ACETATE (Alflorone; F-Cortef; and others)

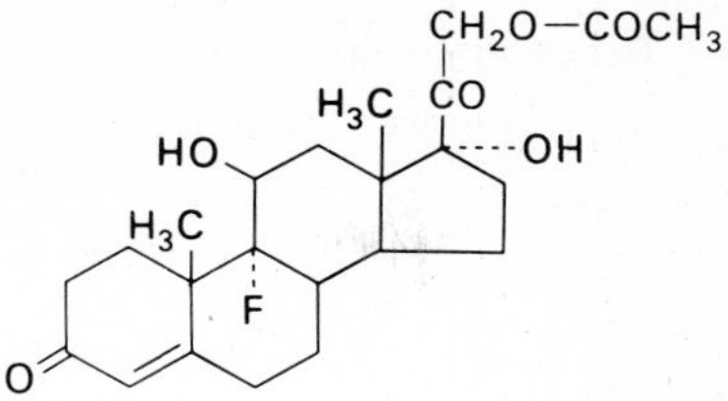

Potent mineral corticoid; may be used in the control of Addison's disease in doses of 0.1 to 0.3 mg daily.

Dose: 0.05% to 0.25% topically.

FLURANDRENOLONE ACETONIDE (Cordran)

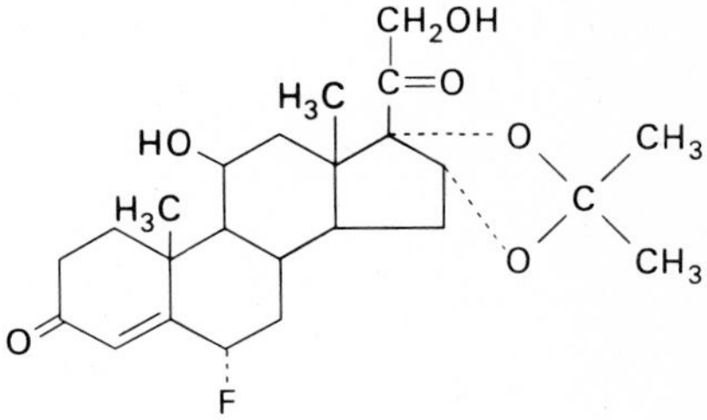

Dose: 0.05% topically 2 to 3 times daily.

MEDRYSONE (HMS)

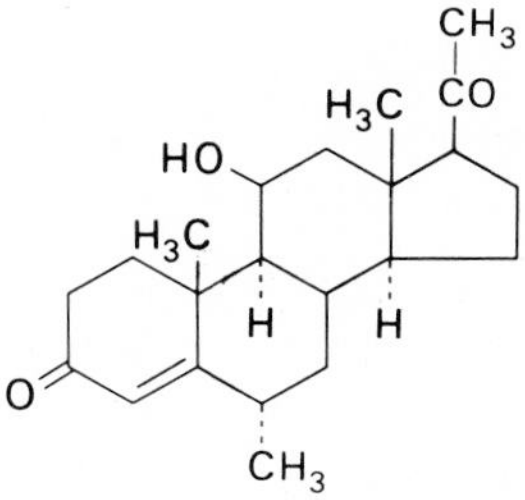

Topical corticoid.
Under investigation.

b. Prednisone, prednisolone, and derivatives (double bond 1-2)

AMCINAFAL

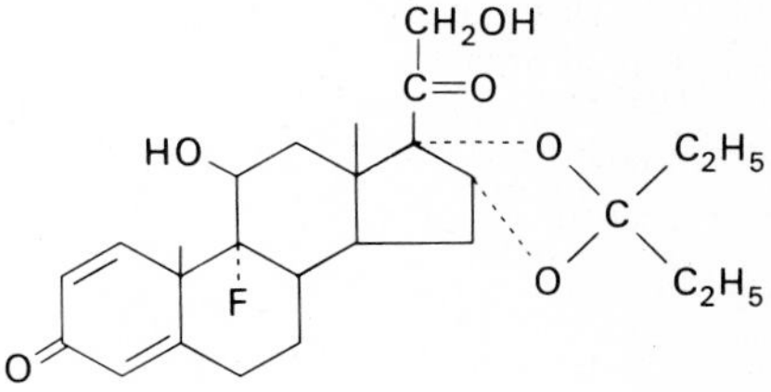

Topical corticoid.
Under investigation.

AMCINAFIDE

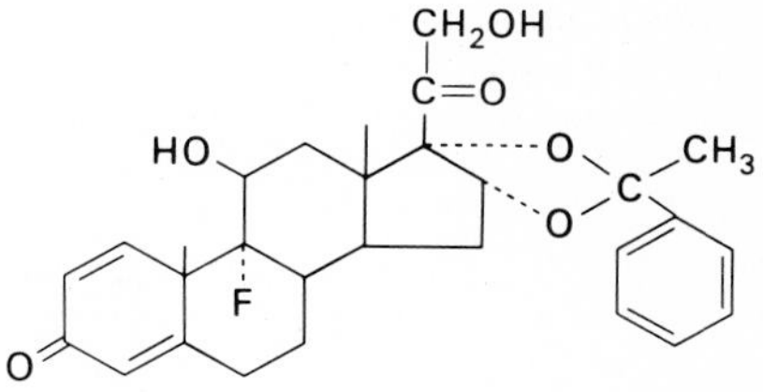

Topical corticoid.
Under investigation.

BETAMETHASONE (Celestone)

Active in small dosage; both sodium retention and increased excretion reported.

Dose: 0.6 to 3 mg daily by mouth.

Betamethasone benzoate
Betamethasone valerate
Betamethasone dipropionate

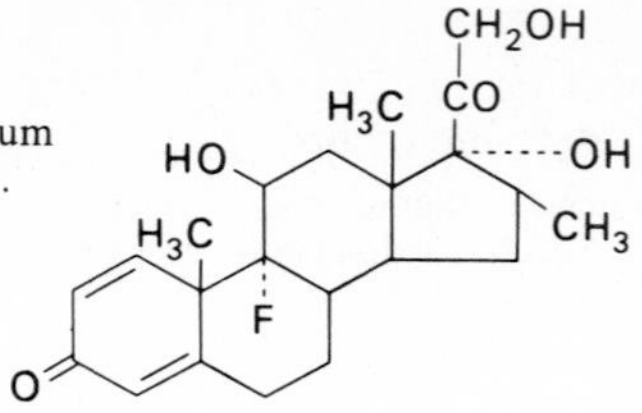

CHLOROPREDNISONE ACETATE

Topical corticoid.
Under investigation.

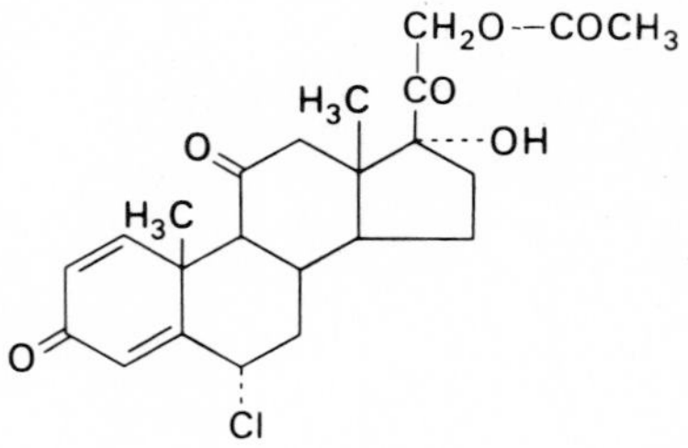

CLOCORTOLONE ACETATE

Under investigation.

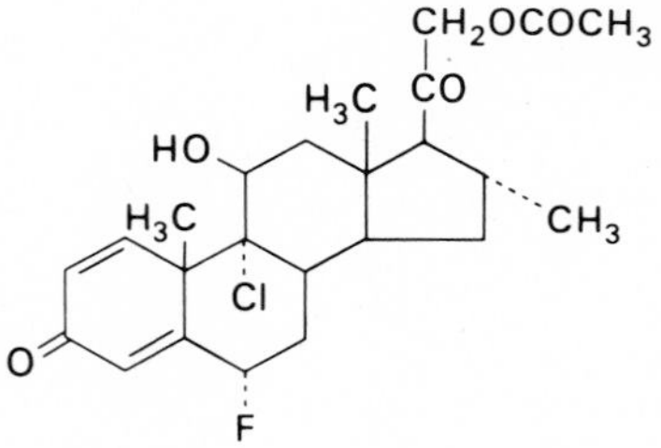

DESCINOLONE ACETONIDE

Topical corticoid.
Under investigation.

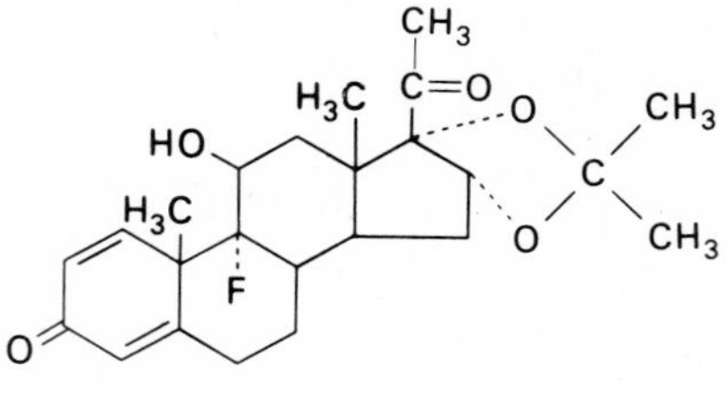

DESONIDE

Topical corticoid.
Under investigation.

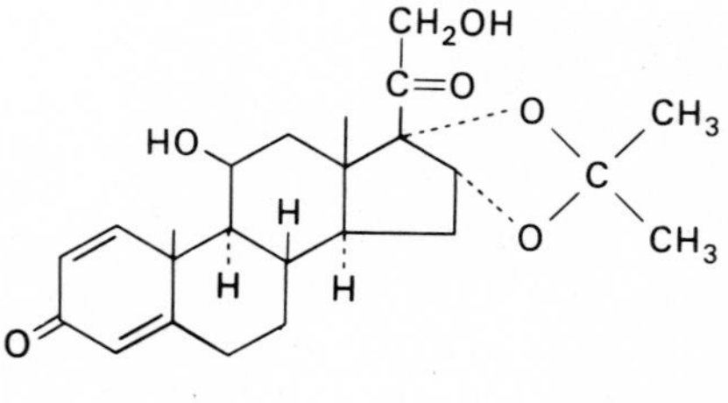

DESOXIMETASONE (Topicort)

Dose: 0.25% topically.

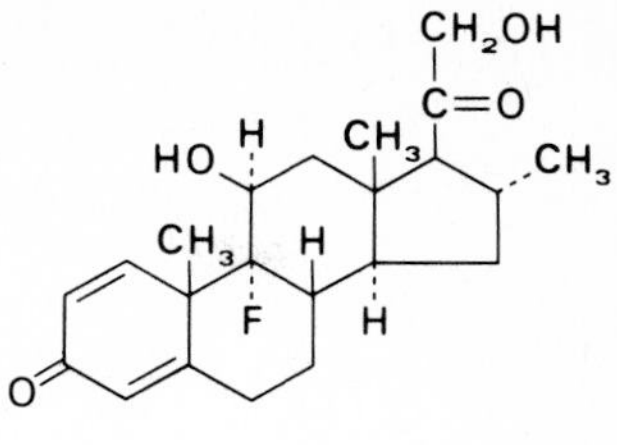

DEXAMETHASONE (Decadron; Deronil)

Dose: 0.75 mg daily by mouth; 0.1% cream or ointment topically.

Dexamethasone phosphate

A water-soluble ester.

Dose: 0.05% ophthalmic; 0.1% topical.

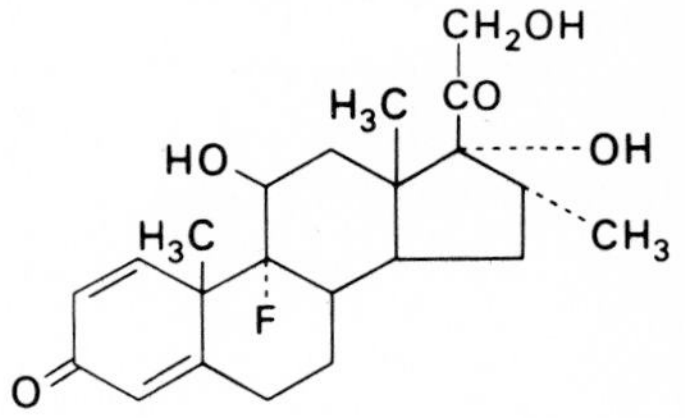

DICHLORISONE ACETATE (Diloderm)

Dose: 0.025% topically.

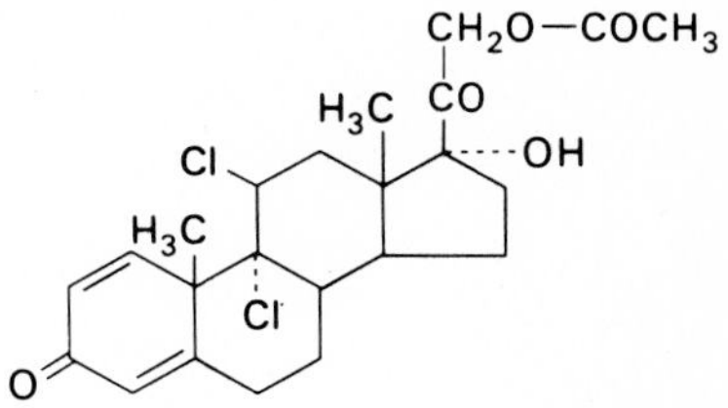

DIFLUPREDNATE

Under investigation.

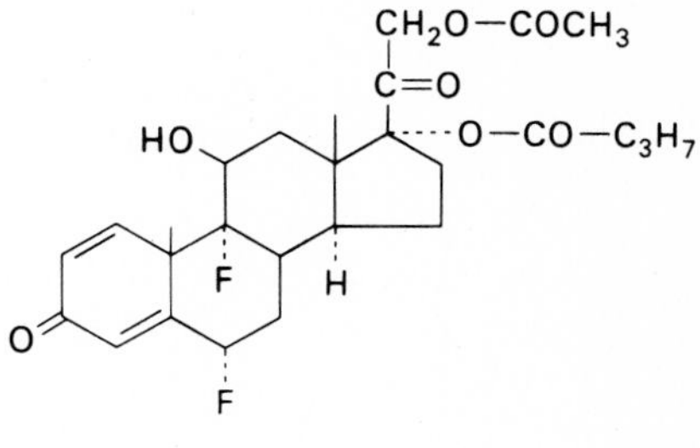

FLUCLORONIDE

Topical corticoid.

Under investigation.

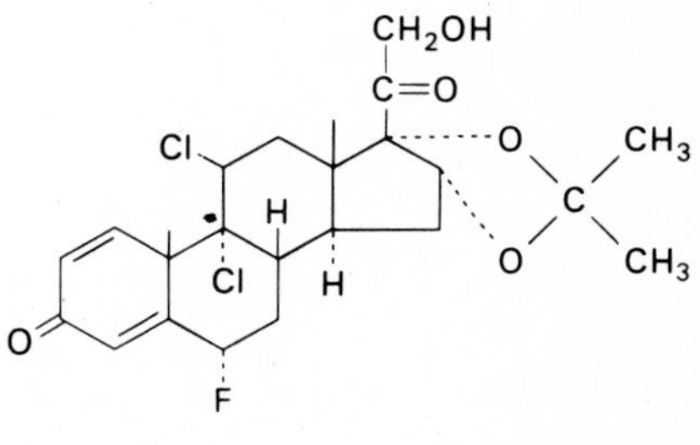

FLUMETHASONE

Under investigation.

Flumethasone pivalate (Locorten)

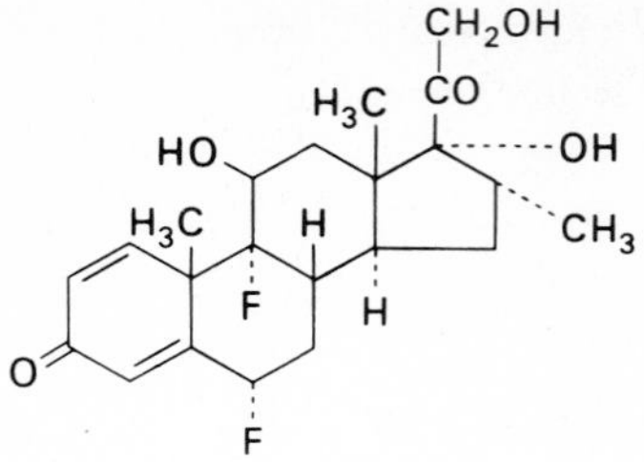

FLUNISOLIDE ACETATE

Topical corticoid.
Under investigation.

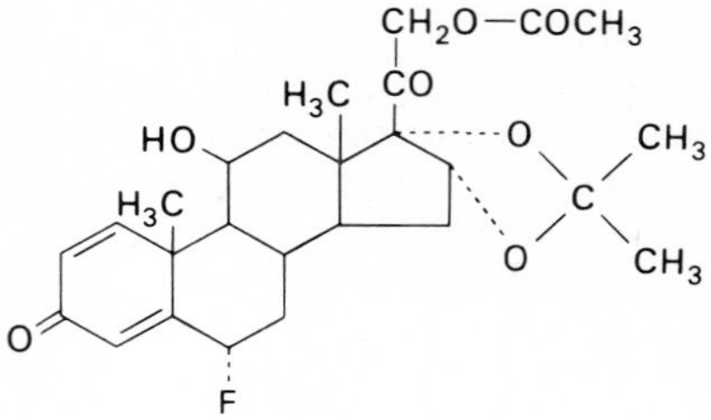

FLUOCINOLONE ACETONIDE (Synalar)

Dose: 0.025% topically.

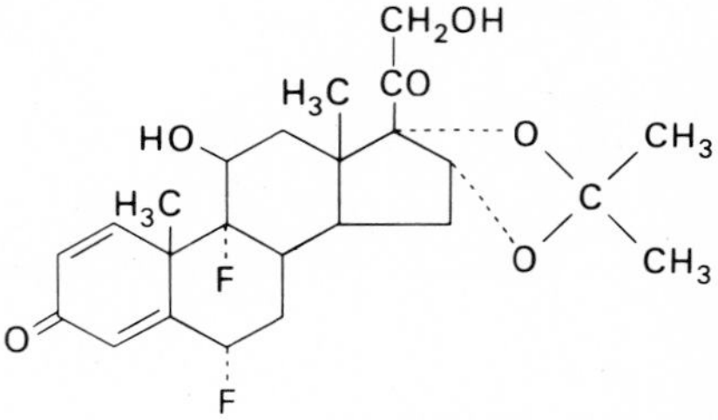

FLUOCINONIDE (Lidex; Synalate)

Dose: 0.01% to 0.025% topically.

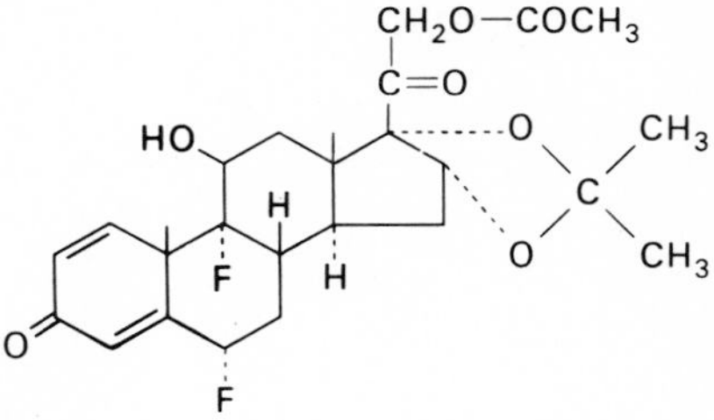

FLUOCORTOLONE

Under investigation.

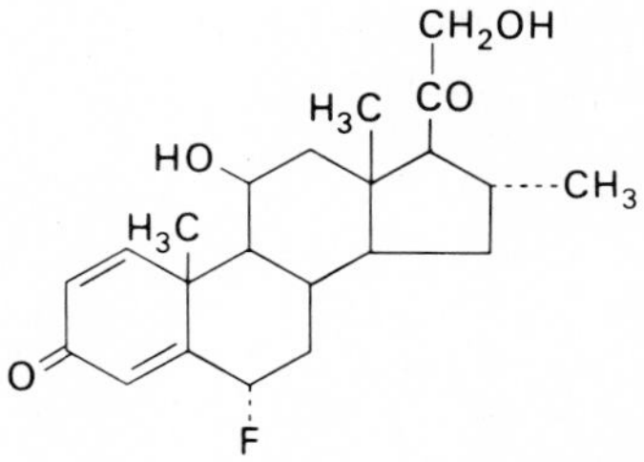

FLUOROMETHOLONE (Oxylone)

Dose: 0.025% topically.

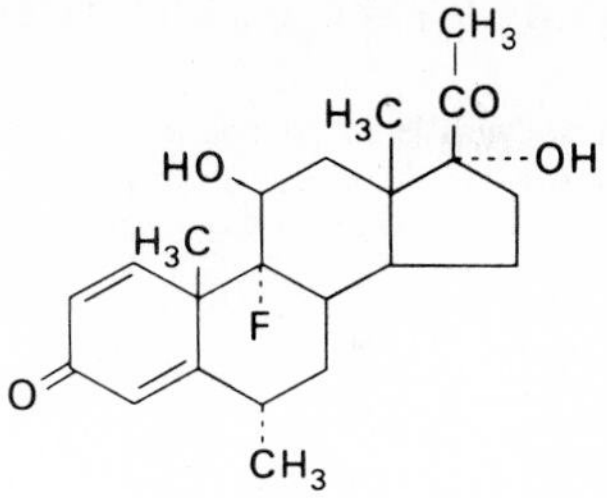

FLUPEROLONE ACETATE (Methral)

Under investigation.

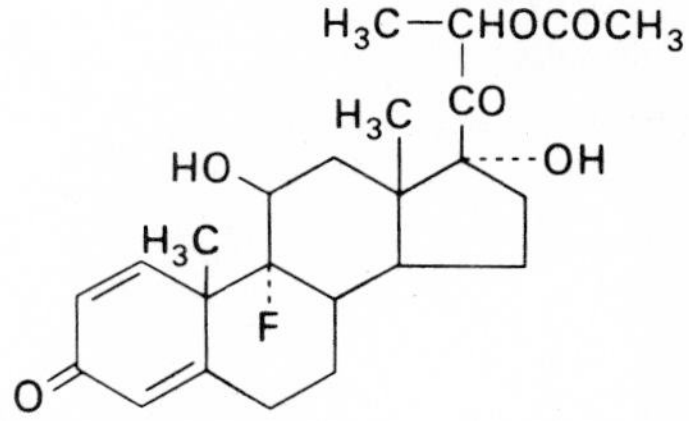

FLUPREDNISOLONE (Alphadrol)

Potent: doses over 6 mg daily may produce side effects.

Dose: 5 to 15 mg by mouth daily.

Fluprednisolone valerate.

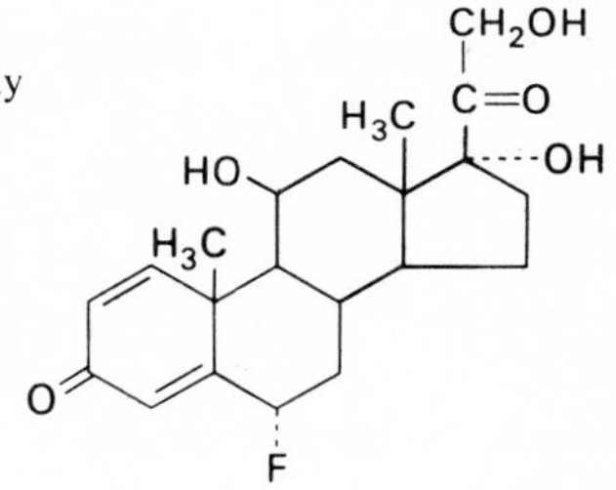

MEPREDNISONE (Betapar)

Under investigation.

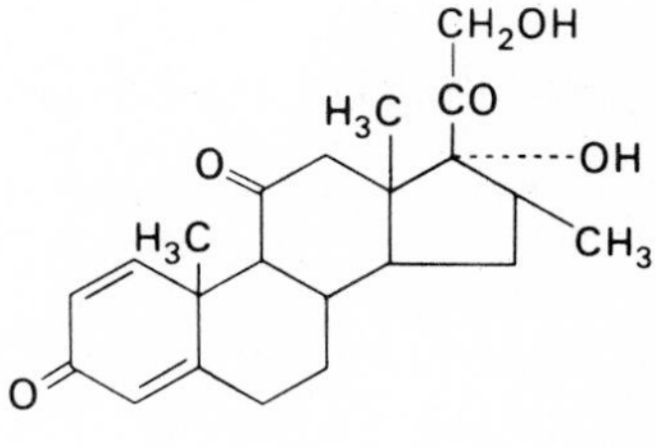

METHYL PREDNISOLONE (Medrol)

Dose: 5 to 50 mg daily by mouth.

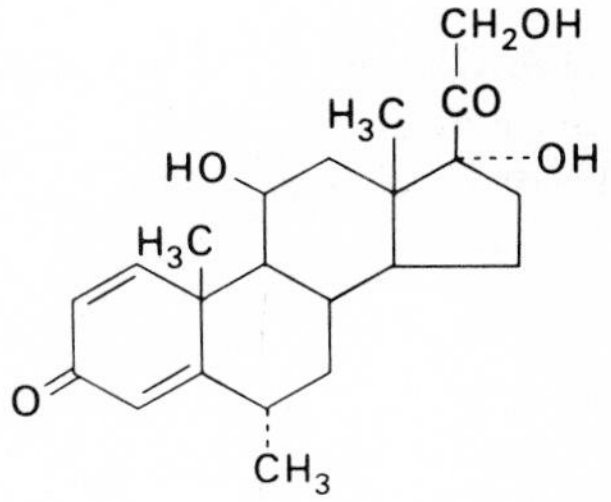

PARAMETHASONE ACETATE (Haldrone; Stemex)

Minimal sodium retention and potassium depletion.

Dose: 2 mg 2 to 3 times a day by mouth.

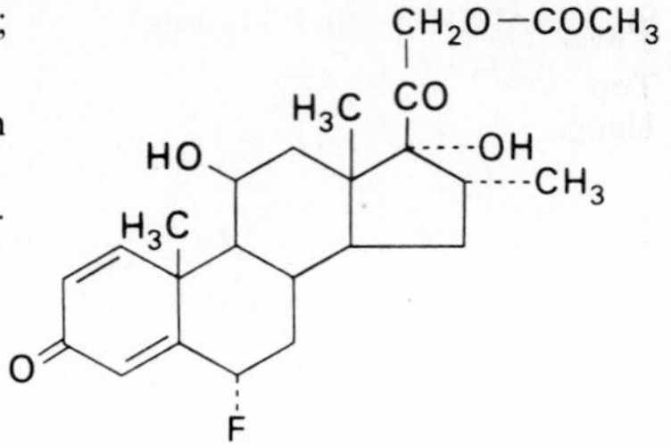

PREDNISOLAMATE
(Deltacortril)

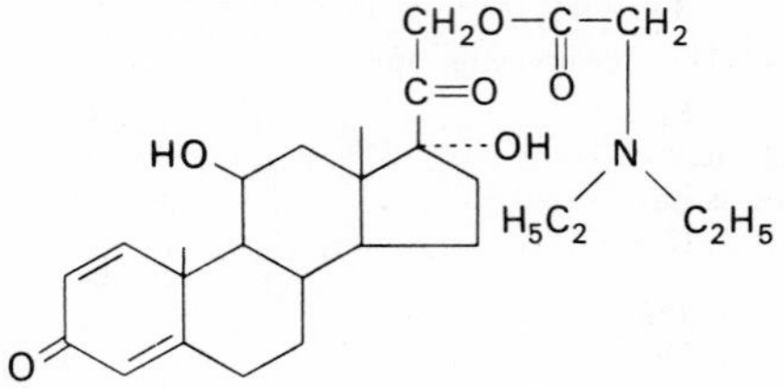

PREDNISOLONE (Delta Cortef; Meticortelone; and others)

Dose: 5 to 50 mg daily by mouth.

Prednisolone acetate (Sterane)

Dose: intramuscularly in doses equivalent to prednisolone.

Prednisolone butylacetate (Hydeltra-T.B.A.)

Dose: intrasynovially in equivalent doses.

Prednisolone phosphate sodium (Hydeltrasol).

Dose: by topical, intramuscular, intravenous, or intrasynovial routes in equivalent doses.

Prednazate (Sixty six-20)

Perphenazine salt of prednisolone hemisuccinate.

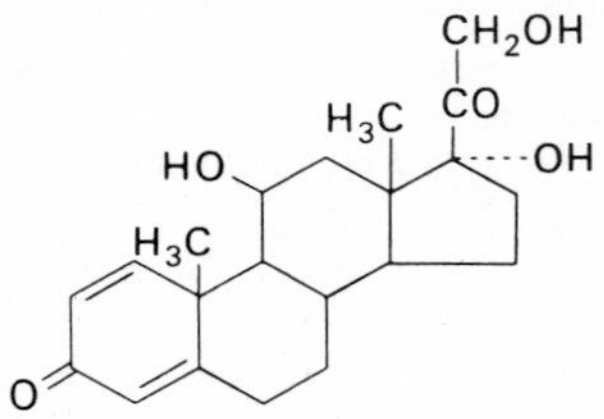

PREDNISONE (Deltasone; Deltra; and others)

Dose: 5 to 50 mg daily by mouth.

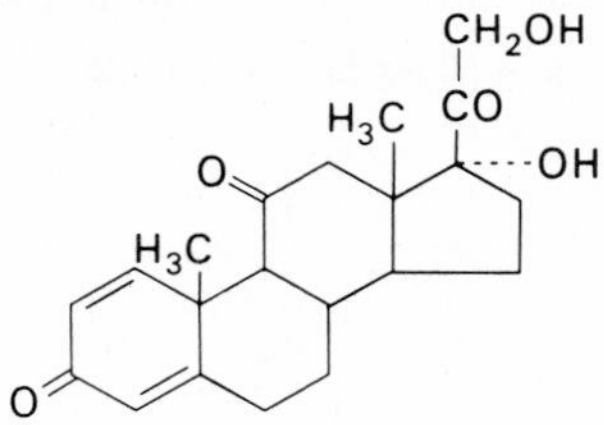

PREDNIVAL

Topical.
Under investigation.

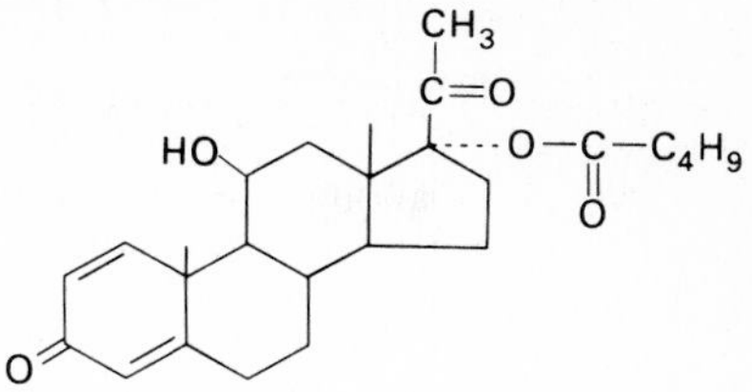

TRIAMCINOLONE (Aristocort; Kenacort)

Produces minimal salt retention. Headache, facial flushing, anorexia, muscular weakness have been noted.

Dose: 1 to 20 mg daily by mouth.

Triamcinolone acetonide (Kenalog)
Dose: 0.1% topically.

Triamcinolone hexacetonide
Triamcinolone diacetate

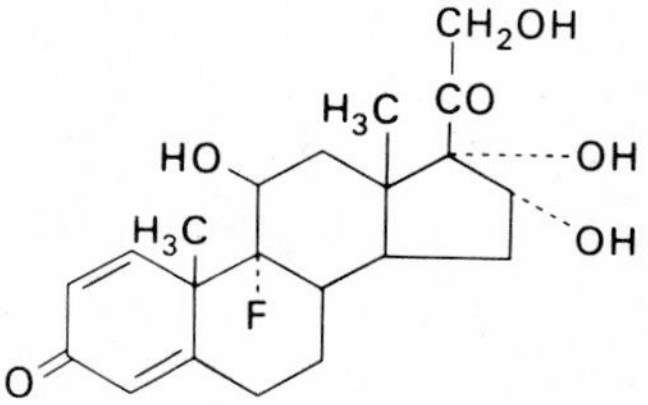

OTHERS

CORTIVAZOL

Under investigation.

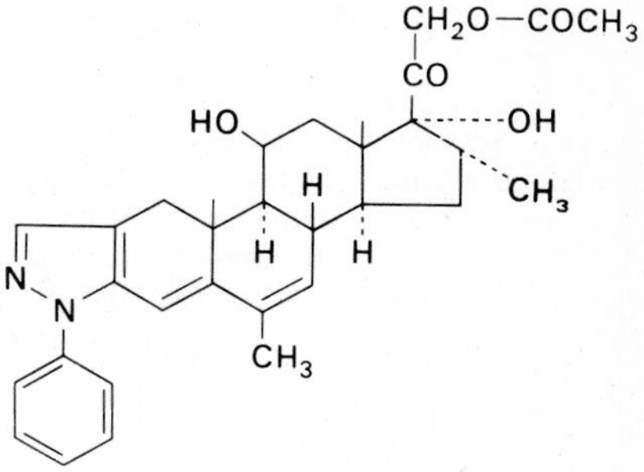

FORMOCORTAL

Topical corticoid.
Under investigation.

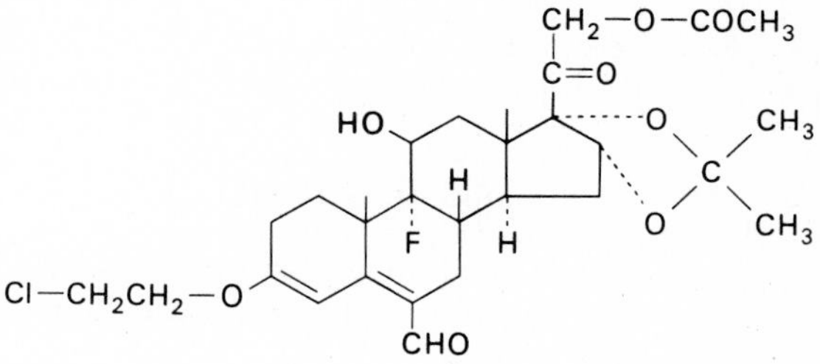

NIVAZOL

Under investigation.

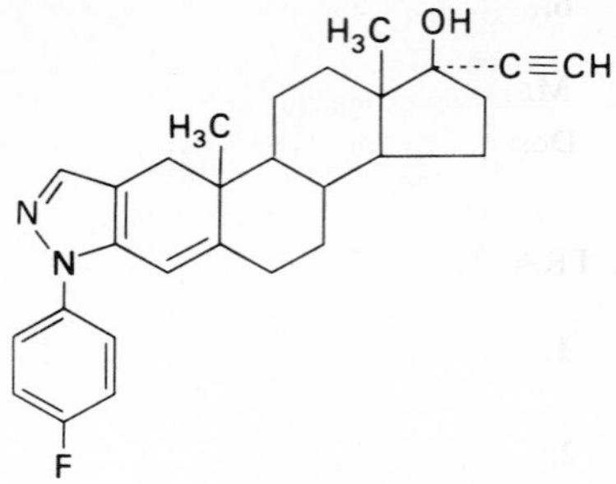

D. Antagonists of Cortical Hormones

METYRAPONE

1. **Chemistry**

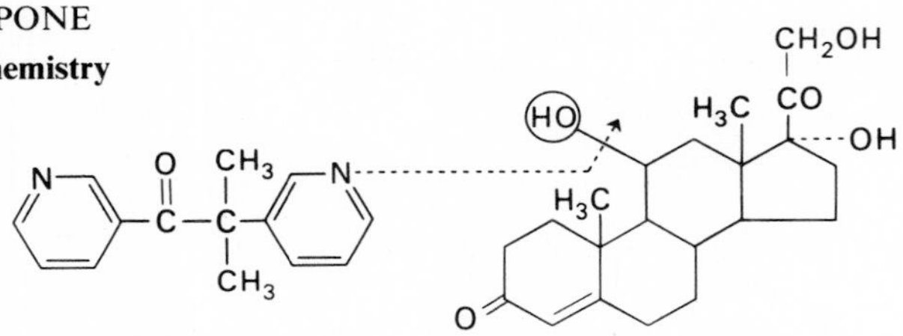

metyrapone hydrocortisone

2. **Action.** a. Inhibits the synthesis (11-β-hydroxylation) of hydrocortisone and aldosterone (and thus tends to induce diuresis).

b. However, deficiency of hydrocortisone results in increased production of ACTH which stimulates production of 11-deoxycorticosterone and 11-deoxyhydrocortisone (mineral corticoids, normally produced only in small amounts). This promotes sodium retention, nullifying the diuresis. (Gaunt, Science, 133:613, 1961.)

3. **Mechanism.** Interferes with formation of 11-β-hydroxylase, needed for 11-β-hydroxylation.

4. **Pharmacodynamics and Toxicity.** Toxicity: vertigo; may precipitate adrenal insufficiency in patients with minimally functioning adrenals.

5. **Uses.** a. Unsatisfactory as a clinical inhibitor of corticoid production.

b. Diagnosis of anterior pituitary function; in deficiency (with normal adrenals) administration fails to increase excretion of deoxysteroids (11-deoxycorticosterone; 11-deoxyhydrocortisone; Reichstein S) measured as 17-hydroxycorticosteroids.

6. Preparation

METYRAPONE DITARTRATE (SU-4885; Metopirone)

Dose: 30 mg per kg body weight in 1,000 ml saline solution intravenously.

TETRACHLORODIPHENYLETHANE

1. Chemistry. Isomer of insecticide (DDD).

2. Action and Mechanism. Causes cell damage with atrophy of adrenal.

3. Use. Toxic but under trial in metastatic adrenal carcinoma.

4. Preparation

MITOTANE (Lysodren)

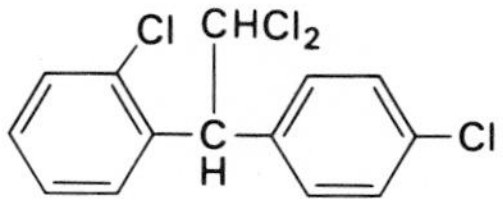

Cl CHCl$_2$ — C(H) — Cl

OTHERS

Amphenone; spironolactone (see Diuretics).

SUMMARY: ADRENAL CORTICAL HORMONES

TYPE	*ACTION AND MECHANISM*	*TOXICITY*	*USE*	*EXAMPLES*
Mineral corticoid	Increases Na reabsorption in distal renal tubules May act by exposing DNA templates	Excessive salt retention, edema, hypertension	Adrenal insufficiency	Desoxycortico-sterone acetate
Glucocorticoid	Gluconeogenesis Other effects on protein, fat, mineral, and other meta-bolism to preserve body's homeostasis Mechanism unknown	Cushing's syndrome	Adrenal insufficiency, antiinflam-matory	Hydrocortisone
Antagonists	Inhibit synthesis (11-β-hydrox-ylation) of normal corti-coids; others then made in excess	Vertigo	Diagnosis of anterior pituitary competence	Metyrapone ditartrate

Reviews

Munson, P. Endocrine pharmacology. Ann. Rev. Pharmacol., 1:315, 1961.

Smelik, P., and Sawyer, C. Pharmacological control of adrenocorticoid and gonadal secretions. Ann. Rev. Pharmacol., 2:313, 1962.

Applezweig, N. Steroid Drugs. New York, McGraw-Hill Book Company, 1962.

Bush, I. Chemical and biological factors in the activity of adrenocortical steroids. Pharmacol. Rev., 14:317, 1962.

Michael, M. Uses and misuses of adrenal corticosteroids. J.A.M.A., 185:280, 1963.

Samuels, L. Actinomycin and its effects. Influence on an effector pathway for hormone control. New Eng. J. Med., 271:1252, 1964.

Ross, E. Aldosterone and its antagonists. Clin. Pharmacol. Ther., 6:65, 1965.

Hechter, O., and Halkerston, I. Effects of steroid hormones on gene regulation and cell metabolism. Ann. Rev. Physiol., 27:133, 1965.

Thorn, G. W. Clinical considerations in the use of corticosteroids. New Eng. J. Med., 274:775, 1966.

Temple, T., and Liddle, G. Inhibitors of adrenal steroid synthesis. Ann. Rev. Pharmacol., 10:199, 1969.

34. Thyroid Hormones and Related Compounds

A. The Thyroid

1. History. a. Murray (1891) introduced endocrine substitution therapy by using sheep thyroid in hypothyroidism.

b. Kendall (1915) identified thyroxine chemically.

2. Chemistry. Iodine-containing thyronines (coupled pairs of iodinated tyrosines).

3. Action. Increases rate of oxidation in tissues; also stimulates cellular amino acid uptake and protein synthesis.

4. Mechanism. a. Controls active phosphorylation in the tissues. Thyroxine, by an active process requiring electron transport, causes swelling of mitochondrial membranes and thus inhibits their ability to "couple" phosphate units to form ATP. The energy which is accordingly not stored as ATP is available and gives increased oxidation in the tissues (Lehninger, Ann. N.Y. Acad. Sci., 86:484, 1960).

b. The fundamental action may be the redirection of high-energy intermediates into the synthesis of protein, probably at the ribosomal level (Rall, 23rd Int. Cong. Physiol., Tokyo, 1965).

c. The "uncoupling" produced by thyroxine differs from that produced by dinitrophenol in that the latter is active in the presence of mitochondrial fragments.

5. Pharmacodynamics. a. Thyroid (dried, powdered gland), levothyroxin, and levotriiodothyronine are satisfactorily absorbed by mouth; racemic thyroxine absorbed erratically.

b. Triiodothyronine provides a somewhat more rapid onset, peak, and cessation of action than thyroid or thyroxine and for this reason may be less satisfactory therapeutically; also it is less bound to serum protein.

6. Toxicity. Overdosage of thyroid substances produces hyperthyroidism.

7. Uses. a. To supply thyroid deficiency in hypothyroidism.

b. Use for other purposes, especially in obesity, common but inadvisable.

8. Preparations

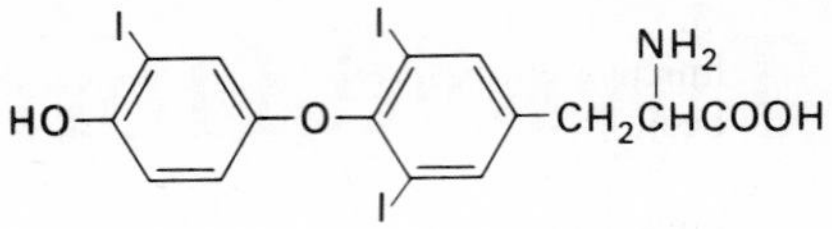

LIOTHYRONINE SODIUM (levotriiodothyronine; Cytomel; T3)

Dose: 5 to 25 mcg daily by mouth, increased as needed.

LIOTRIX (Euthyroid; Thyrolar)

Levothyroxine and liothyronine in a 4:1 mixture.
Dose: 75 to 150 mcg daily by mouth.

THYROID

Contains between 1:1, and 4:1, mixture of levothyroxine:levotriiodothyronine.
Dose: 25 to 200 mg daily by mouth.

THYROGLOBULIN (Proloid, Thyrar)

Preparation of thyroid globulin.
Dose: 25 to 200 mg daily by mouth.

THYROXINE

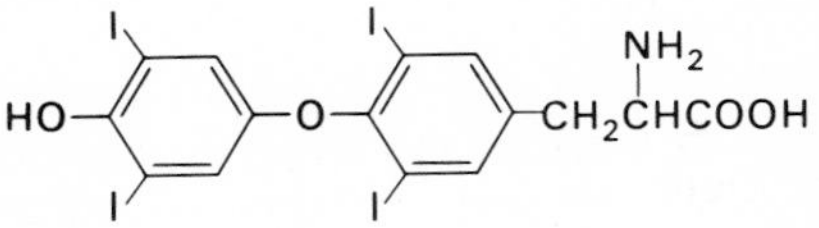

Racemic mixture has no advantage over thyroid and requires intravenous injection for consistent effect.

LEVOTHYROXINE SODIUM (Synthroid; T4)

Levo isomer of thyroxine.
Dose: 0.05 to 0.1 mg daily by mouth, increased as needed.

The dextro isomers of triiodothyronine and thyroxine, and a number of other derivatives and analogues are under study as cholesterol-lowering agents. (See Atherosclerosis.)

B. Antithyroid Substances

Antithyroid substances are used primarily in the treatment of hyperthyroidism, in which there is an excessive production of thyroid hormone. The reason for this excess is not clear. In toxic adenoma it appears to be unrelated to thyrotropic hormone (TSH) but in exophthalmic goiter the clinical condition is closely like that produced by TSH in animals.

Therapy is possible by several antithyroid measures. Thyroidectomy, following preparation by an agent of the thiouracil group and iodine, is commonly used; irradiation by radioactive iodine is an alternative method.

THIOURACIL GROUP.

1. History. a. MacKenzie (1941 and later) showed that sulfonamides, *p*-aminobenzoic acid, and thiourea had antithyroid effects.

b. Astwood (1943) used thiourea in clinical hyperthyroidism.

2. Chemistry. Thiourea and thiouracil derivatives.

3. Action. a. Inhibition of synthesis of thyroid hormones. The appearance of clinical hypothyroidism is delayed for 3 to 6 weeks until preformed hormone has been exhausted.

b. In response to the hypothyroidism, TSH increases and the thyroid becomes large, hyperplastic and vascular.

c. Prior treatment with iodide promotes storage and synthesis and so delays the thiouracil response, but late administration of iodides reverses the increased vascularity (and makes thyroidectomy easier).

4. Mechanism. Prevention of iodination of tyrosine.

Suggested mechanisms:

a. Inhibition of oxidation of iodide to iodine by reduction of free iodine before it can combine with tyrosine:

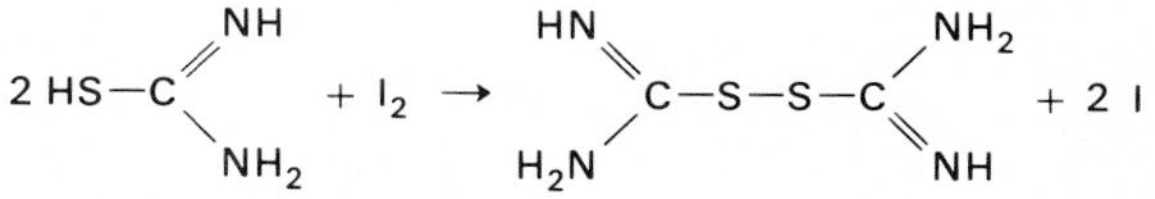

$$2\,HS{-}C(=NH)NH_2 + I_2 \rightarrow (HN{=})(H_2N)C{-}S{-}S{-}C(NH_2)({=}NH) + 2\,I$$

b. Inhibition of thyroid peroxidases.

5. Pharmacodynamics. Oral absorption satisfactory. Moderately rapid excretion necessitates administration 3 or 4 times a day.

6. Toxicity. Thiourea produces allergic reactions and dermatitis; thiouracil produces occasional agranulocytosis; propylthiouracil and subsequent derivatives less toxic.

7. Uses. a. Used in the preparation of patients for thyroidectomy; therapy is continued until hyperthyroidism is controlled which may take 4 to 8 weeks. Iodide is given concurrently during the last 2 or 3 weeks of preparation. (See Iodides.)

b. Thiouracil drugs are also used alone in attempts to induce a permanent remission of hyperthyroidism, but the incidence of success is probably less than 50% even when therapy is continued for a year or more.

c. Therapy should always include observations to detect granulocytopenia quickly if it should appear.

8. Preparations

CARBIMAZOLE (Neomercazole)

Dose: 5 to 10 mg 3 or 4 times a day.

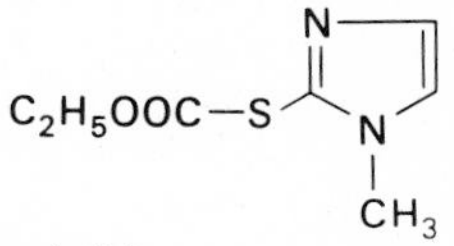

[Structure: $C_2H_5OOC{-}S$ attached to imidazole ring with N and N–CH_3]

IOTHIOURACIL (Itrumil)

Combination of thiouracil and iodine, but advantages doubtful.

Dose: 50 to 100 mg 3 or 4 times a day.

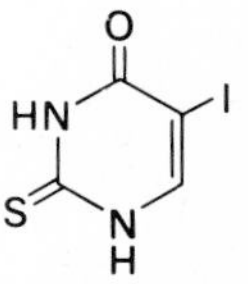

[Structure: pyrimidine ring with O, HN, I, S, N–H]

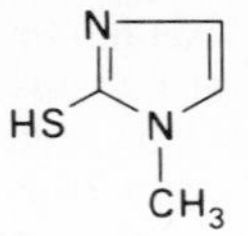

METHIMAZOLE (Tapazole)

Widely used.
Dose: 5 to 10 mg 3 times a day by mouth.

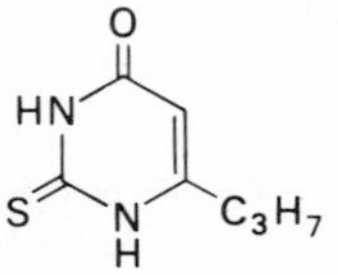

PROPYLTHIOURACIL

Widely used.
Dose: 50 to 100 mg 3 or 4 times a day by mouth.

OBSOLETE

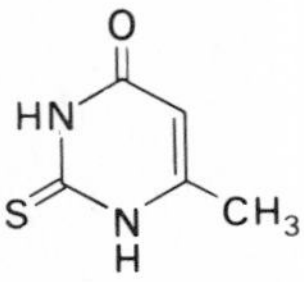

methylthiouracil

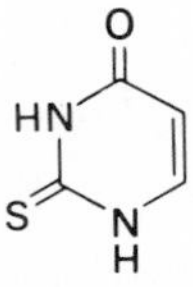

thiouracil

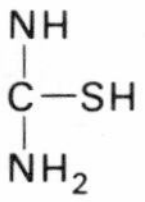

thiourea

C. Iodides

1. History. Used by generations of physicians for an array of unrelated conditions.

2. Chemistry. Most forms of iodine are converted in the body to iodide. The cation is indifferent.

3. Action and Mechanism. a. Constituent of thyroid hormones. Absence of adequate iodine intake responsible for about 90% of cretinism (10% from genetic deficiency of oxidative enzyme for conversion of iodide to iodine).

b. Suppresses hyperthyroidism incompletely, but partial relief continuous. Control may be good in mild disease, but incomplete in severe disease with return of florid signs if therapy is stopped. Inhibits the release of thyroid hormone. Also inhibits the uptake of iodine by the thyroid gland.

c. Fibrolytic ("alterative"). Causes resolution in granulomas, especially syphilis and fungus disease; mechanism obscure. Formerly thought to exert a somewhat similar action in arteriosclerosis.

d. Expectorant. Thins sputum through a gastric reflex plus local irritation or osmotic effects from iodide excreted in sputum.

e. Antiseptic. (See Antiseptics.)

f. Radioactivity carried, as I^{131}.

4. Pharmacodynamics. a. Inorganic iodine compounds well absorbed by mouth.

b. Distributed widely, following the pattern of chloride, and excreted by the kidneys and in other secretions.

5. Toxicity. Iodism, characterized by dermatitis, bronchitis, stomatitis, mental depression.

6. Uses. a. The uses vary according to the different pharmacological actions. Iodides are used for the prophylaxis of endemic goiter and in the treatment or preoperative preparation of patients with hyperthyroidism. In such preparation iodides are usually given after the disease has been nearly controlled by a thiouracil, to induce a reduction of vascularity in the gland.

b. The iodides are also used for their fibrinolytic, expectorant and (iodine) antiseptic actions.

c. Sodium iodide I^{131} has replaced x-ray for the irradiation treatment of hyperthyroidism. I^{131} has a half-life of 8 days and is a desirable alternative to an operation or a thiouracil in adults, especially in poor operative risks. The hazard of carcinogenicity appears to be slight, but it should not be used in pregnant women.

7. Preparations

SODIUM IODIDE (NaI)

Dose: 0.3 gm daily by mouth.

SODIUM IODIDE I^{131}

Dose: 5 to 15 mc by mouth, the exact dose based upon severity of disease, size of gland, and iodine uptake; doses may be as high as 100 mc in carcinoma of the thyroid. Alternatively, treatment may be by multiple doses of 2 to 7 mc at 3- to 4-week intervals.

STRONG IODIDE SOLUTION (Lugol's solution)

Contains 5% iodine and 10% KI.
Dose: 0.3 ml daily by mouth.

TINCTURE OF IODINE

Antiseptic.
Dose: applied topically.

D. Goitrogens

In addition to thiouracil, there are a number of goitrogens that are seldom used clinically. Some are of importance as they may be responsible for endemic goiter in regions where iodine intake is adequate.

THIOCYANATE GROUP

1. History. Barker (1936) noted the goitrogenic activity of thiocyanate in man during treatment for hypertension.

2. Chemistry. The thiocyanate group (pharmacologically) includes thiocyanates, perchlorates, periodates, and related compounds.

3. Action and Mechanism. a. Members of this group produce goiter of the iodine-deficiency type by interfering with the iodine accumulating mechanism of the thyroid.

b. Perchlorate and iodide have similar volumes and may compete for the protein receptor of the "trap," which will chelate ions of this size (Pitt Rivers, Ann. N.Y. Acad. Sci., 86:367, 1960).

4. Uses. Potassium perchlorate is occasionally used as an alternative to a thiouracil derivative, but has been reported to cause agranulocytosis.

5. Preparation

POTASSIUM PERCHLORATE: $KClO_4$
Dose: 200 mg 3 times a day by mouth.

THIOOXAZOLIDINE

1. History. a. Kennedy (1941) showed that rape seed produced goiter in rats.

b. Astwood (1949) identified the responsible agent and showed its presence in various Brassicae: rape, cauliflower, Brussels sprouts, kale, cabbage, turnips, rutabaga.

c. Greer (1959) showed progoitrin relationship.

2. Chemistry. The goitrogenic substance is a cyclized isothiocyanate, L-5-vinyl-2-thiooxazolidine (goitrin), which is formed from a mustard oil glycoside precusor (progoitrin). The process is enzymatic, but will proceed in the intestine even after the food containing it has been cooked, through the influence of alimentary bacteria.

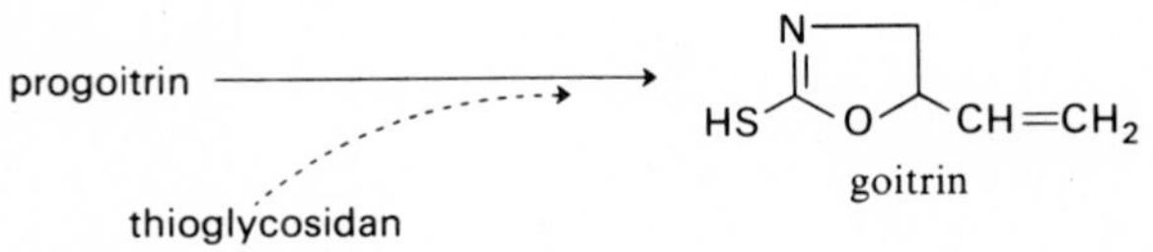

progoitrin → (thioglycosidan) → goitrin [HS–C(=N–CH₂–CH(CH=CH₂)–O) ring]

goitrin

3. Action and Mechanism. a. Goitrin inhibits the production of the thyroid hormone, presumably through the same mechanism by which thiouracil acts, that is, by preventing the iodination of tyrosine.

b. It appears to be responsible for goiter in school children in Tasmania and New Zealand.

OTHER GOITROGENS

AMINOTRIAZOLE

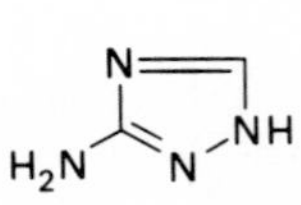

Used as a weed killer; responsible for the "cranberry episode" of 1959 because of goitrogenic, and doubtful carcinogenic, efforts produced by large doses in animals.

[Structure: H_2N, N, NH, N= — aminotriazole]

SUMMARY: THYROID HORMONES AND RELATED COMPOUNDS

TYPE	*ACTION AND MECHANISM*	*TOXICITY*	*USE*	*EXAMPLES*
Thyroid preparations	Increase rate of oxidation in tissues by inhibiting coupling of phosphate units to form ATP	Hyperthyroidism	Hypothyroidism	Levothyroxine sodium
Antithyroid substances	Inhibition of synthesis of thyroid, preventing iodination of tyrosine	Agranulocytosis	Hyperthyroidism	Propylthiouracil
Iodides	Constituent of thyroid hormone	Dermatitis, mental depression	Prevent endemic goiter; suppress hyperthyroidism	Sodium iodide

Reviews

Maloof, F., and Soodak, M. Intermediary metabolism of thyroid tissue and the action of drugs. Pharmacol. Rev., 15:43, 1963.

DeGroot, L. Current views on formation of thyroid hormone. New Eng. J. Med., 272:243, 1965.

Rosenberg, I., and Bastomsky, C. The thyroid. Ann. Rev. Physiol., 27:71, 1965.

Selenkow, H., and Wool, M. Thyroid hormones. Topics Med. Chem., 1:241, 1967.

——— Antithyroid drugs. Topics Med. Chem., 1:273, 1967.

35.
Female Sex Hormones

A. Estrogens

NATURAL ESTROGENS

1. History. a. Allen and Doisy (1923) developed bioassay for estrogens based on rat vaginal smear.

b. Doisy (1928) and Butenandt (1928) isolated estrone from urine; Schwenk and Hildebrandt (1933) reduced estrone to estradiol.

2. Chemistry. a. C-18 steroids derived from perhydrocyclopentenophenanthrene nucleus.

b. Estradiol is the principal natural hormone but exists in the body in equilibrium with estrone, which in turn is converted to estriol for excretion.

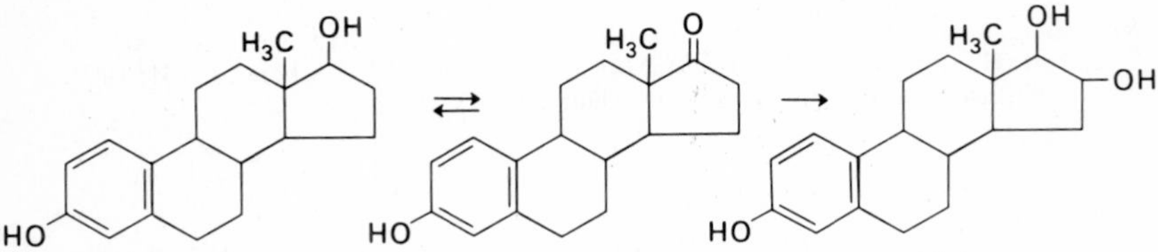

estradiol ⇄ estrone → estriol

c. Formed in the ovary, placenta, adrenal cortex, and Leydig cells; commercially extracted from human or mare urine, or made synthetically.

3. Action. a. Cause the development of secondary sexual characteristics in female.

b. Promote growth of the endometrium; thickening, stratification and cornification of the vagina.

c. Cause growth of the ducts in the mammary gland, but inhibit lactation.

d. Inhibit the anterior pituitary.

e. Cause capillary dilatation, fluid retention, and protein anabolism.

f. Production of estrogens is controlled (increased) by gonadotropins.

4. Mechanism. Estrogens form a complex with cytoplasmic receptor proteins in certain tissues (uterus, vagina, pituitary, estrogen-dependent tumors, breast, and others). The complex then moves into the nucleus and reacts with a gene repressor.

The derepressed gene then guides the manufacture of an RNA polymerase and the resultant effector protein.

5. Pharmacodynamics. a. Absorption good by mouth and after intramuscular injection.

b. Distribution is wide throughout the tissues.

c. Metabolized in the liver and in the intestinal epithelium.

d. Largely degraded in the body with about 10% being excreted as conjugated sterols in the urine.

6. Toxicity. a. Anorexia, nausea, vomiting, proportional to estrogenic potency.

b. Question of carcinogenicity in humans is not settled.

7. Uses. a. Principal use in women is to control menopausal symptoms, hot flushes and later osteoporosis, by inhibition of gonadotropin production.

b. Used in combination with progestins in oral contraceptives.

c. Also used in atrophic vaginitis, and to relieve postpartum breast engorgement, dysmenorrhea, amenorrhea, menorrhagia, and as substitution therapy in ovarian dwarfism.

d. Used in men to control prostatic carcinoma.

8. Preparations

a. Natural estrogens

ESTRADIOL (Dimenformon; Progynon; and others)
Dose: 0.5 mg 3 times a day by mouth.

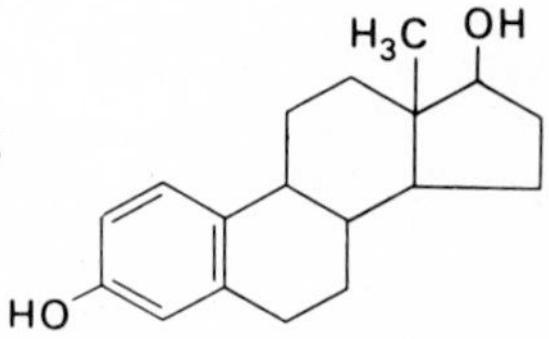

ESTRADIOL BENZOATE

Dose: 1 to 2 mg 2 times a week, reduced to 0.3 to 1 mg after 1 or 2 weeks intramuscularly.

Estradiol cypionate (Depo-testadiol)
Long acting.
Dose: 1 to 5 mg intramuscularly weekly, then every 3 to 4 weeks.

Estradiol dipropionate
Dose: 1 mg weekly intramuscularly.

Estradiol enanthate

Polyestradiol phosphate (Estradurin)
Polymer with protracted effect; used against cancer.
Dose: 40 to 80 mg intramuscularly every 2 to 4 weeks.

Estradiol valerate (Delestrogen)
Dose: 5 mg intramuscularly monthly.

ESTROGENS, CONJUGATED (Premarin; Conestron; and others)
Amorphous conjugated estrogens from urine of pregnant mares.
Dose: 1.25 mg daily by mouth.

ESTRIOL

Dose: 0.1 mg 4 times a day by mouth.

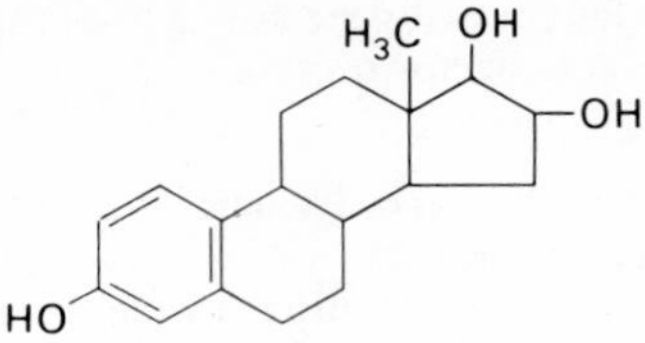

ESTRONE (Theelin and others)

Dose: 1 mg 3 times a day by mouth.

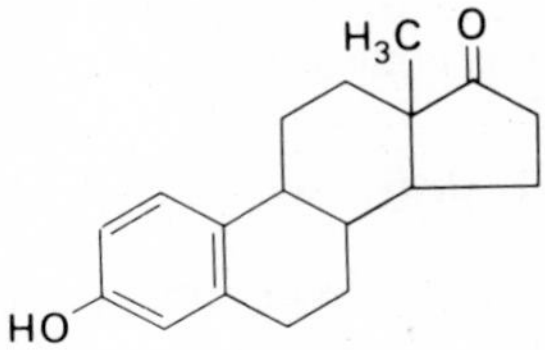

PIPERAZINE ESTRONE SULFATE (Sulestrex)

Dose: 1.5 mg daily by mouth.

b. Semisynthetic derivatives

ETHINYL ESTRADIOL (Estinyl; Feminone; and others)

Improved oral absorption.
Dose: 0.01 to 0.05 mg daily by mouth.

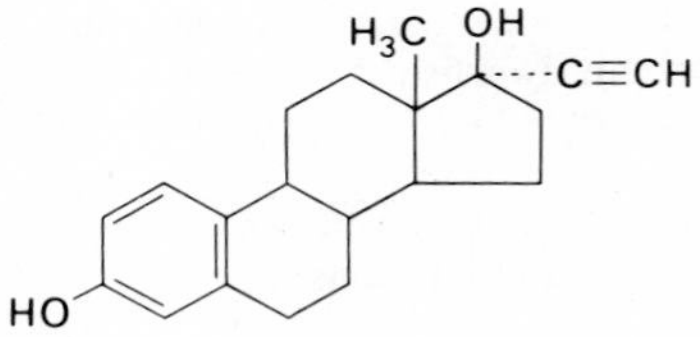

MESTRANOL

Estrogen present with progestins in several antifertility mixtures.

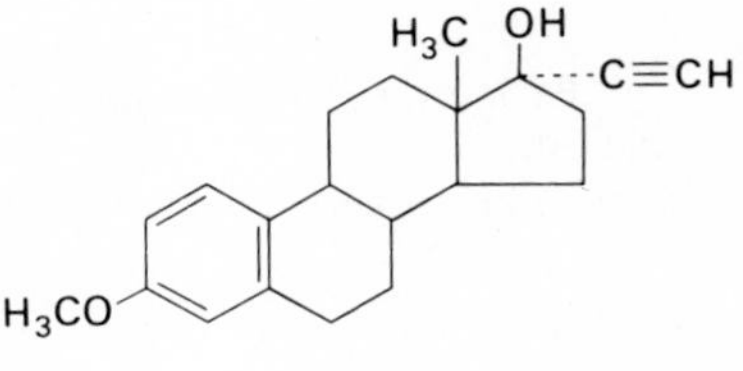

OTHERS

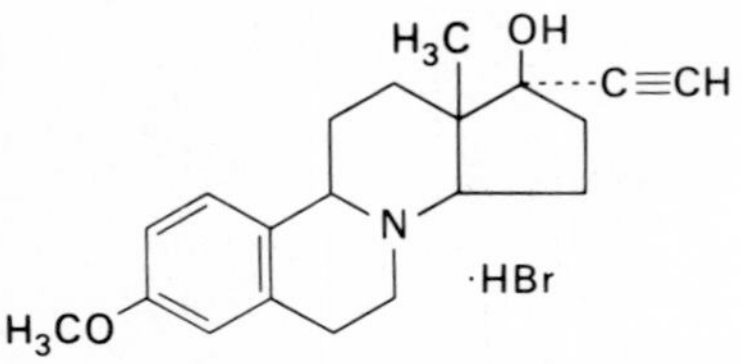

estrazinol HBr

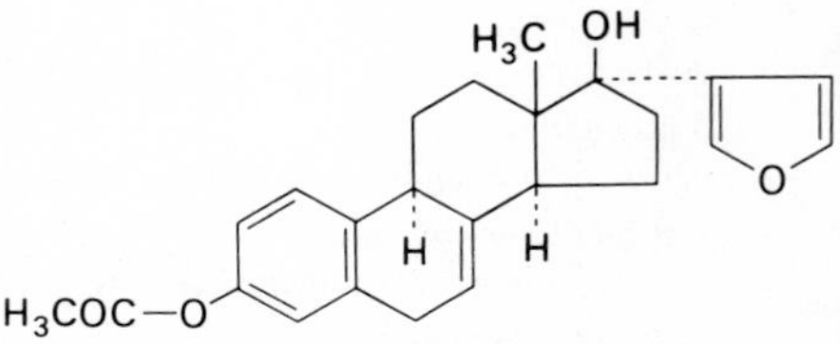

estrofurate

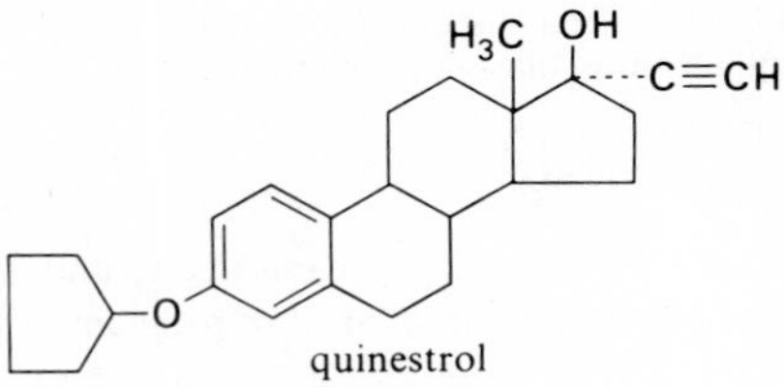

quinestrol

SYNTHETIC ESTROGENS

1. History. Dodds (1938) synthesized diethylstilbestrol.

2. Chemistry. Stilbene derivatives.

3. Action and Mechanism. a. The action of the synthetic estrogens appears to be identical with that of the natural compounds in humans.

b. The mechanism of action is unknown, but the synthetic agents may assume a steroid conformation resembling that of the natural compounds closely enough to activate the appropriate receptors.

4. Pharmacodynamics and Toxicity. a. Absorption satisfactory by mouth.

b. About one third is excreted in conjugated form in the urine.

c. Toxicity may include nausea, vomiting, and headache, but these symptoms result from sudden, high estrogenic levels rather than from qualitative differences from natural estrogens.

d. Vaginal cancer reported in young females whose mothers were treated with Diethylstilbestrol in early pregnancy.

5. Uses. a. Uses are the same as for the natural products.

b. The synthetic compounds have the advantage of cheapness, which is especially important when large doses are used, as in the treatment of prostatic carcinoma.

c. Diethylstilbestrol is used as a morning-after contraceptive (50 to 100 mg per day for 4 to 6 days).

6. Preparations

BENZESTROL

Dose: 2 to 3 mg daily by mouth, reduced as permissible (menopause).

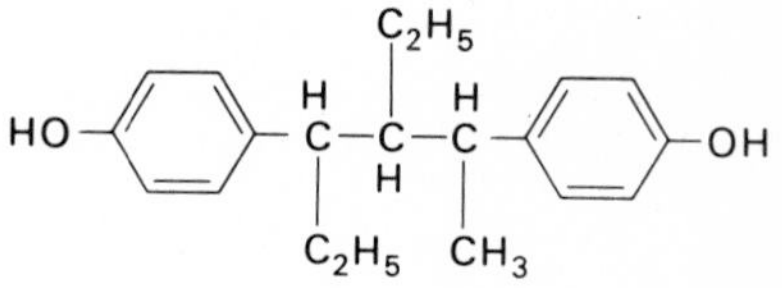

CHLOROTRIANISENE (Tace)

Acts partly as a precursor; effects prolonged because of storage of drug in fat.

Dose: 10 to 25 mg daily by mouth.

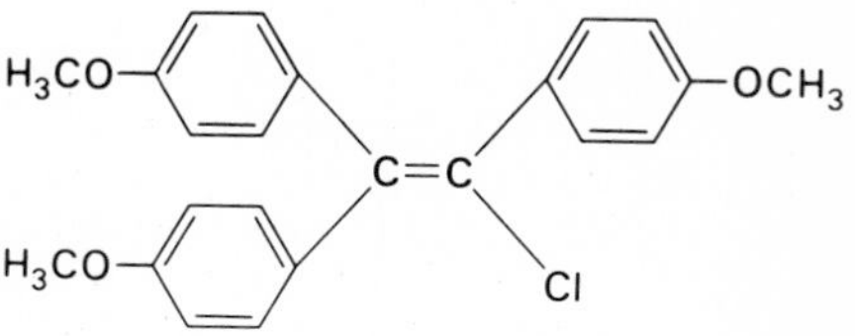

DIETHYLSTILBESTROL (Stilbestrol)

Dose: 0.5 to 1 mg daily by mouth (menopausal); 3 mg or more daily by mouth or by intramuscular injection (prostatic carcinoma).

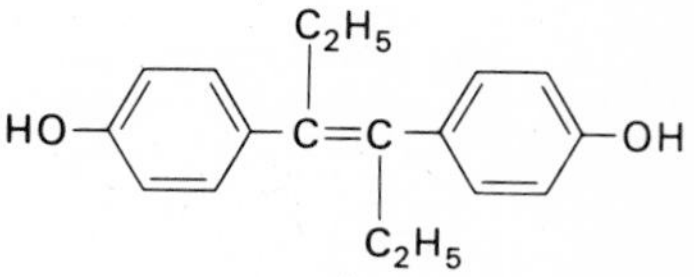

DIETHYLSTILBESTROL DIPHOSPHATE (Stilphostrol)

DIETHYLSTILBESTROL DIPROPIONATE (Dibestil)

DIENESTROL (Synestrol)

Dose: Doses similar to diethylstilbestrol.

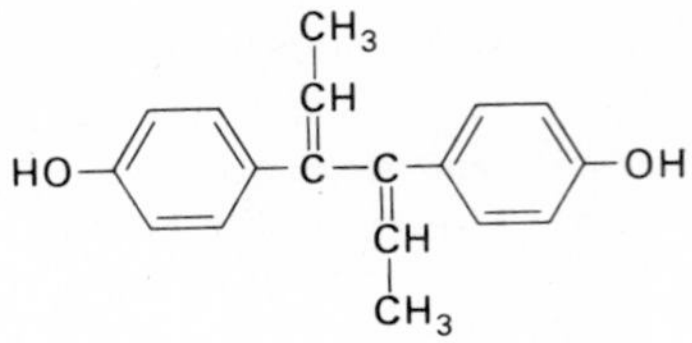

HEXESTROL

Dose: 2 to 3 mg daily by mouth, reduced as permissible (menopausal).

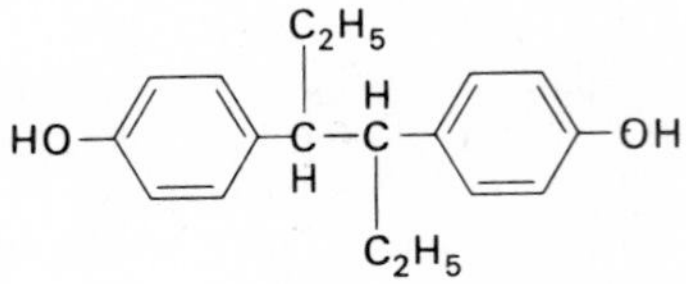

METHALLENESTRIL (Vallestril)

Not a stilbene derivative.
Dose: 6 mg daily by mouth.

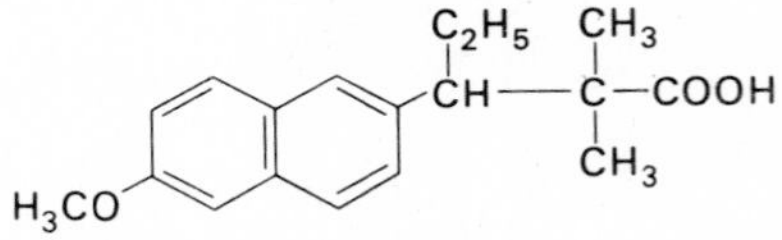

B. Progestins

NATURAL PROGESTINS

1. History. a. Fraenkel (1903) showed that the corpus luteum was necessary for the maintenance of pregnancy.

b. Corner and Allen (1929) prepared effective luteal extracts; progesterone identified (1934).

2. Chemistry. a. Progesterone is a C-21 derivative of cholesterol.

b. Occurs in the corpus luteum, placenta, and adrenal cortex; made commercially by extraction from ovaries or by synthesis.

3. Action. a. Progesterone transforms proliferative uterine endometrium into secretory; induces mammary gland duct development.

b. Causes slight rise in body temperature (mid-cycle temperature increase).

c. Causes mild sodium retention and nitrogen catabolism.

4. Mechanism. It penetrates the cell wall, binds to cytoplasm, and is transported into the nucleus where it may influence RNA synthesis.

5. Pharmacodynamics and Toxicity. a. Is not effective by mouth because of the rapid metabolism in the intestinal epithelium and in the liver.

b. After injection, metabolized in the body to pregnanolones and pregnanediols, and excreted as pregnanediol glucuronide.

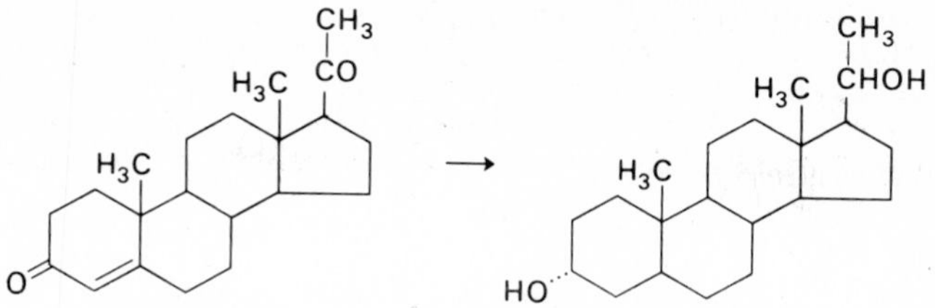

progesterone → pregnanediol

c. Progesterone is nontoxic except for minor nausea.

6. Uses. Progesterone has been used for many years in the treatment of threatened abortion, dysmenorrhea, and functional uterine bleeding; in none of these uses has it proved to be of outstanding value. The synthetic progestins have all but replaced progesterone.

7. Preparation

PROGESTERONE (Lucorteum, Proluton; and others)

Dose: 5 to 10 mg intramuscularly.

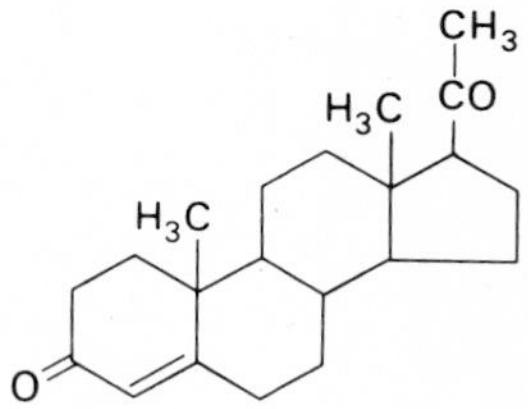

SYNTHETIC PROGESTINS

1. History. a. Inhoffen (1938) and Ruzika synthesized ethisterone.

b. Djerassi (1951) synthesized norethindrone; Colton (1952) synthesized norethynodrel.

c. Pincus (1958), first large scale antifertility demonstrations with preparations containing norethynodrel.

2. Chemistry. Progesterone derivatives with a methyl at 19, or testosterone relatives without a methyl at 19.

3. Action and Mechanism. a. Progestational effects similar to progesterone; some show slight estrogenic, androgenic or corticoid effects as well, and there may be inhibition of gonadotropin production.

b. Norethindrone may produce endometrial hyperplasia if given without periodic interruption.

c. Anticonceptive effects:

a′. Induce and maintain a pseudodecidual endometrium, preventing uterine bleeding; when withdrawn, normal menstrual flow in three days.

b′. Inhibit production of pituitary gonadotropin, preventing ovulation.

c′. Produce tenacious cervical mucus, resistant to passage of sperm.

d′. Addition of estrogen enhances suppression of pituitary.

4. Pharmacodynamics and Toxicity. a. Well absorbed by mouth.

b. Toxicity: may include headache, nausea, chloasma, acne, break-through bleeding, weight gain, loss of libido, all of which disappear when therapy is stopped; cholestatic liver damage (see also side effects of antifertility preparations).

c. Treatment should be stopped if pregnancy supervenes, because of possibility of masculinizing the fetus.

5. Uses. a. Used in threatened and habitual abortion, endometriosis, and menstrual disorders; the effect is more substantial than with progesterone, and there is greater convenience of administration and lower cost.

b. Several compounds, especially the C-19-nor members, are used for maintaining a pseudodecidual endometrium in endometriosis; ovulation and menstruation cease when they are given continuously.

c. Extensively used as antifertility agents.

6. Preparations

a. C-19 derivatives

ALGESTONE ACETOPHENIDE (in Deladroxate)

Dose: 150 mg (+ 10 mg estradiol enanthate) once monthly 8 days after start of menstruation.

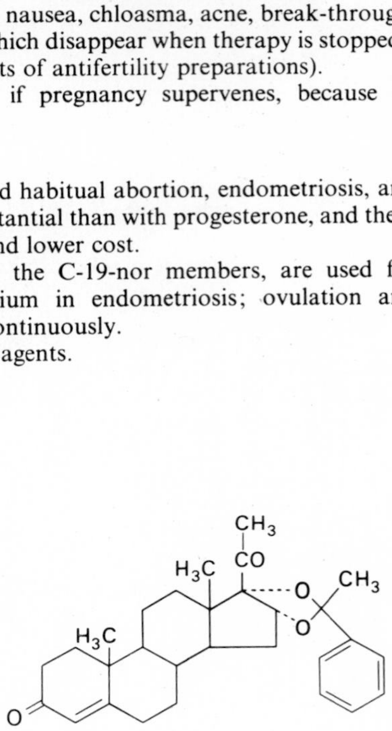

AZACOSTEROL HYDROCHLORIDE

Veterinary (avian) antifertility agent.

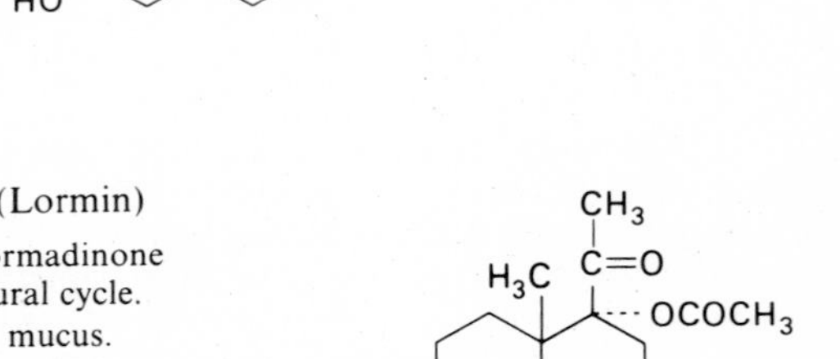

CHLORMADINONE ACETATE (Lormin)

Estrogen for 20 days with chlormadinone during last 5 closely duplicates natural cycle.

May act primarily on cervical mucus.

Has produced mammary masses in dogs; withdrawn from use in certain countries.

Dose: 2 mg daily by mouth.

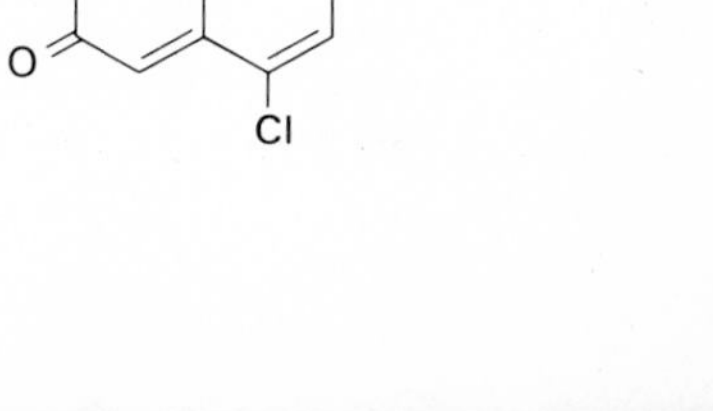

Cismadinone

Cis form.

Delmadinone acetate (Estrex)
Unsaturation at 1–2.

Hydromadinone

CLOGESTONE ACETATE
Under investigation.

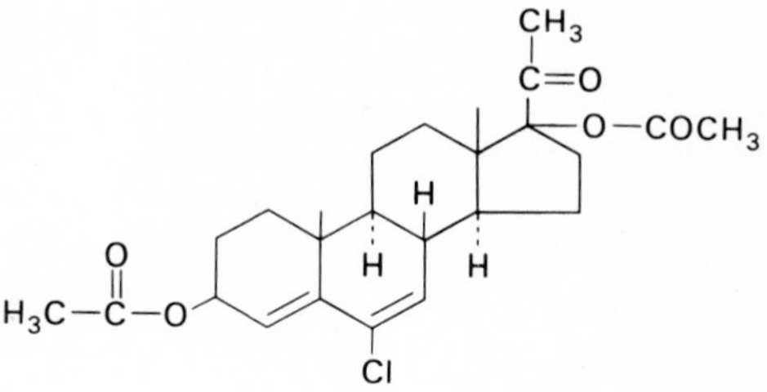

CLOMEGESTONE ACETATE
Under investigation.

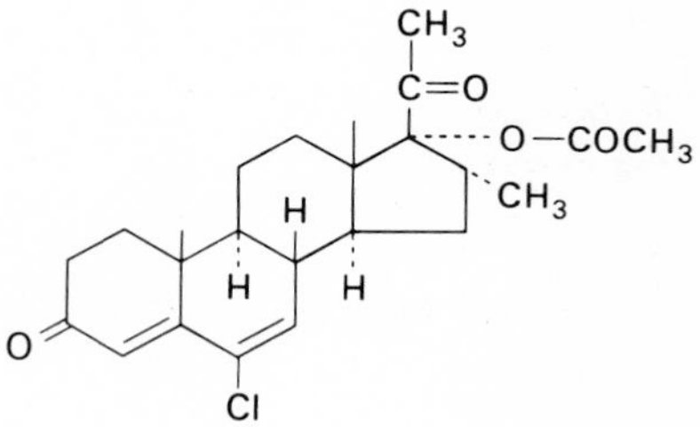

DIMETHISTERONE (in Oracon)
Under investigation.

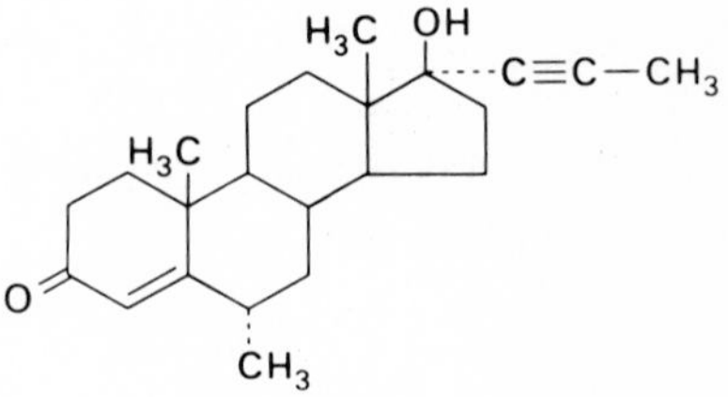

DYDROGESTERONE (Duphaston)

A retroprogesterone; purely progestational; does not inhibit ovulation. Excreted slowly over 48 hours.

Dose: 5 to 20 mg by mouth daily.

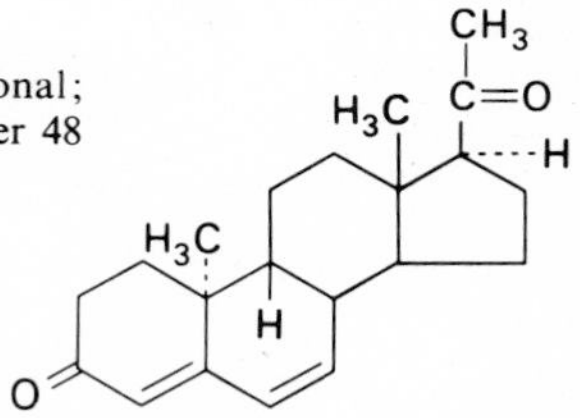

ETHISTERONE (Lutocyclol; Pranone)

Dose: 5 to 10 mg daily by mouth.

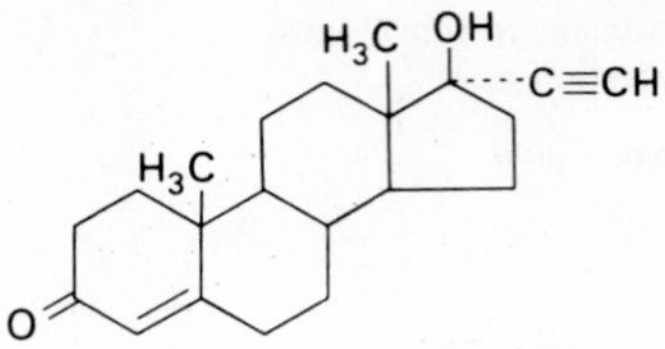

FLUROGESTONE ACETATE (Cronolone)

Under investigation.

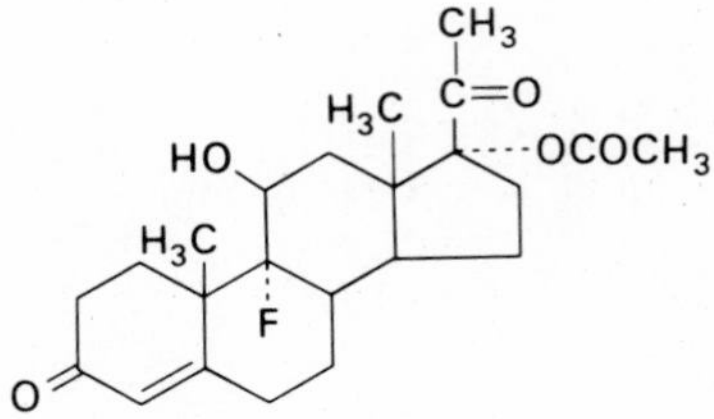

GESTACLONE

Under investigation.

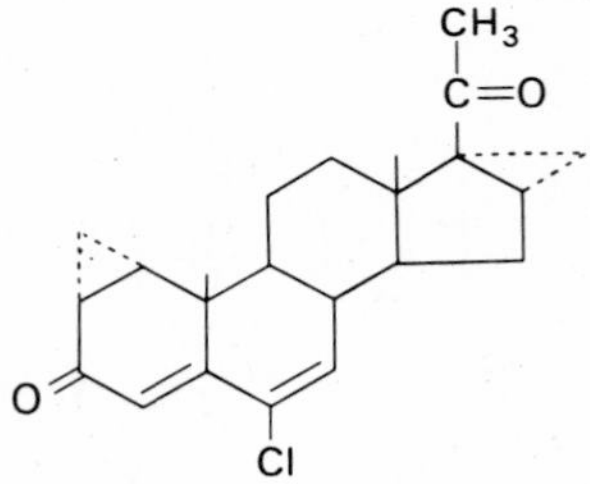

HALOPROGESTERONE (Prohalone)

Under investigation.

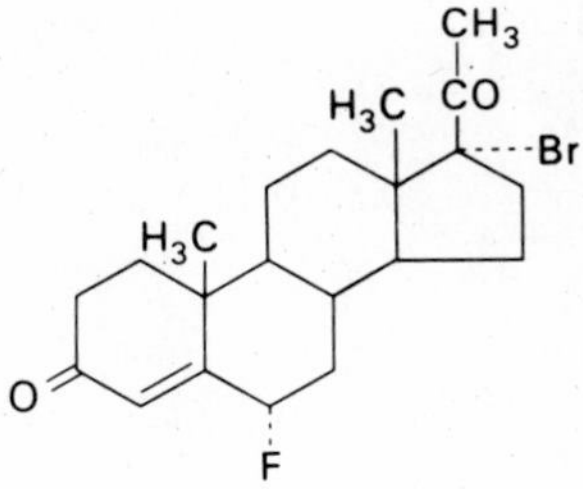

HYDROXYPROGESTERONE CAPROATE (Delalutin)

Long-acting derivative.

Dose: 250 mg once weekly intramuscularly.

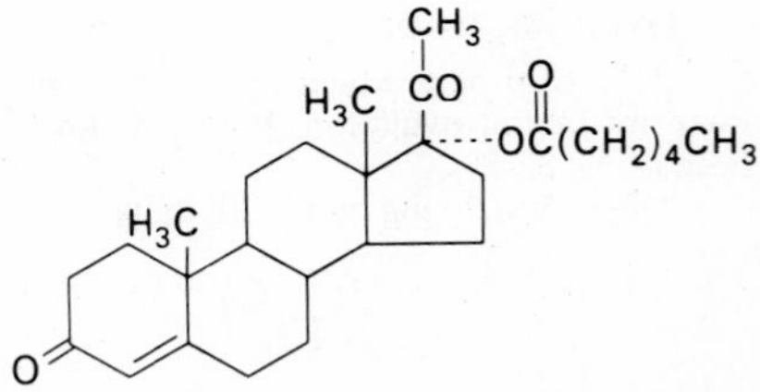

MEDROGESTONE

Dose: 2 mg by mouth.

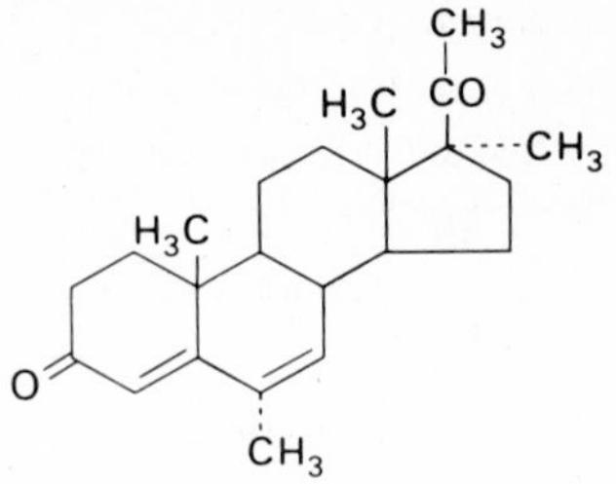

MEDROXYPROGESTERONE ACETATE (Provera)

Said to be most active progestin.

Dose: 2.5 to 10 mg daily by mouth; also depot form 150 mg every 3 months.

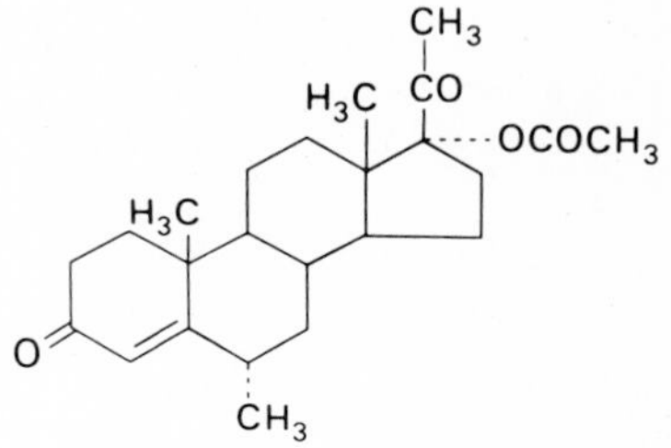

MEGESTROL ACETATE (Volidan)

Claimed to be superior to 19-nor compounds as antifertility agent because of less effect on endometrium and vagina; said to produce a hostile cervical mucus.

Dose: 2 mg daily by mouth.

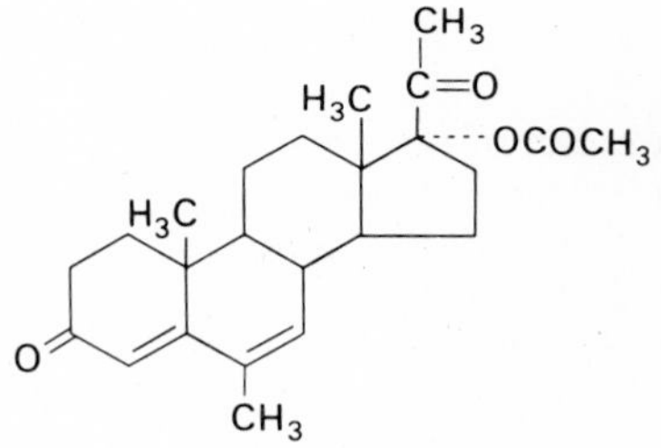

MELENGESTROL ACETATE

Under investigation.

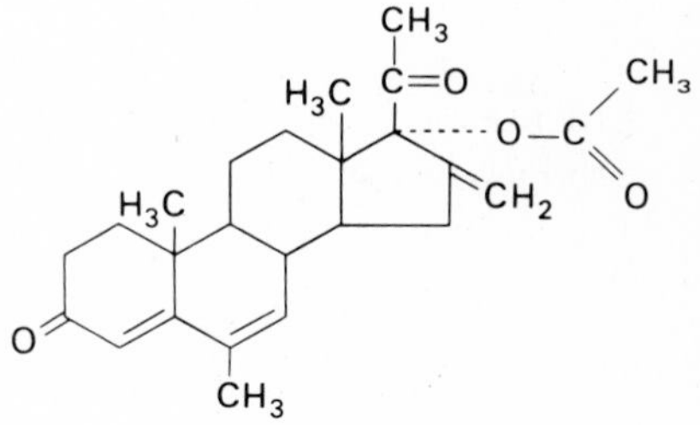

QUINGESTRONE

Under investigation.

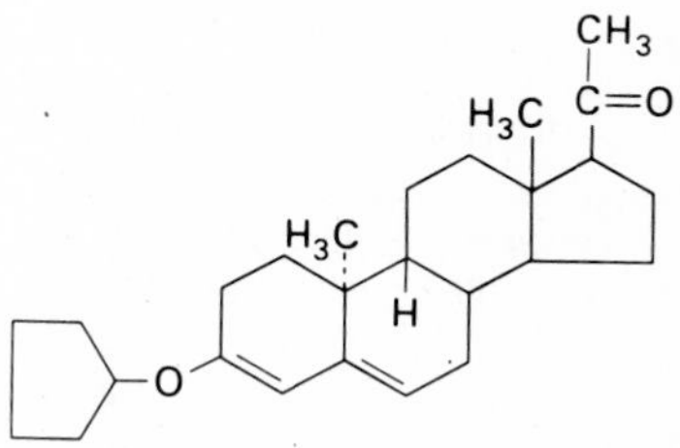

b. C-19-nor derivatives

ALLYLESTRENOL (Gestanon)

Lacks an O at 3 and is claimed to be strongly progestational without side effects.

Dose: 5 mg 1 to 3 times a day by mouth.

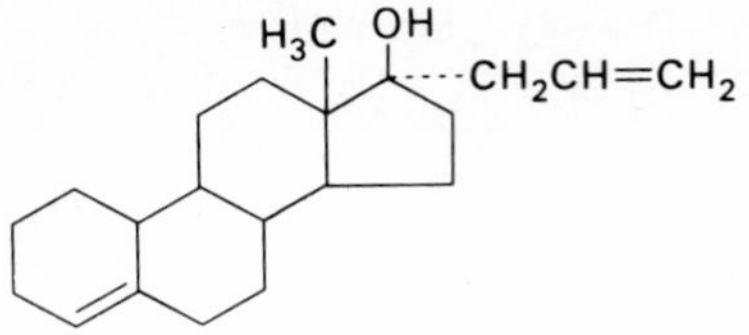

H_3C OH $CH_2CH{=}CH_2$

AMADINONE ACETATE

Under investigation.

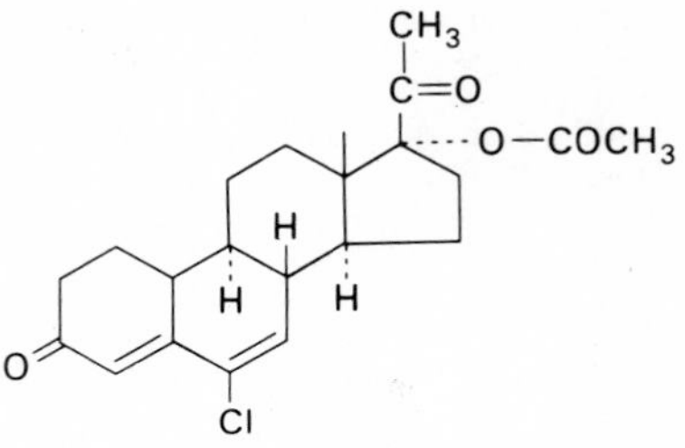

CH_3 C=O O—$COCH_3$ H H H O Cl

CINGESTOL

Under investigation.

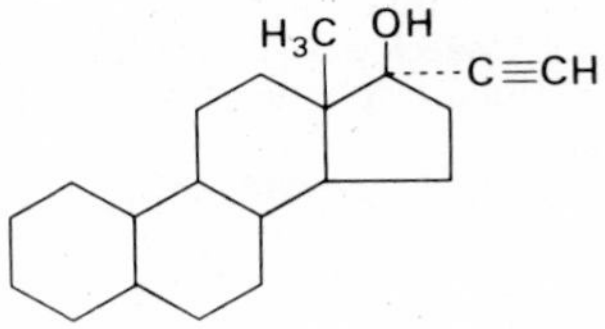

H_3C OH C≡CH

ETHYNERONE

Under investigation.

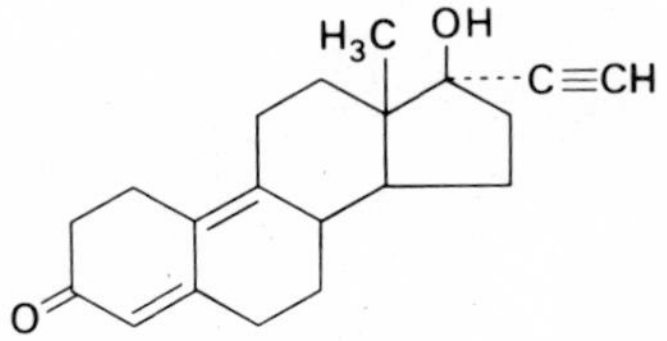

H_3C OH C≡CH O

ETHYNODIOL DIACETATE

Promising antifertility agent (Pincus, Science, 138:439, 1962).

Dose: 1 mg with 0.1 mg mestranol.

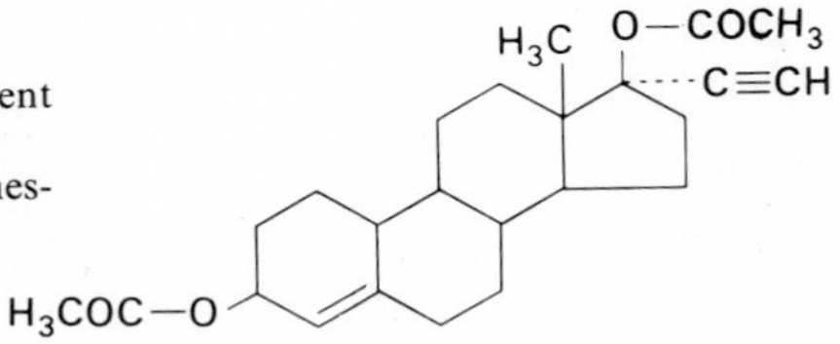

H_3C O—$COCH_3$ C≡CH H_3COC—O

GESTONORONE CAPROATE

Under investigation.

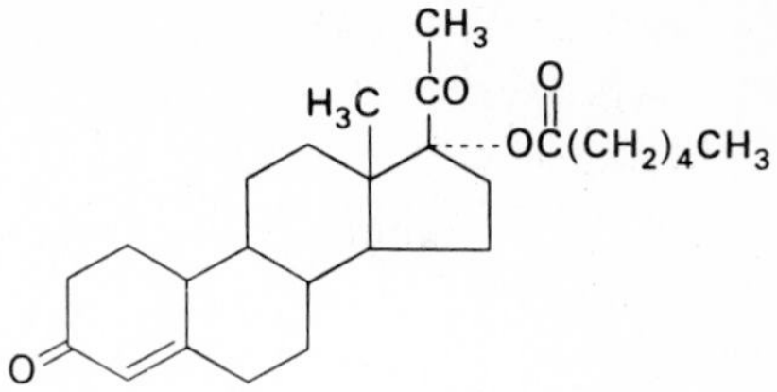

LYNESTRENOL (in Lyndiol)

Progestational; ovulation inhibiting.
Dose: 5 mg (with 0.15 mg mestranol).

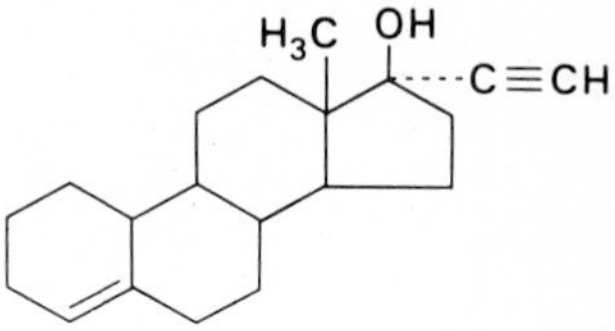

NORETHINDRONE (Norethisterone; Norlutin)

Dose: 10 to 20 mg daily by mouth.

Norethindrone acetate (Norlutate)
Dose: 5 mg daily by mouth.

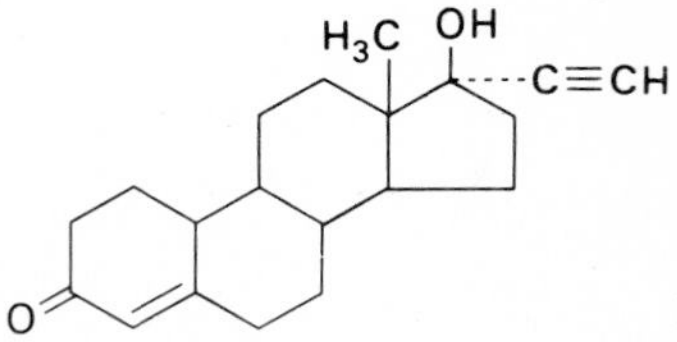

NORETHYNORDREL (component of Enovid)

Dose: 5 to 10 mg daily by mouth.

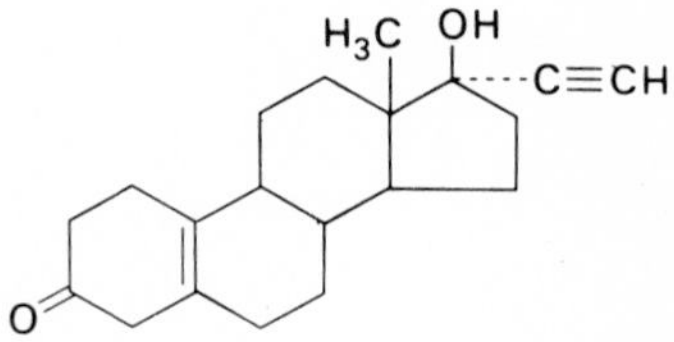

NORGESTREL (in Orval)

Dose: 0.5 mg daily by mouth.

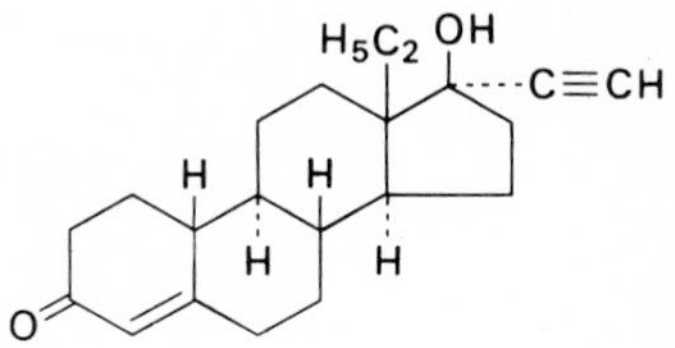

NORGESTERONE (Vestalin)

Under investigation.

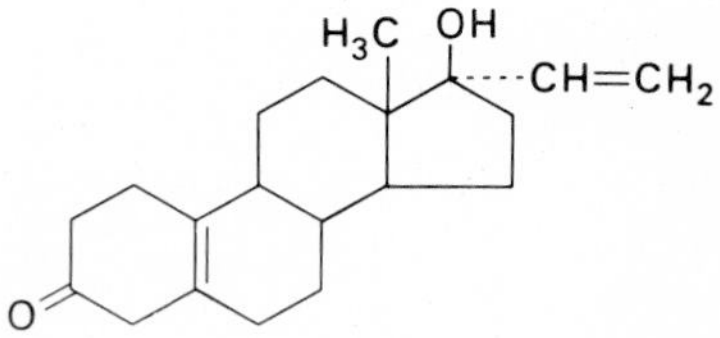

NORVINISTERONE

Under investigation.

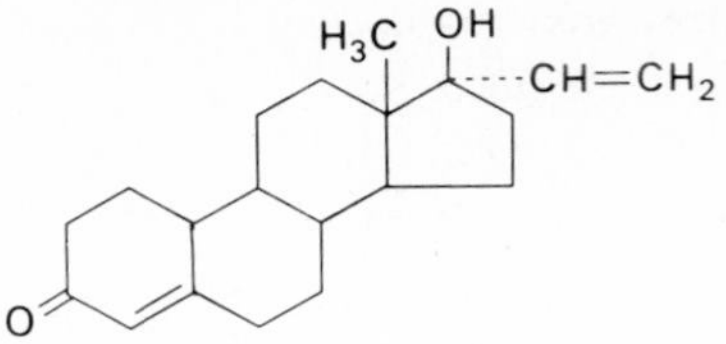

OXOGESTONE

Dose: Under investigation.

Oxogestone phenpropionate

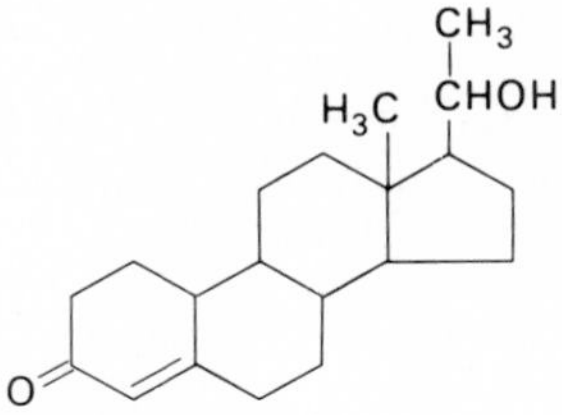

QUINGESTANOL ACETATE

Under investigation.

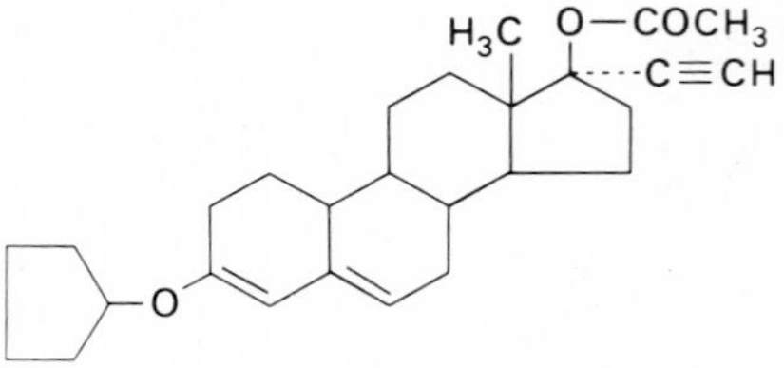

TIGESTOL

Under investigation.

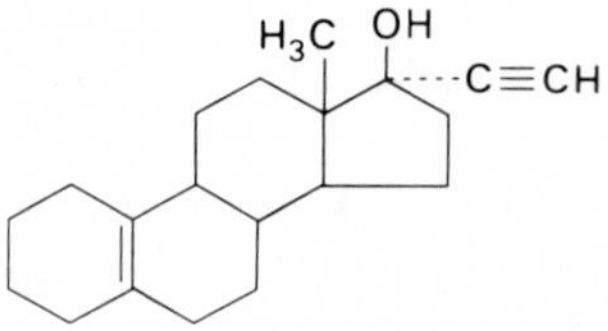

ORAL CONTRACEPTIVES

TRADE NAME	*ESTROGEN*	*PROGESTIN*
	*Combinations**	
Brevicon	35 μg ethinyl estradiol	0.5 mg norethindrone
Demulen	50 μg ethinyl estradiol	1.0 mg ethynodiol diacetate
Enovid 5 mg	75 μg mestranol	5.0 mg norethynodrel
Enovid-E	100 μg mestranol	2.5 mg norethynodrel
Loestrin 1/20	20 μg ethinyl estradiol	1.0 mg norethindrone acetate
Loestrin 1.5/30	30 μg ethinyl estradiol	1.5 mg norethindrone acetate
Lo/Ovral	30 μg ethinyl estradiol	0.3 mg norgestrel
Modicon	35 μg ethinyl estradiol	0.5 mg norethindrone
Norinyl 1/50	50 μg mestranol	1.0 mg norethindrone
Norinyl 1/80	80 μg mestranol	1.0 mg norethindrone
Norlestrin, 1 mg	50 μg ethinyl estradiol	1.0 mg norethindrone acetate
Norlestrin 2.5 mg	50 μg ethinyl estradiol	2.5 mg norethindrone acetate

ORAL CONTRACEPTIVES (cont.)

TRADE NAME	*ESTROGEN*	*PROGESTIN*
	*Combinations** (contd.)	
Ortho-Novum 1/50	50 μg mestranol	1.0 mg norethindrone
Ortho-Novum 1/80	80 μg mestranol	1.0 mg norethindrone
Ortho-Novum 2	100 μg mestranol	2.0 mg norethindrone
Ovcon-35	35 μg ethinyl estradiol	0.4 mg norethindrone
Ovcon-50	50 μg ethinyl estradiol	1.0 mg norethindrone
Ovral	50 μg ethinyl estradiol	0.5 mg norgestrel
Zorane 1/20	20 μg ethinyl estradiol	1.0 mg norethindrone acetate
Zorane 1.5/30	30 μg ethinyl estradiol	1.5 mg norethindrone acetate
Zorane 1/50	50 μg ethinyl estradiol	1.0 mg norethindrone acetate
	Sequentials†	
Norquen; Ortho-Novum SQ	80 μg mestranol	2.0 mg norethindrone
Oracon	100 μg ethinyl estradiol	25 mg dimethisterone
	Minipills‡	
Micronor		35 μg norethindrone
Nor-Q.D.		35 μg norethindrone
Ovrette		75 μg norgestrel

* 1 tablet a day for 20 to 21 days and off for 7 to 8 days.
† Estrogen alone for 2 weeks, followed by combination for 5 to 6 days and off for 7 to 8 days.
‡ 1 tablet a day continuously.

C. Agents for Fertility Inhibition

Many routes to fertility control, by drugs with systemic effects, have been studied experimentally (Jackson, Pharmacol. Rev., 11:135, 1959):

a. By impairment of gametogenesis: Through mitotic damage: e.g., alkylating agents, nitrofurans, colchicine, N,N′-bis-(dichloroacetyl)-1,8-octamethylenediamine.

b. By prevention of ovulation: Through suppression of the gonadotropic activity of the pituitary: e.g., various steroids, but especially progestins (the most practicable agents at present). Through other antigonadotropic agents: e.g., *Lithospermon ruderale* extracts. (See previous section.)

c. By interference before or at implantation: Through damage in oviduct, obstruction in oviduct, or impairment of endometrium: e.g., estrogens or androgens (antiprogestational), ergotoxin, xylohydroquinone, MER-25 (*p*-2-diethylaminoethoxyphenyl-1-phenyl-2-anisyl ethanol).

d. By interference with gestation: Through interference with the growth of the embryo: e.g., desoxypyridoxine, folic acid antagonists, azaserine, DON.

e. By degeneration of corpus luteum (?): prostaglandins.

INVESTIGATIONAL AGENTS

BOXIDINE

See also under Inhibitors of Cholesterol Synthesis.

Under investigation.

F_3C–(biphenyl)–O–CH_2CH_2–N(pyrrolidine)

N,N′BIS(DICHLORACETYL)-1,8-OCTAMETHYLENE DIAMINE (WIN-18446)

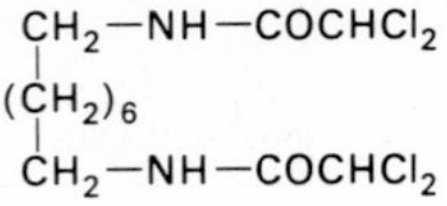

Arrests spermatogenesis without affecting Leydig cells; effect reversible. In trials in humans, 1 gm per day halted production of sperm (Potts, Fed. Proc., 20:418, 1961) but produced severe flushing when patients consumed alcohol.

$CH_2-NH-COCHCl_2$
$(CH_2)_6$
$CH_2-NH-COCHCl_2$

p-2-DIETHYLAMINOETHOXYPHENYL-1-PHENYL-2-ANISYL ETHANOL (MER-25)

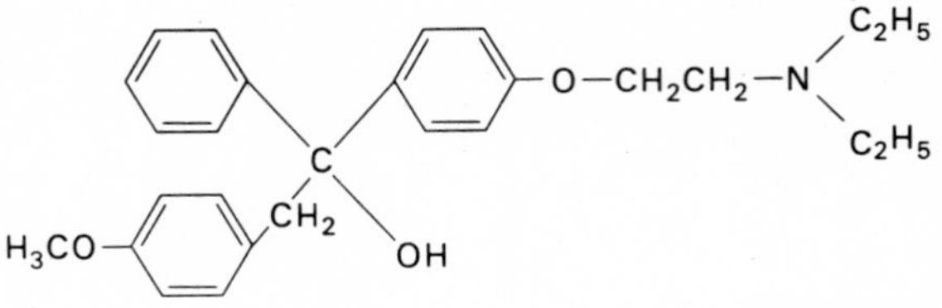

Related to estrogen, chlorotrianisene, and may act as a competitor. Under investigation.

H_3CO CH_2 C OH $O-CH_2CH_2-N$ C_2H_5 C_2H_5

1-(N,N-DIETHYLCARBAMYLMETHYL)-2,4-DINITROPYRROLE (ORF-1616)

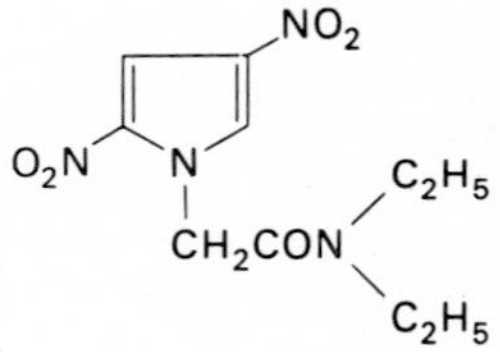

Inhibits sperm production in rats about 3 weeks after administration.

NO_2 O_2N N CH_2CON C_2H_5 C_2H_5

trans-1-(P-β-DIMETHYLAMINOETHOXYPHENYL-1,2-DIPHENYLBUT-1-ENE) (ICI 46,474)

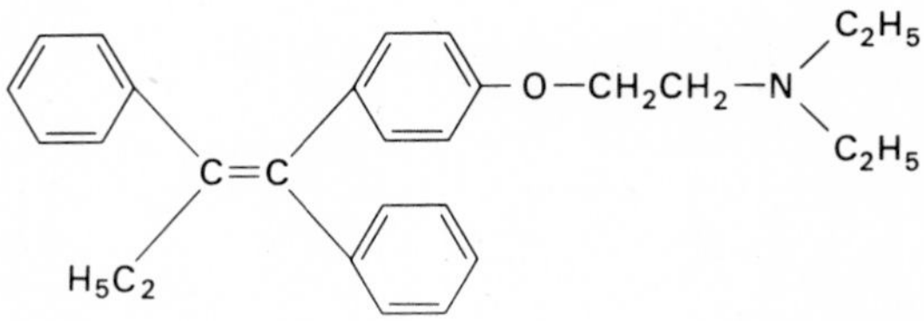

Prevents implantation in rats.

$O-CH_2CH_2-N$ C_2H_5 C_2H_5 C=C H_5C_2

METALLIBURE (Aimax; 1-α-Methylallylthiocarbamoyl-2-methylthiocarbamoylhydrazine; Ayerst 61122)

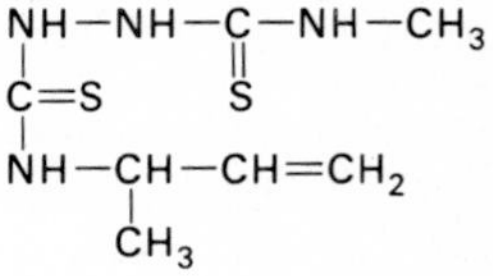

Ovulation inhibitor.

$NH-NH-C(=S)-NH-CH_3$
$C=S$
$NH-CH(CH_3)-CH=CH_2$

2-(*p*-(6-METHOXY-2-PHENYLINDEN-3-YL)-PHENOXY)-TRIETHYLAMINE HYDROCHLORIDE (U-11,555A)

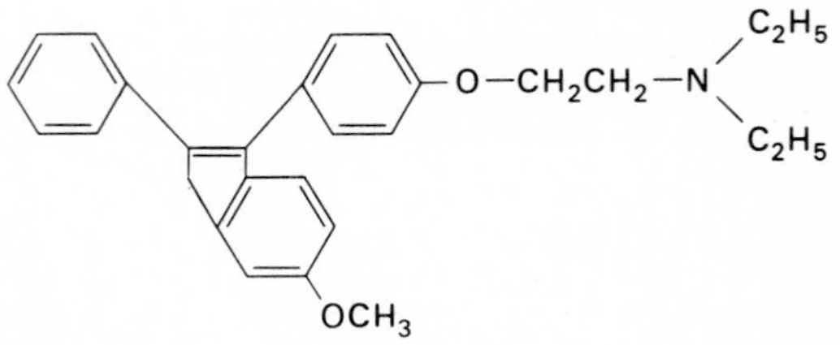

Inhibits fertility during tubal transport in the rat and during implantation in the rabbit. Also suppresses spermatogenesis in the rat by hypophyseal inhibition. Produces toxic skin reaction in man.

$O-CH_2CH_2-N$ C_2H_5 C_2H_5 OCH_3

2-METHYL-3-ETHYL-4-PHENYL-Δ-4-CYCLOHEXENECARBOXYLIC ACID (ORF 3858)

Prevents implantation in rabbit and primate.

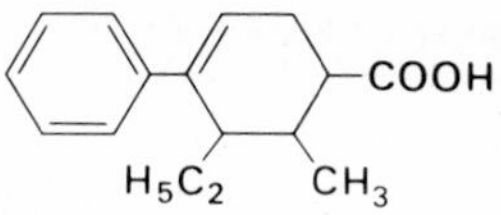

NAFOXIDINE HYDROCHLORIDE (U-11100A)

Potent antifertility agent in animals; reported to inhibit implantation. Has been tried against renal cancer.

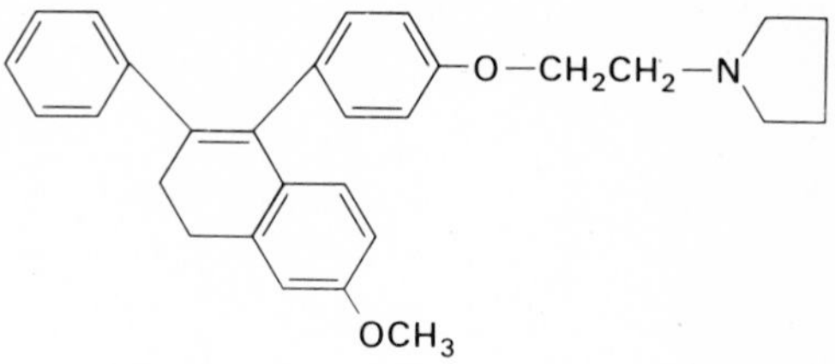

D. Agents for Fertility Increase

In ovulation failure a number of agents may induce maturation of the follicle and ovulation (Tyler, J.A.M.A. 205:16, 1968). They are in general antiestrogens.

CLOMETHERONE

Estrogen antagonist.

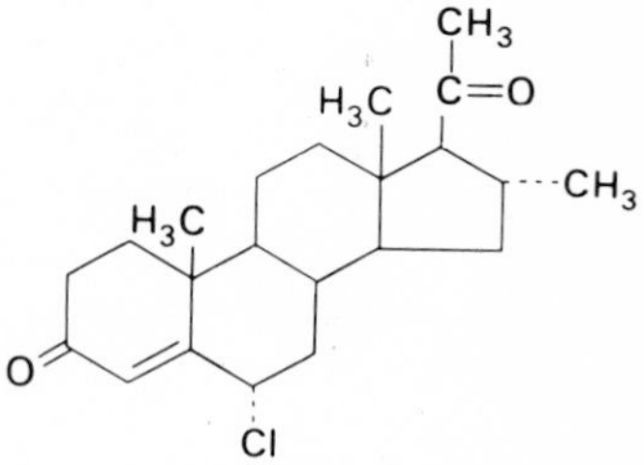

CLOMIPHENE CITRATE (Clomid; MRL/41)

An analogue of chlorotrianisene. In humans, stimulates the anovulatory ovary to secrete estrogen, and acts on the hypothalamus to produce and release gonadotropins; induces ovulation. Multiple births have followed use.

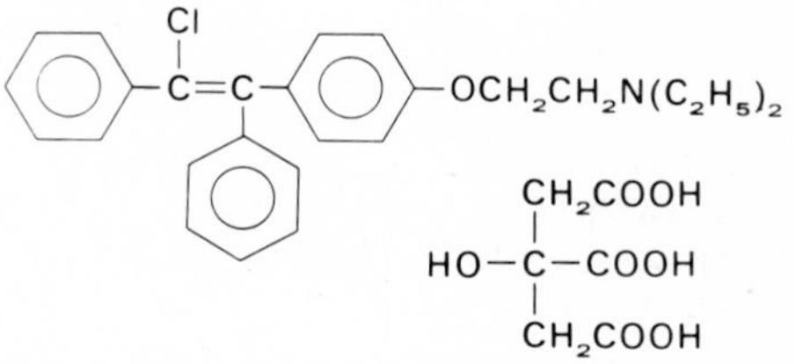

Although not as toxic as triparanol, ovarian enlargement, ascites, and blurred vision have been reported.

Dose: 50 to 100 mg for 5 days by mouth.

Transclomiphene
Cisclomiphene

EPIMESTROL

May induce ovulation in women having anovulatory cycles.

Under investigation.

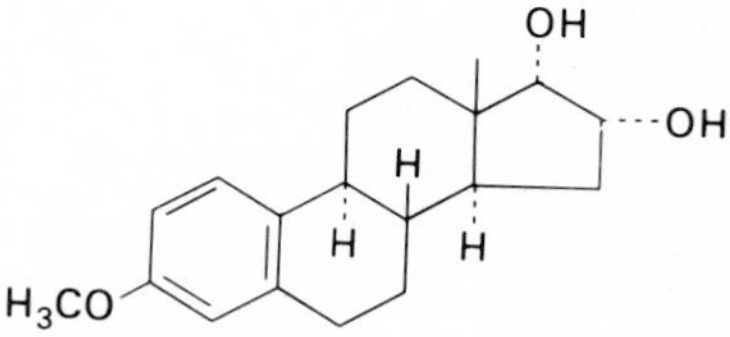

TAMOXIFEN CITRATE

$$(CH_3)_2NCH_2O-C_6H_4-C(C_6H_5)=C(C_6H_5)-C_2H_5 \cdot HO-C(CH_2COOH)(COOH)-CH_2COOH$$

MENOTROPINS

See Nonpituitary Gonadotropins.

E. Nonsteroid Luteal Factors

RELAXIN

1. Chemistry. Polypeptide produced by the corpus luteum of pregnancy (extracted from the ovaries of pregnant sows).

2. Action and Mechanism. a. Causes relaxation of guinea pig symphysis pubis by proliferation of capillaries and dissolution of collagen.

b. Also inhibits uterine contractions in experimental animals and may relax the cervix; does not antagonize oxytocin.

3. Pharmacodynamics and Toxicity. Not absorbed by mouth. Nontoxic except in pork sensitivity.

4. Uses. To halt premature labor and to facilitate cervical softening at labor. Actual clinical usefulness doubtful and uncertain.

5. Preparation

RELAXIN (Cervilaxin)

Dose: 20 mg every 4 hours intramuscularly.

SUMMARY: FEMALE SEX HORMONES

TYPE	*ACTION AND MECHANISM*	*TOXICITY*	*USE*	*EXAMPLES*
Natural estrogens	Promote growth of endometrium, mammary ducts, vaginal cornification	Anorexia nausea, vomiting	Menopause, atrophic vaginitis, contraception	Estradiol
Synthetic estrogens	Same	Same	Same	Diethylstilbestrol

SUMMARY: FEMALE SEX HORMONES (cont.)

TYPE	*ACTION AND MECHANISM*	*TOXICITY*	*USE*	*EXAMPLES*
Natural progestins	Induces secretory endometrium	Minor	Habitual abortion	Progesterone
Synthetic progestins	Same Inhibit anterior pituitary May affect uterine mobility and cervical mucus	Androgenic side effects, thrombosis	Menstrual disorders, endometriosis, contraception	Norethynodrel
Fertility inducers	Induce ovarian maturation and ovulation	Multiple births	Infertility	Clomiphene

Reviews

Gaunt, R., Chart, J., and Renzi, A. Interactions of drugs with endocrines. Ann. Rev. Pharmacol., 3:109, 1963.
Fridhandler, L., and Pincus, G. Pharmacology of reproduction and fertility. Ann. Rev. Pharmacol., 4:177, 1964.
Tyler, E. Antifertility agents. Ann. Rev. Pharmacol., 7:381, 1967.
Rudel, H., and Martinez-Manautau, J. Oral contraceptives. Topics Med. Chem., 1:339, 1967.
Fox, B., and Fox, M. Biochemical aspects of the actions of drugs on spermatogenesis. Pharmacol. Rev., 19:21, 1967.
Jackson, H., and Schnieden, H. Pharmacology of reproduction and fertility. Ann. Rev. Pharmacol., 8:467, 1968.
Segal, S. Research in fertility inhibition. New Eng. J. Med., 279:364, 1968.
Kalman, S. Effects of oral contraceptives. Ann. Rev. Pharmacol., 9:363, 1969.
Drill, V. (ed). Antifertility drugs. Fed. Proc., 29:1209, 1970.
Jensen, E. V., and DeSombre, E. R. Ann. Rev. Biochem., 41:203, 1972.

36.
Androgens and Anabolic Agents

A. Androgens

TESTOSTERONE AND DERIVATIVES

1. History. a. John Hunter (1771) transplanted testes into hens, producing masculinity, in the first published demonstration of hormone action; Barthold (1849) showed that transplantation of testes into castrated roosters restored male characteristics.

b. Butenandt (1931) isolated androsterone from urine and used the capon comb test; Laqueur (1935) isolated testosterone; Butenandt (1935) and Ruzika (1935) synthesized testosterone.

2. Chemistry. a. The androgens are C-19 steroids.

b. Testosterone is made in the interstitial (Leydig) cells of the testes; androgens are also made in the adrenal cortex (primary source in females), in cells near the ovarian hilus and in the placenta. Commercial source, cholesterol and other plant sterols.

3. Action. a. Androgen is formed in the fetal testes by the influence of maternal gonadotropin; this causes descent of the testes; subsequently little androgen is formed until puberty.

b. At puberty the hypophysis stimulates, through LH and FSH together, the interstitial cells to produce androgen again, with resultant development of the testes and secondary sexual characteristics.

c. In the adult male, androgens maintain the testes (including spermatogenesis) and accessory structures (seminal vesicles and prostate) and secondary masculine characteristics. Androgens also inhibit the anterior pituitary.

d. Androgens stimulate protein anabolism (retention of nitrogen). The anabolic effect may be assayed by the production of hypertrophy of the levator ani in a castrate rat.

4. Mechanism. a. Testosterone is reduced in the target tissue to dihydrotestosterone. The latter binds to the protein in the cytoplasm and is transferred into the nucleus.

b. In the nucleus dihydrotestosterone causes increased synthesis of specific RNA and protein.

5. Pharmacodynamics. a. Testosterone is absorbed by mouth but is ineffective because of rapid metabolism in the intestine and liver. Methyltestosterone is well absorbed and effective orally or sublingually.

b. Testosterone is inactivated in the liver, and excreted as androsterone, androstanediol and other 17-ketosteroids.

c. Methyltestosterone produces creatinuria but no increase in 17-ketosteroid excretion.

6. Toxicity. Acne, baldness, testicular inhibition, priapism, cholestatic hepatitis (methyltestosterone); sodium and water retention; hypercalcemia, especially in immobilized patients. Prolonged use may produce impotence and azoospermia in male and masculinization in female.

7. Uses. a. Testosterone has limited use in hypogonadism, cryptorchidism and possibly the male climacteric.

b. It has greater use in treating breast engorgement, cancer of the female breast, and possibly dysmenorrhea.

c. It has been replaced by synthetic androgens for producing a positive nitrogen balance in debilitated states.

8. Preparations

TESTOSTERONE

Dose: 10 to 100 mg intramuscularly (aqueous suspension).

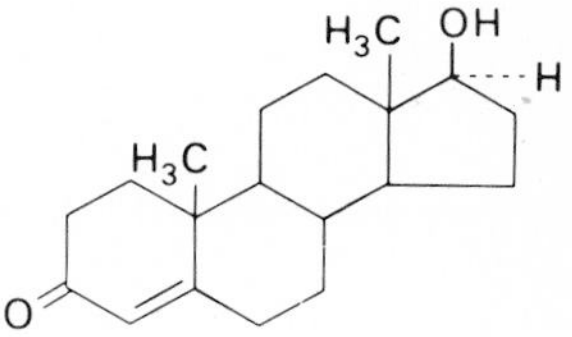

TESTOSTERONE PROPIONATE (Oreton; Perandren)

Dose: 10 to 50 mg daily or every other day intramuscularly; maintenance may be obtained from 5 to 25 mg daily buccally.

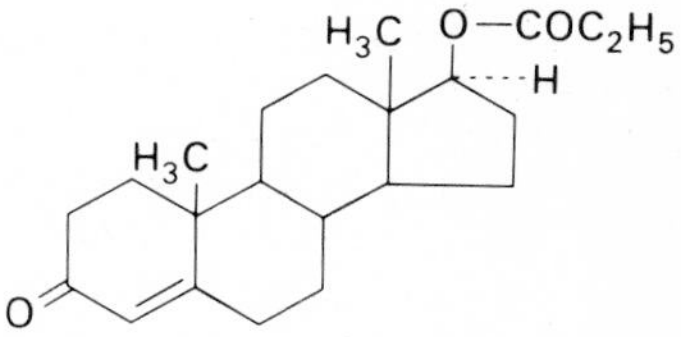

Testosterone cypionate (Depo-testosterone)

Dose: 10 to 50 mg every 1 to 2 weeks intramuscularly.

Testosterone propionate

Testosterone enanthate (Delatestryl)

Dose: 100 to 500 mg every 2 to 4 weeks intramuscularly.

Testosterone phenylacetate (Perandren phenylacetate)

Testosterone ketolaurate

METHYLTESTOSTERONE (Metandren; Oreton M)

Substitution (CH_3) prevents biotransformation in tissues, but may produce hepatotoxicity.

Dose: 5 to 25 mg daily by mouth.

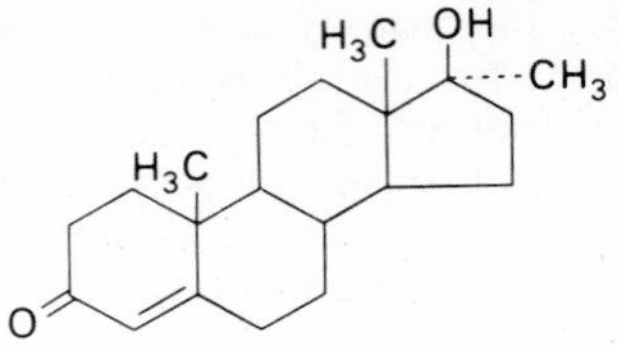

MESTEROLONE (Proviron)

Oral androgen.

Dose: 50 to 100 mg daily by mouth.

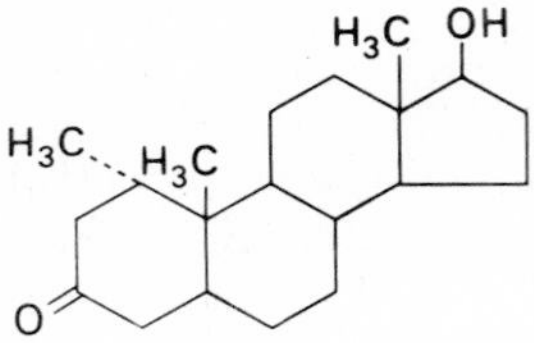

B. Anabolic Androgens

1. Chemistry. Testosterone relatives.

2. Action. Differ from testosterone in relative enhancement of anabolic effects over androgenic effects.

3. Mechanism. a. Steroid is bound in euchromatin portion of nucleus of cells of target organs.

b. It there stimulates the rate of RNA synthesis.

c. Result is increased protein manufacture.

4. Pharmacodynamics. Qualitatively similar to testosterone. Usually effective orally.

5. Toxicity. Intrahepatic cholangitis with dilatation of the canaliculi and parenchymal cell damage in the liver have been reported from norethandrolone (Marquardt, J.A.M.A., 175:851, 1961).

6. Uses. a. The principal use of the primarily anabolic steroids is to promote nitrogen retention and weight gain in undernourished patients, especially the elderly and those with chronic disease.

b. Also used for suppression of cancer of the breast in premenopausal women.

7. Preparations

a. Primarily used for anabolic effect

BOLANDIOL DIPROPIONATE

Under investigation.

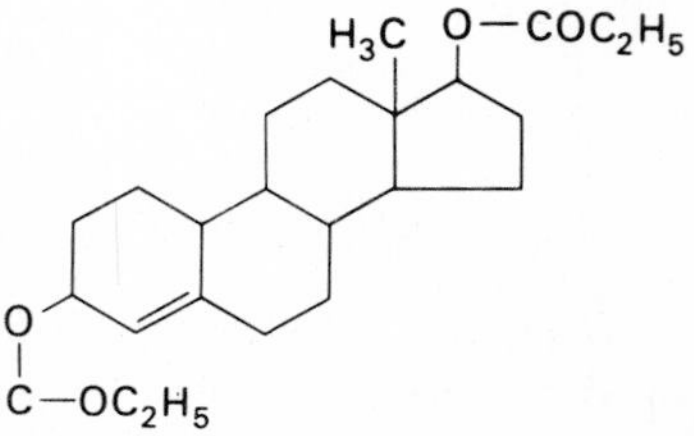

Bolasterone

Dose: 1 to 2 mg by mouth daily.

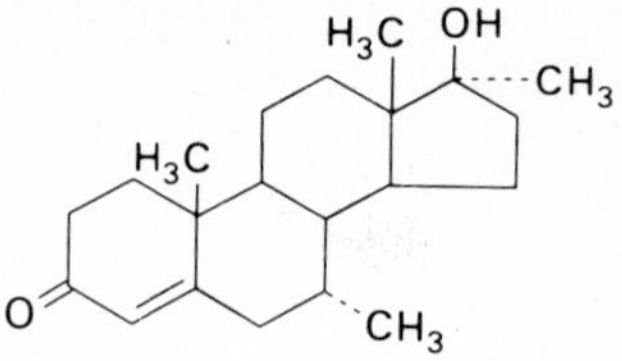

Bolenol

Under investigation.

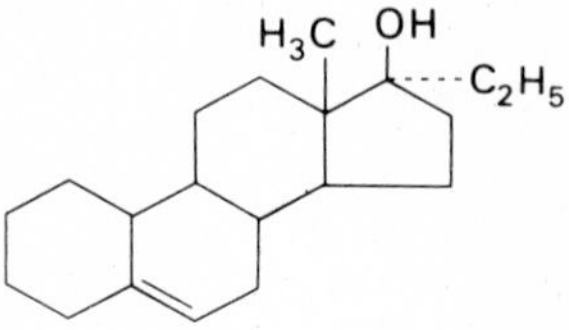

Boldenone undecylenate (Parenabol)

Under investigation.

$O{-}CO{-}(CH_2)_8{-}CH{=}CH_2$

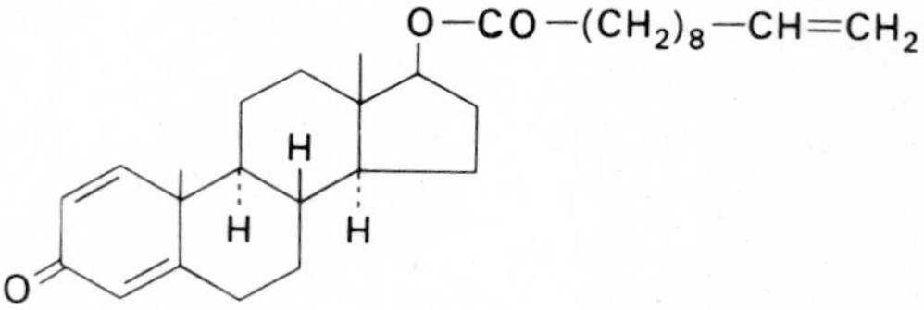

Bolmantalate

Under investigation.

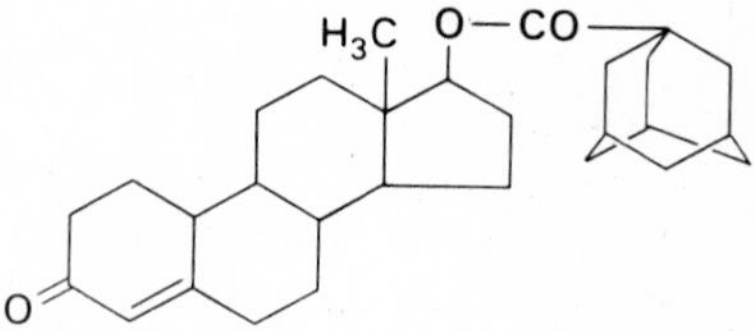

Ethylestrenol (Maxibolin)

Dose: 4 mg by mouth daily.

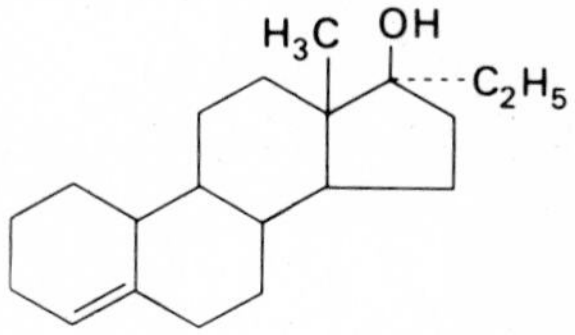

Fluoxymesterone (Halotestin; Ultranden)

Mildly androgenic but strongly anabolic; F increases potency about 5 times.

Dose: 4 to 10 mg daily by mouth.

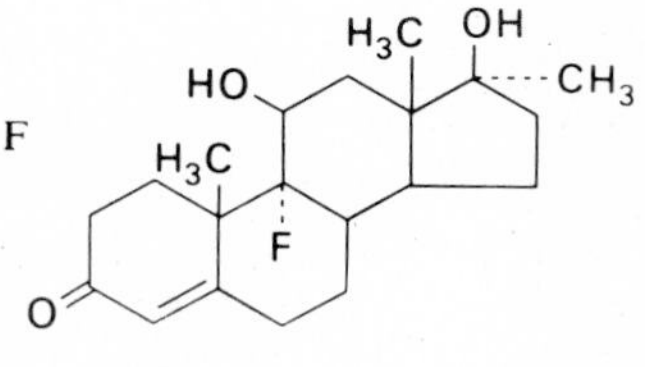

METHANDRIOL (Stenediol)

Mildly androgenic but strongly anabolic.

Dose: 25 mg 2 to 5 times a week by mouth, sublingually or intramuscularly.

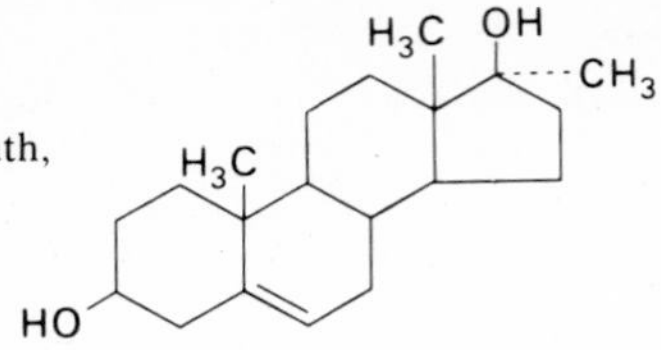

METHANDROSTENOLONE (Dianabol)

Oral anabolic agent.

Dose: 5 mg daily by mouth.

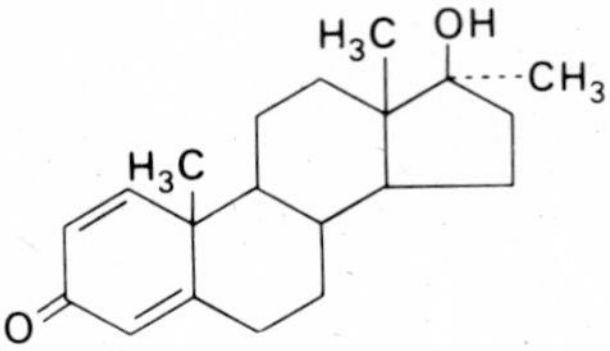

METHENOLONE ENANTHATE (Primobolan)

Methenolone acetate

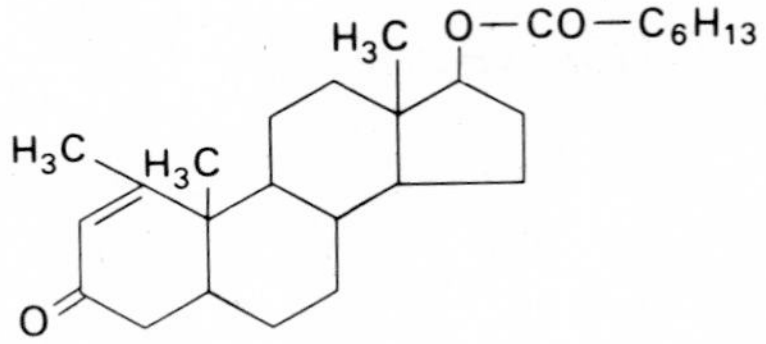

MIBOLERONE

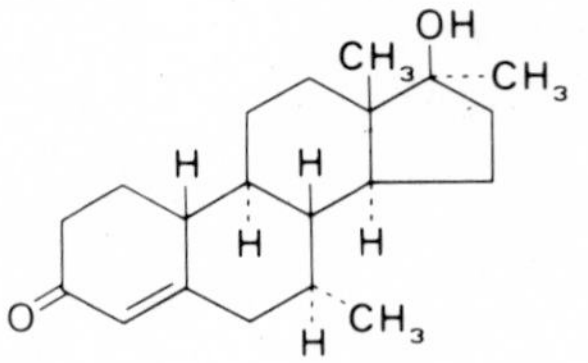

NANDROLONE CYCLOTATE

NANDROLONE DECANOATE (Deca-Durabolin)

Mildly androgenic but strongly anabolic; long acting.

Dose: 50 to 100 mg once a month intramuscularly.

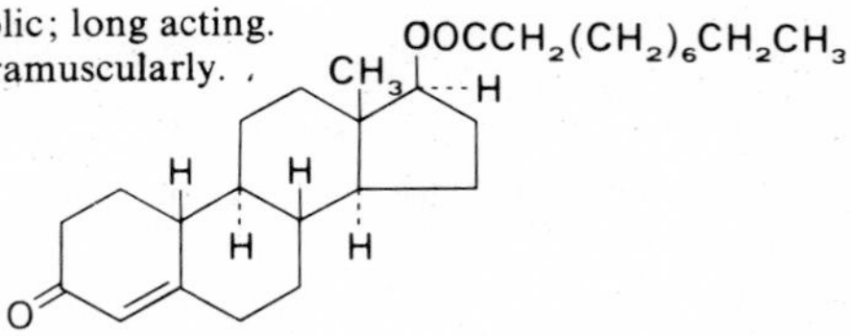

NANDROLENE PHENPROPIONATE (Durabolin)

NORBOLETHONE (Genabol)

Under investigation.

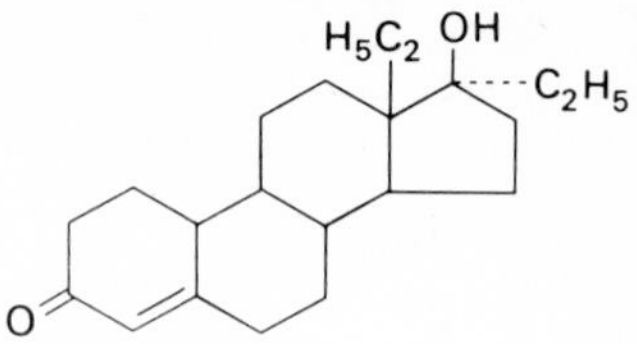

NORETHANDROLONE (Nilevar)

Mildly androgenic but strongly anabolic.

Dose: 30 to 50 mg daily orally or intramuscularly.

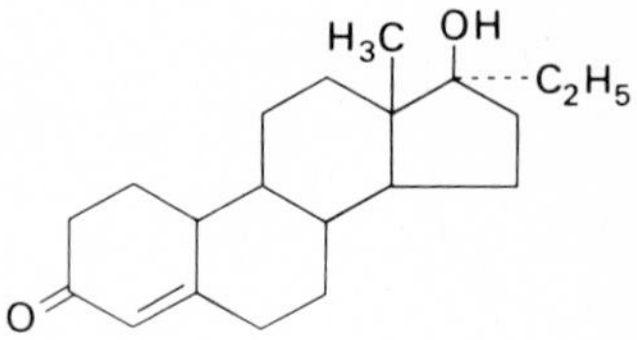

NORMETANDRONE (Orgasteron)

Under investigation.

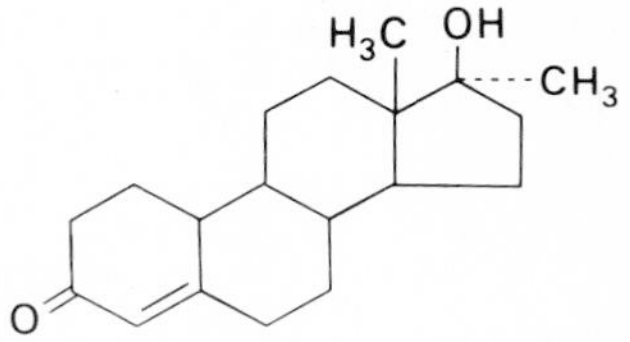

OXANDROLONE (Anavar)

Under investigation.

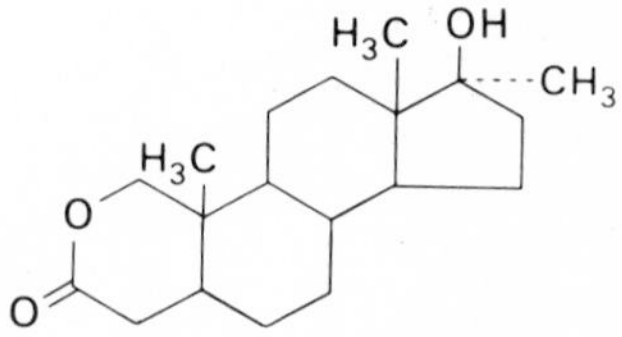

OXYMETHOLONE (Adroyd)

Effective orally; about half as androgenic as testosterone.

Dose: 2.5 to 5 mg 3 times a day by mouth.

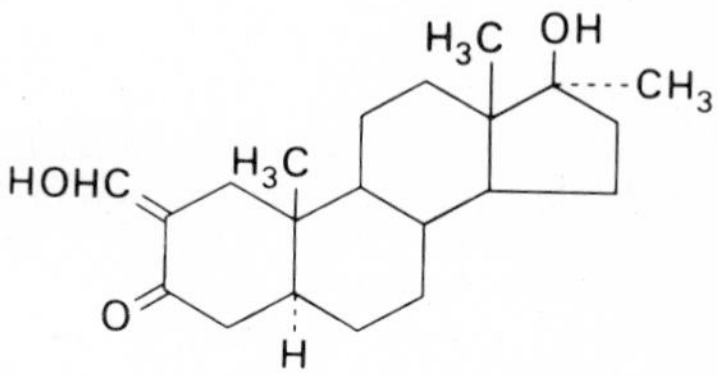

QUINBOLONE

Under investigation.

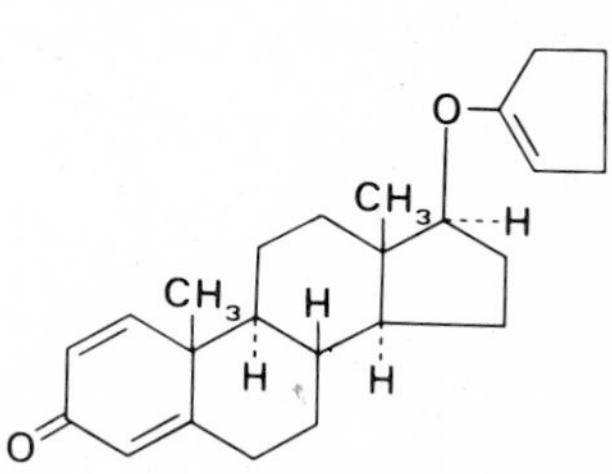

SILANDRONE

Under investigation.

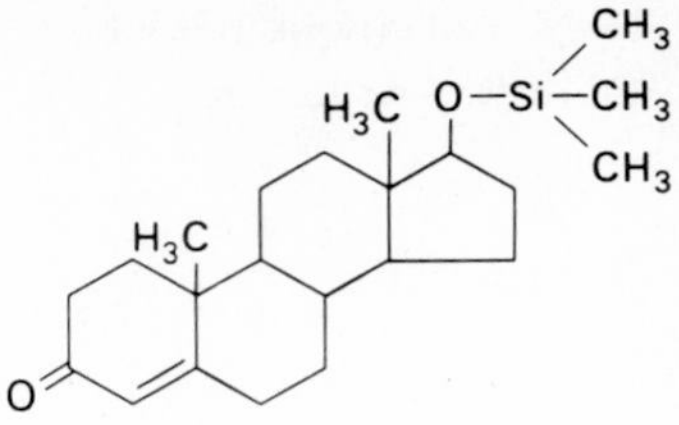

STANOZOLOL (Winstrol)

Dose: 2 mg 3 times a day by mouth, before meals.

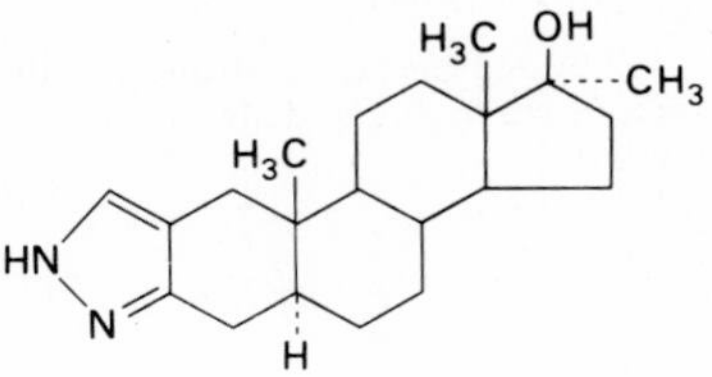

STENBOLONE ACETATE

Under investigation.

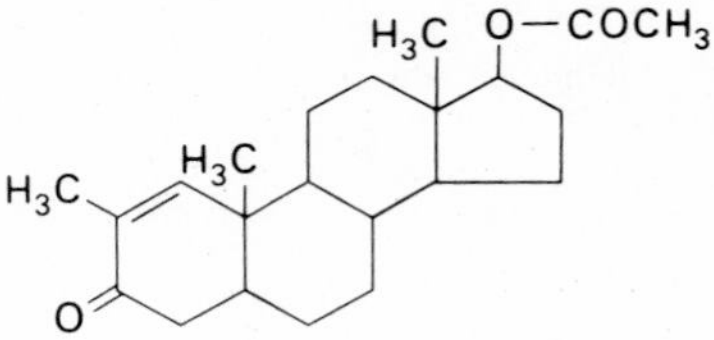

TIBOLONE

Under investigation.

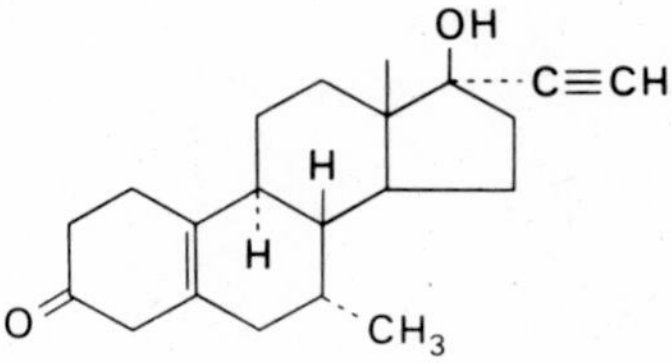

ZERANOL

Resorcylic acid lactone from *Gibberella zaea*. Promotes N and Ca retention in cattle after implant.

Under investigation.

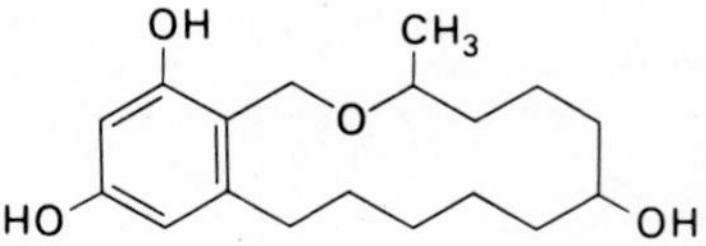

b. Primarily used for anticancer effect

CALUSTERONE (Methosarb)

Under investigation.

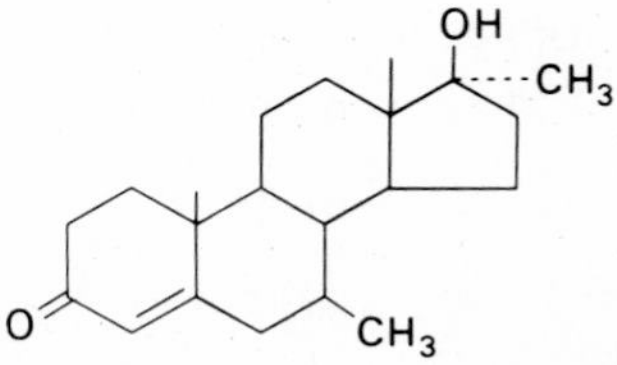

DROMOSTANOLONE PROPIONATE (Drolban)

Less virilizing than testosterone; used in metastatic carcinoma of the breast.

Dose: 100 mg 3 times a week intramuscularly.

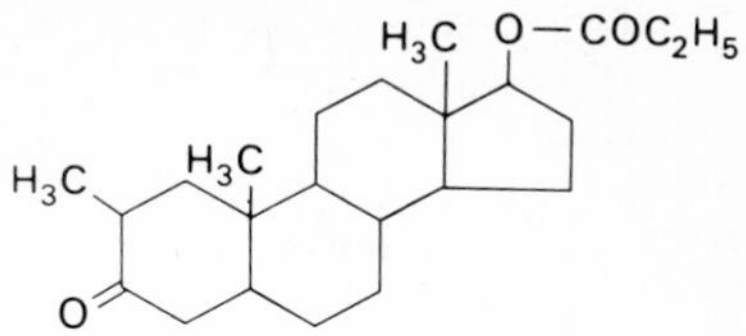

METRENOLONE

Antineoplastic and androgenic.
Under investigation.

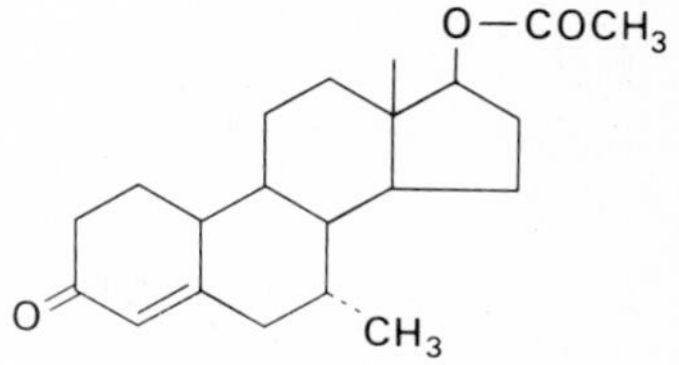

STANOLONE (Neodrol)

Used especially for suppression of carcinoma of the breast; virilization may appear.

Dose: 100 mg daily intramuscularly.

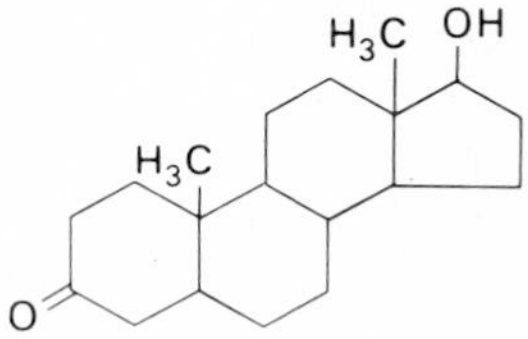

TESTOLACTONE (Teslac)

Antineoplastic. Does not cause masculinization or increased sex desire. Does not stimulate erythropoiesis.

May cause edema, nausea, vomiting, hypercalcemia.

Dose: 150 mg 3 times a week orally or intramuscularly.

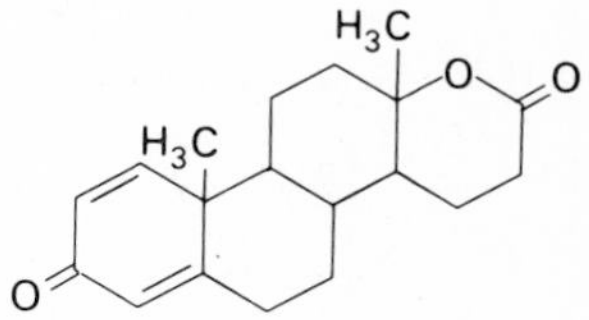

TRESTOLONE ACETATE (Teslac)

Antineoplastic and androgenic.
Under investigation.

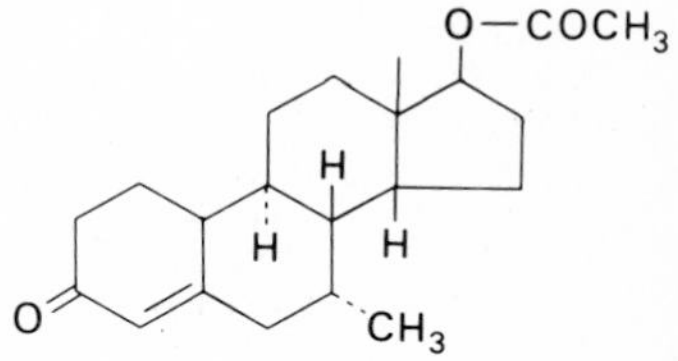

C. Other Steroids

ANTIANDROGENIC STEROIDS

Potential use in cancer of the prostate, male contraception, and depressives of male sexual behavior.

CYPROTERONE ACETATE

Potent antiandrogen. Under investigation.

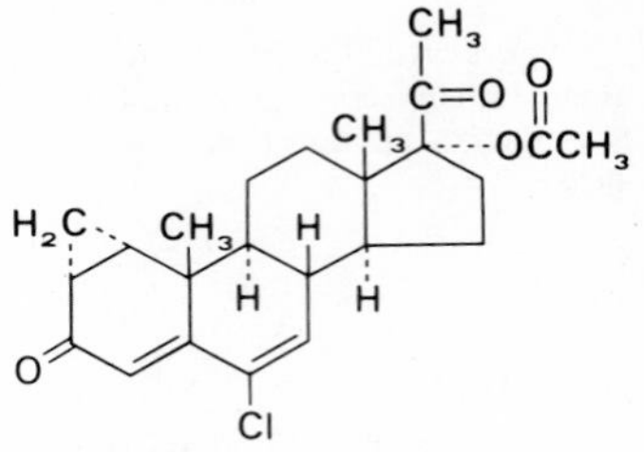

OTHERS

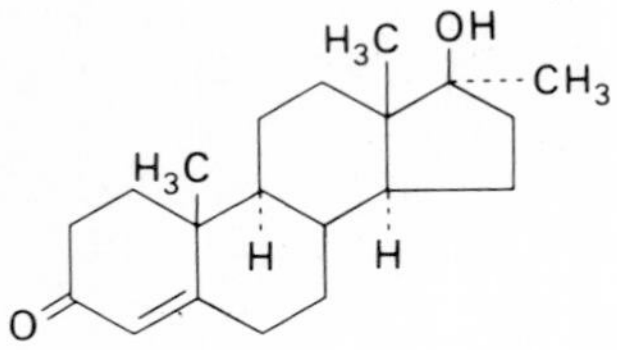

benorterone

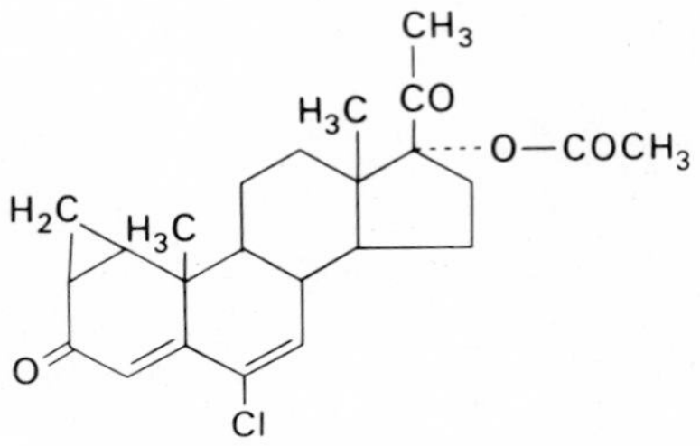

clanterone acetate

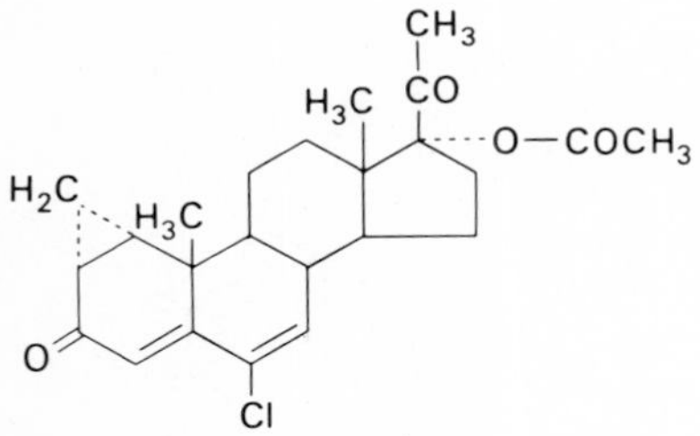

cyproterone

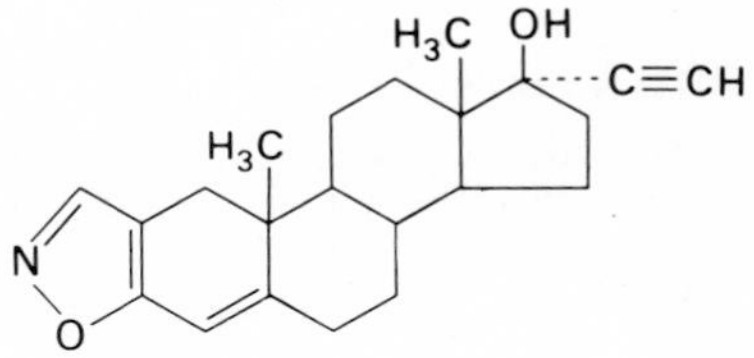

danazol

SUMMARY: ANDROGENS AND ANABOLIC AGENTS

TYPE	ACTION AND MECHANISM	TOXICITY	USE	EXAMPLES
Androgens	Maintain testes and secondary sex characteristics Anabolic	Acne, bladness, sodium retention, hypercalcemia	Breast engorgement, female breast cancer	Testosterone
Anabolic androgens	Anabolic effects enhanced	Similar	Weight gain in undernourished patients	Norethandrolone
Anabolic antineoplastic	Similar	Similar	Female breast cancer	Testolactone

Review

Short, R. V. Reproduction. Ann. Rev. Physiol., 29:373, 1967.

37. Agents in Diabetes Mellitus

A. Insulin

1. History. a. Von Mering and Minkowski (1890) showed that extirpation of the pancreas gave diabetes; Laguesse (1893) showed that ligation of the pancreatic duct gave acinar atrophy; DeMeyer (1909) proposed the name "insuline" for the islet hormone.

b. Banting and Best (1921) made islet extracts containing insulin; Abel (1926) crystallized insulin; Sanger (1955) determined the formula.

2. Chemistry. a. Protein composed of two chains of amino acids linked by two disulfide bridges; mol. wt. about 6,000 (Sanger, Science, 129:1340, 1959).

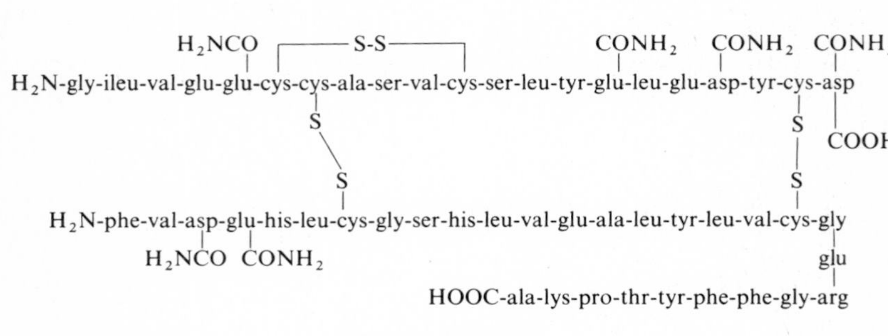

insulin (beef)

b. Crystalline insulin contains 24 units per mg.

3. Action. a. Insulin is secreted by the beta islet cells of the pancreas in response to a rise in blood sugar; it then acts to lower the blood sugar by promoting peripheral utilization of glucose and limiting hepatic release.

b. It thus assists in the maintenance of blood sugar in the normal range, and prevents glycosuria and ketosis.

4. Mechanism. a. The insulin receptor, localized in the cell membrane, has been purified, characterized, and the kinetics of binding defined (Cuatrecasas, Fed. Proc., 32:1838, 1973).

b. The principal mechanism of action appears to be the facilitation of the penetration of glucose through cell membranes (primarily skeletal muscle cells), probably including membranes of subcellular organelles (Edelman, Nature, 197: 878, 1963). This action is antagonized by growth hormone and adrenal corticoids.

c. Insulin also enhances amino acid uptake and protein synthesis while inhibiting protein degradation.

5. Role in Disease. In juvenile diabetes, a hereditary disease, the insulin synthesis and secretion is absent. In diabetes that develops in the mature person, the production of insulin may be normal but the beta cells fail to respond rapidly to the stimulation by glucose with secretion. In either case there is an inadequate insulin secretion resulting in hyperglycemia, hyperlipemia, ketonemia, and azoturia. Administration of insulin corrects these symptoms.

6. Pharmacodynamics. a. Insulin, as protein, is normally digested rather than absorbed when given by mouth.

b. After injection it is rapidly destroyed in the tissues, presumably by a proteolytic enzyme that breaks down both insulin and glucagon.

7. Toxicity. The principal hazard from insulin is hypoglycemia, with sweating, dizziness, impaired judgment, unconsciousness, and convulsions; occasional allergic hypersensitivity.

8. Uses. a. Insulin is used for the control of diabetes mellitus.

b. Limited use for the production of hypoglycemic shock in psychoses and for stimulation of the appetite.

c. Three types of insulin preparations are available:

a′. *Rapid:* Acts immediately; lasts about 6 to 14 hours. For the control of severe, labile diabetics and diabetic emergencies.

b′. *Intermediate:* Onset 2 to 4 hours; duration 12 to 24 hours. For the control of most diabetics requiring insulin (obese diabetics are better treated by dietary limitation in most cases). The preparation should give adequate control of blood sugar during the daytime when food is periodically eaten, yet be less active during the night so that the patient is not hypoglycemic in the morning.

c′. *Long*: Onset in 6 to 8 hours; duration 24 to 48 hours. For use in mild diabetes; in severe diabetes a dose adequate to control daytime hyperglycemia is likely to produce hypoglycemia the next morning, but may be used in such patients in smaller dosage, supplemented by a more quickly acting insulin.

9. Preparations

a. Rapid

INSULIN, INJECTION (Iletin)

INSULIN, NEUTRAL

INSULIN ZINC, PROMPT (Semilente Insulin, Semilente Iletin)

b. Intermediate

INSULIN, DALANATED

INSULIN, GLOBIN ZINC

INSULIN, ISOPHANE (NPH Iletin)

INSULIN ZINC (Lente Insulin, Lente Iletin)

c. Long

INSULIN PROTAMINE ZINC

INSULIN ZINC, EXTENDED (Ultralente Insulin, Ultralente Iletin)

B. Other Hypoglycemic Agents

SULFONYLUREA GROUP

1. History. a. Janbon (1942) showed that isopropylthiodiazylsulfanilamide produced hypoglycemia.

b. Loubatières (1942) introduced carbutamide, the forerunner of present clinical compounds.

2. Chemistry. Sulfonylureas derived from isopropylthiodiazylsulfanilamide.

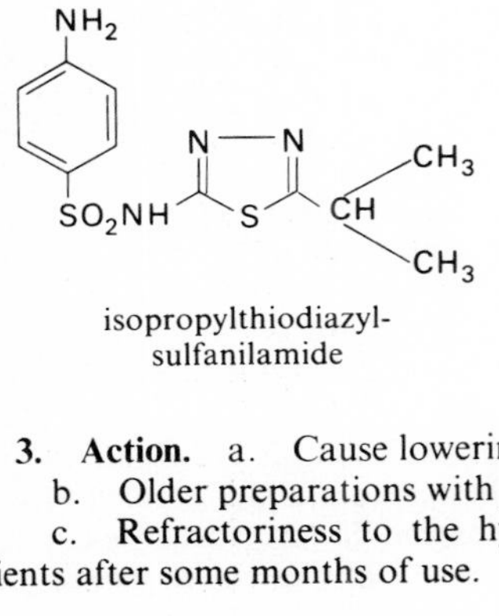

NH_2 / SO_2NH / N—N / S / CH / CH_3 / CH_3

isopropylthiodiazyl-sulfanilamide

NH_2 / $SO_2NH—C(=O)—NH—C_4H_9$

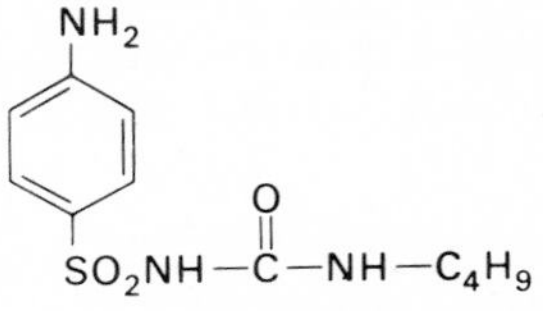

carbutamide

3. Action. a. Cause lowering of blood sugar.

b. Older preparations with *p*-amino group were antibacterial.

c. Refractoriness to the hypoglycemic action occurs in 5% to 10% of patients after some months of use.

4. Mechanism. Primary action may be to free endogenous insulin from protein-bound complexes in the pancreatic β cells, the plasma, and the tissues.

5. Pharmacodynamics. a. Well absorbed by mouth in two to four hours.

b. Tolbutamide rapidly destroyed in the body (half-life of 4 hours); chlorpropamide excreted almost completely unchanged over four days giving prolonged effect. Metahexamide also long acting.

c. Maximal stimulation of the β cells may be produced by small doses; effect not increased by larger doses.

6. Toxicity. a. Carbutamide is not used in the United States because of fever, rash, and hepatitis.

b. Tolbutamide may cause indigestion, urticaria; flushing after alcohol; cholestatic jaundice; thrombocytopenia, agranulocytosis, increased mortality from heart disease. Chlorpropamide may produce nausea, vomiting, neurological disturbances, and cholestatic jaundice. Also it can produce hypoglycemia, which is unlikely with tolbutamide, but has been reported in elderly patients on irregular diets.

7. Uses. a. Tolbutamide should be used only in adult-onset diabetes that cannot be adequately controlled by diet and in which the use of insulin is impractical. True value and safety are in doubt.

b. The status of chlorpropamide and the other preparations is uncertain, but they are best limited to older, mild or moderate diabetics who can be freed from insulin injections entirely by their use.

c. Inadequate in severe or childhood diabetes because pancreas incapable of producing adequate insulin. No advantage if insulin still required (except that reduced insulin may be continued during initiation of treatment).

8. Preparations

ACETOHEXAMIDE (Dymelor)

Dose: 250 mg by mouth initially; increased as needed up to 1.5 gm.

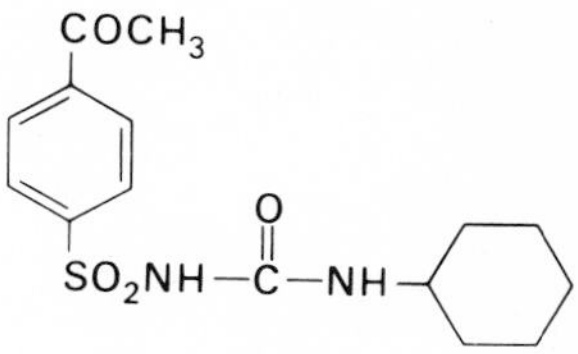

GLYPINAMIDE (Parinase)

Dose: 100 to 500 mg daily by mouth in a single dose.

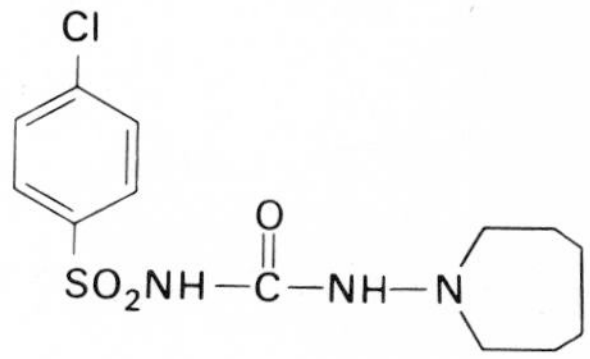

CHLORPROPAMIDE (Diabinese)

Dose: 0.5 gm by mouth initially, then 0.1 daily, gradually increasing to 0.25 gm once daily over 6 to 8 weeks time, by mouth. Phenformin may be added if dose of more than 0.25 gm daily required (Beaser, Clin. Pharmacol. Ther., 2:157, 1961).

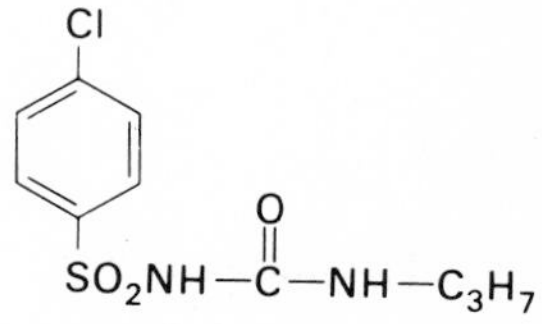

TOLAZAMIDE (Tolinase)

Dose: Up to a maximum of 3 gm daily.

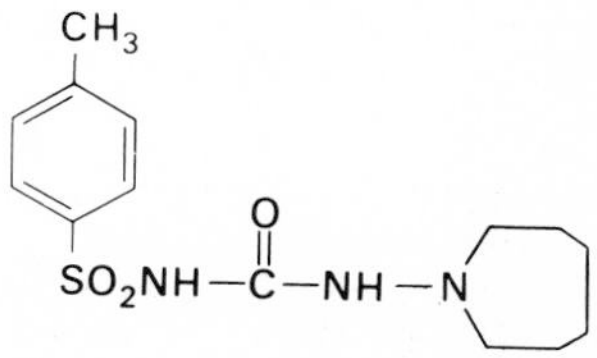

TOLBUTAMIDE (Orinase)

Dose: 1 gm 2 or 3 times a day by mouth.

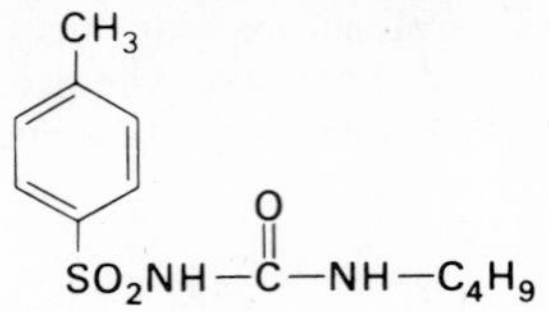

CH_3 … $SO_2NH{-}C(=O){-}NH{-}C_4H_9$

OTHERS

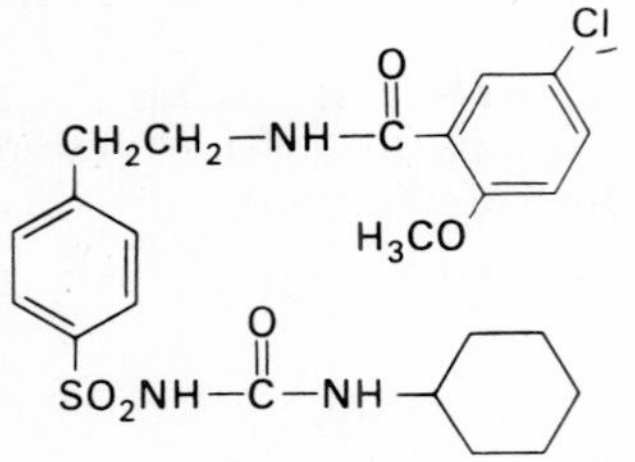

glyburide

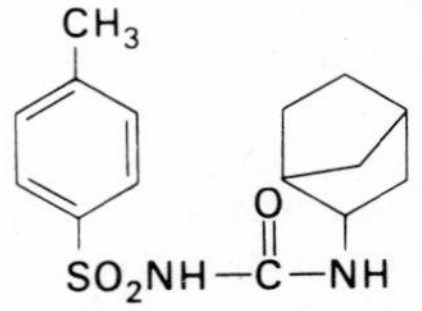

glibornuride

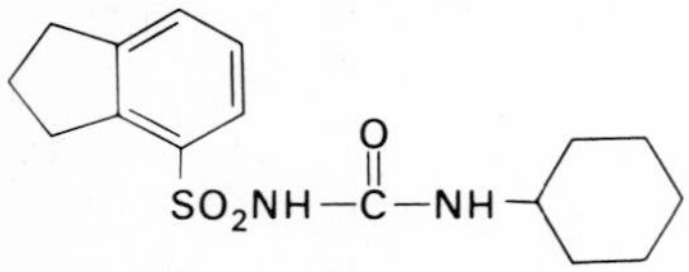

glyhexamide (Subose)

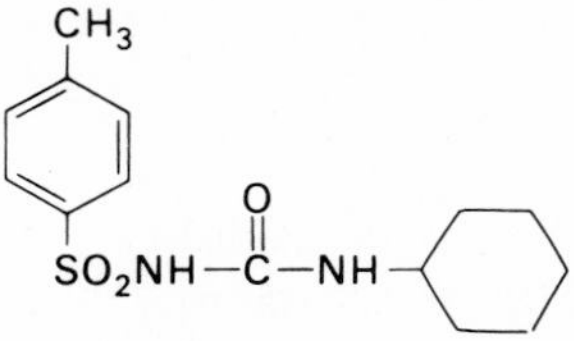

glycyclamide

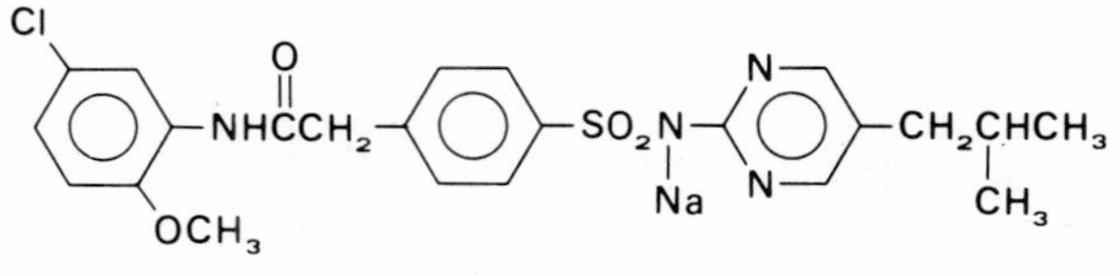

glicentanile sodium

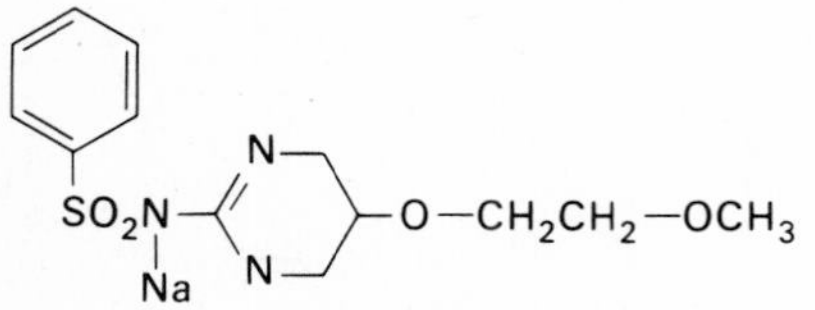

glymidine sodium (Redul)

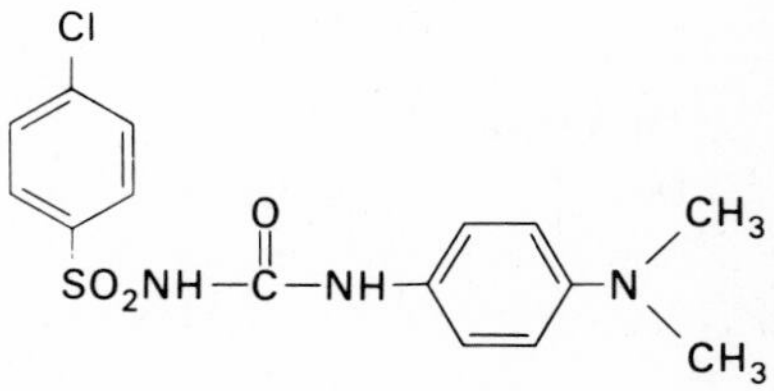

glyparamide

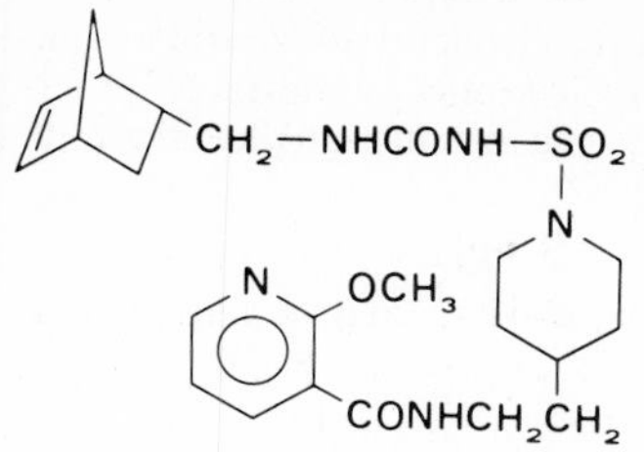

gliamilide

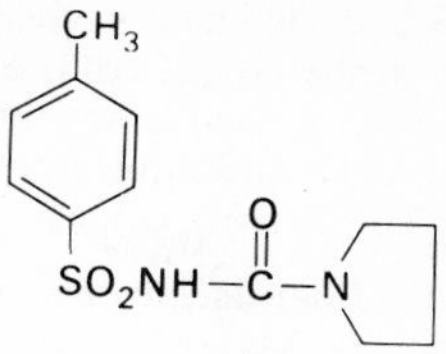

tolpyrramide

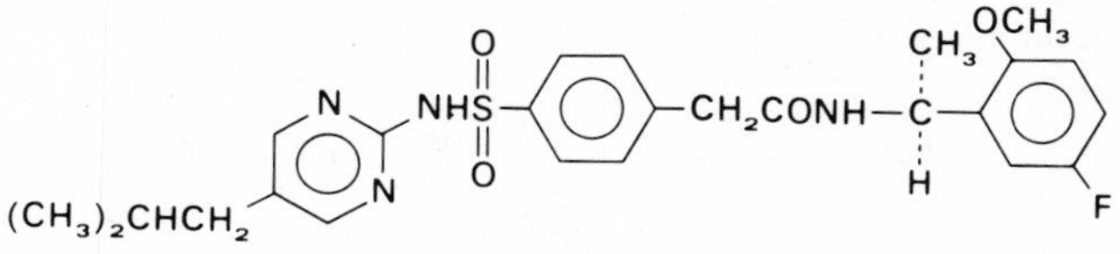

gliflumide

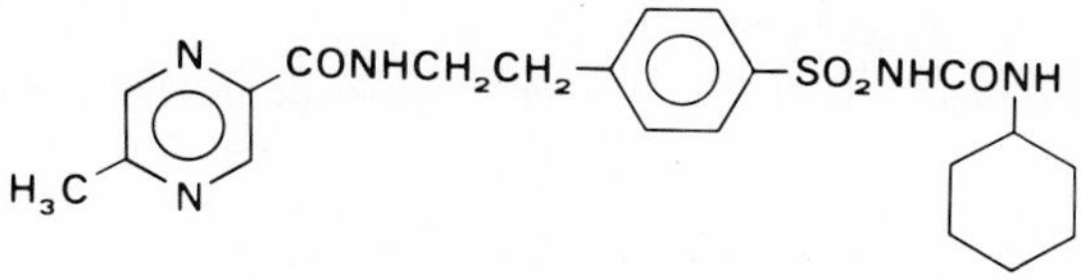

glipizide (glibenese)

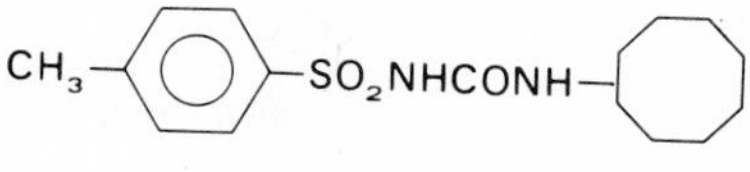

glyoctamide

BIGUANIDE GROUP

1. History. Unger (1957) showed hypoglycemic effect of phenformin in animals; Pomeranze (1957) introduced it clinically.

2. Chemistry. Biguanide derivatives. Phenformin exists as a monobasic cyclic cation at the pH of body fluids.

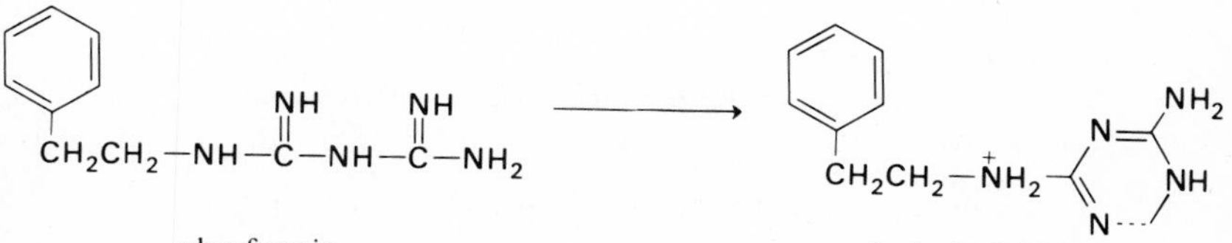

phenformin

(in body fluids)

3. Action and Mechanism. a. Increase the peripheral utilization of glucose; active in the absence of the pancreas or the liver; little effect in normals.

b. Enhance anaerobic glycolysis (lactic acid production), decrease gluconeogenesis and inhibit intestinal absorption.

4. Pharmacodynamics. Absorbed well by mouth. Maximal activity in about four hours. Major portion excreted in 24 hours.

5. Toxicity. a. Anorexia, nausea, vomiting, diarrhea frequent (probably of central origin) but minimized by low dosage with gradual increase.

b. Hypoglycemia rare, but acidosis and ketosis may appear without glycosuria (accumulation of lactic acid from exercise, lactacidosis).

6. Uses. a. May be used as insulin or sulfonylurea replacement or supplement in severe as well as mild adult diabetes.

b. May supplement insulin in childhood diabetes.

c. Because of toxicity (lactacidosis) use severely restricted.

7. Preparations

PHENFORMIN HYDROCHLORIDE (DBI)

Dose: 25 mg 2 times a day by mouth (initial); increased slowly to 25 to 50 mg 2 or 3 times a day.

OTHERS

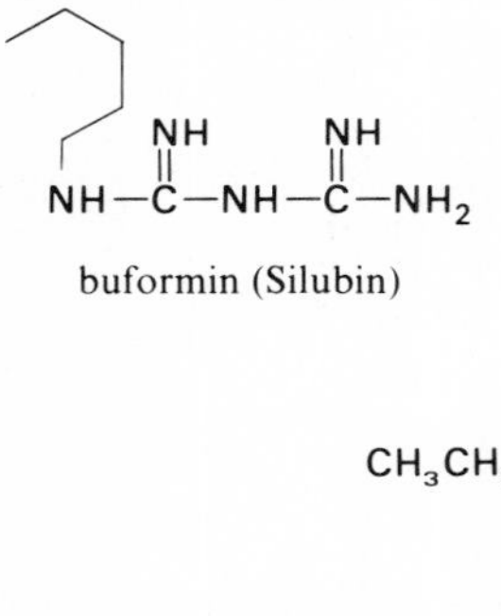

$$\text{(butyl)}-NH-\overset{NH}{\overset{\|}{C}}-NH-\overset{NH}{\overset{\|}{C}}-NH_2$$

buformin (Silubin)

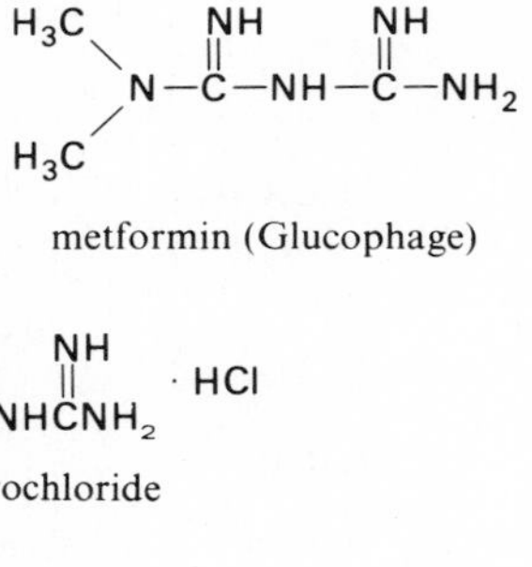

$$(H_3C)_2N-\overset{NH}{\overset{\|}{C}}-NH-\overset{NH}{\overset{\|}{C}}-NH_2$$

metformin (Glucophage)

$$CH_3CH_2CH_2CH_2NH\overset{CH_3CH_2N}{\overset{\|}{C}}NH\overset{NH}{\overset{\|}{C}}NH_2 \cdot HCl$$

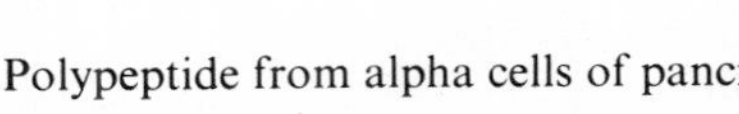

etoformin hydrochloride

C. Agents Producing Hyperglycemia

GLUCAGON

1. Chemistry. Polypeptide from alpha cells of pancreatic islets.

```
      NH2
      |
his-ser-glu-gly-thr-phe-thr-ser-asp-tyr-ser-lys-tyr-leu
                                                     |
                                                    ser
                                                     |
thr-asp-met-leu-tyr-glu-val-phe-asp-glu-ala-arg-arg-asp
    |               |               |
    NH2             NH2             NH2
```

2. Action. a. Raises blood sugar by increasing breakdown of glycogen to glucose in the liver.

b. May be a physiological antagonist to insulin, liberated and acting during hypoglycemia (Foa).

c. Is an inotropic and chronotropic agent on the heart, resembling epinephrine.

3. Mechanism. a. Stimulates synthesis of cyclic AMP and thus activates liver phosphorylase, which is the rate-limiting enzyme in the glycogen-glucose conversion.

b. Through the activation of phosphorylase, facilitates breakdown of glycogen to glucose in liver (like epinephrine), but not in muscle (unlike epinephrine).

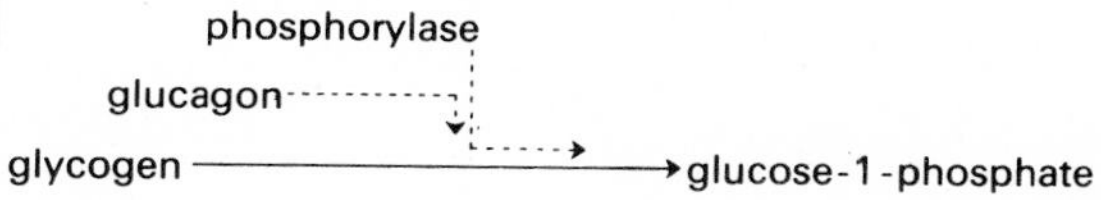

phosphorylase

glucagon ┈┈→

glycogen ——→ glucose-1-phosphate

4. Pharmacodynamics and Toxicity. a. Not active by mouth.

b. May produce mild nausea and vomiting, but apparently of low general toxicity and not sensitizing.

5. Uses. a. Alternative to glucose in insulin reactions with unconsciousness (especially in insulin shock therapy) because easier to administer; patients recover consciousness in 5 to 20 minutes and then should be fed.

b. Experimental in glycogen storage disease (von Gierke's) where glycogen is not broken down with normal ease; result only partially satisfactory.

c. Has been tried in heart failure (20 to 45 mg intravenously) but produces severe nausea.

6. Preparation

GLUCAGON HYDROCHLORIDE

Dose: 0.5 to 2 mg subcutaneously or intramuscularly.

OTHER AGENTS

a. Hypoglycemic

PHLORIDZIN

Glycoside from the root bark of certain fruit trees. Acts by interfering with the reabsorption of glucose by the proximal tubules in the kidney, and thus produces glycosuria. Of experimental interest only.

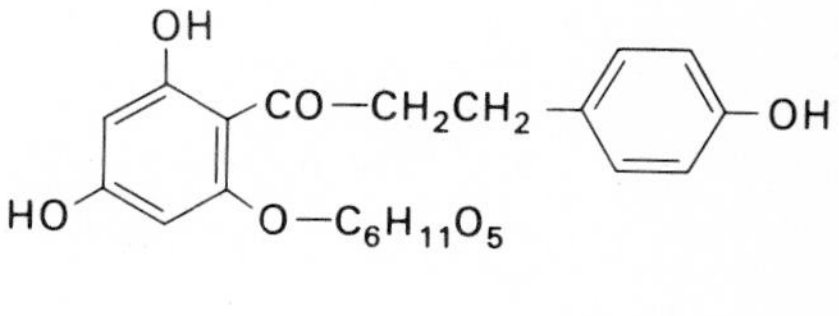

OH; HO; $CO-CH_2CH_2-$(phenyl)$-OH$; $O-C_6H_{11}O_5$

HYPOGLYCINS A and B

Plant amines capable of producing experimental hypoglycemia.

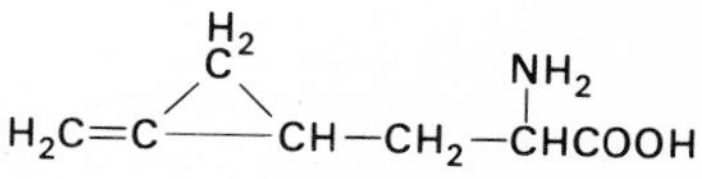

H_2 C; NH_2

$H_2C{=}C$—$CH-CH_2-CHCOOH$

hypoglycin A

DIAZOXIDE

Used orally as an antihypoglemic (See Thiazides).

b. Hyperglycemic

ALLOXAN

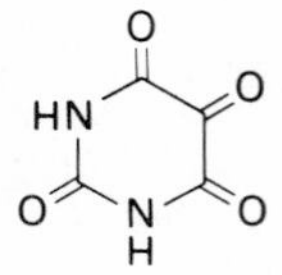

Dunn (1943) showed that alloxan could destroy the β cells of the pancreatic islets. It apparently acts by attaching to SH groups and lowering the blood glutathione; its action is prevented by such glutathione sources as glutathione itself, and cysteine.

STREPTOZOCIN

Acts similarly to Alloxan (see Cancer Chemotherapy).

D. Sweetening Agents

1. Uses. Sweetening agents are useful to increase the palatability of low caloric or low carbohydrate diets and so may be useful in the treatment of diabetes or obesity.

2. Preparations

ASPARTAME

Artificial sweetener.

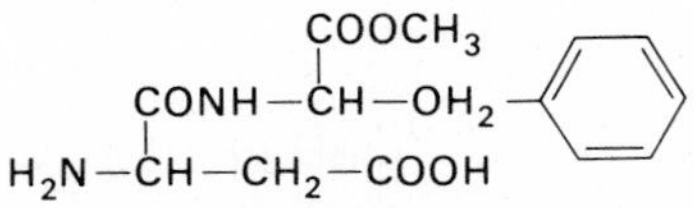

SACCHARIN SODIUM

Dose: 15 mg by mouth as desired; nontoxic.

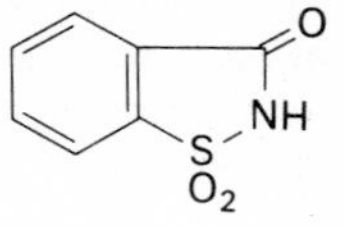

CYCLAMIC ACID

CYCLAMATE SODIUM OR CALCIUM (Sucaryl)

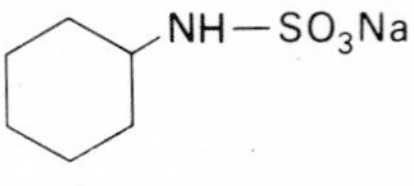

Ten % sodium or calcium saccharin added to overcome bitterness.

Withdrawn because of experimental cancer in rats, and chromosome breaks in rat and human cells in vitro.

SUMMARY: AGENTS IN DIABETES MELLITUS

TYPE	*ACTION AND MECHANISM*	*TOXICITY*	*USE*	*EXAMPLES*
Insulin	Lower blood sugar by facilitating penetration of glucose into cells	Hypoglycemia	Diabetes mellitus	Lente insulin

SUMMARY: AGENTS IN DIABETES MELLITUS (contd.)

TYPE	*ACTION AND MECHANISM*	*TOXICITY*	*USE*	*EXAMPLES*
Sulfonylurea insulin substitutes	Lower blood sugar by releasing insulin from beta cells of islets	Urticaria, jaundice, agranulocytosis, Increased mortality from heart disease	Adult-onset diabetes	Chlorpropamide
Biguanide insulin substitutes	Increase peripheral utilization of insulin	Nausea, diarrhea, hypoglycemia, lactacidosis	Adult diabetes	Phenformin HCl
Hyperglycemic agents	Facilitates breakdown of glycogen to glucose in liver	Nausea, vomiting	Hypoglycemia	Glucagon HCl
Sweetening agents	Low calorie sweeteners	Minor (except cyclamates)	Dietary agents	Saccharin sodium

Reviews

Levine, R., and Berger, S. Orally active hypoglycemic substances and the rationale of their use. Clin. Pharmacol. Ther., 1:227, 1961.

Butterfield, W., and Mahler, R. "Hypoglycemic Agents in Diabetes Mellitus," in Recent Advances in Pharmacology, 3rd ed., Robson, J., and Stacey, R. (eds.), Boston, Little, Brown, 1962.

Duncan, L., and Clarke, B. Pharmacology and mode of action of the hypoglycaemic sulphonylureas and diguanides. Ann. Rev. Pharmacol., 5:151, 1965.

Singer, D., and Hurwitz, D. Long-term experience with sulfonylureas and placebo. New Eng. J. Med., 277:450, 1967.

Davidoff, F. Oral hypoglycemic agents and the mechanism of diabetes mellitus. New Eng. J. Med., 278:148, 1968.

38.
Parathyroid Hormone and Calcium Metabolism

A. Calcium Metabolism

1. Chemistry. a. Normal diet contains about 1 gm of calcium daily.

b. Exists in blood about one-half ionized (active) and one-half bound to protein (inactive), but in equilibrium.

2. Action

a. Calcium is required for the following purposes:

a′. Construction and maintenance of the bony skeleton.

b′. Contraction of skeletal and cardiac muscle.

c′. Nerve conduction; decreased calcium increases irritability and may produce tetany.

d′. Maintenance of membrane permeability; decreased calcium increases permeability; partial mechanism for effects on muscle contraction and nerve transmission.

e′. Blood coagulation; necessary for conversion of prothrombin to thrombin.

b. Calcium in the blood has a partially reciprocal status with phosphorus, and is influenced by the presence of vitamin D and parathyroid hormone.

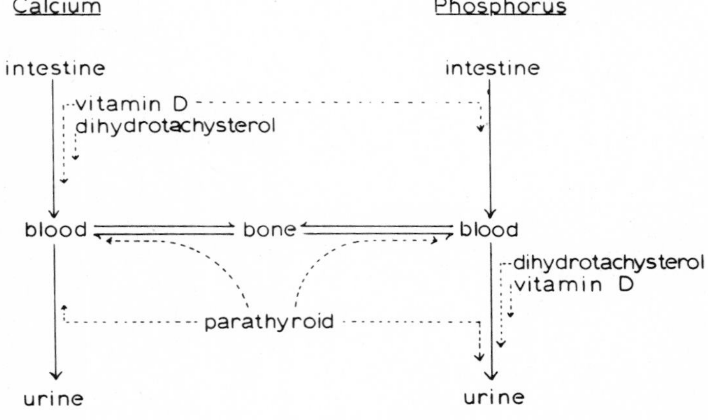

3. Role in Disease. a. Hypercalcemia: May be produced by hyperparathyroidism, hypervitaminosis D or dihydrotachysterol, physical immobilization; characterized by anorexia, nausea, polyuria, headache, kidney stones, tissue calcification.

b. Hypocalcemia: May be produced by hypoparathyroidism, severe vitamin D deficiency, steatorrhea, hypoproteinemia, low calcium intake, chronic renal disease; characterized by tetany, cataract, coarse skin, nails, and hair.

4. Pharmacodynamics. a. Absorbed in the upper gastrointestinal tract; absorption promoted by vitamin D and to a minor extent by dihydrotachysterol; absorption also promoted by an acid medium and low P content of the food, diminished by fat, oxalates, Mg, K.

b. Excretion 30% or more in urine, balance in stool.

5. Toxicity. Production of hypercalcemia relatively easy with vitamin D, dihydrotachysterol, or parathyroid.

6. Uses. a. Medicinal calcium is used to supplement that of the diet during pregnancy and lactation, where the requirement rises to 2 or 3 gm daily.

b. In hypocalcemic tetany it should be given intravenously at once to relieve symptoms, and orally to supplement dihydrotachysterol or other therapy as long as the condition persists.

c. The absorption of calcium may be facilitated by reducing the P content in the bowel, either by reducing the intake, or by simultaneous administration of $Al(OH)_3$ which forms insoluble P salts.

7. Preparations

CALCIUM CARBONATE
(See Antacids)

CALCIUM CHLORIDE
(See Diuretics)

CALCIUM GLUBIONATE (Neo-Calglucon)

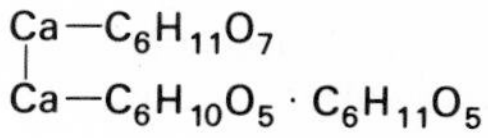

$$\begin{array}{l} Ca-C_6H_{11}O_7 \\ | \\ Ca-C_6H_{10}O_5 \cdot C_6H_{11}O_5 \end{array}$$

Contains 6% calcium.
Dose: 15 ml of 10% solution by mouth 3 times a day.

CALCIUM GLUCEPTATE

Dose: 5 to 20 ml of 23% solution intravenously.

CALCIUM GLUCONATE

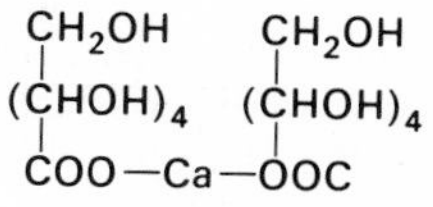

$$\begin{array}{ccc} CH_2OH & & CH_2OH \\ | & & | \\ (CHOH)_4 & & (CHOH)_4 \\ | & & | \\ COO & -Ca- & OOC \end{array}$$

Contains 9% calcium.

Dose: 5 to 30 gm daily by mouth, or 10 to 20 ml of 10% solution intramuscularly or intravenously.

CALCIUM LACTATE

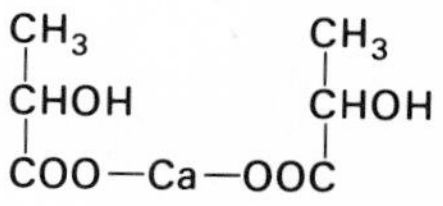

$$\begin{array}{ccc} CH_3 & & CH_3 \\ | & & | \\ CHOH & & CHOH \\ | & & | \\ COO & -Ca- & OOC \end{array}$$

Contains 13% calcium.
Dose: 5 to 30 gm daily by mouth.

CALCIUM LEVULINATE $(CH_3-CO-CH_2-CH_2-COO)_2Ca$

Contains 13% calcium.
Dose: 5 to 10 ml of 10% solution intravenously.
4 to 5 gm powder 3 times a day orally.

CALCIUM PHOSPHATE DIBASIC: $CaHPO_4$

Contains 30% calcium.
Dose: 4 to 8 gm daily by mouth.

B. Parathyroid Hormone

1. History. a. Gley (1891) showed that extirpation of parathyroids produced tetany.

b. McCollum and Voegtlin (1908) demonstrated relationship to calcium metabolism; mechanism studied by Albright (1929 and later).

c. Hanson (1924) and Collip (1926) prepared extracts; Rasmussen (1961) determined structure.

2. Chemistry. a. Polypeptide containing 84 residues of 17 amino acids; mol. wt. of about 9,500.

b. Of the 84 amino acids, 34 appear to be necessary for activity, 50 others to stabilize.

3. Action

a. Raises blood calcium and lowers blood phosphorus by:

a′. Mobilizing P and Ca from bone to blood by stimulating osteoclasts; mechanism involves production of lactate or citrate in bone.

b′. Repressing tubular reabsorption of P but increasing that of Ca in the kidney.

c′. Promoting absorption of calcium from the intestine.

b. Secretion of parathyroid hormone controlled by the blood level of Ca or P; not influenced by the pituitary.

4. Mechanism. Regulation of transport of divalent ions across membranes, especially mitochondrial membranes, probably by increasing cyclic AMP.

5. Role in Disease. a. Hyperparathyroidism: Parathyroid tumors may produce excessive parathyroid hormone with resultant mobilization of calcium from bone and decalcification, nephrocalcinosis from the increased level of Ca, and anorexia and muscular weakness. The blood Ca is high; the P low. Treatment is by surgical removal of the tumor.

b. Hypoparathyroidism: Parathyroid deficiency may be idiopathic, or the result of surgical removal incident to thyroidectomy. It is characterized by the signs of hypocalcemia: tetany, trophic changes in the lens, nails, and skin, and a low Ca with a raised P in the blood. Treatment is by calcium administration (intravenously in acute tetany) and dihydrotachysterol or vitamin D. Therapy should be controlled so that Ca is barely present in the urine (slight cloud with Sulkowitch test).

6. Pharmacodynamics. a. Effective only after parenteral injection.

b. Action delayed until 4 hours after administration; duration 24 hours.

c. Effect is transient with present preparations, disappearing after 3 or 4 weeks of administration, presumably because of the development of antibodies to (contaminating?) foreign protein.

7. Toxicity. Excessive dosage may produce hypercalcemia.

8. Uses. a. There is little rational use for present preparations, except temporarily in occasional patients unresponsive to hypercalcemic steroids.

b. Synthetic hormone (consisting of the active 1–34 amino acids) is available for investigation.

9. Preparation

PARATHYROID INJECTION (Parathormone)
(1 u = approx. 0.4 mcg bovine parathyroid hormone)
Dose: 100 to 300 units subcutaneously.

C. Calcitonin

1. History. Discovered by Copp (1962).

2. Chemistry. A series of related polypeptides secreted by parafollicular cells in the thyroid in man and in the ultimobranchial body in most vertebrates.

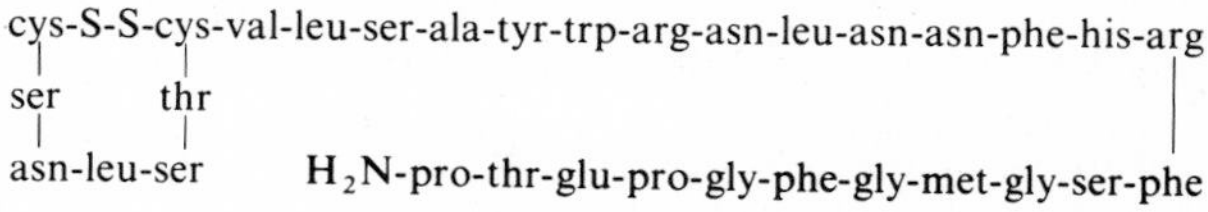

```
cys-S-S-cys-val-leu-ser-ala-tyr-trp-arg-asn-leu-asn-asn-phe-his-arg
 |       |                                                       |
ser     thr                                                      |
 |       |                                                       |
asn-leu-ser      H2N-pro-thr-glu-pro-gly-phe-gly-met-gly-ser-phe
```

porcine calcitonin

3. Bioassay. Activity compared with the British Medical Research Council (MRC) standard and expressed as MRC unit; 1 MRC u = 4 μg pure porcine calcitonin.

4. Action. a. Lowers blood calcium by inhibiting bone resorption.

b. Increases excretion of calcium and phosphate in urine and lowers blood PO_4.

5. Toxicity. Nausea, irritation at the site of injection, allergic reactions.

6. Uses. Drug of choice in Paget's disease. May be useful in hyperparathyroidism.

7. Preparation

CALCITONIN-SALMON (Calcimar)

Synthetic polypeptide consisting of 32 amino acids, same sequence as in the natural product; in 16% gelatin solution.

Dose: 100 MRC u daily subcutaneously or intramuscularly.

D. Hypercalcemic Steroids

VITAMIN D

1. History. a. Mellanby (1919) showed that experimental rickets could be prevented by cod liver oil; Huldschinsky (1919) showed that ultraviolet light was also effective.

b. McCollum (1922) separated vitamin A and D effects.

c. Hess (1924) and Steenbock (1924) irradiated food containing ergosterol, thus producing vitamin D.

2. Chemistry. a. Ultraviolet irradiation of various steroid precursors produces hypercalcemic compounds; vitamin D generic term for the active group.

b. Ergosterol is the most important commercial precursor; 7-dehydrocholesterol is the normal precursor in the body; the active products are calciferol and vitamin D_3, respectively:

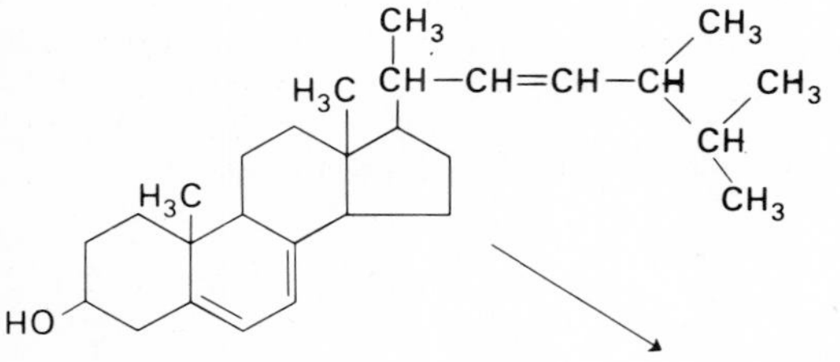

CH_3 CH_3 H_3C CH—CH=CH—CH CH_3 CH H_3C CH_3 HO

ergosterol

CH_3 CH_3 H_3C CH—CH=CH—CH CH_3 CH H_2C CH_3 HO

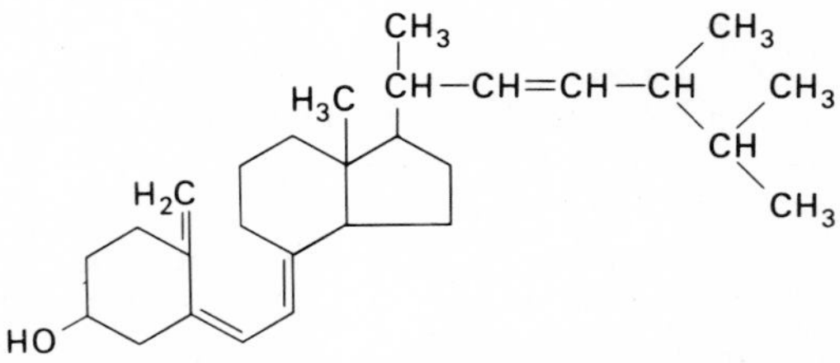

calciferol (vitamin D_2)

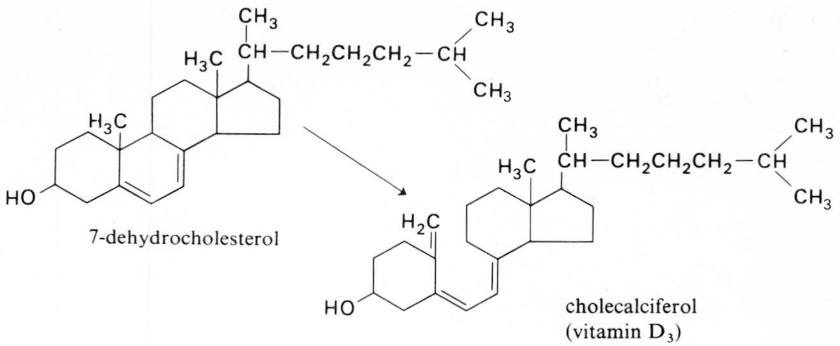

7-dehydrocholesterol

cholecalciferol
(vitamin D_3)

3. Action. a. In man vitamin D_2 and D_3 possess the same antirachitic property.

b. Primary actions: a′. increase intestinal absorption of calcium.

b′. Promote Ca mobilization from bone.

c′. Promote reabsorption of Ca and PO_4 in the kidney (larger doses increase PO_4 excretion).

d′. Essential for the function of parathyroid.

4. Mechanism. a. Vitamin D is inactive, the active form is 1,25-OH-D_3. The conversion occurs in the liver (cholecalciferol-25-hydroxylase) and in the kidney (25-hydroxycholecalciferol-1-hydroxylase).

b. The RNA directs the synthesis of the enzyme system responsible for the metabolic activation of vitamin D.

5. Pharmacodynamics and Toxicity. a. Well absorbed by mouth.

b. Pharmacologically inactive except for influence on Ca and P metabolism.

c. Large doses may mobilize Ca from bone, probably as the result of the increased P excretion, producing rarefaction of the bone hypercalcinemia, and metastatic calcification elsewhere (especially nephrocalcinosis).

6. Uses. a. For the treatment and prevention of rickets, where a vitamin D deficiency prevents adequate absorption of Ca, with resultant improper calcification of epiphyseal bone and bony deformities.

b. Also in osteomalacia (adult rickets of the Orient) and hypoparathyroidism.

7. Preparations

CHOLOCALCIFEROL

ERGOCALCIFEROL (calciferol; vitamin D_2; Drisdol)

Dose: 1,000 to 50,000 IU daily by mouth (rickets); 50,000 to 150,000 IU daily by mouth (hypoparathyroidism). (1 IU = 0.025 μg of vitamin D_3.)

SYNTHETIC OLEOVITAMIN D (solution of calciferol or activated 7-dehydrocholesterol in oil; Viosterol in oil)

Doses as for calciferol.

FISH LIVER OILS (often fortified with calciferol and containing vitamin A)

Doses equivalent to those for calciferol.

DIHYDROTACHYSTEROL

1. Chemistry. UV irradiation of ergosterol produces tachysterol as well as calciferol; then reduced to isomeric dihydro forms.

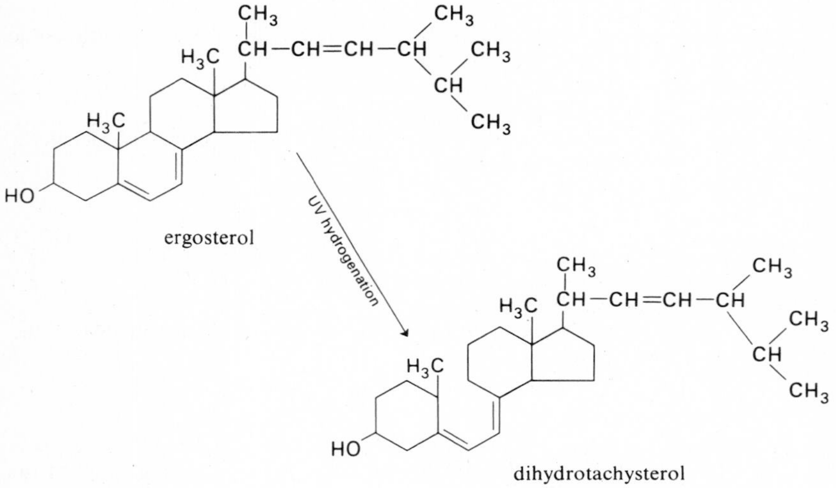

ergosterol

UV hydrogenation

dihydrotachysterol

2. Action. Similar to those of vitamin D, but proportionately more increase in P excretion and less effect on Ca absorption. Effective in mobilizing calcium from the bone.

3. Pharmacodynamics and Toxicity. a. Adequately absorbed by mouth.

b. Excessive dosage produces hypercalcemia, similar to that from excessive vitamin D, with anorexia, loss of weight, and occasionally kidney stones.

4. Uses. To raise and maintain serum calcium in hypocalcemic tetany.

5. Preparation

DIHYDROTACHYSTEROL (Hytakerol)

Dose: Initial: 0.8 to 2.4 mg/day; maintenance: 0.2 to 1.0 mg/day.

E. Phosphorus Metabolism

1. Action

a. Phosphorus is involved in several physiological processes:

a′. Bone formation and maintenance.

b′. Phosphorylation in metabolic processes; high energy phosphate is the fuel of the body (ATP).

c′. Synthesis of phospholipids; nucleic acids.

d′. Buffering action of salts in various body fluids.

b. The adult requires about 1.5 gm of P daily; in pregnancy and lactation the amount rises to 2.5 to 3 gm.

c. The control of P absorption and metabolism are discussed under Calcium.

2. Role in Disease. a. Hyperphosphatemia: may result from vitamin D excess, hypoparathyroidism, renal failure.

b. Hypophosphatemia: may result from vitamin D deficit, hyperparathyroidism, steatorrhea.

3. Uses. It is rarely necessary to administer phosphorus since the dietary intake is ordinarily adequate.

SUMMARY: PARATHYROID HORMONE AND CALCIUM METABOLISM

TYPE	*ACTION AND MECHANISM*	*TOXICITY*	*USE*	*EXAMPLES*
Calcium preparations	Raise calcium level in body	Minor	Dietary supplement, hypocalcemic tetany	Calcium gluconate
Parathyroid hormone	Mobilizes calcium from bone	Anorexia, nephrocalcinosis	None	Parathyroid injection
Calcitonin	Lowers blood Ca by inhibiting bone resorption	Under study	Osteoporosis?	Calcitonin
Vitamin D	Increases absorption of Ca and P from intestine	Metastatic calcification	Rickets, osteomalacia hypoparathyroidism	Ergocalciferol
Dihydrotachysterol	Similar	Similar	Hypoparathyroidism	Dihydrotachysterol

Reviews

Munson, P. Endocrine pharmacology. Ann. Rev. Pharmacol., 1:315, 1961.

Arnaud, C., Tenenhouse, A., and Rasmussen, H. Parathyroid hormone. Ann. Rev. Physiol., 29:349, 1967.

Foster, G. Calcitonin (Thyrocalcitonin). New Eng. J. Med., 279:349, 1968.

Copp, D. Calcitonin and parathyroid hormone. Ann. Rev. Pharmacol., 9:327, 1969.

39. The Vitamins

The vitamins are essential nutrients which do not give energy but are required in small amounts for normal metabolism. They are relatively simple organic compounds, originally thought by Funk (1911) to be "vital amines," hence the name "vitamin." Most have been synthesized, but for normal persons foods remain the cheapest and most desirable sources.

Most vitamins act physiologically by being integral parts of coenzymes. In enzymatic reactions the apoenzyme determines the substrate specificity, but may have a coenzyme associated with it which determines the chemical nature of the reaction.

VITAMIN A

1. History. a. Stepp (1909), Osborne and Mendel (1911), Hopkins (1912), McCollum (1914), Drummond (1925) all demonstrated variously that butter fat contained an unknown growth factor for animals, absent from lard, called vitamin A.

b. Moore (1930) showed that carotene had vitamin A activity; Karrer (1931) determined the structure and (1936) synthesized vitamin A.

2. Chemistry. a. Carotenes (α, β, γ) and cryptoxanthin are fat-soluble lipochromes formed in plants and diatoms.

b. They are converted into vitamin A (the active form) in the intestinal mucosa or liver (man) of animals.

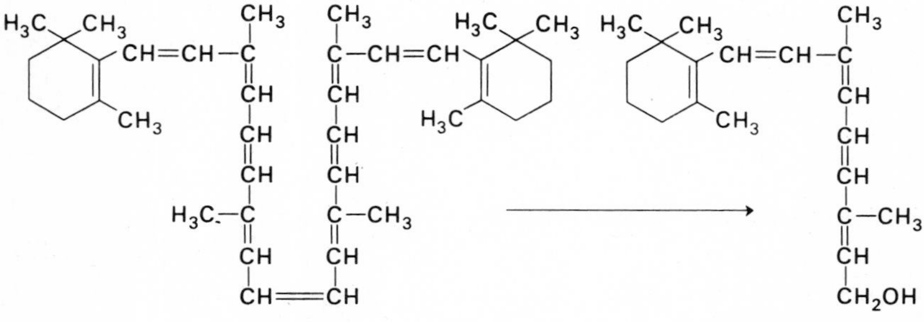

carotene → vitamin A

c. Dietary sources of carotene or vitamin A include: vegetables, butter (20 units/gm), eggs, milk (1 unit/gm); fish liver oils.

3. Action and Mechanism. a. Maintains the integrity of epithelium by preventing metaplasia to the stratified squamous type. May act by stabilizing SH groups in protein and maintaining normal amounts of mucoprotein, glycoprotein, and keratoprotein in epithelial structures; effect may be by release of a protease in cells.

b. Promotes cyclic resynthesis of visual purple. Vitamin A is converted enzymatically to retinaldehyde, which then reacts with the protein, opsin, forming rhodopsin (visual purple). Rhodopsin is converted into retinene by light (in the most sensitive chemical reaction known: 1 quantum of light changes 1 molecule and a change of 8 or 9 quanta can be discerned), and is then regenerated from retinene in the absence of light.

c. Beta carotene protects against sunlight damage in erythropoetic porphyruria.

4. Role in Disease. Deficiency of vitamin A may produce:

a. Hyperkeratosis, a condition in which the skin is horny and rough, especially around the hair follicles, and xerophthalmia, in which metaplasia of the cornea and conjunctiva may produce ulceration and necrosis.

b. Night blindness, in which decreased formation of rhodopsin reduces vision, especially in poor light.

5. Pharmacodynamics. a. Absorption is good by mouth, best from an aqueous medium.

b. Distribution wide; stored in the liver.

c. Vitamin A may be assayed chemically (spectrophotometrically) or biologically (growth rate in rats). One unit = 0.6 mcg.

6. Toxicity. Overdosage gives hypervitaminosis A, characterized by anorexia, irritability, pruritis, alopecia, cracked lips, hepatomegaly, and periosteal thickening.

7. Uses. a. To prevent or cure vitamin A deficiency producing hyperkeratosis, xerophthalmia, night blindness.

b. Normal requirement: 5,000 IU daily; prophylactic supplement: 3,000 to 5,000 IU daily.

c. Therapeutic dosage: 5,000 to 10,000 IU daily; in steatorrhea, or other deficiency of fat absorption, up to 50,000 IU daily.

8. Preparations

a. Vitamin A and related compounds

TRETINOIN (retinoic acid, RetinA)

Keratolytic agent used in acne. Under investigation.

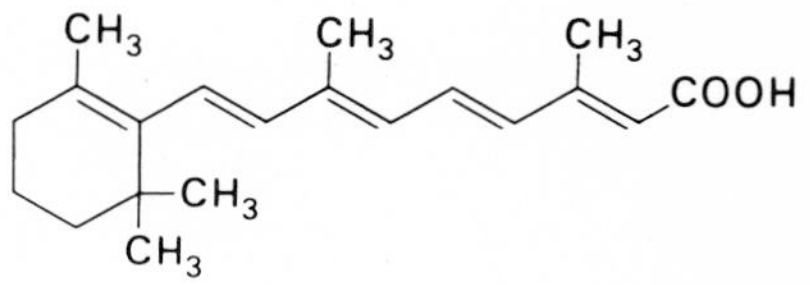

CH_3 CH_3 CH_3 COOH CH_3 CH_3

VITAMIN A: contains 50,000 IU per gm.

Vitamin A, water-miscible: contains 50,000 IU per gm.

b. Preparations containing vitamins A and D

COD LIVER OIL

Contains 850 IU per gm.

HALIBUT LIVER OIL

Contains 5,000 or 25,000 IU per gm.

PERCOMORPH LIVER OIL

Contains 60,000 IU per gm.

THIAMIN

1. History. a. Adm. Takaki (1884) showed that beriberi was caused by eating polished rice; Eijkman that the polyneuritis of chickens was due to polished rice and preventable by rice bran.

b. Jansen and Donath (1926) isolated and crystallized thiamin; Williams (1936) synthesized it.

2. Chemistry. a. Pyrimidine-thiazole derivative; water-soluble; moderately heat-stable.

b. Dietary sources include: yeast, whole grains (germ and outer layers of seeds, nuts, legumes), pork, liver, muscle, eggs.

3. Action and Mechanism. a. Constituent of cocarboxylase, which is essential for the anaerobic decarboxylation of pyruvic acid to acetate, and hence for proper carbohydrate metabolism (Peters, 1936):

thiamin + pyrophosphate (ATP)

↘

cocarboxylase + Mg + carboxylase
(coenzyme) (enzyme)

pyruvic acid ⟶ acetate

b. Thiamin diphosphate (pyrophosphate) is also a coenzyme in the reactions of transketolation that occur in the direct oxidative pathway for glucose metabolism.

c. May be a coenzyme in a system activating pyruvate for participation in many reactions; may be an inhibitor of cholinesterase.

4. Role in Disease. Deficiency causes beriberi, characterized by apathy, weakness, polyneuritis, edema, heart failure (high output); alcoholic neuritis (Wernicke's) usually beriberi.

5. Pharmacodynamics and Toxicity. a. Absorption excellent by all routes.

b. Distribution wide; excretion rapid and renal (practically quantitative in a nondeficient person).

c. Toxicity is nil except for occasional allergic hypersensitivity.

6. Uses. a. To prevent and cure beriberi or the thiamin deficiency element in multiple deficiencies.

b. Possibly of limited use to stimulate the appetite; incidental mosquito and flea repellent.

c. Normal requirement: 2 mg daily (0.5 mg, children; 3 mg, pregnant and nursing women).

d. Therapeutic dosage: 2 to 10 mg (of little value to increase dose above 10 mg owing to rapid excretion).

7. Preparations

THIAMIN HYDROCHLORIDE (Aneurin)

Dose: 1 mg to 10 mg daily by mouth, subcutaneously, intramuscularly, or intravenously.

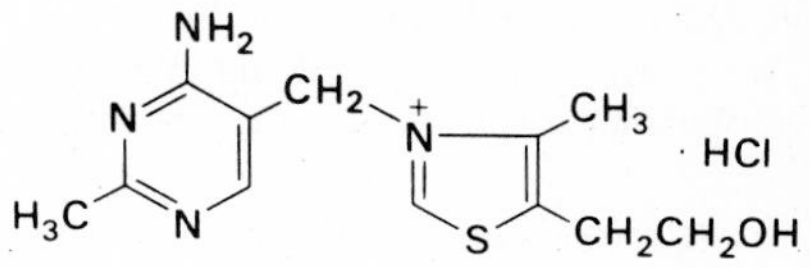

WHEAT GERM

Contains 1 mg per 100 mg.

YEAST, DRIED (Brewers' yeast)

Contains 10 mg per 100 mg.

8. Antithiamin Substances

PYRITHIAMINE

Experimental antagonist requiring 5 times the concentration of thiamin.

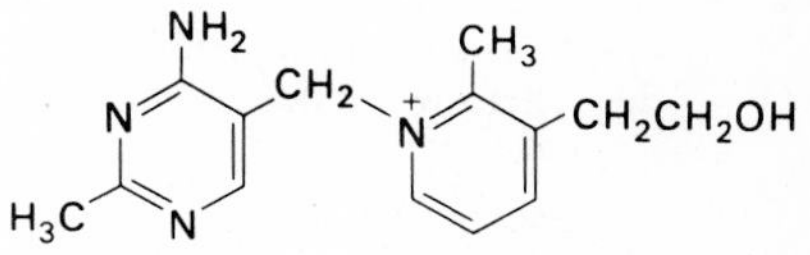

OXYTHIAMINE

Thiamin antagonist.

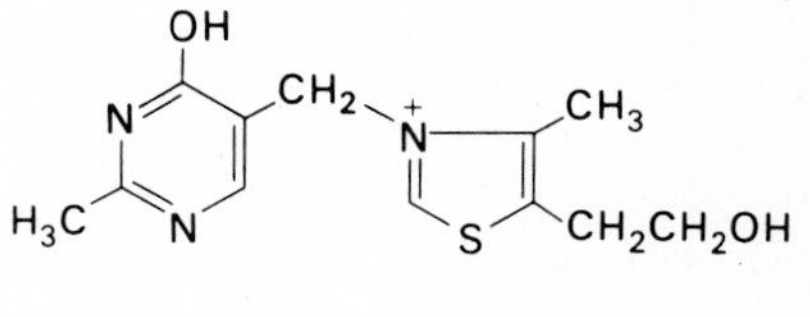

NATURAL THIAMINASES

In fish fed to foxes, giving deficiency; in bracken eaten by horses, giving staggers; curable by thiamin.

NIACIN

1. History. a. Goldberger (1925) produced black tongue in dogs, and pellagra in man, by diet deficient in "PP" factor.

b. Spies (1935) found that yeast extracts contained the PP factor and cured black tongue.

c. Elvehjem (1937) identified nicotinic acid amide as the essential agent.

2. Chemistry. a. Nicotinic acid (niacin) functions in the body as the amide.

b. Water-soluble, heat-stable; not closely related to nicotine.

c. Dietary sources include: yeast, wheat germ, green leafy vegetables, legumes; liver, kidney, muscle, milk, fish.

3. Action and Mechanism. a. Essential component of coenzymes I and II (diphosphopyridine nucleotide (DPN); triphosphopyridine nucleotide (TPN)).

b. Both enzymes serve as hydrogen acceptors and donors in oxidation-reduction reactions of the citric acid cycle and in carbohydrate, fat, and protein metabolism.

c. Niacin (not niacinamide) is a vasodilator.

4. Role in Disease. a. Deficiency causes pellagra, characterized by glossitis, dermatitis, and encephalopathy.

b. Deficiency of the niacin precursor, tryptophan, in the diet, and an inhibitory factor in corn (maize), may also be factors.

5. Pharmacodynamics. a. Absorption is good by mouth.

b. Distribution is wide; excretion is in the urine, largely as combination products such as trigonelline.

6. Toxicity. a. Nil except for vascular effects: transient "nitritoid" flushing.

7. Uses. a. In the prevention and treatment of pellagra.

b. Also in angina, migraine, Ménière's disease as a vasodilator; in atherosclerosis as a cholesterol lowering agent.

c. Normal requirement: 25 mg daily.

d. Therapeutic dosage: 100 to 500 mg daily.

8. Preparations

NIACIN (nicotinic acid)

Dose: 25 mg or more 4 times a day by mouth.

COOH
N

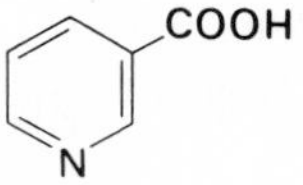

NIACINAMIDE (nicotinic acid amide)

Dose: 25 mg or more 4 times a day by mouth.

$CONH_2$
N

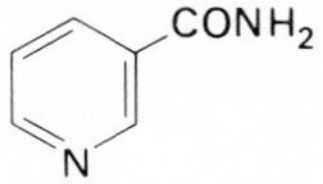

NADIDE (Enzopride)

Diphosphopyridine nucleotide; tried in alcoholism.
Dose: Under investigation.

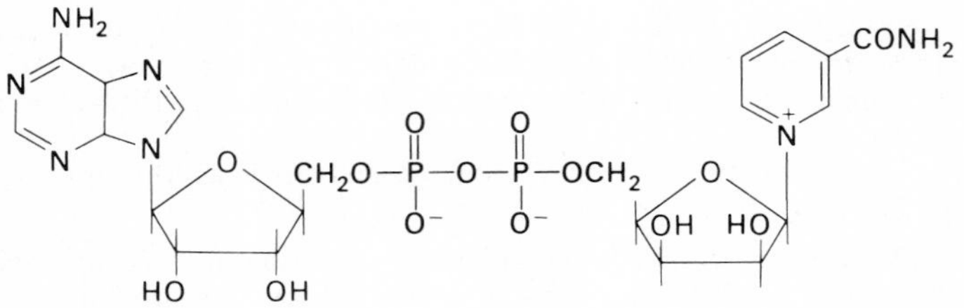

NH_2 N N N N O $CH_2O-\overset{O}{\overset{\|}{P}}-O-\overset{O}{\overset{\|}{P}}-OCH_2$ O^- O^- O HO OH OH HO $CONH_2$ $\overset{+}{N}$

RIBOFLAVIN

1. **History.** a. Blyth (1879) identified riboflavin as a yellow pigment in milk.

b. Emmet and Luros (1919) showed it to have a growth promoting action in rats.

c. Sebrell and Butler (1938) demonstrated its use in cheilosis.

2. **Chemistry.** a. A heat-stable flavin riboside; constituent of flavin adenine dinucleotide.

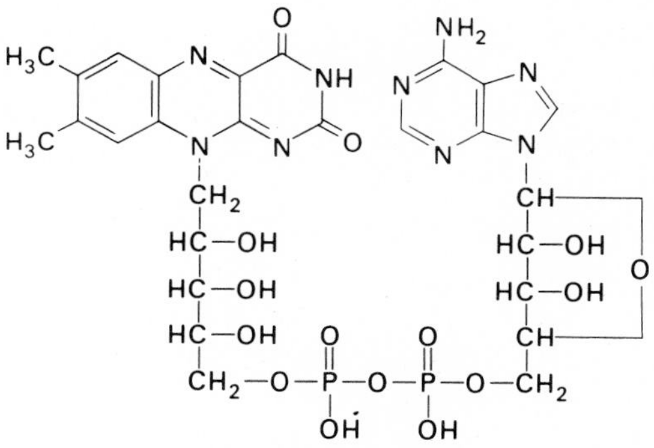

flavin adenine dinucleotide

b. Dietary sources include yeast, wheat germ, green vegetables, liver, milk, eggs, cheese, muscle.

3. **Action and Mechanism.** a. As riboflavin phosphate, or riboflavin adenine nucleotide, acts as a coenzyme in enzyme systems for hydrogen transport in the Krebs cycle, degradation of fatty acids, oxidation of pyruvic acid in the nervous system, and others.

b. The apoenzymes include Warburg's yellow enzyme, the diaphorases, cytochrome C reductase, xanthine oxidase.

4. **Role in Disease.** Deficiency causes cheilosis, glossitis, keratitis; however, these states are not as severe as would be expected from the ubiquitous involvement of the coenzyme.

5. **Pharmacodynamics and Toxicity.** Absorption easy by mouth. Distribution wide; excess is excreted in the urine. There is no apparent toxicity.

6. **Uses.** a. Replacement therapy in states of riboflavin and general B complex deficiencies.

b. Normal requirement: 2 mg per day (2.5 mg in pregnancy). Therapeutic: 2 to 15 mg.

7. Preparations

RIBOFLAVIN

Dose: 5 mg daily by mouth.

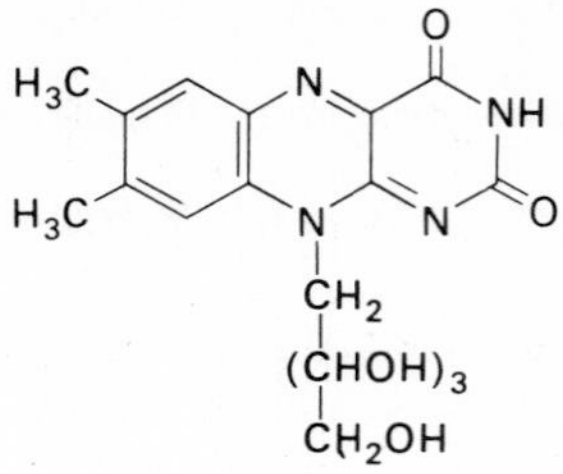

METHYLOL RIBOFLAVIN
(Hyflavin)

A mixture of methylol derivatives.

Dose: 10 mg subcutaneously or intramuscularly.

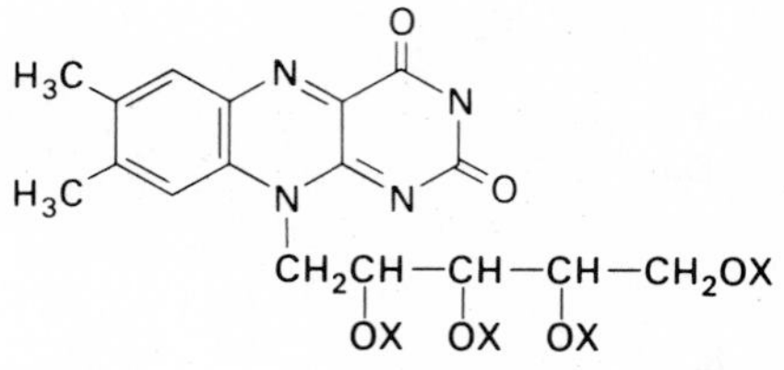

X = H, CH_2OH

PYRIDOXINE

1. History. György (1935) showed that deficiency produced rat dermatitis.

2. Chemistry. a. Occurs in nature as a mixture of three related pyridine derivatives; interconversion carried out in the body.

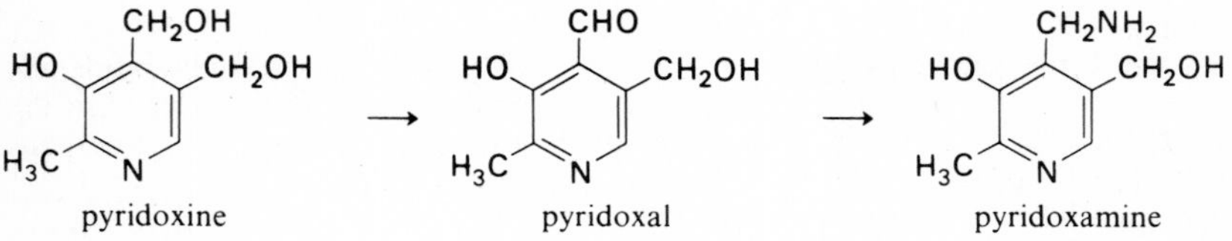

pyridoxine → pyridoxal → pyridoxamine

b. Dietary sources include yeast, rice bran, wheat germ, crude cane molasses, liver.

3. Action and Mechanism. a. In the active forms of phosphorylated pyridoxal or pyridoxamine, an essential coenzyme in enzyme systems for the decarboxylation, transamination, and racemization of amino acids.

b. May also assist in the transport of amino acids across membranes, in the synthesis of unsaturated fatty acids, and in the conversion of tryptophan to nicotinic acid.

4. Role in Disease. a. Deficiency causes dermatitis, convulsive seizures, anemia, variously in different species; not a prominent deficiency in man.

b. Carbazides, such as isoniazid, and EDTA may induce pyridoxine deficiency.

5. **Pharmacodynamics and Toxicity.** Absorption, distribution, and excretion are satisfactory. Toxicity is nil.

6. **Uses.** a. Presumably should be useful in recognized deficiencies.
b. Prophylactically in treatment with isoniazid or hydralazine.
c. For treatment of pyridoxine-responsive anemia, a rare disease.
d. Has been tried with dubious results in parkinsonism, vomiting of pregnancy.

7. **Preparation**

PYRIDOXINE HYDROCHLORIDE (Vitamin B_6)
Dose: 10 mg daily by mouth.

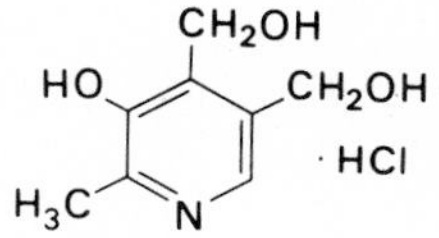

CH_2OH / HO / CH_2OH / $\cdot HCl$ / H_3C / N

8. **Antipyridoxine Substances**

DESOXYPYRIDOXINE
Used experimentally.

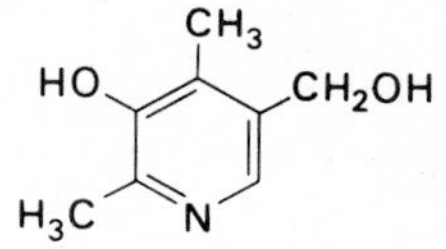

CH_3 / HO / CH_2OH / H_3C / N

PANTOTHENIC ACID

1. **History.** a. Williams (1933) noted it to be a growth factor essential for yeast.
b. Woolley (1939) and Jukes (1939) showed that the chick antidermatitis factor was pantothenic acid.
c. Williams (1939) determined the structure; Stiller (1940) synthesized it.

2. **Chemistry.** a. A labile oil, but with a stable Ca salt; dextro isomer active.
b. Dietary sources include yeast, rice bran, wheat bran, crude cane molasses, liver, egg yolk.

3. **Action and Mechanism.** Constituent of coenzyme A which is involved in the synthesis of acetylcholine and other acetylations, in the first step of the Krebs cycle, and in fatty acid metabolism and amino acid synthesis.

4. **Role in Disease.** a. Deficiency causes chick dermatitis and CNS degeneration, rat adrenal necrosis and alopecia, and dog liver degeneration.
b. In man, CNS changes have been reported after the administration of a pantothenic antagonist.

5. **Pharmacodynamics and Toxicity.** Absorption, distribution, and excretion are satisfactory. Toxicity is nil.

6. **Uses.** Not defined. Normal requirement: 5 mg daily. Therapeutic: 10 to 50 mg daily.

7. Preparations

PANTOTHENIC ACID

Dose: 50 mg by mouth daily.

$$HOCH_2-C(CH_3)_2-CH(OH)-C(=O)-NH-CH_2CH_2-COOH$$

PANTHENOL (pantothenyl alcohol; constituent of Zentinic)

DEXPANTHENOL (Ilopan, Motilyn)

Alcohol analogue of d-pantothenic acid readily converted into pantothenic acid in body, and thus claimed to result in formation of extra acetylcholine and smooth muscle stimulation. Advised in prevention and treatment of intestinal atony, especially after abdominal operations, but evidence for mechanism and effectiveness or superiority over neostigmine or bethanecol poor. Reported to have caused respiratory depression when given within an hour after succinylcholine.

Dose: 250 to 500 mg every 2 to 6 hours intramuscularly for abdominal distention or paralytic ileus.

$$HOCH_2-C(CH_3)_2-CH(OH)-C(=O)-NH-CH_2CH_2CH_2OH$$

8. Antipantothenic Acid Substances

METHYLPANTOTHENIC ACID

Experimental antagonist.

BIOTIN

1. History. a. Bateman (1910) and Boas (1927) showed that high concentrations of egg white were toxic; Eakin (1940) showed this to be due to glycoprotein, avidin.

b. Kögl and Tönnis (1936) obtained a yeast growth factor from egg yolk and named it biotin.

c. György (1940) showed that biotin prevented the egg white injury.

d. Du Vigneaud (1942) determined the structure, and Harris (1943) synthesized biotin.

2. Chemistry. a. An organic acid; dextro form active.

b. Dietary sources include yeast, grains, nuts, vegetables, fruits, liver, kidney, heart, egg yolk, milk, chicken, sea food (ubiquitous in nature); also synthesized by alimentary bacteria.

3. Action and Mechanism. Essential action is as the coenzyme of carboxylation and transcarboxylation processes (Knappe, Ann. Rev. Biochem., 39:757, 1970).

4. Role in Disease. a. Is a growth factor for bacteria.

b. Prevents the spectacle eye of rats produced by avidin.

c. Deficiency may produce a seborrheiclike dermatitis in man.

5. Pharmacodynamics and Toxicity. Absorption, distribution, and excretion apparently satisfactory. Toxicity is nil.

6. Uses. a. Not defined. Normal and therapeutic requirements not defined.
b. Deficiency in rats controlled by minute doses, i.e., 0.1 mcg.

7. Preparation

BIOTIN

Not available for drug use.

$CH_2CH_2CH_2CH_2COOH$

8. Antibiotin Substances

BIOTIN SULFONE

DESTHIOBIOTIN

H_3C $CH_2CH_2CH_2CH_2CH_2COOH$

ASCORBIC ACID

1. History. a. Jacques Cartier (1536) treated scurvy with infusions of pine needles; Lind (1747) showed the efficacy of lime juice.

b. Szent-Györgyi (1928) isolated ascorbic acid from the adrenal, and recognized its action in 1932. King and Waugh (1932) isolated hexuronic acid and identified it with vitamin C.

2. Chemistry. a. Forms an oxidation-reduction system with dehydroascorbic acid; levo form active.

CH_2OH ascorbic acid ⇌ CH_2OH dehydroascorbic acid

ascorbic acid

dehydroascorbic acid

b. Dietary sources include: peppers, oranges, lemons, limes, tomatoes, grapefruit, cabbage, other vegetables and fruits; nondietary sources include: adrenal cortex, pituitary, corpus luteum.

3. Action and Mechanism. a. A strong reducing substance and probably helps to maintain oxidation-reduction conditions appropriate for many enzymatic activities.

b. Probably required for the metabolism of tyrosine.

c. Apparently is involved in the maintenance of collagen in mesenchymal tissues.

4. Role in Disease. Deficiency causes scurvy, characterized by weakening of the intercellular cement substance, especially of capillaries, connective tissue, and bone.

5. Pharmacodynamics and Toxicity. a. Absorption by mouth is good; distribution is wide; it is partly excreted in the urine (25 to 50 mg daily).

b. Toxicity is unknown.

6. Uses. To prevent or treat scurvy. Normal requirement: 30 mg per day. Therapeutic dosage: 100 mg per day.

7. Preparations

ASCORBIC ACID (vitamin C)

Dose: 10 to 50 mg daily by mouth.
Lemon juice and spinach: 60 mg per 100 ml or gm.
Orange juice: 50 mg per 100 ml.
Tomato juice: 30 ml per 100 ml.

VITAMIN E

(d and dl alpha tocopherol and other derivatives.)

1. History. a. Evans (1922) showed that deficiency in rats produced sterility.

b. Synthesized by Karrer (1938).

2. Chemistry. a. Most active of over 100 related compounds of the series.

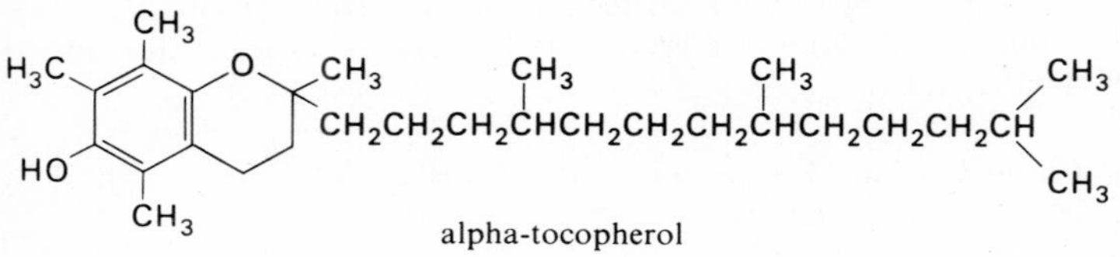

alpha-tocopherol

b. Dietary sources include: leafy green vegetables, wheat germ oil. In almost all plants and animals.

3. Action and Mechanism. a. Essential action unknown.

b. An antioxidant, possibly active within cells.

4. Role in Disease. Deficiency produces germinal atrophy and abortion in rats, defective embryonic development in chicks, and muscular dystrophy in rabbits.

5. Pharmacodyamics and Toxicity. Not well understood. Apparently non-toxic.

6. Uses. a. Has been tried in habitual abortion and muscular dystrophy, but the results are equivocal.

b. Requirements: not known.

7. Preparations

ALPHA-TOCOPHEROL (vitamin E)

Dose: 50 to 100 mg daily by mouth.

TOCOPHERSOLAN

Water-miscible derivative.

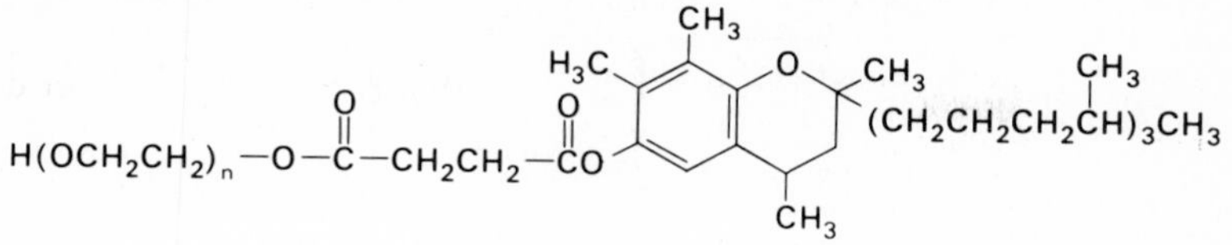

$$H(OCH_2CH_2)_n{-}O{-}\overset{O}{\overset{\|}{C}}{-}CH_2CH_2{-}\overset{O}{\overset{\|}{C}}O$$

CH_3 H_3C O CH_3 CH_3 $(CH_2CH_2CH_2\overset{|}{C}H)_3CH_3$ CH_3

MULTIVITAMIN PREPARATIONS

Preparations, usually capsules, containing varying quantities of most of the better known vitamins, are in wide use. In most cases this represents a waste of expensive drugs. However, at times such preparations may be indicated, as in persons on highly restricted reducing diets. When used for such prophylactic purposes, the content of the various vitamins should be related to the normal requirements for the different substances.

Actual therapeutic need for multiple vitamin supplements, as in the multiple deficiencies usual in pellagra, may also be met by multivitamin preparations, but administration of proper amounts of the agents specifically needed is ordinarily more rational.

1. Preparations

DRIED YEAST, or WHEAT GERM

Sources of the vitamin B complex.

Dose: 30 gm or more daily by mouth.

HEXAVITAMIN CAPSULES, or TABLETS (N.F.)

Contain: vitamin A 1.5 mg, vitamin D 10 mcg, ascrobic acid 75 mg, thiamin hydrochloride 2 mg, riboflavin 3 mg, nicotinamide 20 mg.

Dose: 1 or 2 tablets daily by mouth.

SUMMARY: THE VITAMINS

TYPE	*ACTION AND MECHANISM*	*TOXICITY*	*USE*	*EXAMPLES*
Vitamin A	Prevents metaplasia of epithelium Promotes resynthesis of visual purple	Anorexia, periosteal thickening	To prevent or cure deficiency	Vitamin A
Thiamin	Constituent of cocarboxylase	Minor	Beriberi	Thiamin HCl
Nicotinic acid	Constituent of coenzymes I, II	Flushing	Pellagra, vasodilator	Niacin
Riboflavin	Constituent of flavin adenine nucleotide	Minor	To prevent or cure deficiency	Riboflavin

(cont.)

SUMMARY: THE VITAMINS (contd.)

TYPE	*ACTION AND MECHANISM*	*TOXICITY*	*USE*	*EXAMPLES*
Pyridoxine	Coenzyme for decarboxylation, transamination	Minor	None	Pyridoxine HCl
Vitamin C	Maintains oxidation reduction status	Minor	Scurvy	Ascorbic acid

Review

Olson, J. The metabolism of vitamin A. Pharmacol. Rev., 19:559, 1967.

40. Agents in Nutrition

A. Nutrition

1. Average Diet. The usual diet in the United States is composed somewhat as follows (adult men):

Carbohydrates	about 1,700 calories
Proteins	about 350 calories
Fats	about 1,200 calories
Minerals and vitamins	0 calories
Total	3,250 calories

2. Carbohydrates. a. Supply a ready source of fuel for the body's energy requirements, and certain items for synthesis.

b. Provide about 50% to 60% of the dietary calories. Of these about two thirds come from cereals and about one third from sugars.

3. Proteins. a. Supply materials for synthesis and energy.

b. Provide about 10% to 20% of the dietary calories. Actual protein need, however, is only about one half of this amount, i.e., in the neighborhood of 45 gm daily.

c. The following essential amino acids are required for protein synthesis:

tryptophan	250 mg per day	valine	800 mg per day
phenylalanine	1,100 mg per day	methionine	1,100 mg per day
lysine	800 mg per day	leucine	1,100 mg per day
threonine	500 mg per day	isoleucine	700 mg per day

4. Fats. a. Supply richest energy source to the dietary.

b. Contribute up to 40% of the calories in the usual diet.

c. Usually about 70% animal fat.

B. Special Nutritional Agents

GLUCOSE

Glucose is a common medical source of carbohydrate. Dietary intake may be supplemented by parenteral administration in ill patients, as in unconsciousness, vomiting, intestinal obstruction, and postoperative states.

1. Preparation

DEXTROSE (glucose)

Dose: 1,000 ml of 5% or 10% solution intravenously (provides 200 or 400 calories).

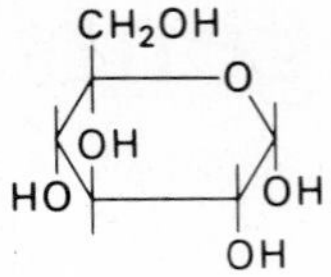

FRUCTOSE

Fructose is partially metabolized as such, and since it does not require insulin, has been used in diabetics. However, as it is extensively converted to glucose, the advantage is not a practicable one.

1. Preparation

FRUCTOSE (levulose)

Dose: 1,000 ml of 1% solution intravenously.

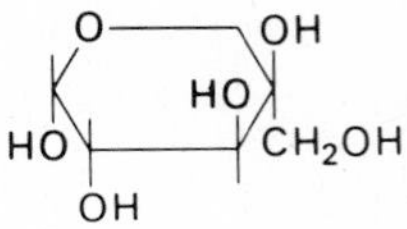

GLUCUROLACTONE

This is a soluble form of glucuronic acid, an essential unit of collagen. For this reason it has been administered in arthritis and collagen diseases; however, it is of doubtful merit.

1. Preparation

GLUCUROLACTONE (Glucurone)

Dose: 500 mg 4 times a day by mouth.

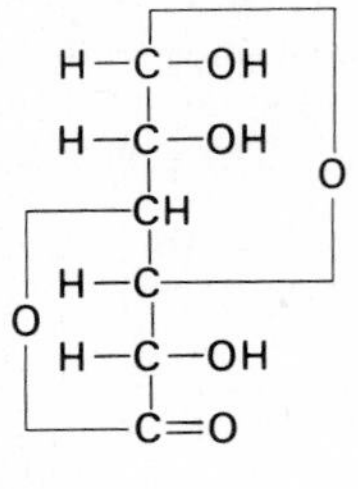

PROTEIN HYDROLYSATES

1. Chemistry. Acid or enzymatic hydrolysates of casein, lactalbumin, plasma, or other proteins in which the protein molecules have been reduced to short polypeptides and amino acids, which are nonantigenic.

2. Uses. a. To supply "protein" when there is interference with intake, digestion, or absorption, as after operations or in severe illness.

b. Preparations often contain glucose to supplement the calories.

c. Usually given intravenously, but may also be given orally, as for allergic infants.

3. Preparations

PROTEIN HYDROLYSATES, INTRAVENOUS (Amigen; Parenamine; and others)
Dose: 1,000 ml intravenously (6% solution).

PROTEIN HYDROLYSATES, ORAL (Caminoids, Aminonat)
Dose: 50 gm or more daily in divided doses by mouth.

PROTEIN HYDROLYSATE, LOW PHENYLALANINE (Lofenlac)
A processed casein hydrolysate low in phenylalanine, and including fat, carbohydrate, vitamins, and minerals for use in children with phenylketonuria.

GLUTAMIC ACID AND ARGININE

1. Actions. Amino acids involved in the removal of the NH_3 from the blood by the liver; mechanisms not fully understood.

2. Pharmacodynamics and Toxicity. Apparently well handled and nontoxic.

3. Uses. a. In hepatitis there may be a failure in the production of urea from ammonia, with resultant rise in blood ammonia, and signs of encephalopathy. Removal of ammonia by the administration of glutamic acid and arginine appears to be of some clinical value. An intestinal antibiotic, such as neomycin, may assist by inhibiting production of NH_3 in the bowel (Silen, Postgrad. Med., 28:445, 1960).

b. Glutamate is also used to enhance the flavor of certain foods, especially meats.

4. Preparations

SODIUM GLUTAMATE (Glutavene)

Dose: 29 gm in 1,000 ml of dextrose solution intravenously.

$$\begin{array}{l} \quad\;\; NH_2 \\ \quad\;\; | \\ CH_2-CH-COOH \\ | \\ CH_2-COONa \end{array}$$

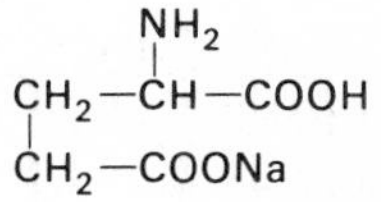

ARGININE HYDROCHLORIDE (Argivene)

Dose: 20 gm in 1,000 ml of dextrose solution intravenously.

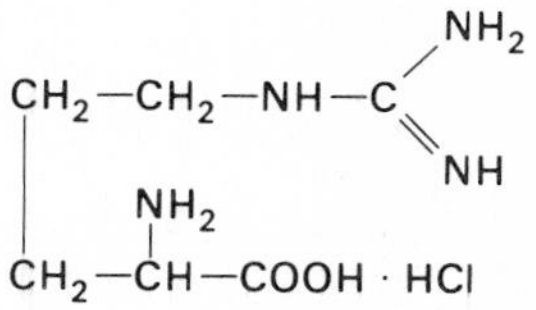

ARGININE GLUTAMATE (Modumate)

Dose: 100 ml of prepared solution (containing 13.5 gm arginine; 11.5 gm glutamic acid) in 1,000 ml of dextrose solution intravenously.

$$\begin{array}{l} CH_2-CH_2-NH-C(=NH)-NH_2 \\ | \\ CH_2-CH(NH_2)-COOH \cdot HCl \end{array}$$

POTASSIUM AND MAGNESIUM ASPARTATES (Spartase)

Nonessential amino acid claimed to relieve fatigue; evidence inconclusive.

Dose: 1 gm orally twice a day.

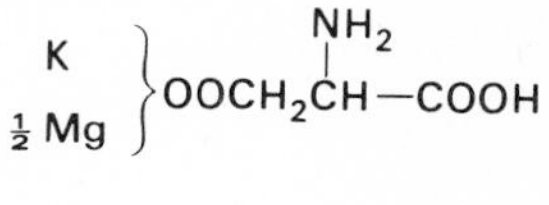

$$\left.\begin{array}{l} K \\ \tfrac{1}{2}\,Mg \end{array}\right\} OOCH_2CH(NH_2)-COOH$$

HOMOGENIZED FATS

1. Chemistry. Emulsions of coconut oil, peanut oil, or other oils with particle size of about 1 micron, suitable for intravenous injection.

2. Action. Supply energy source.

3. Pharmacodynamics and Toxicity. a. Adequately utilized when administered intravenously.

b. May produce immediate "colloid" reaction, with chest pain, dyspnea, flushing, urticaria, chills, fever; or delayed "overloading" syndrome with chills, fever, abdominal pain, hepatomegaly with fatty infiltration of the liver, coagulation defects with thrombocytopenia and bleeding.

4. Uses. To supply concentrated energy source in severe illness or malnutrition.

5. Preparation

COTTONSEED OIL EMULSION (Lipomul)
Dose: 250 ml or more of 15% emulsion daily intravenously; contains 4% dextrose.

INTRAVENOUS FAT EMULSION (Intralipid)
From soybean.

OTHER AGENTS

CHOLINE
Formerly used in fatty infiltration of the liver.

GLYCINE
Formerly used in myasthenia gravis (obsolete).

HISTIDINE
Formerly used in peptic ulcer (obsolete).

INOSITOL
Formerly used as a lipotropic agent.

LYSINE
Proposed in liver disease.

METHIONINE
Formerly used in liver damage.

SUMMARY: AGENTS IN NUTRITION

TYPE	*ACTION AND MECHANISM*	*TOXICITY*	*USE*	*EXAMPLES*
Carbohydrate	Calorie source	Minor	Parenteral alimentation	Dextrose
Protein	Protein source	Minor	Parenteral or oral alimentation	Protein hydrolysates

SUMMARY: AGENTS IN NUTRITION (contd.)

TYPE	*ACTION AND MECHANISM*	*TOXICITY*	*USE*	*EXAMPLES*
Fat	Calorie source	Chest pain, urticaria, hepatomegaly	Parenteral alimentation	Cottonseed oil emulsion

41. Sympathetic Stimulants or Adrenergic Agents

A. Natural Sympathetic Stimulants

NOREPINEPHRINE AND EPINEPHRINE

1. History. a. Oliver and Schäfer (1895) showed that adrenal extracts could produce hypertension; Abel and Crawford (1897) partially isolated epinephrine from such extracts; Takamine and Aldrich (1901) completed the isolation.

b. Elliot (1904) proposed that epinephrine might be the sympathetic transmitter, but Barger and Dale (1910) showed that other amines (anticipating norepinephrine) produced some of the effects of sympathetic stimulation.

c. Cannon sought to explain the presence of opposing excitatory and inhibitory effects of sympathetic stimulation on the basis of two types of transmitter, sympathins E and I.

d. Von Euler (1946) showed norepinephrine to be the principal transmitter; Tullar (1949) isolated the active levo isomer using chromatography.

2. Chemistry. Derivatives of catecholethylamine. Commercial products are now made synthetically.

3. Action. a. Norepinephrine is the principal product released by stimulation of sympathetic nerves, while under ordinary conditions epinephrine is the principal product of the adrenal medulla.

b. The general effects produced are those of sympathetic stimulation which may include: dilated pupils, viscid saliva, relaxed bronchi, sweating, tachycardia, increased cardiac output, vasoconstriction (except coronaries), increased blood pressure, inhibited alimentary peristalsis and secretion, and relaxed bladder.

c. Norepinephrine is, in the main, liberated close to effector cells; its principal peripheral effects are on arterioles, particularly in the large skeletal muscle mass; the result of the vasoconstriction is a maintained or increased blood pressure. Like epinephrine, it increases cardiac rate and output.

d. Epinephrine is liberated mainly by the adrenal and its effects are more diffuse as it is carried to all cells. It increases the heart rate and the cardiac output and is constrictor to the vessels of the skin and mucous membranes, but dilates the vascular bed of skeletal muscle, which reduces its hypertensive effects as compared to norepinephrine. It is a potent bronchial dilator, and produces various metabolic effects, especially glycogenolysis which raises blood sugar.

4. Mechanism and Physiology

a. Synthesis

a′. Precursor amino acids (phenylalanine or tyrosine) enter the sympathetic nerve fiber, cells of the adrenal medulla or other chromaffin cells, or nerve cells of the brain.

b′. Synthesis proceeds in the presence of ATP, Mg^{++}, and the appropriate enzymes as follows:

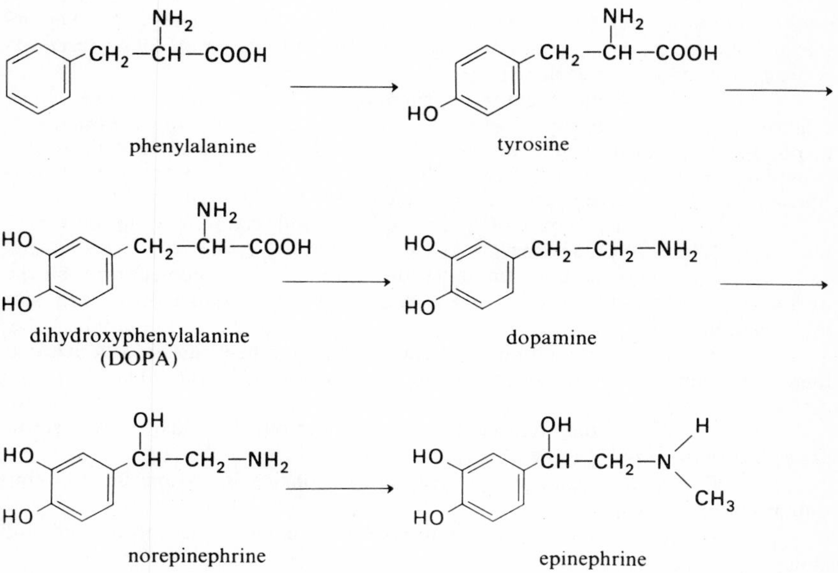

phenylalanine → tyrosine →

dihydroxyphenylalanine (DOPA) → dopamine →

norepinephrine → epinephrine

c′. In sympathetic nerve fibers the resultant catecholamines are present in part as dopamine (about 50%), and the synthesis terminates in norepinephrine, much of which is stored with ATP and a binding protein in vesicles near the tip of the axon. Presumably the same is true in brain cells, but in the adrenal medulla the synthesis proceeds in large part (about 80%) to epinephrine except in the presence of a pheochromocytoma.

b. Release.

a′. When sympathetic nerves are stimulated, norepinephrine is released, probably from both the vesicles and the cytoplasm. Some enters the cleft between the tip of the nerve and the receptor on the adjacent cell, and crosses to and stimulates the latter.

b′. Excess norepinephrine returns in part to intracellular storage, or is destroyed, that within the nerve fiber by deamination in mitochondria by MAO (monoamineoxidase), and that in the cleft by COMT (catechol-O-methyltransferase) (Weiner, Ann. Rev. Pharmacol., 10:273, 1970).

c′. Destruction of circulating epinephrine is primarily by COMT in the liver and in the environment of receptors.

c. Receptors

a′. Catecholamine reaching a receptor stimulates the adenyl cyclase attached to the receptor to increase (or decrease) the conversion of ATP to cyclic AMP. The latter then incites a physical response by altering intracellular kinases, phosphorylases, and probably permeability of cell membranes to Ca^{++}. Excess cyclic AMP is inactivated by phosphodiesterase, which together with adenyl cyclase thus constitute a balancing mechanism (Sutherland, Pharmacologist, 12:33, 1970, and J.A.M.A., 214:1280, 1970).

b′. There are at least two types of receptors:

a″. Alpha receptors: Generally excitatory (vasoconstriction), but may be inhibitory (relax intestine); respond strongly to norepinephrine and epinephrine; blocked by α-blocking adrenolytic agents. Stimulation of alpha receptors probably causes a fall in cyclic AMP.

b″. Beta receptors: Generally inhibitory (relax intestine; vasodilation in muscle) but may be excitatory (increase heart rate and contractility); respond to epinephrine or isoproterenol; blocked by β-blocking adrenolytic agents. Stimulation of beta receptors produces also metabolic effects (hyperglycemia, hyperlipemia, increased oxygen consumption), mediated through cyclic AMP.

c″. The nature of central and metabolic receptors is not known.

d. Effects of other agents

a′. Amphetamine stimulates the synthesis of norepinephrine, blocks its destruction by MAO, favors its release, and inhibits its reuptake, thus strengthening its action.

b′. Reserpine inhibits the uptake of norepinephrine into vesicles; it therefore accumulates in the cytoplasm and is destroyed by MAO, thus reducing its action.

c′. Ephedrine: Releases norepinephrine but also has a direct stimulatory action on alpha and beta receptors.

d′. MAO inhibitors protect norepinephrine in cytoplasm and thus enhance the catecholamine effect.

e′. Cocaine inhibits the reuptake of norepinephrine into the cell, and thus enhances the effect (cocaine sensitization).

f′. Theophylline inhibits phosphodiesterase; glucagon and thyroxine stimulate adenyl cyclase; each therefore augments receptor effects.

g′. Ergotoxin blocks alpha receptors, leaving the inhibitory possibilities of beta receptors exposed. Stimulation may then reverse a previously overriding excitatory response (ergotoxin reversal).

h′. The pressor effect of catecholamines may be enhanced after sympathetic denervation, presumably because few receptors have been preempted by any slow basal release of norepinephrine, and all are therefore available for stimulation.

i′. Tachyphylaxis is a phenomenon of decreasing effect with succeeding doses. This is presumably the result of the exhaustion of stored norepinephrine, or the brief or long occupation of receptors by agents like norepinephrine or ephedrine (not epinephrine), which occlude access of fresh catecholamine.

j′. It has been suggested that adrenergic fibers first release acetylcholine at many endings, which in turn releases norepinephrine (Burn, Advances Pharmacol., 1:2, 1962; Koelle, Nature, 190:208, 1961).

5. Pharmacodynamics. a. The catecholamines are ineffective when given by mouth, presumably because of destruction by catechol oxidases and other enzymes in the intestine.

b. After injection their effects are transient because of rapid destruction in the circulation by other enzymes or by conjugation. The principal steps involved are described by Kopin (Science, 131:1372, 1960), as follows:

epinephrine (HO, HO, $CHOH\,CH_2NHCH_3$)

COMT 70% → metanephrine (H_3CO, HO, $CHOH\,CH_2NHCH_3$) → Urine: free and conjugated = 45±%

metanephrine → 25% → 3-methoxy-4-OH mandelic acid (VMA) (H_3CO, HO, $CHOH\,COOH$)

epinephrine → 25% MAO → 3,4-dihydroxy mandelic aldehyde (HO, HO, $CHOH\,CHO$) → 25% aldehyde dehydrogenase → 3-methoxy-4-OH mandelic acid (VMA)

epinephrine → free and conjugated = 5±%

c. Both norepinephrine and epinephrine follow the same pathways. The methoxy derivatives retain partial biological activity (Champagne, Science, 132:419, 1960).

6. Toxicity. a. Norepinephrine has been reported to cause focal myocarditis, but the only common toxic manifestation is local tissue necrosis at the site of an intravenous injection. Local infiltration with a sympatholytic agent such as phentolamine or piperoxane may alleviate the pain and damage.

b. Epinephrine may cause trembling, pallor, and nervousness, even in therapeutic dosage; cardiac arrhythmias with large doses.

c. Pheochromocytomas are tumors of the adrenal medulla or other chromaffin tissue which elaborate catechol amines, especially norepinephrine, and produce hypertension, remediable by removal of the secreting tissue.

7. Uses. a. Norepinephrine is used to support the blood pressure in shock and sometimes during spinal anesthesia. It is given by slow intravenous drip, with the rate controlled by the blood pressure. When the infusion is stopped the blood pressure usually falls abruptly, a matter of some clinical difficulty. Norepinephrine should then be replaced by metaraminol, mephentermine, or another pressor amine which can release norepinephrine from stores.

b. Epinephrine is used to relieve sensitivity phenomena in allergic states, especially anaphylaxis and the bronchospasm of asthma. The bronchial relaxation is from beta receptor stimulation, but this beneficial effect is augmented by the alpha stimulation which provided decongestion by reducing vessel size. It is also used to stimulate the heart in complete heart block or acute stoppage of the heart, and in solution with local anesthetics to limit the spread of the anesthetic.

8. Preparations

DOPAMINE

In investigational use in congestive heart failure.

Dose: 100 mcg per minute intravenously.

HO, HO, $CH_2CH_2-NH_2$

EPINEPHRINE HYDROCHLORIDE (adrenalin)

Dose: 0.1 to 1 ml of 1:1,000 solution subcutaneously (after injection the site should be massaged to assure absorption); also as an aerosol inhalation; and as suspensions in oil intramuscularly.

Epinephryl borate (Eppy)

HO, HO, OH, $CH-CH_2-N$, H, CH_3, $\cdot HCl$

LEVARTERENOL BITARTRATE (norepinephrine; levo-arterenol; Levophed)

Dose: 2 to 4 mcg per minute by intravenous drip.

HO, HO, OH, $CH-CH_2-NH_2$, $\cdot C_4H_6O_6$

LEVODOPA (dihydroxyphenylalanine; L-dopa; Dopar; Larodopa)

The precursor of dopamine; can pass through the blood-brain barrier rectifying any deficiency of dopamine in the substantia nigra of patients with parkinsonism; or may adjust any imbalance between dopamine and acetylcholine.

HO, HO, $CH_2-CH-NH_2$, COOH

Side effects include anorexia; nausea, dyskinesia and choreiform movements (may be neutralized with pyridoxine, but effect of levodopa correspondingly decreased; avoid polyvitamin preparations with pyridoxine), granulocytopenia, orthostatic hypotension (gradual disappearance), arrhythmias (may control with propranolol without affecting antiparkinson action), hallucinations and ideas of reference.

Dose: 1 gm 3 to 6 times a day by mouth.

CARBIDOPA (Lodosyn)

HO, HO, CH_3, $CH_2-C-COOH \cdot H_2O$, $NHNH_2$

Peripheral decarboxylase inhibitor. Slows down conversion of levodopa, thus allowing more to enter the brain.

ADRENALONE
For ophthalmological use.

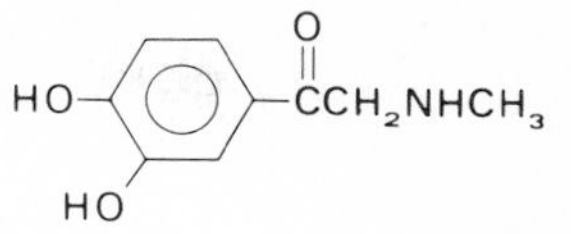

HO, HO, O, CCH_2NHCH_3

OXIDOPAMINE

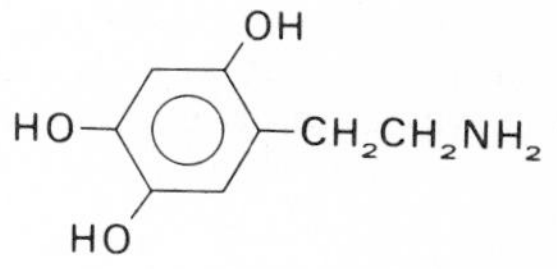

OH, HO, HO, $CH_2CH_2NH_2$

TYRAMINE
Pharmacological tool.

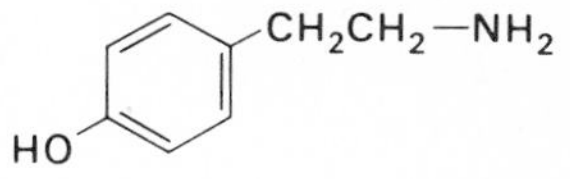

HO, $CH_2CH_2—NH_2$

B. Sympathomimetic Amines

A large number of compounds, mostly synthetic, but some naturally occurring, resemble norepinephrine and epinephrine both chemically and in the actions they produce; they are therefore called sympathomimetics.

1. Chemistry. Chemical structure and characteristics of activity can be correlated to some extent, as follows:

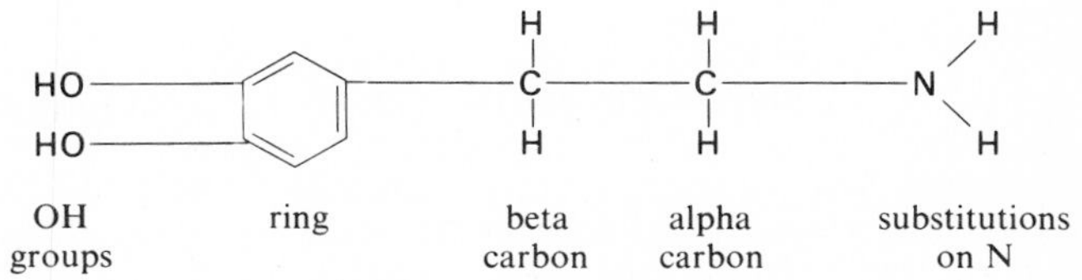

HO, HO, H, C, H, H, C, H, N, H, H

OH groups | ring | beta carbon | alpha carbon | substitutions on N

Prototype: dihydroxyphenylethylamine (dopamine)

a. Hydroxyl groups: There may be 0, 1, or 2 OH groups with changes only in the quantitative activity of the compound; the fewer the OH groups, the more resistant it is to destruction. Therefore, compounds without OH groups produce more long lasting effects, and are more effective by mouth; meta and para OH groups contribute to direct action.

b. Ring: The benzene ring may be replaced by cyclohexyl, naphthalene, or other rings, or by aliphatic chains, with maintenance of the sympathomimetic effect.

c. Beta carbon: The presence of an OH group on this C contributes to a direct action on the receptor; however, other substitutions, such as a CH_3 on the alpha C, may interfere with direct action, even in the presence of the beta OH.

d. Alpha carbon: Substitution on the alpha C retards destruction of phenol (not catechol) compounds and thus contributes to prolonged action.

e. Substitutions on the N: The character of direct action on the receptor is apparently influenced by these substitutions. Thus, the unsubstituted norepinephrine acts directly on alpha receptors; the methyl-substituted epinephrine stimulates both alpha and beta receptors; and isopropyl-substituted isoproterenol stimulates beta receptors.

2. Mechanism and Action. a. The mechanism by which the sympathomimetic amines act has long been puzzling, though it seems clear that their action, in the main, depends upon the presence of the natural sympathetic stimulants, which in some way act more effectively in the presence of the mimetic compounds.

b. The current view is that the principal action is to release the natural compounds from their storage sites, along with some degree of direct action on the receptor (Trendelenburg, J. Pharmacol. Exp. Ther., 138:170, 1962).

c. A former view was that the enzymes responsible for the inactivation of the natural compounds could be decreased through the utilization of the mimetic compounds as substrates, thus allowing the natural compounds to act longer and more effectively.

EPHEDRINE

1. History. Chen and Schmidt (1923) introduced the old Chinese drug into the United States.

2. Chemistry. a. Lacks OH groups on the ring, and is "fully substituted" in the ethylamine chain.

b. Produced by plants of the genus *Ephedra*, but commercial production is by synthesis.

3. Action. a. Ephedrine exhibits most of the effects of sympathetic stimulation in some degree, but resembles epinephrine more than norepinephrine.

b. Blood pressure may be moderately raised, and the heart rate and cardiac output increased; bronchi are relaxed; pupils are somewhat dilated; the alimentary tract is inhibited. However, glycogenolysis is not produced.

c. Moderate central stimulation, much more pronounced than the minor effects from epinephrine.

4. Mechanism. a. Mechanism assumed to be release of stored catecholamines, but also some direct action on the receptors.

b. Tachyphylaxis occurs; cocaine does not potentiate.

5. Pharmacodynamics. a. Differs from epinephrine in being effective orally and in producing effects lasting a few hours, rather than minutes.

b. Conjugation occurs but about 40% of the compound appears unchanged in the urine.

6. Toxicity. The principal side actions are the result of the central stimulatory effects: vertigo, nervousness, insomnia.

7. Uses. a. Ephedrine is used extensively in asthma to produce continued bronchial dilatation.

b. It has been largely replaced by relatives with less central effect as a vasoconstrictor and cardiac stimulant; and by drugs with more central effect when such stimulation is desired.

8. Preparations

EPHEDRINE SULFATE (ma huang)

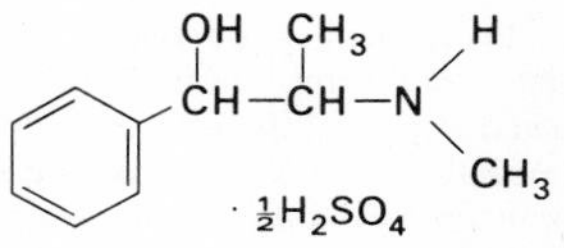

Dose: 25 mg every 3 to 4 hours by mouth; 1% solution in the nose as a decongestant.

OH CH$_3$ H

CH—CH—N

CH$_3$

$\cdot \frac{1}{2}H_2SO_4$

Racephedrine hydrochloride (Vaponephrin)
Racemic ephedrine.
Dose: 25 to 50 mg by mouth; 2.25% aerosol by inhalation.

PSEUDOEPHEDRINE HYDROCHLORIDE (Sudafed; Isoephedrine)

Isomer presumed to have less central nervous system but maintained bronchial effect.
Dose: 30 mg every 3 hours by mouth.

ANALOGUES WITH VASCULAR AND BRONCHIAL EFFECTS

In a large group of sympathomimetics generally resembling ephedrine vascular and bronchial effects are prominent but central effects are minimal.

1. Preparations

a. Catechol, phenol, and methoxy derivatives

DIHYDROXYPHENYLAMINOBUTANOL
Bronchodilator.
Dose: By inhalation.

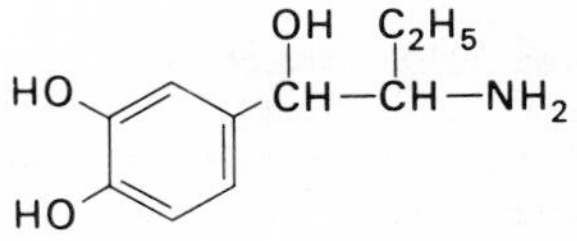

OH C$_2$H$_5$

HO CH—CH—NH$_2$

HO

CLOPRENALINE HYDROCHLORIDE
Bronchodilator.

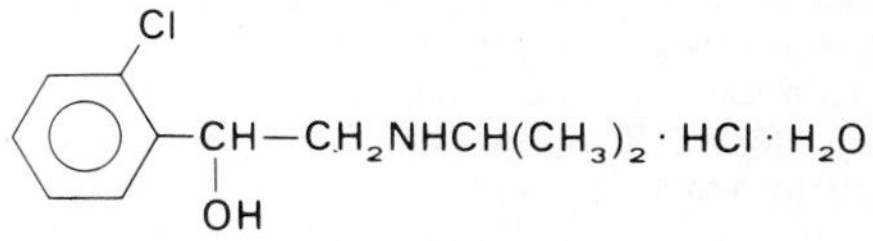

Cl

CH—CH$_2$NHCH(CH$_3$)$_2$ · HCl · H$_2$O

OH

HYDROXYAMPHETAMINE HYDROBROMIDE (Paredrine)

Used as a nasal decongestant and mydriatic.
Dose: 1% solution in the nose or eye.

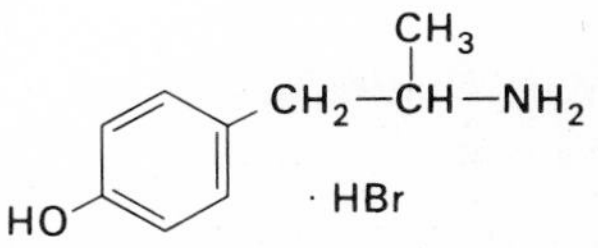

CH$_3$

CH$_2$—CH—NH$_2$

· HBr

HO

METARAMINOL BITARTRATE
(Aramine)

Used as a nasal decongestant, and in shock (see Agents in Shock) where it may produce strong and prolonged increase in BP.

Dose: 0.25 % solution in the nose; 2 to 10 mg subcutaneously or intramuscularly.

$HO-C_6H_4-CH(OH)-CH(CH_3)-NH_2 \cdot C_4H_6O_6$

METHOXAMINE HYDROCHLORIDE
(Vasoxyl)

Produces a good rise in BP, and unlike most other sympathomimetics, the heart is slowed, apparently reflexly; free of central stimulation. Used in shock and the hypotension accompanying spinal anesthesia.

Dose: 10 mg intramuscularly; 5 mg intravenously.

$H_3CO-C_6H_3(OCH_3)-CH(OH)-CH(CH_3)-NH_2 \cdot HCl$

METHOXYPHENAMINE HYDROCHLORIDE
(Orthoxine)

Produces good bronchodilatation with minimal vasopressor effects; used in asthma.

Dose: 50 mg every 4 hours by mouth.

$C_6H_4(OCH_3)-CH_2-CH(CH_3)-N(H)CH_3 \cdot HCl$

NORDEFRIN HYDROCHLORIDE
(Cobefrin)

Vasoconstrictor for infiltration anesthesia.

Dose: 1:10,000 solution.

$(HO)_2C_6H_3-CH(OH)-CH(CH_3)-NH_2 \cdot HCl$

PHENYLEPHRINE HYDROCHLORIDE
(Neosynephrine)

Produces good local vasoconstriction, fair bronchodilatation; used as a nasal decongestant and to sustain BP during spinal anesthesia. Oral effect questionable.

Dose: 50 mg every 3 hours by mouth; 10 mg subcutaneously; 0.25 % solution in the nose.

$HO-C_6H_4-CH(OH)-CH_2-N(H)CH_3 \cdot HCl$

b. Phenyl derivatives

AMIDEPHRINE MESYLATE

Vasoconstrictor and nasal decongestant.

Under investigation.

$CH_3SO_2-HN-C_6H_4-CH(OH)-CH_2-N(H)CH_3 \cdot (CH_3)_2SO_4$

ETAFEDRINE HYDROCHLORIDE (Nethamine)

Dose: 50 mg by mouth.

$C_6H_5-CH(OH)-CH(CH_3)-N(C_2H_5)(CH_3) \cdot HCl$

MEPHENTERMINE SULFATE (Wyamine)

Used as a nasal decongestant and to raise the BP in shock or during spinal anesthesia.

Dose: 15 mg intravenously; volatile base by inhalation.

$C_6H_5-CH_2-C(CH_3)_2-N(H)(CH_3) \cdot \frac{1}{2}H_2SO_4$

PHENYLPROPANOLAMINE HYDROCHLORIDE (Propadrine)

Produces vascular and bronchial effects with little if any central effect. Used in asthma and as a nasal decongestant, both locally and by mouth.

Dose: 25 mg every 4 hours by mouth; 1 % solution in the nose.

$C_6H_5-CH(OH)-CH(CH_3)-NH_2 \cdot HCl$

PHENYLPROPYLMETHYLAMINE HYDROCHLORIDE (Vonedrine)

Formerly used as a volatile nasal decongestant; now obsolete. Note unusual CH_3 substitution on beta C.

$C_6H_5-CH(CH_3)-CH_2-N(H)(CH_3) \cdot HCl$

c. Saturated ring derivatives

CYCLOPENTAMINE HYDROCHLORIDE (Clopane)

Used as a nasal decongestant.

Dose: 0.5 % solution in the nose.

$C_5H_9-CH_2-CH(CH_3)-N(H)(CH_3) \cdot HCl$

PROPYLHEXEDRINE (Benzedrex)

Useful nasal decongestant.

Volatile base by inhalation.

$C_6H_{11}-CH_2-CH(CH_3)-H(H)(CH_3)$

d. Aliphatic derivatives

ISOMETHEPTENE HYDROCHLORIDE, or other salts (Octin)

Used to relax spasm in the alimentary or urinary tracts.

Dose: 100 mg every hour orally or intramuscularly.

$(CH_3)(H_3C)C{=}CH-CH_2-CH_2-CH(CH_3)-N(H)(CH_3) \cdot HCl$

METHYLAMINOHEPTANE HYDROCHLORIDE (Oenethyl)

Vasoconstrictor.

Under investigation.

$H_3C-(CH_2)_4-CH(CH_3)-N(H)(CH_3) \cdot HCl$

METHYLHEXANEAMINE
(Forthane)

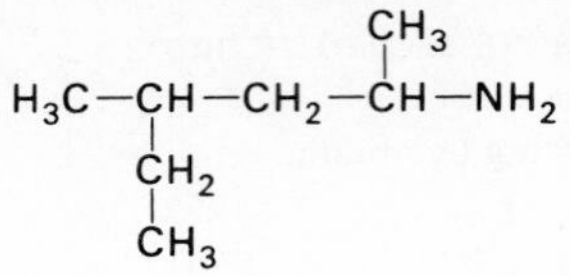

Used as a nasal decongestant.

Dose: Volatile base (as carbonate) by inhalation.

$$H_3C-CH(CH_2CH_3)-CH_2-CH(CH_3)-NH_2$$

OCTODRINE (in Vaporpac)

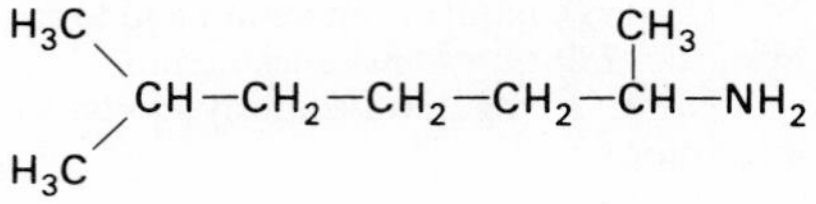

Vasoconstrictor and local anesthetic.

Under investigation.

$$(H_3C)_2CH-CH_2-CH_2-CH_2-CH(CH_3)-NH_2$$

TUAMINOHEPTANE SULFATE
(Tuamine)

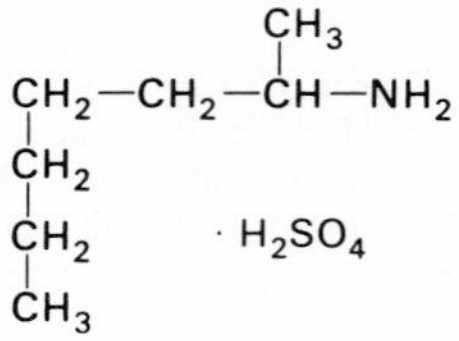

Used as a nasal decongestant.

Dose: 1 % solution in the nose, or volatile base by inhalation.

$$CH_3-CH_2-CH_2-CH_2-CH_2-CH(CH_3)-NH_2 \cdot H_2SO_4$$

e. Heterocyclic derivatives

METIZOLINE HYDROCHLORIDE (Elsyl)

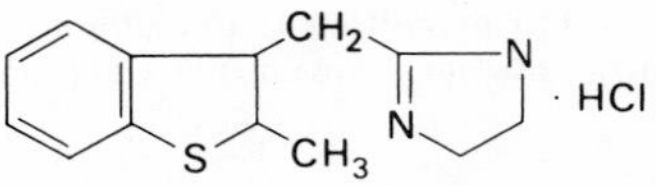

Nasal decongestant.

Under investigation.

NAPHAZOLINE HYDROCHLORIDE
(Privine)

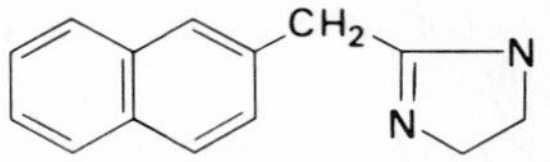

Produces strong local vasoconstriction in the nose and is an effective nasal decongestant. However, there may be rebound congestion upon withdrawal, and bizarre central stimulation with wakefulness and crawling skin. Note the engagement of the ethylamine side chain in an imidazole ring.

Dose: 0.05 % solution in the nose.

OXYMETAZOLINE HYDROCHLORIDE
(Afrin)

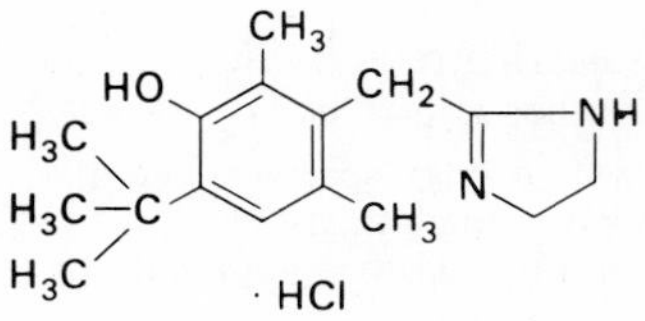

Nasal decongestant.

Dose: 0.5 % as nasal spray.

TETRAHYDROZOLINE HYDROCHLORIDE
(Tyzine)

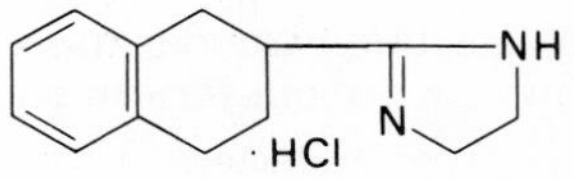

Used as a nasal decongestant.

Dose: 0.1 % solution in the nose.

TRAMAZOLINE HYDROCHLORIDE

Nasal decongestant.
Under investigation.

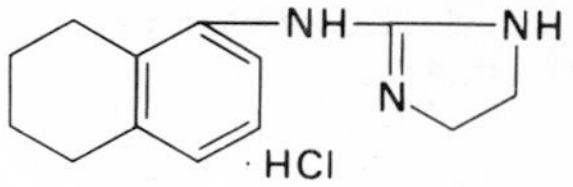

XYLOMETAZOLINE (Otrivin)

Used as a nasal decongestant; relatively free of side effects.

Dose: 0.1% solution in the nose.

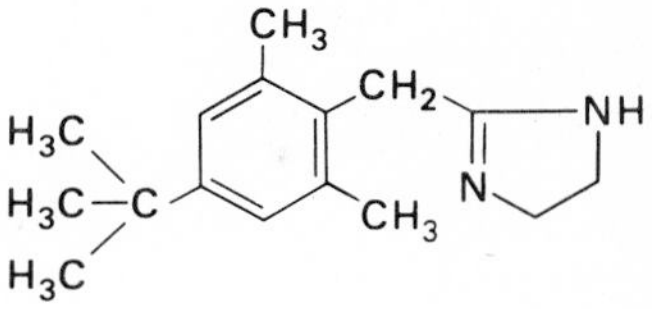

AMPHETAMINE AND ANALOGUES WITH CENTRAL EFFECTS

Members of another group of sympathomimetics resemble ephedrine, but show increased central effects. The prototype, amphetamine, was recognized by Alles (1933) as having this potentiality.

1. Chemistry. Phenylethylamines with an α CH_3 substitution and no β substitution.

2. Action and Mechanism. a. The amphetamines produce vascular effects similar to those of ephedrine, but their principal interest is their potent central stimulation with wakefulness and a heightened mood.

b. The mechanism and receptors involved in the central effects are not understood.

3. Pharmacodynamics. Amphetamine and methamphetamine are well absorbed after oral administration and in general resemble ephedrine.

4. Toxicity. a. The central effects may lead to much more striking side effects than from ephedrine.

b. Although tremendous doses may be tolerated in narcolepsy, overdosage ordinarily causes troublesome nervousness, insomnia, and if extreme, hallucinations and exhaustion.

c. Addiction to the amphetamines is not uncommon; tolerance may develop until as much as 1 or 2 gm daily may be taken in frequent doses ("jolts"). Physical dependence apparently does not develop.

5. Uses. a. The amphetamines are used to produce wakefulness, to reverse fatigue, and in depressed psychic states (see Stimulants).

b. As respiratory stimulants in barbiturate poisoning.

c. In obesity because of their anorexic effect (see Agents in Nutrition and Obesity).

6. Preparations

AMPHETAMINE SULFATE (Benzedrine)

Dose: 5 to 10 mg 1 to 3 or more times daily by mouth; 5 to 10 mg subcutaneously.

$C_6H_5-CH_2-CH(CH_3)-NH_2 \cdot H_2SO_4$

Dextroamphetamine sulfate (Dexedrine)

The dextro isomer of amphetamine, which may allow a greater CNS action.

Dose: 2.5 to 5 mg 1 to 3 times daily by mouth.

METHAMPHETAMINE HYDROCHLORIDE (Desoxyn; Methedrine; and others)

Dose: 2.5 mg 1 to 3 times daily by mouth.

$C_6H_5-CH_2-CH(CH_3)-N(H)(CH_3) \cdot HCl$

APPETITE SUPPRESSANTS

1. Chemistry. Derivatives or relatives of amphetamine.

2. Action and Mechanism. Presumed to be appetite depressant, or "anorexic," but actual effect probably central stimulation, which may distract the patient from eating and encourage dietary cooperation.

3. Pharmacology and Toxicity. In general, relatively harmless except for associated sleeplessness and palpitation.

4. Uses. a. May encourage an obese patient to follow diet more closely; true anorexic effect very limited.

b. Therapy should be before meals, and not late in the day, to avoid insomnia.

5. Preparations

a. Amphetamine type

AMPHECHLORAL (Acutran)

Dose: 7.5 mg 3 times a day by mouth.

$C_6H_5-CH_2-CH(CH_3)-N{=}CH-CCl_3$

AMPHETAMINE SULFATE (Benzedrine)

Amphetamine "carboxy-phen" (in Bontril)

Dextroamphetamine sulfate (Dexedrine)

See preceding section.

Levamphetamine succinate (Cydril)

Dose: 7 mg 3 times a day by mouth.

$C_6H_5-CH_2-CH(CH_3)-NH_2 \cdot H_2SO_4$

BENZPHETAMINE (Didrex)

Dose: 25 to 50 mg 1 or 2 times daily by mouth.

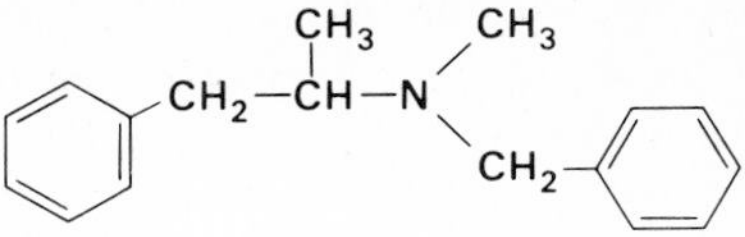

FENFLURAMINE HYDROCHLORIDE

Dose: 120 mg daily by mouth.

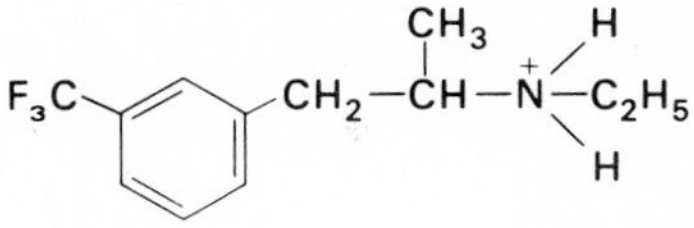

MEFENOREX HYDROCHLORIDE (Anexate; Pondinol)

Under investigation.

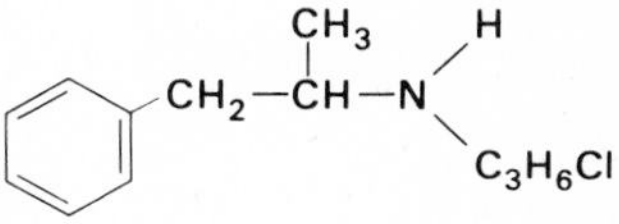

METHAMPHETAMINE HYDROCHLORIDE (Desoxyn; and many others)

Dose: 2.5 to 5 mg 3 times a day by mouth (none after late afternoon).

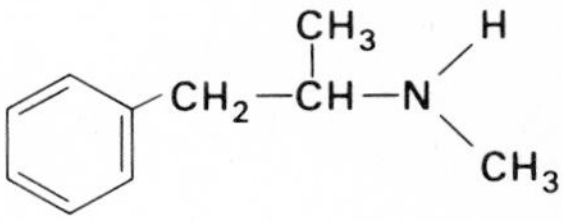

PHENTERMINE HYDROCHLORIDE (Wilpo)

Dose: 8 mg before meals by mouth.

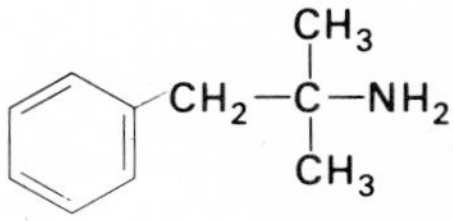

Chlorphentermine (Pre-sate) (para-Cl deriv.)
Clortermine hydrochloride (Voranil) (ortho-Cl deriv.)
Mephentermine
Phentermine (Ionamin)
Dose: 15 to 30 mg once daily by mouth.

OTHERS

Amfepentorex; clobenorex; cloforex; etolorex; fenisorex; formetorex; fenpropex; furfenorex; ortetamine; pentorex.

b. *Related types*

AMINOREX

May cause pulmonary vascular hypertension.
Dose: 7.5 mg 3 times a day by mouth. Withdrawn.

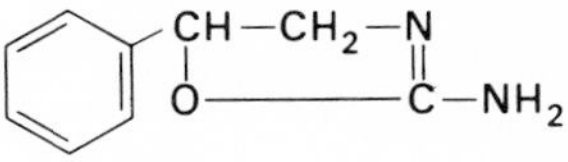

CLOMINOREX

Dose: Under investigation.

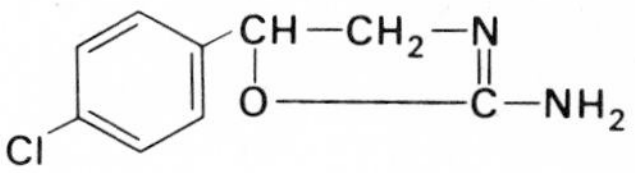

DIETHYLPROPION (Tepanil)
Dose: 25 mg 3 times a day by mouth.

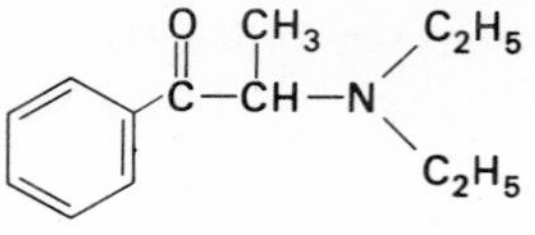

FLUDOREX
Dose: Under investigation.

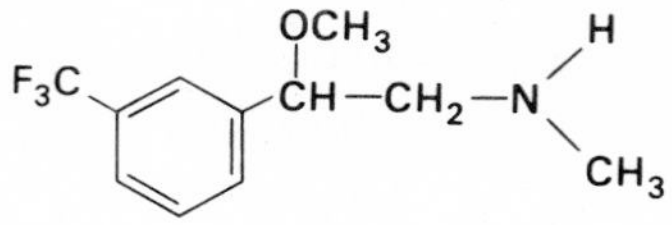

FLUMINOREX
Dose: Under investigation.

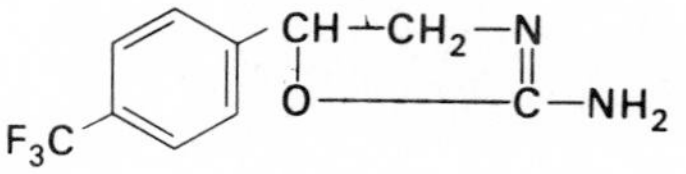

PHENDIMETRAZINE (Plegine)
Dose: 35 mg 3 times a day by mouth.

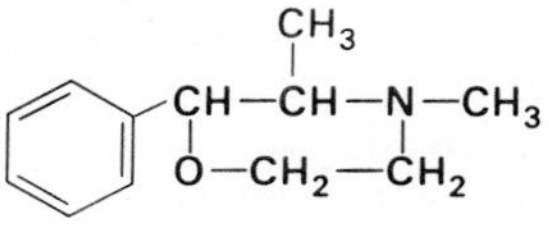

PHENMETRAZINE HYDROCHLORIDE (Preludin)

Reported to be more potent than diethylpropion, but to produce more CNS effects.

Dose: 25 mg 2 or 3 times a day by mouth.

Levophenmetrazine hydrochloride (Myludin)

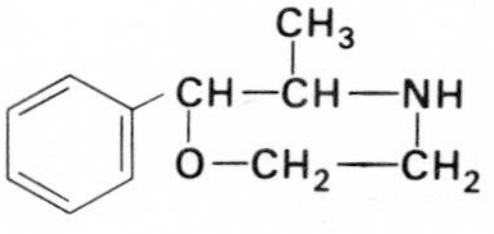

PYROVALERONE HYDROCHLORIDE

Dose: Under investigation.

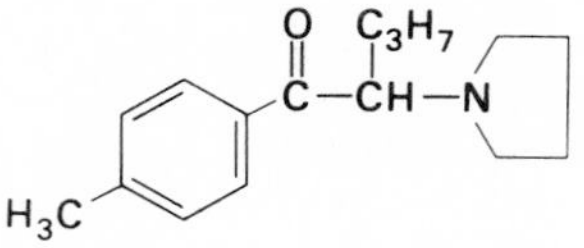

C. Isoproterenol Group

1. Chemistry. a. Comprises a large number of synthetic isopropyl analogues of the sympathomimetic amines.

b. May or may not have OH substitutions on the benzene ring, but all have OH on the beta carbon of the side chain and an isopropyl, or equivalent, on the amine N.

c. Although isoproterenol has been isolated from tissues, a normal physiological role is questionable.

2. Action and Mechanism. a. Bronchodilation, inotropic and chronotropic effects on the heart, vasodilatation of skeletal, renal, and mesenteric vessels, uterine relaxation.

b. Active in epinephrine-fast patients.

c. Relatively pure stimulants of beta receptors.

d. Some members may show a papaverinelike action directly on vascular and other smooth muscle (Lish, J. Pharmacol., 129:191, 1960).

3. Pharmacodynamics and Toxicity. a. Variably absorbed by mouth; excreted slowly, partly in conjugated form. Metabolic fate presumably similar to that of epinephrine.

b. Large doses may cause palpitation, tachycardia, arrhythmias, especially after parenteral injection, hypotension, tremulousness, insomnia.

4. Uses. a. Bronchodilators in asthma.

b. Useful in heart block, including urgent Stokes-Adams attacks.

c. Used as vasodilators in peripheral vascular disease: intermittent claudication, Raynaud's disease, thromboangitis obliterans.

d. Certain members have been used to relax the uterus in dysmenorrhea and threatened abortion. Final assessment of the clinical value of these agents has not been made.

5. Preparations

a. Isoproterenol and analogues with bronchial effects

ISOETHARINE (Dilabron)

Dose: 1.75% solution by aerosol inhalation; 5 to 10 mg orally in enteric coating.

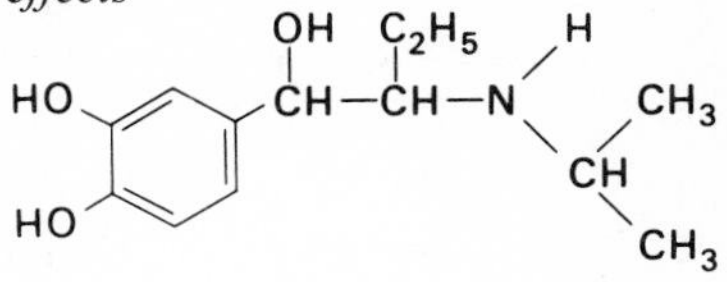

ISOPROTERENOL HYDROCHLORIDE or SULFATE (Isuprel; Isonorin; Aludrine; and others)

Dose: 0.5 ml of an 0.5% solution nebulized for oral inhalation (acute asthma); 15 mg sublingually 4 times a day (milder asthma); 0.02 to 0.15 mg subcutaneously or by intravenous drip cautiously (heart block, or bronchospasm during anesthesia).

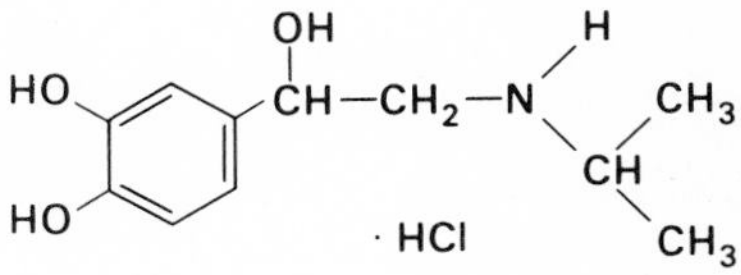

PROTOCHYLOL (Caytine)

Dose: 2 mg 3 times a day by mouth; 0.1 to 0.5 mg subcutaneously or intramuscularly.

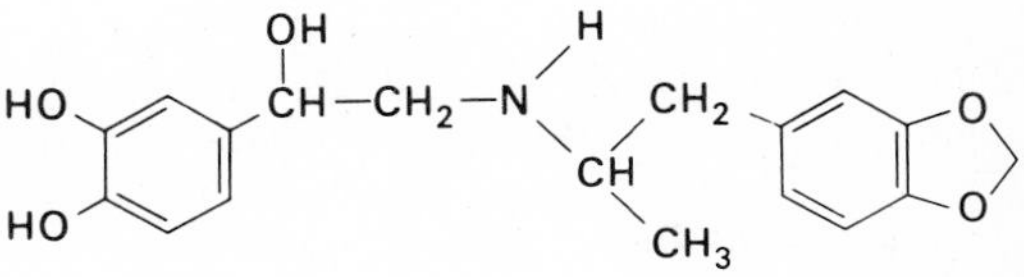

OTHERS

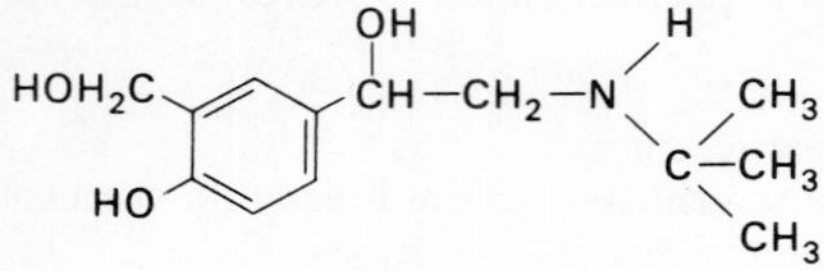

albuterenol

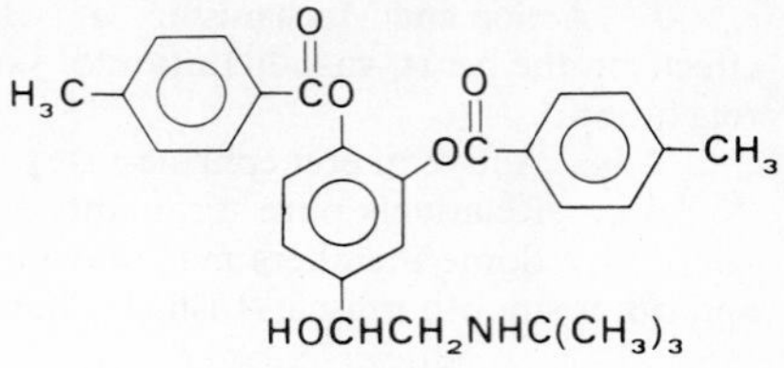

bitolterol

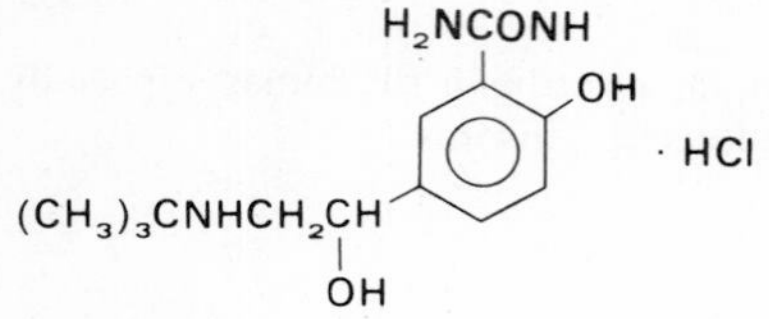

carbuterol hydrochloride

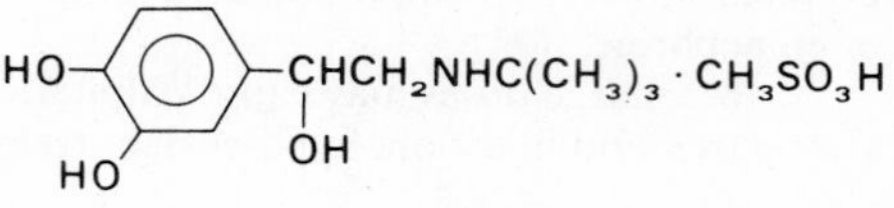

colterol mesylate

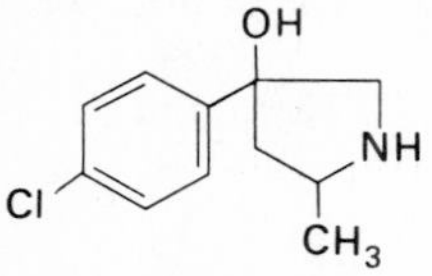

cycloterenol

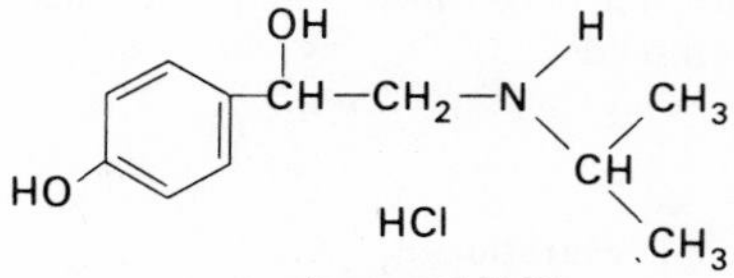

deterenol HCl

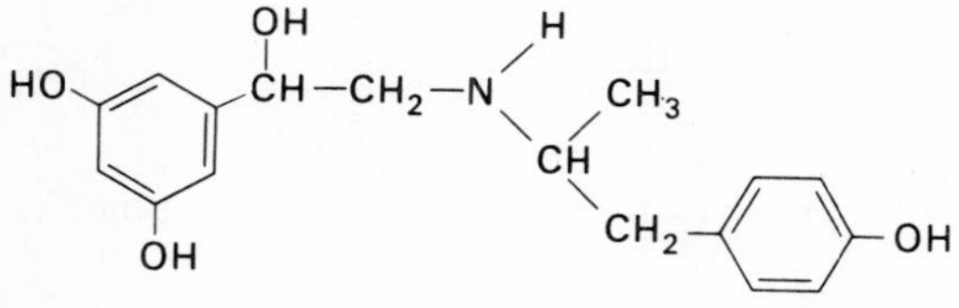

fenoterol

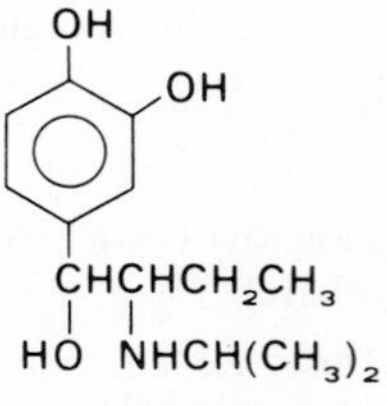

isoetharine

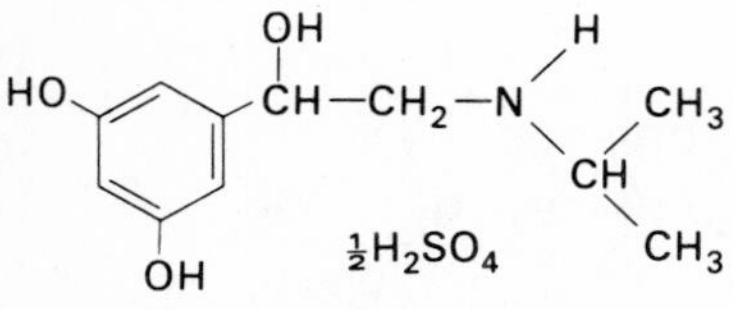

metaproterenol sulfate (Alupent)

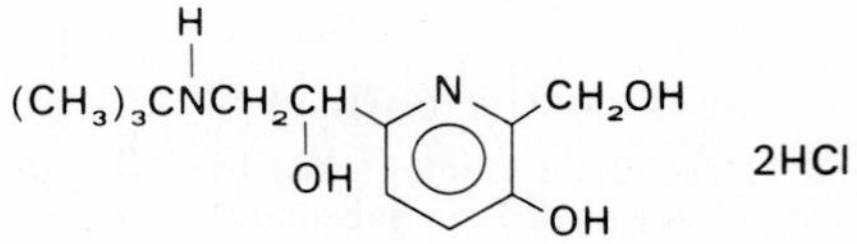

pirbuterol hydrochloride

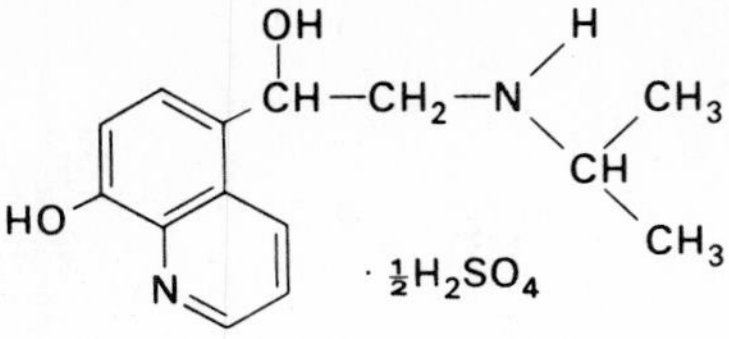

quinterenol sulfate

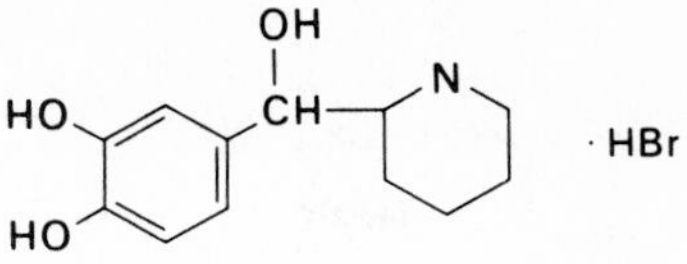

rimiterol HBr

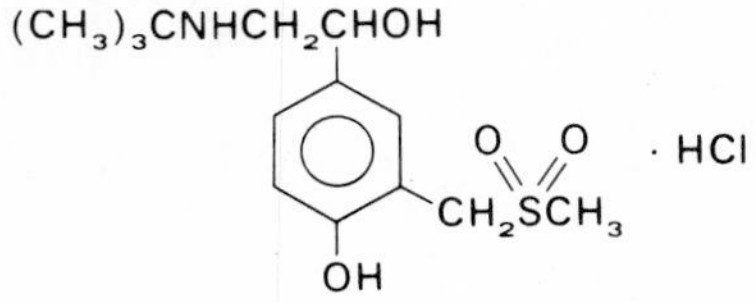

sulfonterol hydrochloride

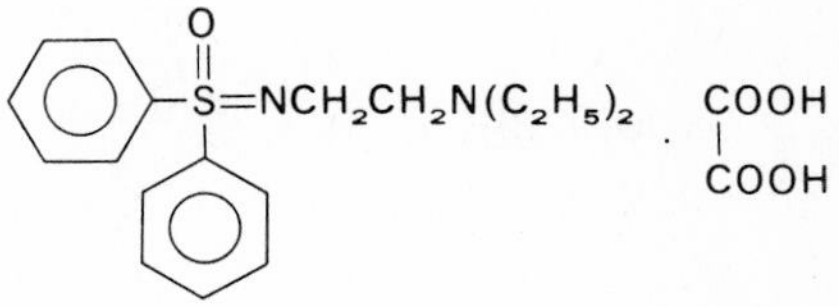

suloxifen oxalate

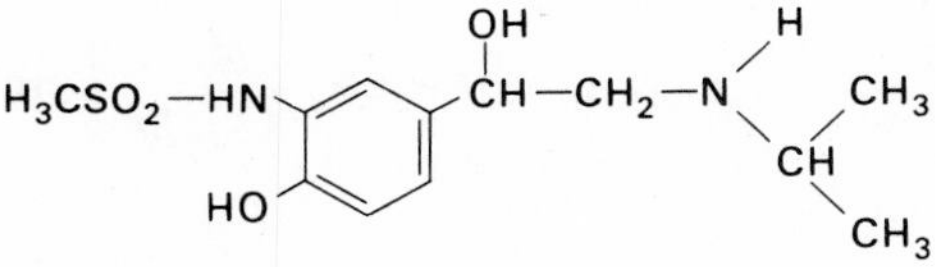

soterenol

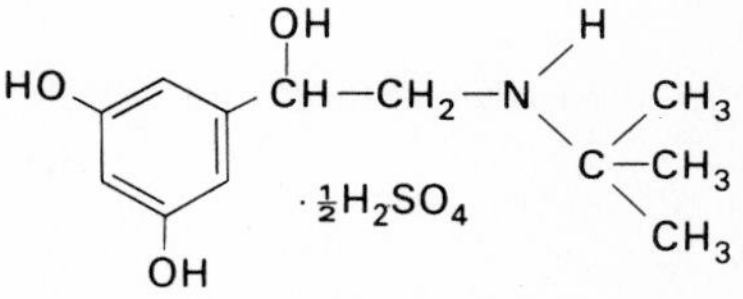

terbutaline sulfate

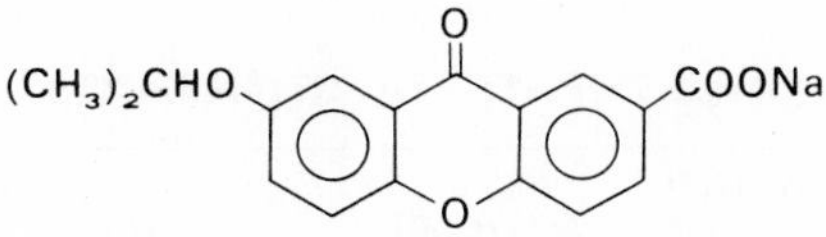

xanoxate sodium

b. Analogues with vascular or uterine effects

CINNAMEDRINE (in Midol)
Uterine antispasmodic.

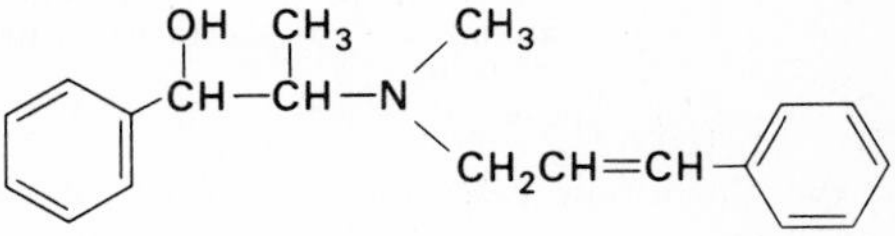

ISOXUPRINE HYDROCHLORIDE (Vasodilan)

Dose: 10 to 20 mg 3 or 4 times a day by mouth.

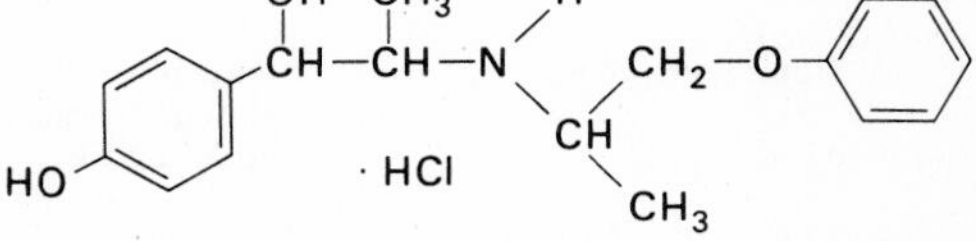

NYLIDRIN HYDROCHLORIDE (Arlidin)

Dose: 6 mg 3 times a day by mouth.

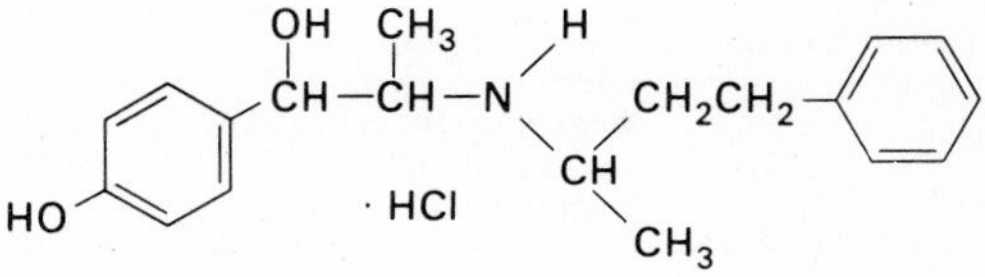

OTHERS

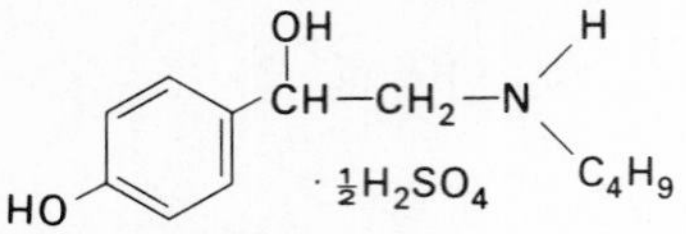

bamethan sulfate (Vasculat)

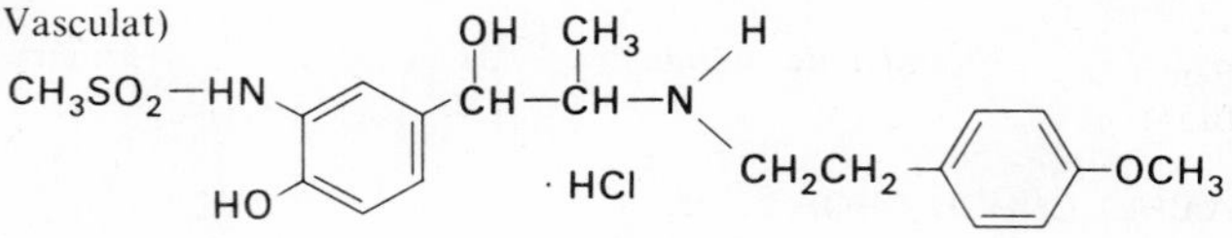

mesuprine HCl

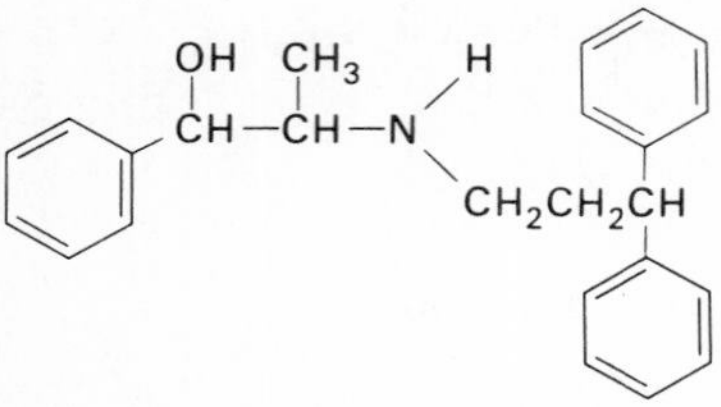

prenylamine (Segontin)

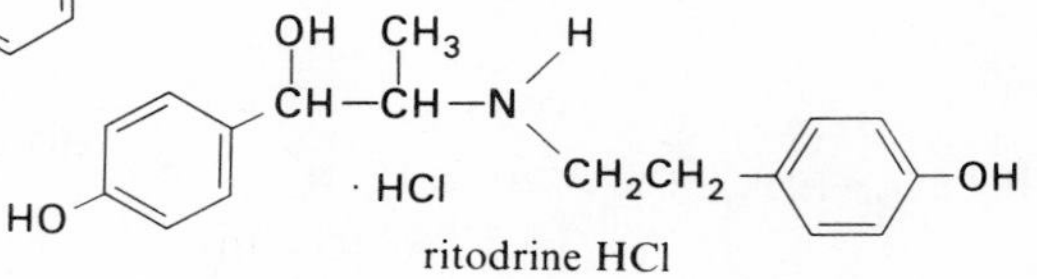

ritodrine HCl

SUMMARY: SYMPATHETIC STIMULANTS

TYPE	*ACTION AND MECHANISM*	*TOXICITY*	*USE*	*EXAMPLES*
Natural catecholamines	Sympathetic receptor stimulation: vasoconstriction, bronchodilation glycogenolysis	Tissue necrosis (norepinephrine), trembling, tachycardia	Allergy, shock	Epinephrine HCl
Sympathomimetic amines (ephedrine)	Release of stored norepinephrine	Nervousness, insomnia	Allergy, nasal decongestion	Ephedrine sulfate
Sympathomimetic amines (amphetamine)	Same	Same, plus hallucinations and addiction	To reverse fatigue, appetite suppression	Amphetamine sulfate
Sympathomimetic amines (isoproterenols)	Broncho-dilatation Vasodilatation Uterine relaxation from beta receptor stimulation	Tachycardia, hypertension	Allergy, peripheral vascular disease, uterine relaxant	Isoproterenol sulfate

Reviews

Modell, W. Status and prospect of drugs for overeating. J.A.M.A., 173:1131, 1960.

Zaimis, E. Pharmacology of the autonomic nervous system. Ann. Rev. Pharmacol., 4:365, 1964.

Wurtman, R. Catecholamines. New Eng. J. Med., 273:637, 1965.

Modell, W., and Hussar, A. Dextroamphetamine sulfate and the eating and sleeping patterns of schizophrenics. J.A.M.A., 193:275, 1965.

Ferry, C. The autonomic nervous system. Ann. Rev. Pharmacol., 7:185, 1967.

Bloom, F., and Giarman, N. Physiologic and pharmacologic considerations of biogenic amines in the CNS. Ann. Rev. Pharmacol., 8:229, 1968.

Andén, N., Carlsson, A., and Häggendal, J. Adrenergic Mechanisms. Ann. Rev. Pharmacol., 9:119, 1969.

Aviado, D. Sympathomimetic drugs. Charles C Thomas, Publisher, Springfield, Ill. 1970.

Calne, D. L-Dopa in the treatment of parkinsonism. Clin. Pharmacol. Ther., 11:789, 1970.

McDowell, F., and others. Symposium on levodopa in Parkinson's disease. Clin. Pharmacol. Ther., 12:317, 1971.

42. Sympathetic Depressants and Adrenolytic Agents

Sympathetic depressants and adrenolytic agents interfere with the transmission of postganglionic sympathetic impulses. This transmission may be impaired by events in the nerve fiber, as by exhaustion of norepinephrine stores, or by blockage of the sympathetic receptors.

I. ALPHA RECEPTOR BLOCKERS

Alpha blockers prevent the normal pressor effects of norepinephrine, especially arteriolar constriction.

A. Ergot Alkaloids

1. **History.** Dale (1906) showed that ergotoxine would reverse the pressor effect of epinephrine on the blood pressure in animal preparations.

2. **Chemistry.** Lysergic acid derivatives; polypeptide side chain necessary for adrenergic blocking activity. (See Smooth Muscle Stimulants.)

3. **Action and Mechanism.** a. A number of ergot alkaloids produce "ergotoxine reversal" of the hypertensive effects of epinephrine in experimental preparations. However, they are also direct stimulants of smooth muscle, which tends to cause vasoconstriction and increased blood pressure. In man the pressor effects outweigh the sympatholytic effects and the net result is pressor.

b. With hydrogenated ergot alkaloids, however, central sympatholytic effects, from depression of the vasomotor center, may be evident in man.

c. The mechanism of reversal by ergotoxine is presumed to be its successful competition with epinephrine for alpha (pressor) receptors, thus excluding pressor effects, but exposing depressor effects.

4. **Uses.** Ergotoxine reversal has no clinical application.

B. Benzodioxanes

PIPEROXAN

1. **History.** Fourneau and Bovet (1933) synthesized series.

2. Chemistry. Substituted phenoxyethylamines and benzodioxanes.

3. Action and Mechanism. a. Piperoxan produces a transient (15 minute) reversal of hypertension from norepinephrine or epinephrine (injected or the result of a pheochromocytoma). In normotensives it produces vasoconstriction and hypertension.

b. This adrenergic blockade has usually been assumed to be the result of fixation of the adrenolytic agent on pressor receptors, preventing the access of the catecholamines.

4. Pharmacodynamics and Toxicity. a. Piperoxan is maximally effective only after intravenous injection.

b. It may produce frequent and unpleasant tachycardia, hyperpnea, and precordial distress.

5. Uses. Piperoxan was formerly used in a diagnostic test for pheochromocytoma, but has been replaced by more satisfactory agents (especially phentolamine) and is no longer marketed.

6. Preparation

PIPEROXAN

Obsolete.

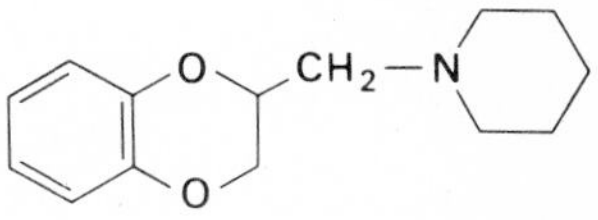

O CH_2—N

O

C. Dibenamines (Phenoxybenzamine)

1. History. Eisleb (1930) synthesized series; Nickerson and Goodman (1947) described adrenergic blocking action.

2. Chemistry. Dibenzylamines; phenoxybenzamine also related to the benzodioxanes.

3. Action and Mechanism. a. Dibenamine is a potent sympatholytic, but unlike the benzodioxanes the action is prolonged and irreversible, and hypotensive effects appear in normals. It also produces antihistaminic effects, and central stimulation.

b. Phenoxybenzamine produces a much more pure sympatholytic effect; it is also a potent antihistamine.

c. The adrenergic blockage is presumed to be the result of fixation to the alpha receptors.

4. Pharmacodynamics and Toxicity. a. Effective orally; phenoxybenzamine quickly, dibenamine only after 1 or 2 hours, presumably denoting alteration to an active compound.

b. Dibenamine produces severe side effects: vomiting, miosis, local irritation, postural hypotension, and bizarre psychic effects (confusion of time and space). The others are much better tolerated.

5. Uses. a. Phenoxybenzamine is used to improve the circulation in peripheral vascular disease.

b. Extensive use in shock (see Agents Used in Shock).

6. Preparations

DIBENAMINE

Not used clinically.

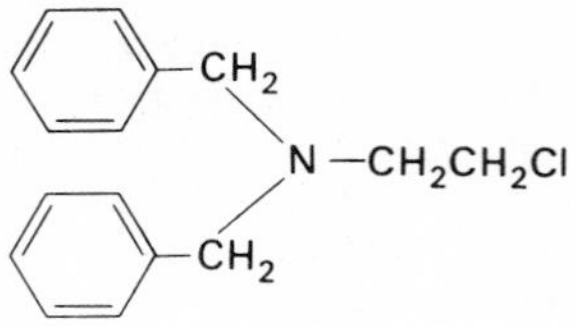

CH_2 / $N-CH_2CH_2Cl$ / CH_2

PHENOXYBENZAMINE HYDROCHLORIDE (Dibenzyline)

Dose: 10 to 60 mg daily by mouth.

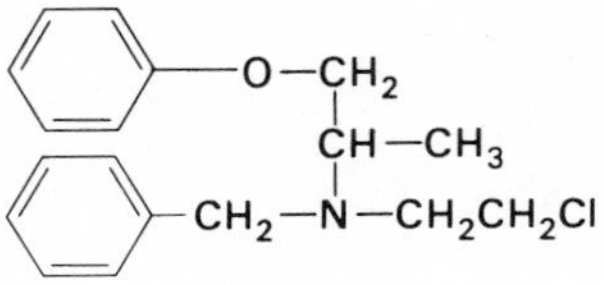

$O-CH_2$ / $CH-CH_3$ / $CH_2-N-CH_2CH_2Cl$

D. Azapetine

AZAPETINE PHOSPHATE (Ilidar)

Has been used to produce a "bloodless" field in surgery and for peripheral vascular disease.

Dose: 25 mg 3 times a day by mouth.

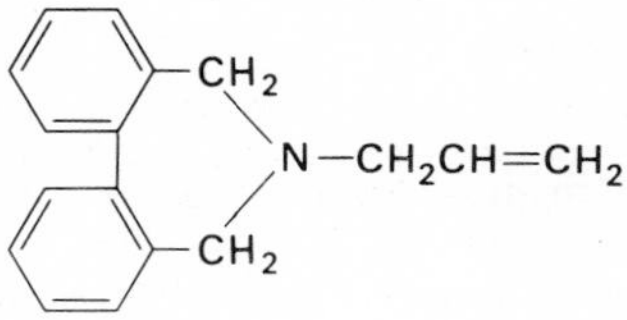

CH_2 / $N-CH_2CH{=}CH_2$ / CH_2

E. Benzazolines (Tolazoline and Phentolamine)

1. History. a. Hartmann and Eisler (1939) synthesized the early members.

b. Chess and Yonkman (1946) recognized sympatholytic activities.

2. Chemistry. Show chemical relationships to sympathomimetics (naphazoline) and histamine.

3. Action and Mechanism. a. The principal effect of each drug is dilation of peripheral arterioles, presumably from competitive interference at the pressor receptors.

b. Tolazoline and, to a lesser extent, phentolamine also show histaminergic, cholinergic, and even sympathomimetic actions.

4. Pharmacodynamics and Toxicity. a. The drugs are absorbed by mouth; effects last 3 to 8 hours.

b. Tolazoline may produce a variety of side effects, mostly autonomic: crawling skin, gooseflesh, flushing, sweating, apprehension, audible peristalsis, increased gastric acidity, dizziness, nausea, headache, congested nose, and postural hypotension; the side effects of phentolamine are less prominent.

5. Uses. a. To produce vascular relaxation in Raynaud's disease, gangrene, causalgia, trench foot, and other peripheral vascular disease. At best, effectiveness is not outstanding.

b. Phentolamine is a preferred agent in the diagnosis of phenochromocytoma and has replaced the less reliable piperoxan; hypertension resulting from the presence of catechol amines is temporarily abated by receptor block. When hypertension is not present, an attack may be precipitated by methacholine or histamine, which stimulate the adrenal tumor to release pressor amines, but the procedure carries danger of the production of excessive hypertension.

6. Preparations

FENSPIRIDE HYDROCHLORIDE

Bronchodilator and alpha blocker. Under investigation.

CH_2CH_2-N N O O

TOLAZOLINE HYDROCHLORIDE (Priscoline)

Dose: 25 mg 4 times a day by mouth.

CH_2 N N

PHENTOLAMINE HYDROCHLORIDE (Regitine)

Dose: 50 mg 4 times a day by mouth; or, in the diagnosis of pheochromocytoma, 5 mg intramuscularly or intravenously proceeded and followed by serial blood pressure measurements, a sharp fall being compatible with tumor.

H_3C $N-CH_2$ N HN HO

II. BETA RECEPTOR BLOCKERS

1. History. Dichloroisoproterenol noted as β blocking agent by Powell and Slater (1958).

2. Chemistry. Derivatives of isoproterenol; or, phenyloxypropanolamines.

3. Action and Mechanism. a. Block β receptors; this decreases inotropic, chronotropic, and metabolic effects on the heart, and may stop arrhythmias produced by excess epinephrine.

b. The need of the heart for O_2 may be decreased, preventing angina.

c. Propranolol also has a quinidine and local anesthetic effect on the heart (sotalol does not), which may stop arrhythmias.

4. Pharmacodynamics and Toxicity. a. Most absorbed orally, but some may be given parenterally.

b. Toxicity includes gastrointestinal effects, CNS depression, skin rashes; bradycardia, hypotension, congestive failure may result from negative inotropic and chronotropic effects.

c. Pronethalol may be neoplastic in mice.

5. Uses. a. Antiarrhythmic in various conditions including digitalis or epinephrine toxicity and ventricular arrhythmias.

b. May relieve angina pectoris.

6. Preparations

a. Isoproterenol derivatives

DICHLOROISOPROTERENOL (DCI)

Use limited to laboratory.

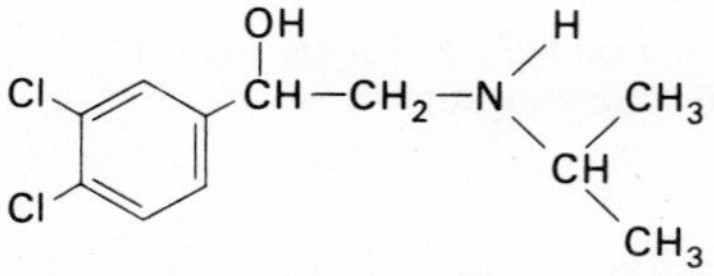

Cl, Cl; OH; CH—CH_2—N; H; CH_3; CH; CH_3

PRONETHALOL (nethalide; Alderlin)

Dose: 50 to 100 mg by mouth 3 times a day; 0.5 to 1 mg per kg body weight intravenously. Discontinued.

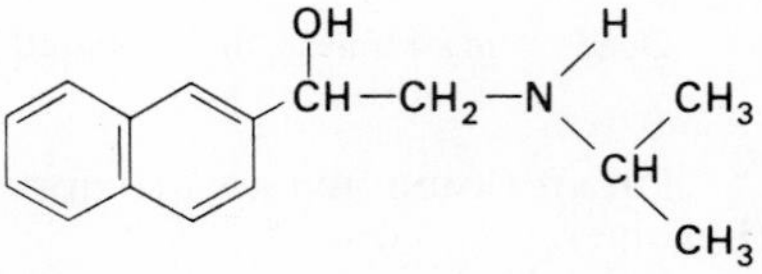

OH; CH—CH_2—N; H; CH_3; CH; CH_3

SOTALOL

Dose: 4 mg intravenously.

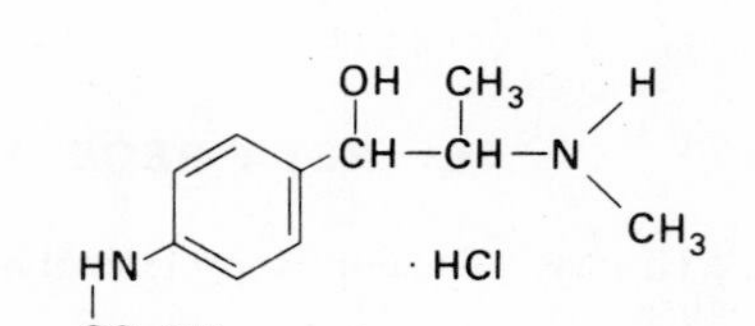

OH; CH—CH_2—N; H; CH_3; CH; CH_3; HN; SO_2CH_3

OTHERS

H_3CO; OH CH_3; CH—CH—N; H; CH_3; C—CH_3; CH_3; OCH_3

butoxamine

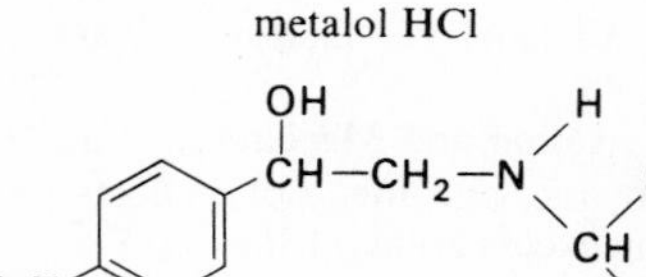

OH CH_3; CH—CH—N; H; CH_3; · HCl; HN; SO_2CH_3

metalol HCl

OH; CH—CH_2—N; H; CH_3; CH; CH_3; O_2N

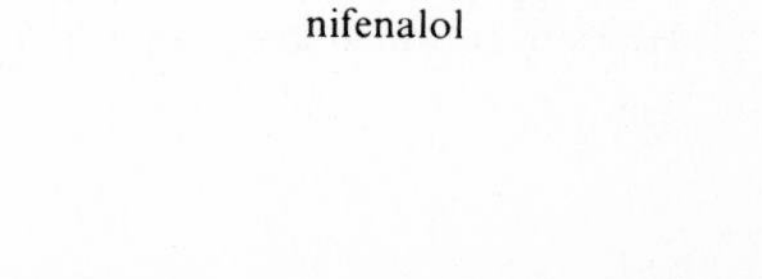

nifenalol

b. Phenyloxypropanolamines

ALPRENOLOL HYDROCHLORIDE (Aptine)

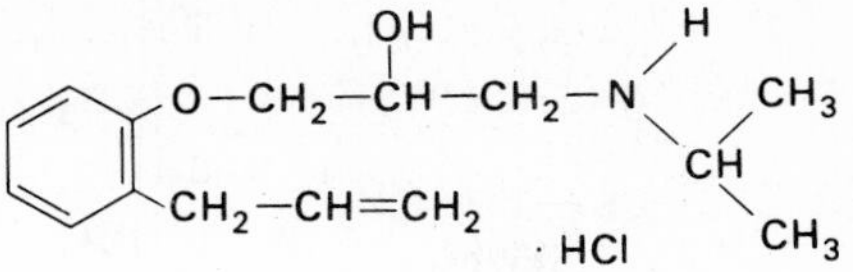

Dose: 100 mg 4 times a day by mouth; 1 mg per minute for 12 to 20 minutes intravenously.

PROPRANOLOL HYDROCHLORIDE (Inderal)

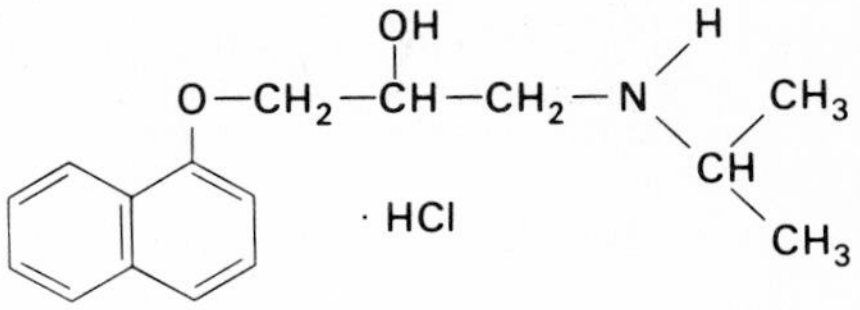

Used in arrhythmias, and hypertension.

Dose: 10 to 30 mg 3 to 4 times a day by mouth; or 1 to 3 mg slowly intravenously.

OTHERS

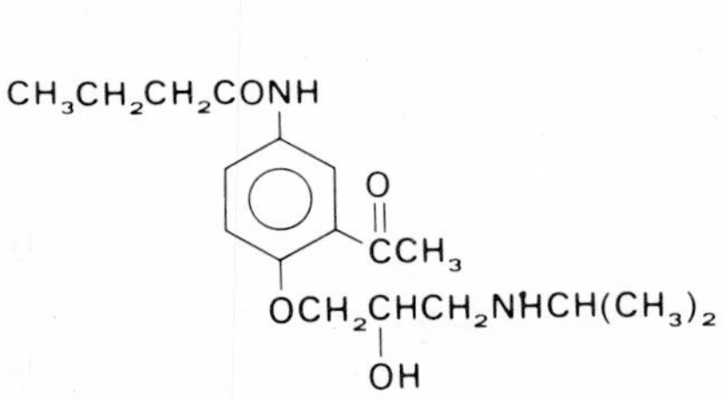

acebutol

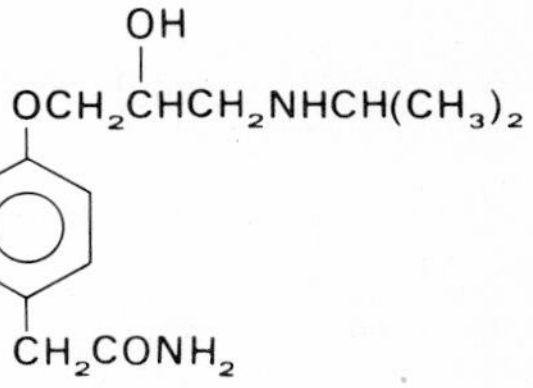

atenolol

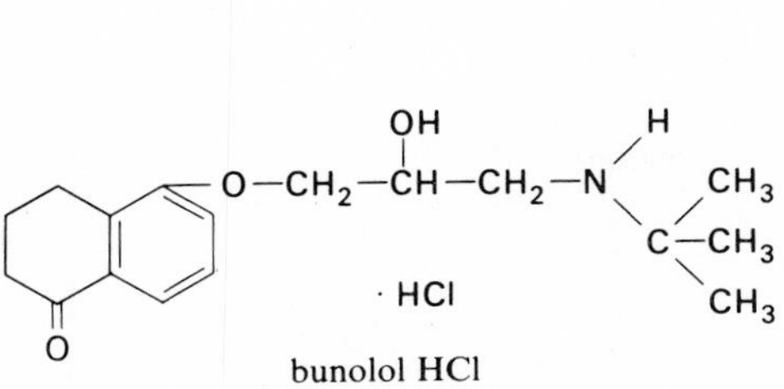

· HCl

bunolol HCl

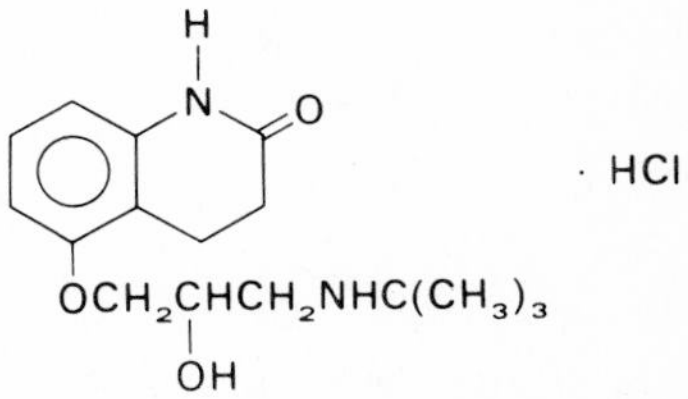

carteolol hydrochloride

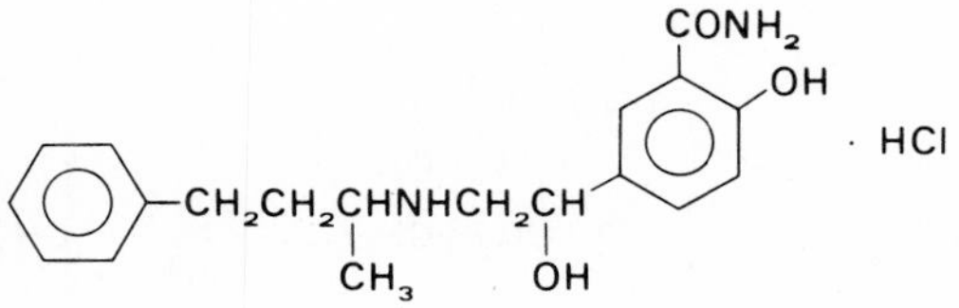

labetalol hydrochloride

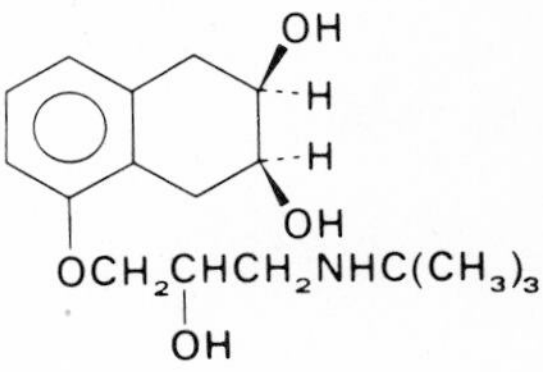

oxprenolol (Trasicor)

pamatolol sulfate

pindolol (Visken)

practolol

timolol maleate

tiprenolol HCl

xipranolol

SUMMARY: SYMPATHETIC DEPRESSANTS AND ADRENOLYTIC AGENTS

TYPE	*ACTION AND MECHANISM*	*TOXICITY*	*USE*	*EXAMPLES*
Ergot alkaloids	Ergotoxin reversal from alpha block	Uterine contracture	Laboratory use only	Ergotoxin
Benzodioxanes	Hypotension from alpha block	Tachycardia, hyperpnea	Obsolete for diagnosis of pheochromocytoma	Piperoxan
Dibenamines	Same	Vomiting, postural hypotension, bizarre psychic effects	Shock	Phenoxybenzamine HCl
Benzazolines	Same	Crawling skin, flushing, headache, hypotension	Peripheral vascular disease; diagnosis of pheochromocytoma	Phentolamine HCl
Beta blockers	Decreases inotropic effects on heart Local anesthetic	Rashes, bradycardia, hypotension	Arrhythmias, angina pectoris	Propranolol HCl

Reviews

Volle, R. Pharmacology of the autonomic nervous system. Ann. Rev. Pharmacol., 3:129, 1963.

Copp, F. Adrenergic neurone blocking agents. Advances Drug Res., 1:161, 1964.

Epstein, S., and Braunwald, E. Beta-adrenergic receptor blocking drugs. New Eng. J. Med., 275:1106, 1966.

Moran, N. New adrenergic blocking drugs. Bull. N.Y. Acad. Sci., 139:541, 1967.

Ahlquist, R. Agents which block adrenergic beta receptors. Ann. Rev. Pharmacol., 8:259, 1968.

Ghouri, M., and Haley, T. Structure action relationships in the adrenergic blocking agents. J. Pharm. Sci., 58:511, 1969.

Dollery, C., Paterson, J., and Conolly, M. Clinical pharmacology of beta-receptor-blocking agents. Clin. Pharmacol. Ther., 10:765, 1969.

43. Parasympathetic Stimulants or Cholinergic Agents

The natural mediator or stimulant at postganglionic parasympathetic endings is acetylcholine. It is also the mediator at certain sympathetic endings (sweat glands, some blood vessels). A large number of other substances, natural and synthetic, may also produce the effects of parasympathetic stimulation, either by acting directly upon the receptors or by inactivating acetylcholinesterase and thus allowing the natural acetylcholine longer tenure at the receptor.

A. Acetylcholine

1. History. a. Acetylcholine synthesized (1866); Hunt (1906) recognized it in the adrenal medulla.

b. Loewi (1921) demonstrated the presence of a parasympathetic transmitting substance (Vagusstoff) which was soon identified as acetylcholine. Dale, and in more recent years Nachmansohn, emphasized and clarified its function.

2. Chemistry. Acetylcholine is an ester of acetic acid and choline.

$$\underset{\text{acetate}}{CH_3COO^-} + \underset{\text{choline}}{HO{-}CH_2CH_2{-}\overset{+}{N}(CH_3)_3} \longrightarrow \underset{\text{acetylcholine}}{H_3C\overset{O}{\overset{\|}{C}}{-}O{-}CH_2CH_2{-}\overset{+}{N}(CH_3)_3}$$

3. Action. a. The general effects produced by parasympathetic stimulation from the natural release of acetylcholine include contracted pupils, salivation, slowed heart, constricted bronchi, increased peristalsis, and dilated splanchnic vessels.

b. When acetylcholine is injected subcutaneously in moderate dosage an almost alarming reaction takes place. After a few moments the skin flushes, sweat, saliva and tears pour forth, and the subject apprehensively clutches his chest as bronchial constriction and cardiac slowing appear; in about 5 minutes the maelstrom is over, usually without sphincter relaxation. This reaction is quite different from the mild, relaxed postprandial state of natural stimulation of the parasympathetic system, but the difference is largely a matter of degree.

c. Injected acetylcholine reaches principally the postganglionic receptors only, so ganglionic and myoneural signs are minimal.

4. Mechanism. a. In the transmission of a parasympathetic impulse, acetylcholine is liberated from the nerve endings, crosses to and stimulates the appropriate receptors, and then is quickly hydrolyzed by acetylcholine esterase. The situation is thus parallel to that at the sympathetic nerve endings, except for the presence of only a single transmitter, receptor, and destructive enzyme (other choline esterases present in the body are not of importance at the cholinergic junction); however, the destruction of acetylcholine is much more rapid than the corresponding inactivation of norepinephrine.

b. Acetylcholine stimulates the receptor by depolarizing its surface.

a′. In the resting state the receptor mechanism is polarized (90 millivolts) because of different concentrations of Na^+ outside the cell and K^+ inside the cell.

b′. With the arrival of a nerve impulse at a synapse, acetylcholine (ACh) is released from storage vesicles into a narrow cleft (200Å) between the cells. A flux of ions across the cleft then carries Na^+ into the distal cell until the charges are balanced; stimulation then occurs.

c′. Excess acetylcholine is immediately hydrolyzed by acetylcholine esterase (AChE), and K^+ ions leave the cell, reestablishing polarization.

d′. Finally, the ions are returned to their resting position by active transport and the cycle is complete.

e′. Stimulation may result not only from the presence of acetylcholine, but from other choline esters or other direct stimulants; from the presence of AChE inhibitors (presuming the constant liberation of small amounts of ACh); or from other alteration of the electrical charge or ion concentration.

5. Pharmacodynamics, Toxicity, and Uses. Acetylcholine is unstable (hygroscopic) chemically and too abrupt and fleeting for satisfactory therapeutic use.

B. Other Direct Cholinergics

A number of other compounds, both synthetic and natural, resemble acetylcholine in being direct stimulants of cholinergic receptors. All are choline esters, or contain in their molecules what appear to be choline ester equivalents (except possibly pilocarpine).

SYNTHETIC CHOLINE ESTERS

1. History. Series introduced by Hunt who synthesized methacholine and Simonart (1932) who used it clinically.

2. Chemistry. Chemical structure and characteristics of activity may be correlated to a considerable extent. The following points are relevant to therapeutic compounds:

$$H_3C-\overset{\overset{O}{\|}}{C}-O-\underset{\underset{H}{|}}{\overset{\overset{H}{|}}{C}}-\underset{\underset{H}{|}}{\overset{\overset{H}{|}}{C}}-\overset{+}{N}(CH_3)_3$$

acetyl   beta carbon   alpha carbon   substitutions on N

a. Acetyl group: Substitution of the acetyl by carbamate blocks the hydrolytic activity of acetylcholinesterase and produces compounds of long action.

b. Beta carbon: Substitution prevents the molecule from being attacked by nonspecific esterases and it therefore gains the receptor area more satisfactorily; also, the molecule no longer appears to fit at the ganglionic or neuromuscular receptors, thus limiting the action to postganglionic receptors.

c. Alpha carbon: Substitutions tend to increase the nicotinic effect.

d. Substitutions on N: Substitutions of larger groups for CH_3 diminish or alter the cholinergic response, but involvement of the N in a ring is compatible with activity.

3. Action and Mechanism. a. Produce postganglionic parasympathomimetic effects, similar to acetylcholine but usually prolonged; principal desired effect usually smooth muscle stimulation.

b. Some also mimic effects of acetylcholine at ganglia or striated muscle.

4. Pharmacodynamics and Toxicity. Most poorly absorbed. Side effects include intestinal cramping and excessive sweating, bradycardia, hypotension.

5. Uses. To stimulate intestinal peristalsis, as in postoperative ileus, and to induce micturition.

6. Preparations

ACETYLCHOLINE CHLORIDE
Dose: 1% ophthalmic solution.

METHACHOLINE CHLORIDE (Mecholyl)

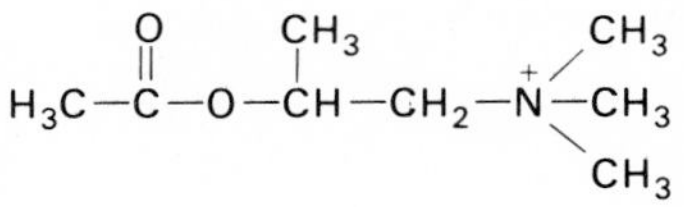

$$H_3C-\overset{\overset{O}{\|}}{C}-O-\overset{\overset{CH_3}{|}}{CH}-CH_2-\overset{+}{N}(CH_3)_3$$

Actions postganglionic only, but brief, and injection required. Formerly used to slow the heart in paroxysmal tachycardia, to stimulate intestinal peristalsis, and to promote micturition. Intravenous administration dangerous: cardiac arrest, asthma. Obsolete.

CARBACHOL CHLORIDE (Doryl)

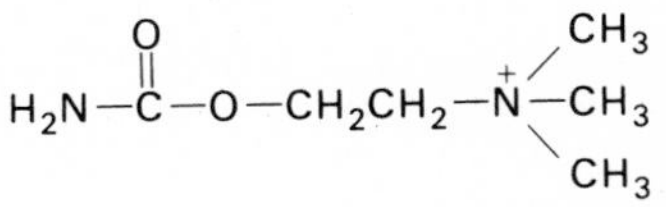

$$H_2N-\overset{\overset{O}{\|}}{C}-O-CH_2CH_2-\overset{+}{N}(CH_3)_3$$

Produces ganglionic and muscular effects as well as postganglionic. Formerly used to induce micturition. Obsolete, except in eyedrops.

Dose: 0.75 to 3.0% ophthalmic solutions.

BETHANECHOL CHLORIDE (Urecholine)

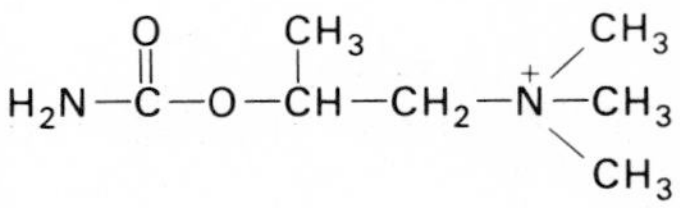

$$H_2N-\overset{\overset{O}{\|}}{C}-O-\overset{\overset{CH_3}{|}}{CH}-CH_2-\overset{+}{N}(CH_3)_3$$

Prolonged action, with effects limited to postganglionic. Useful for the relief of acute urinary retention, and of chronic retention from ganglionic inhibitors in hypertensive patients. It has also been used in paralytic ileus, and to provoke emptying of the stomach after vagotomy. May produce sweating and other parasympathetic side effects.

Dose: 5 to 30 mg by mouth; 3 to 5 mg subcutaneously.

PILOCARPINE

1. History. Isolated in 1871.

2. Chemistry. Tertiary amine obtained from the Brazilian shrub, *Pilocarpus Jaborandi*, or prepared synthetically.

3. Action and Mechanism. a. Produces strong postganglionic stimulation and slight ganglionic stimulation.

b. Stimulates salivary and bronchial secretions; produces sweating and increased peristalsis; may improve drainage from anterior chamber of the eye in glaucoma.

c. The mechanism is direct cholinergic receptor stimulation.

4. Pharmacodynamics and Toxicity. a. Pilocarpine is absorbed well by mouth or by injection.

b. Overdosage causes diarrhea, pulmonary edema, cardiac arrest, collapse (antidote: atropine, and vice versa).

5. Uses. a. Principal use is in the treatment of chronic, simple glaucoma (wide or open angle), where there is inadequate drainage of aqueous humor from the anterior chamber of the eye through the canal of Schlemm, with resultant increased intraocular tension and optic atrophy. Pilocarpine constricts the pupil and dilates the canal, relieving the situation; carbonic anhydrase inhibitors may also be used (in angle closure, or narrow angle, glaucoma, surgery is required rather than miotics).

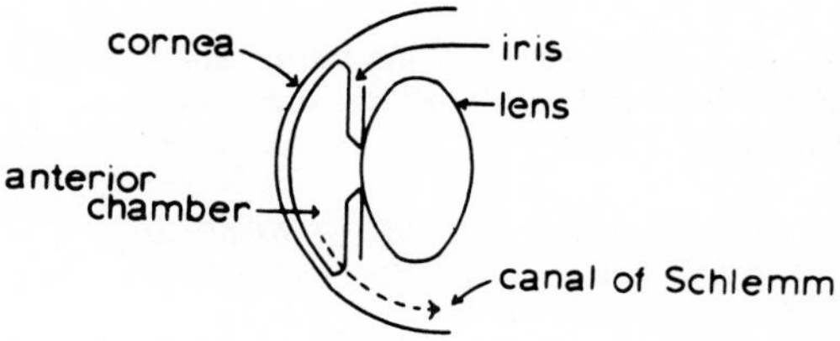

b. Formerly used as a diaphoretic, but the production of intense sweating for the removal of toxins from the body is seldom if ever advisable.

6. Preparation

PILOCARPINE NITRATE

Dose: 0.5% to 4% solution in the eye; 3 to 30 mg by mouth or subcutaneously.

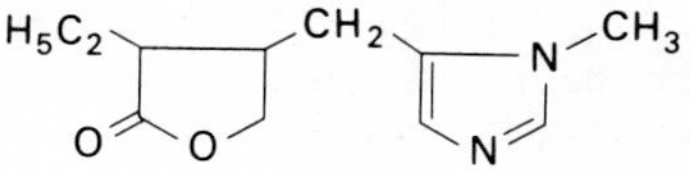

PILOCARPINE HYDROCHLORIDE

OTHER ALKALOIDS

MUSCARINE

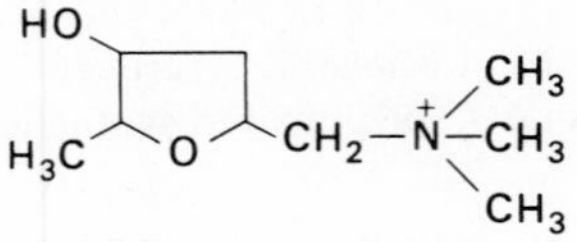

The natural cholinergic substance in *Amanita muscaria*, the fly agaric mushroom; described in 1811; early lent its name to postganglionic parasympathetic stimulation ("muscarine effect"). Correct formula and isomeric state not defined until 1958. Poisoning uncommon but may produce psychotic states; atropine an effective antidote for peripheral effects. (Not to be confused with *Amanita phalloides*, which causes gastroenteritis after some hours delay, and late hepatic and renal necrosis.)

No clinical use.

ARECOLINE

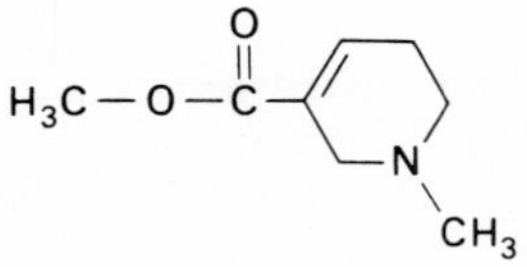

Alkaloid present in the betel nut. The seed is commonly chewed with lime in Southeast Asia and produces red teeth and saliva, and a feeling of well-being.

ACECLIDINE (Glaucostat)

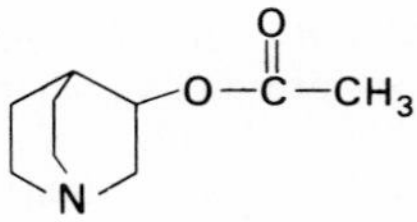

Dose: 0.5 to 2% solution in the eye to reduce intraocular pressure.

C. Cholinesterase Inhibitors

Inhibitors of acetylcholinesterase accentuate the effect of acetylcholine at receptors by sparing the transmitter from immediate destruction.

1. Chemistry. a. Cholinesterase inhibitors are esters (or organic phosphates) having steric forms related to acetylcholine. The reaction of inhibitor with acetylcholinesterase (AChE) is similar to that between acetylcholine and the enzyme:

$$\text{Inhibitor (ester)} + \text{AChE} \rightarrow \text{AChE:Ester}$$
$$\text{AChE:Ester} \rightarrow \text{AChE} + \text{acid} + \text{alcohol}$$

b. When both steps occur, the inhibition is rapid, fleeting, and reversible. When only the first step occurs, and AChE combines with the inhibitor but then cannot split it, the action is slow, prolonged, and irreversible as the AChE is permanently removed from availability. The carbamic esters are examples of the first type; the organic phosphates of the second type.

D. Carbamic Esters

PHYSOSTIGMINE

1. History. The Calabar bean (Esere bean), seed of *Physostigma venenosum*, has been used in primitive African societies for trial by ordeal; if vomited up, so that symptoms were aborted, the verdict was not guilty.

2. Chemistry. An alkaloid.

3. Action and Mechanism. a. A potent postganglionic stimulant (stronger than pilocarpine) which also produces minor stimulation at other cholinergic endings.

b. Actions include: miosis, bradycardia, increased intestinal motility.

4. Pharmacodynamics and Toxicity. a. Absorbed well; actions last 3 or 4 hours.

b. Side effects may include muscular weakness, nausea and vomiting, CNS stimulation, bronchospasm; neutralized by atropine.

5. Uses. Principal use is as a miotic; when solutions are dropped in the eye the pupil is constricted and intraocular tension decreased. It is therefore of use in glaucoma, to break up synechia, and to oppose atropine mydriasis.

6. Preparation

PHYSOSTIGMINE SALICYLATE (Eserine)
Dose: 0.1% to 1% solution in the eye.

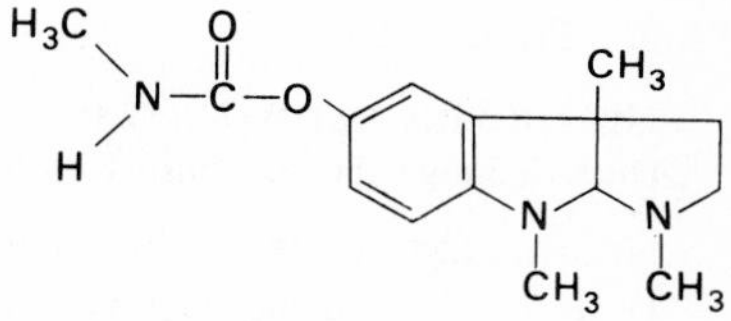

H_3C, H — N—C(=O)—O— (ring); CH_3; N—CH_3, N—CH_3

PHYSOSTIGMINE SULFATE

NEOSTIGMINE

1. History. a. Walker (1931) reported the effectiveness of physostigmine in myasthenia gravis.

b. Aeschlimann and Reinert then showed the greater effectiveness of the derived neostigmine.

2. Chemistry. Neostigmine differs from physostigmine in two important respects:

a. Instead of being a simple amine, the N is present in a quaternary ion, which retards hydrolysis and so gives a longer effect; penetration into cells is also retarded.

b. It possesses an effective "choline portion" which actively stimulates the receptor, as well as a "carbamic portion" which blocks AChE.

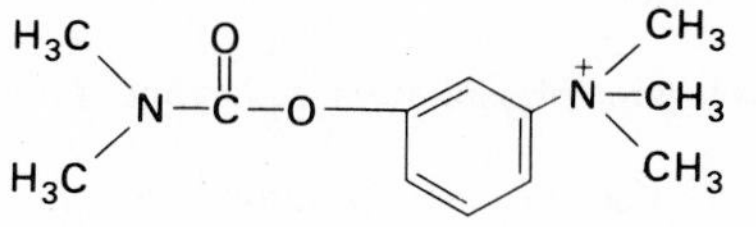

H_3C, H_3C — N—C(=O)—O— (ring) — $\overset{+}{N}$(CH_3)$_3$

carbamic portion (blocks AChE) "choline" portion (stimulates receptor)

neostigmine

3. Action and Mechanism. Acts potently on both postganglionic and myoneural endings, producing respectively: bradycardia, sweating, stimulation of intestine, bladder, and other smooth muscle; stimulation of striated muscle (fasciculation).

4. Pharmacodynamics and Toxicity. a. Absorbed erratically; little known about metabolic fate.

b. Overdosage may produce sweating, bradycardia, bronchial constriction, weakness, and paralysis.

5. Uses. a. Effective as a peristaltic stimulant in paralytic ileus and morphine constipation; also in urinary retention.

b. Used as a test of early pregnancy by inducing menstruation in a nonpregnant person; the test is not altogether reliable; assumed to be based on rectification of a diminished responsiveness to acetylcholine.

c. Uses on striated muscle (myasthenia gravis; curare antidote) are considered under Myoneural Agents.

6. Preparations

NEOSTIGMINE METHYLSULFATE
Dose: 0.5 mg subcutaneously or intramuscularly.

NEOSTIGMINE BROMIDE (Prostigmine)
Dose: 15 mg by mouth (see Myoneural Agents).

OTHER RELATED AGENTS

DEMECARIUM BROMIDE (Humorsol)

Chemically two molecules of neostigmine with a decamethylene chain interposed. Used as a long acting miotic in glaucoma and accommodative esotropia.

Dose: 0.25% solution locally in the eye.

$$(H_3C)_3\overset{+}{N}-C_6H_4-\overset{O}{\overset{\|}{C}}-O-\underset{}{\overset{CH_3}{\overset{|}{N}}}-(CH_2)_{10}-\overset{CH_3}{\overset{|}{N}}-O-\overset{O}{\overset{\|}{C}}-C_6H_4-\overset{+}{N}(CH_3)_3$$

See also ambenonium, benzpyrium, edrophonium, and pydidostigmine under Myoneural Agents.

E. Organic Phosphates

1. Chemistry. Organic phosphates (see Myoneural Agents for greater detail).

2. Action and Mechanism. a. Organic phosphates inhibit acetylcholinesterase irreversibly and produce what may be described as acetylcholine poisoning; the general actions are described under Myoneural Agents.

b. Local application in the eye, however, results in only the postganglionic effect of miosis and allows use for this restricted purpose.

3. Pharmacodynamics and Toxicity. a. Systemic effects are avoided by local use.

b. Ciliary spasm may be an annoying side effect; corneal ulcers have resulted from the irritating qualities of isofluorophate.

4. Uses. In wide angle glaucoma to give prolonged miosis.

5. Preparations

ISOFLUROPHATE (DFP; Floropryl)

Somewhat capricious; occasionally intraocular tension may be raised. Oily vehicle unpleasant.

Dose: 0.1% in the eye.

$$(H_7C_3-O)(C_3H_7-O)P(=O)F$$

ECHOTHIOPHATE IODIDE (Phospholine)

Claimed to be somewhat more reliable than isoflurophate. Water soluble.

Dose: 0.25% solution in the eye.

$$(H_5C_2-O)(C_2H_5-O)P(=O)-S-CH_2CH_2-\overset{+}{N}(CH_3)_3$$

SUMMARY: PARASYMPATHETIC STIMULANTS OR CHOLINERGIC AGENTS

TYPE	*ACTION AND MECHANISM*	*TOXICITY*	*USE*	*EXAMPLES*
Direct cholinergics	Stimulate cholinergic receptors producing salivation, bradycardia, bronchoconstriction, increased peristalsis, miosis	Intestinal cramping, sweating	Paralytic ileus, inability to void	Bethanechol
Cholinesterase inhibitors	Preserve acetylcholine, allowing above effects	Muscular weakness, bronchospasm	Miotic	Physostigmine

Reviews

Waser, P. Chemistry and pharmacology of muscarine, muscarone and some related compounds. Pharmacol. Rev., 13:465, 1961.

de Robertis, E. Histophysiological aspects of signal transmission in the nervous system. Triangle, 5:76, 1961.

Nachmansohn, D. Nerve activity explained by biochemical analysis. J.A.M.A., 179:639, 1962.

Koelle, G. A new general concept of the neurohumoral functions of acetylcholine and acetylcholinesterase. J. Pharm. Pharmacol., 14:65, 1962.

——— Handbuch der experimentellen Pharmakologie, Vol. 15. Berlin, Springer-Verlag, 1963.

44. Parasympathetic Depressants or Anticholinergic Agents

1. PARASYMPATHETIC DEPRESSANTS

Parasympathetic depressants interfere with the transmission of postganglionic parasympathetic impulses. So far as is known, the interference is based on receptor competition.

Reduction of parasympathetic impulses may also be produced by interruption of transmission in ganglia (see Ganglionic Agents).

A. Belladonna Alkaloids

ATROPINE AND SCOPOLAMINE

1. History. a. Solanaceae actions known in antiquity; used in medieval Italy to dilate pupils attractively, hence belladonna.

b. Mein (1832) isolated atropine; Ladenburg (1880) made semisynthetic homatropine. Schmidt (1890) isolated scopolamine.

2. Chemistry. a. Esters of amino alcohols with an organic acid.

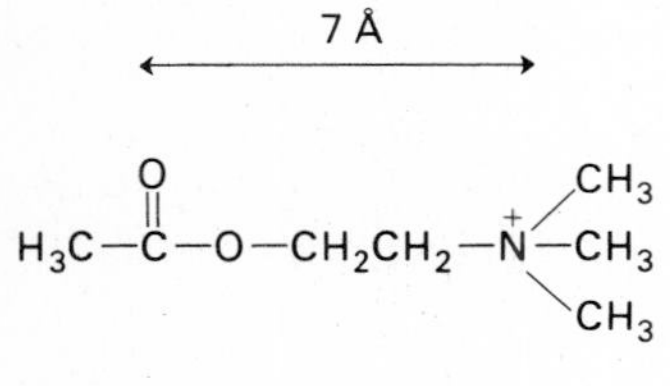

7 Å

$$H_3C-\overset{O}{\overset{\|}{C}}-O-CH_2CH_2-\overset{+}{N}(CH_3)_3$$

acetylcholine

7 Å

$$HOH_2C(C_6H_5)CH-\overset{O}{\overset{\|}{C}}-O-CH\langle(CH_2-CH)_2\rangle N-CH_3 \;(\text{bridged by } CH_2-CH_2)$$

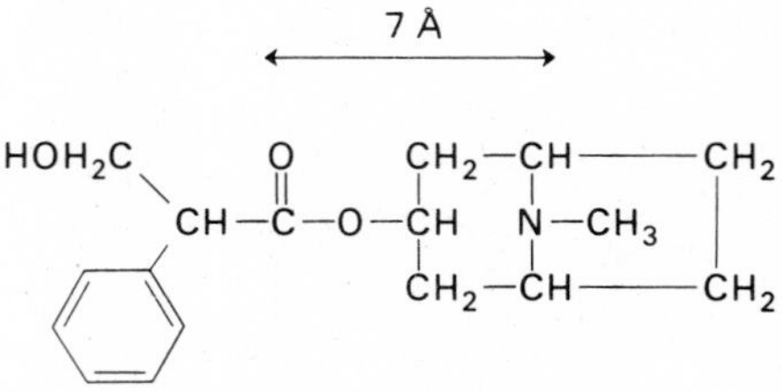

tropic acid (organic acid) | tropine (amino alcohol)

atropine

b. Structure allied to acetylcholine; critical distance of 7Å between choline N and carboxy C same, but acid moiety lengthened.

c. Botanical derivation:

FAMILY	SPECIES	CRUDE DRUGS	PRINCIPAL ALKALOIDS
Solanaceae (potato)	Atropa belladonna	belladonna	*l*-hyoscyamine
	Hyoscyamus niger	hyoscyamus	*dl*-hyoscyamine (atropine)
	Datura stramonium	stramonium	*l*-scopolamine
	Scopolia, and others		

d. Atropine is the racemic mixture of *d*- and *l*-hyoscyamine, usually prepared by racemization of the *l*-form, or by synthesis. It has the advantage of greater stability than the pure *l*-form.

3. Action. a. Act peripherally to produce parasympathetic inhibition, characterized by tachycardia, dilated pupils, a dry skin, mouth, bronchial tree, and stomach, relaxation of alimentary and bronchial smooth muscle.

b. Atropine acts centrally in larger doses to produce what appears to be excitement, but which actually may be a depression of inhibitions, as with alcohol.

c. Scopolamine produces stronger central effects than atropine, with marked depression; sometimes hallucinations.

d. Both atropine and scopolamine depress basal ganglia.

4. Mechanism. a. Agents of the belladonna group attach themselves to the postganglionic receptors and thus prevent the access of acetylcholine. The attachment is primarily by the amino alcohol portion; there may be transitory stimulation of the receptor during attachment. Most of the group are not easily dislodged and the action tends to be moderately prolonged.

b. It is not clear why the atropine group of drugs attach primarily to the postganglionic receptors, and not to ganglionic or striated muscle receptors (except after very large doses; 40 ×). It may be that they do not penetrate to the latter sites, for when atropine is given intraarterially they may be stimulated. Or it may be that the receptors are slightly different.

5. Pharmacodynamics. a. Absorption by mouth is reasonably good; effects after oral or parenteral administration are manifest in a few minutes to half an hour and last 4 to 6 hours.

b. Distribution is wide; urinary excretion of about one third of the administered compound, together with other metabolic products, is uneventful.

6. Toxicity. Dangerous toxicity is rare, but side effects, consisting of amplifications of the normal effects, are frequent: dry mouth, difficulty in reading (dilated pupils and paralyzed accommodation), difficulty in urination (especially older men).

7. Uses

a. Atropine has wide applications:

a′. Antispasmodic: To relax smooth muscle in the alimentary and biliary tracts (as in peptic ulcer); in the urinary tract (as in the tenesmus of infection); in the uterus (as in dysmenorrhea); in the bronchi (as in asthma).

b′. Antisecretory: To reduce sweating (as in night sweats); to reduce salivary and bronchial secretions (during anesthesia); to reduce gastric secretion (in ulcer).

c′. Mydriatic: To dilate the pupil and paralyze accommodation, for examinations and postoperatively.

d′. Cardiac stimulant: To increase heart rate by vagal inhibition (as in bradycardia with syncope).

e′. Central "antispasmodic" effect: To reduce tremor and rigidity (as in parkinsonism).

b. Scopolamine is used principally for central effects: To reduce tremor and rigidity in parkinsonism; as a sedative, often in connection with morphine (twilight sleep); as a preanesthetic medication; in motion sickness.

8. Preparations

a. Natural products

ATROPINE SULFATE

Dose: 0.5 mg by mouth or subcutaneously.

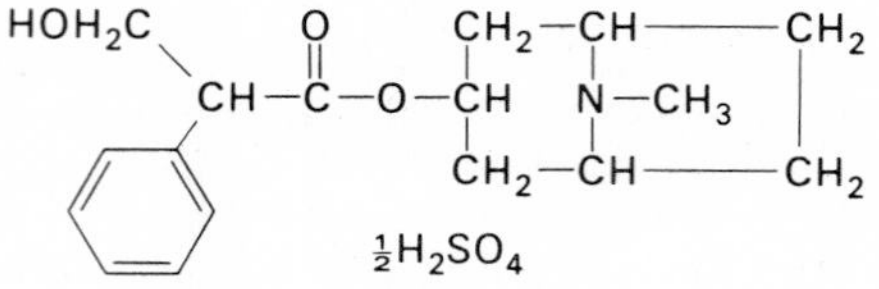

SCOPOLAMINE HYDROBROMIDE (hyoscine)

Dose: 0.5 mg by mouth or subcutaneously.

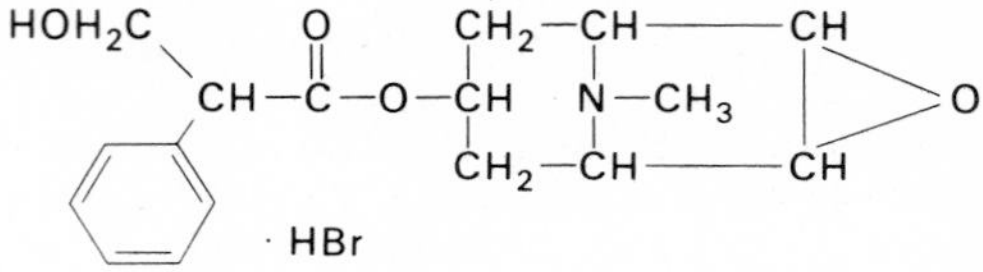

BELLADONNA EXTRACT

Dose: 15 mg by mouth.

TINCTURE OF BELLADONNA

Dose: 0.5 ml every 4 hours by mouth or as needed.

b. Quaternized derivatives

METHSCOPOLAMINE BROMIDE (Pamine, and others)

Alimentary antispasmodic with some ganglionic as well as postganglionic effects (quaternized N).

Dose: 2.5 to 5 mg every 4 hours by mouth; 0.25 to 1 mg subcutaneously.

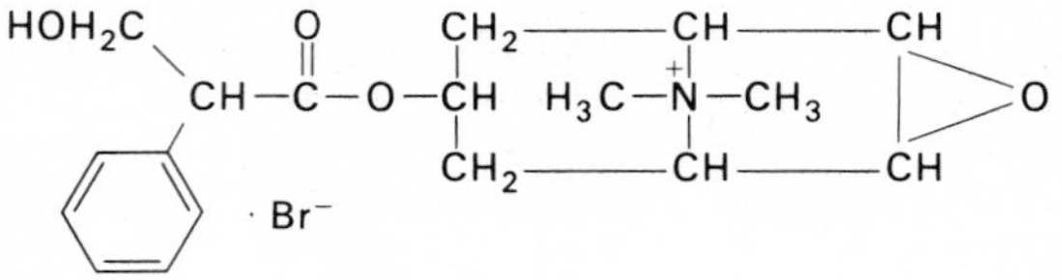

METHYLATROPINE NITRATE (Metropine)

Dose: 1 to 2 mg by mouth every 3 to 4 hours.

B. Smooth Muscle Antispasmodics

A myriad of synthetic or semisynthetic atropine derivatives and relatives are used to relax smooth muscle.

1. Chemistry. The compounds run from those with a complicated tropine or scopine base, like homatropine, to simpler analogues (in which the N of the base may or may not be quaternized) as in the early anticholinergic adiphenine.

2. Action and Mechanism. a. Antispasmodic and antisecretory effects similar to atropine.

b. Some also produce slight ganglionic inhibition at tolerable dosage, with enhancement of the antisecretory effect on gastric acid. Quaternization increases the ganglionic action and decreases CNS effects.

c. Many of the simpler compounds, especially those in which the N is not quaternized, also act directly on smooth muscle to relax it (musculotropic or anti-barium action).

3. Pharmacodynamics and Toxicity. In general resemble atropine.

4. Uses. As antispasmodics and antisecretory agents, particularly for the alimentary tract, and to a lesser extent for the urinary tract.

5. Preparations

a. Esters of tropine or scopine bases (resemble the natural alkaloids in general structure)

ANISOTROPINE METHYLBROMIDE (Valpin)

Resembles homatropine.

Dose: 10 mg by mouth every 4 hours.

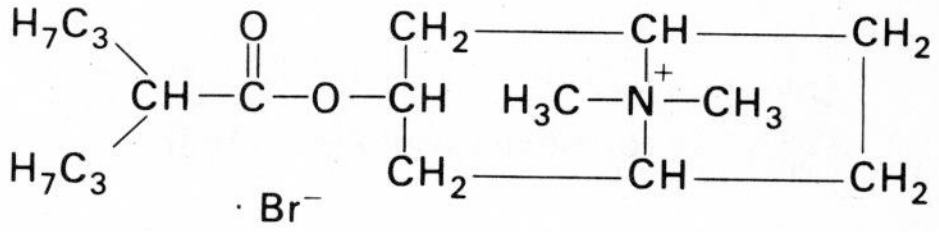

H_7C_3, H_7C_3 — CH—C(=O)—O—CH (CH_2—CH—CH_2; H_3C—N^+—CH_3; CH_2—CH—CH_2) · Br^-

HOMATROPINE METHYLBROMIDE (Novatrin, and others)

An alimentary antispasmodic with minimal side effects; also used as a mydriatic.

Dose: 2.5 mg every 4 hours by mouth.

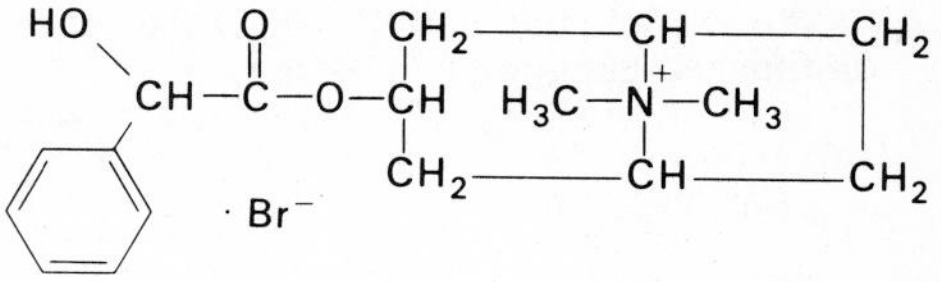

HO, phenyl — CH—C(=O)—O—CH (CH_2—CH—CH_2; H_3C—N^+—CH_3; CH_2—CH—CH_2) · Br^-

OTHERS

HOH_2C, phenyl — CH—C(=O)—O—CH (CH_2—CH—CH_2; O=N—CH_3; CH_2—CH—CH_2)

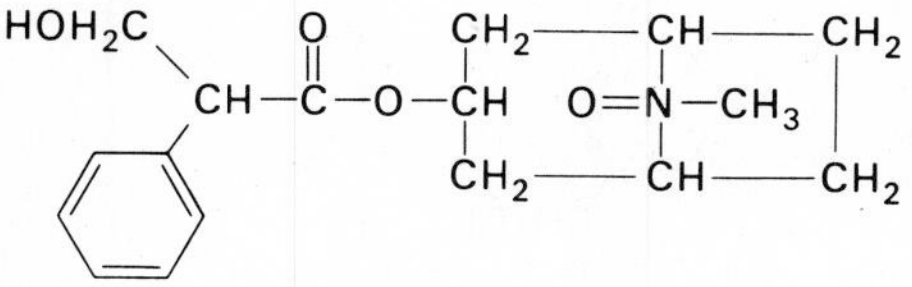

atropine oxide HCl (Genatropine; Xtro)

clidinium Br (Quarzan)

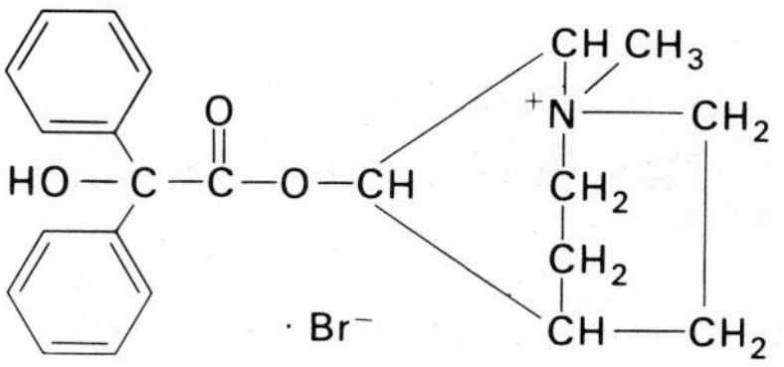

HO—C(diphenyl)—C(=O)—O—CH (CH CH_3; $^+$N—CH_2; CH_2; CH_2; CH—CH_2) · Br^-

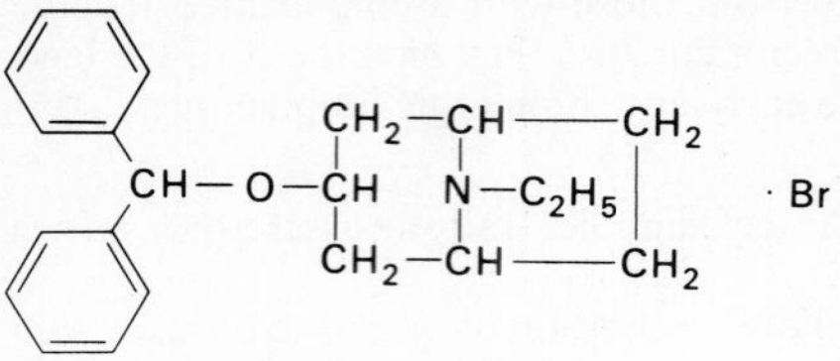

ethylbenztropine Br
(Panolid)

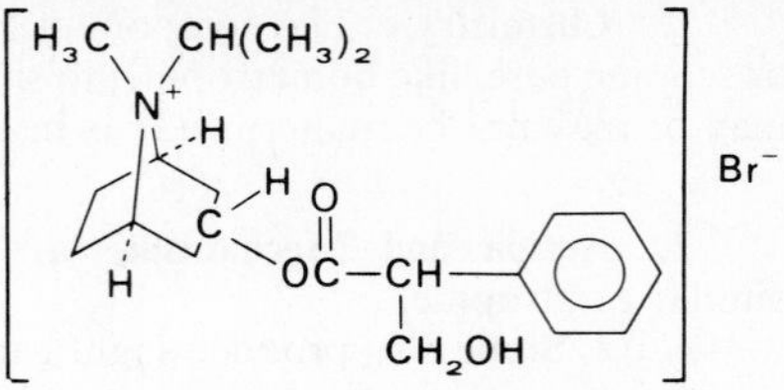

ipratropium bromide (Atrovent)

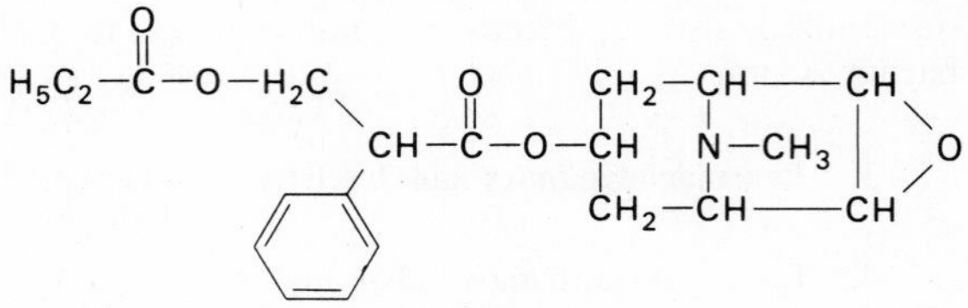

poskine

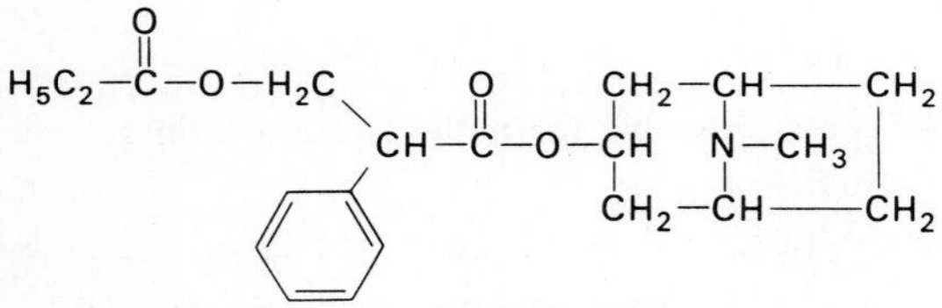

propionyl atropine (Prampine)

b. Esters of simple bases with trivalent nitrogen (accentuated musculotropic, diminished ganglionic, actions)

ADIPHENINE HYDROCHLORIDE (Trasentine)

Dose: 75 mg every 3 hours orally. Little used.

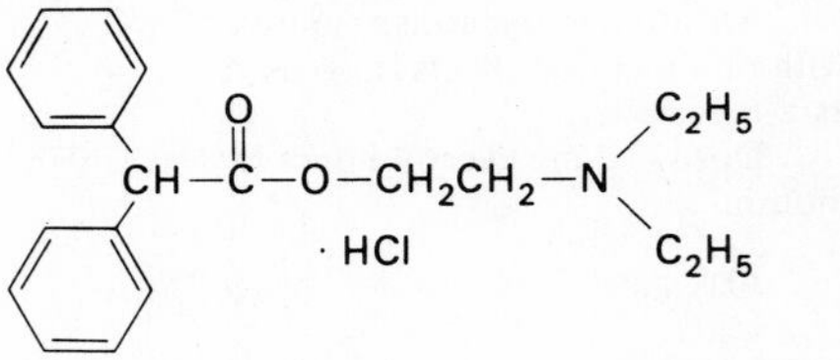

AMOLANONE HYDROCHLORIDE (Amethone)

Also a local anesthetic.
Dose: 50 mg every 4 hours by mouth.

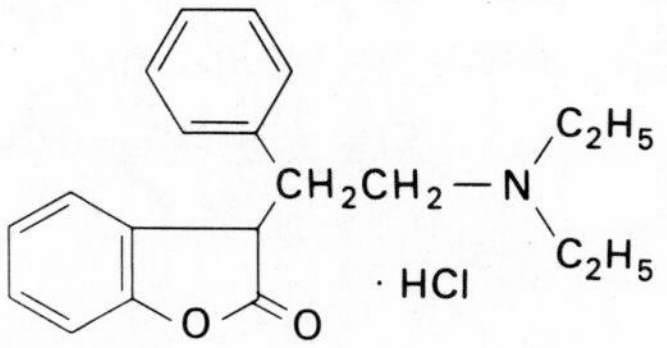

AMPROTROPINE (Syntropan)

Dose: 50 mg every 4 hours by mouth.

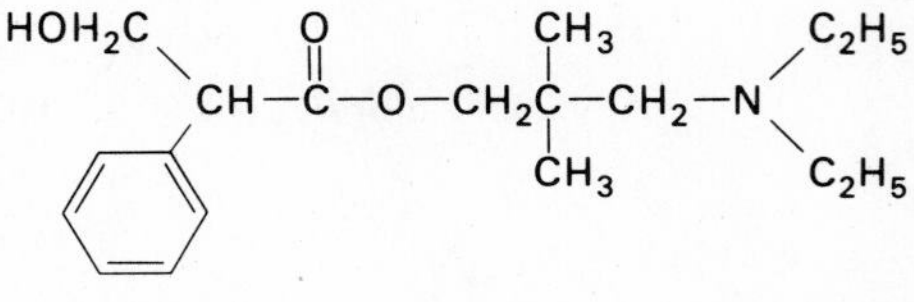

CARBATRINE (Pavatrine)

Dose: 125 mg every 3 hours by mouth. Relatively weak.

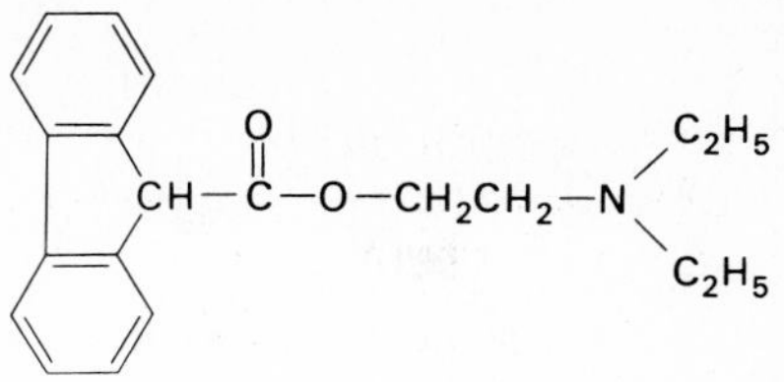

DICYCLOMINE HYDROCHLORIDE (Bentyl)

Claimed to be only musculotropic and therefore not to cause urinary retention and to be safe in glaucoma.

Dose: 10 mg every 4 hours by mouth.

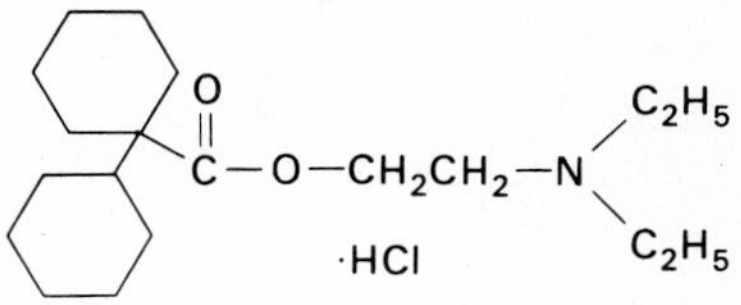

OXYPHENCYCLIMINE HYDROCHLORIDE (Daricon)

Long acting.

Dose: 10 mg every 4 to 12 hours by mouth.

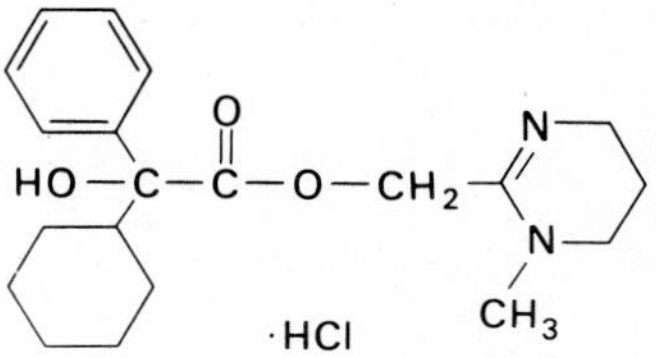

PIPERIDOLATE HYDROCHLORIDE (Dactil)

Less potent than atropine; toxicity low.

Dose: 50 mg every 4 hours by mouth.

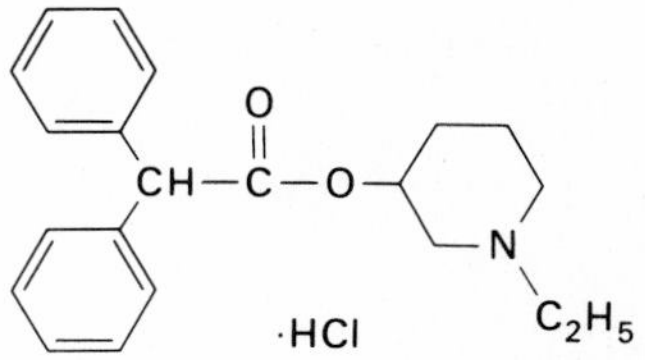

THIPHENAMIL HYDROCHLORIDE (Trocinate)

Dose: 200 to 300 mg 4 times a day by mouth.

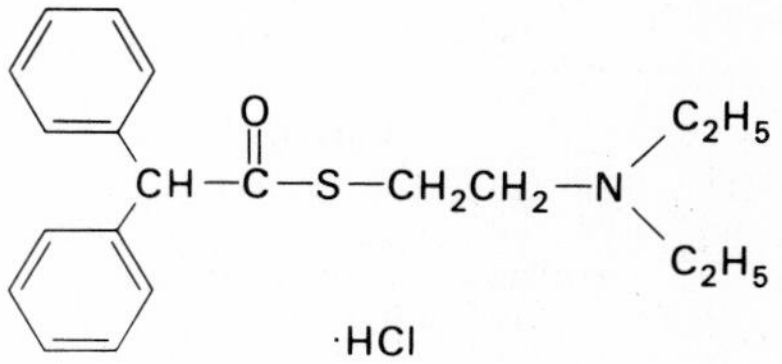

OTHERS

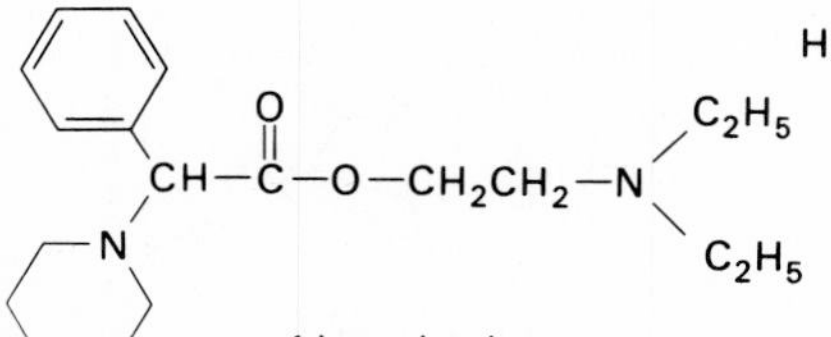

bietamiverine

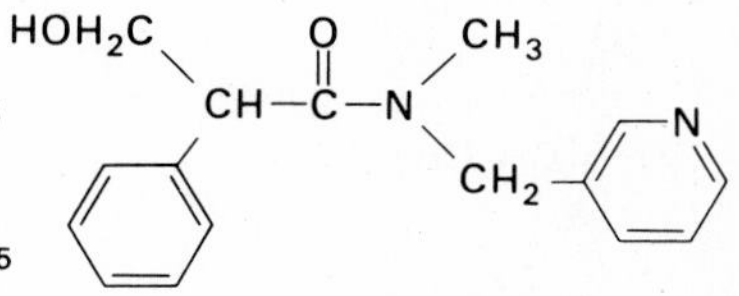

bimetremide

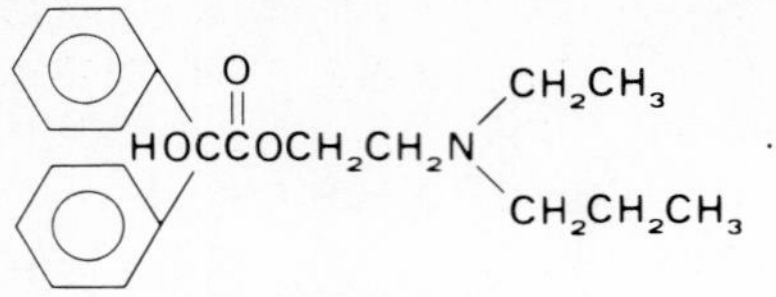

benapryzine hydrochloride

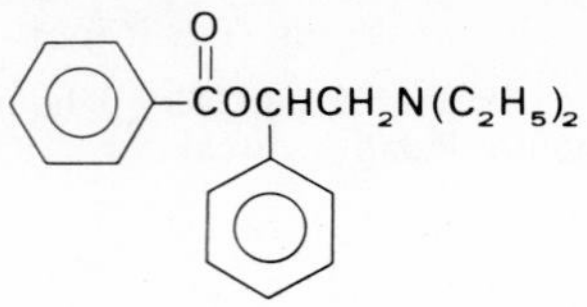

elucaine

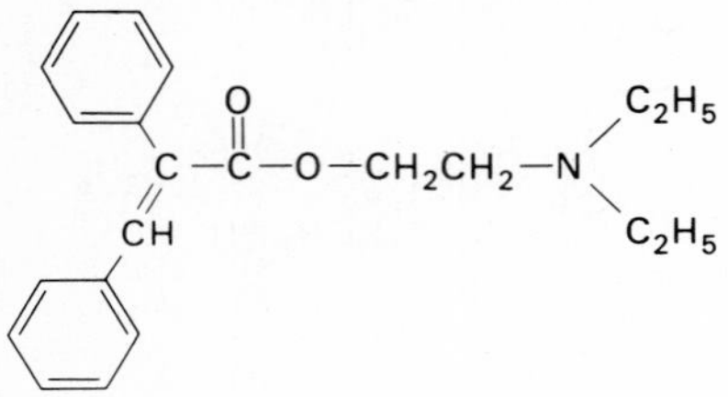

cinnamaverine

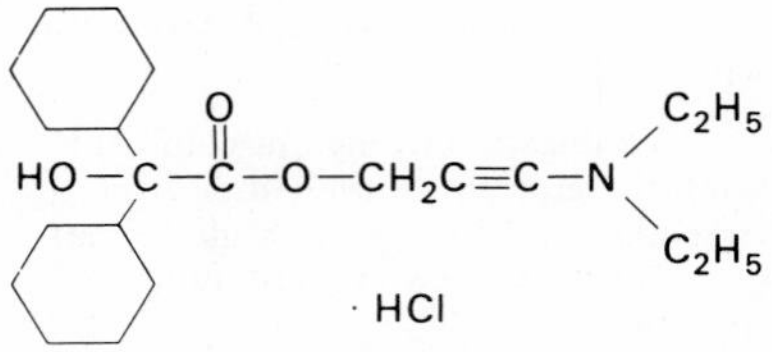

cyclonylamine HCl

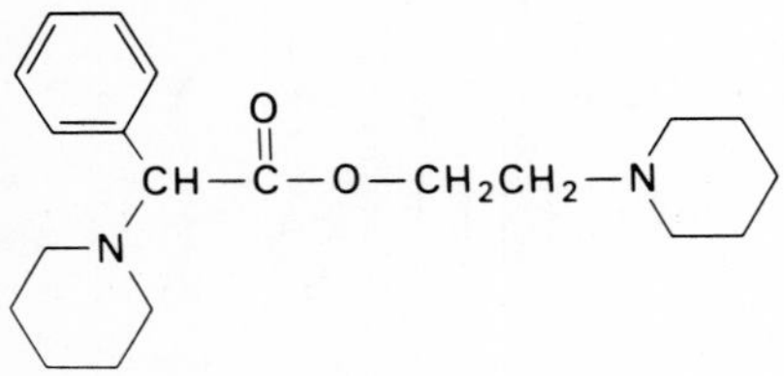

dipiproverine

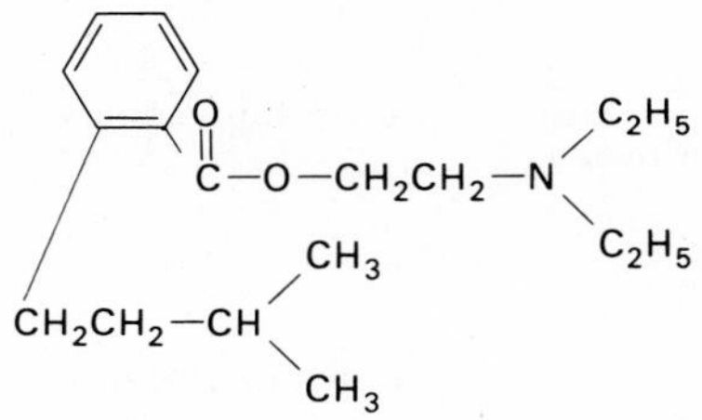

isomylamine HCl (Neurylan)

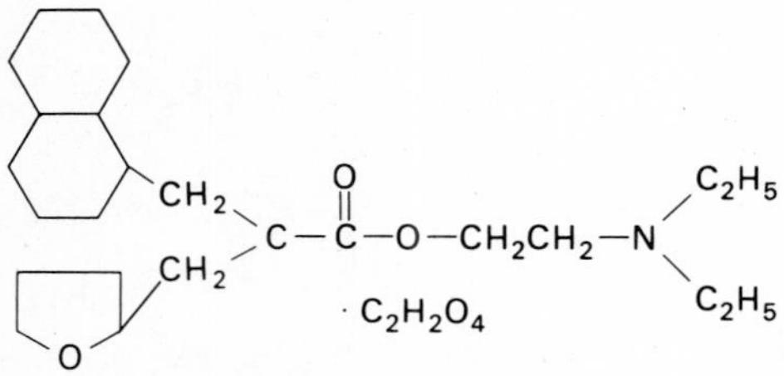

nafronyl oxalate (Praxilene)
(vasodilator)

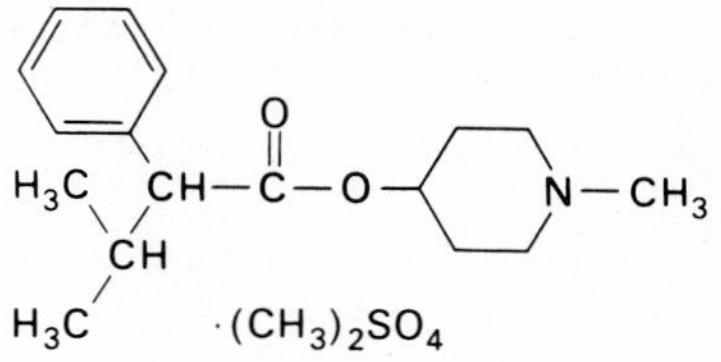

pentapiperide mesylate (Quilene)

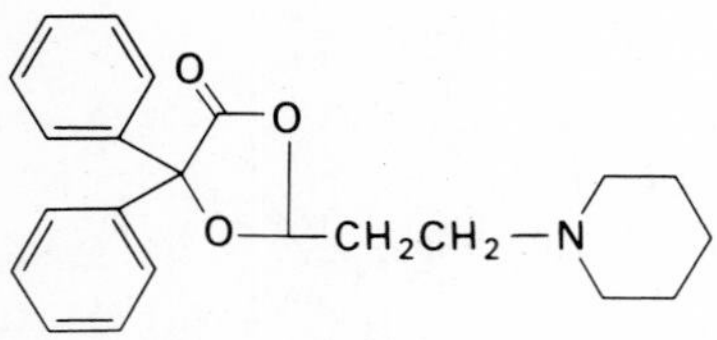

pipoxolan HCl (Rowa)

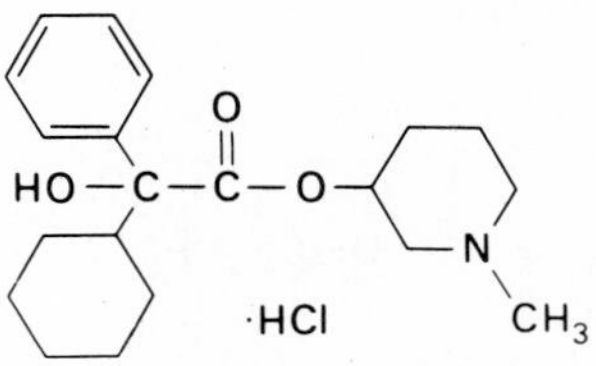

propenzolate HCl (Delinal)

c. Esters of simple bases with quaternary nitrogen (accentuated ganglionic effects; absence of musculotropic and central effects; absorption incomplete; excretion rapid)

GLYCOPYRROLATE
(Robinul)

Dose: 1 mg 3 times a day by mouth.

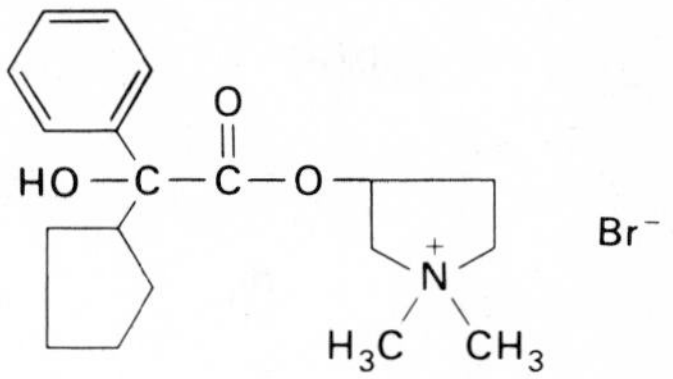

MEPENZOLATE METHYLBROMIDE
(Cantil)

Claim greater activity on colon.
Dose: 25 mg every 4 hours by mouth.

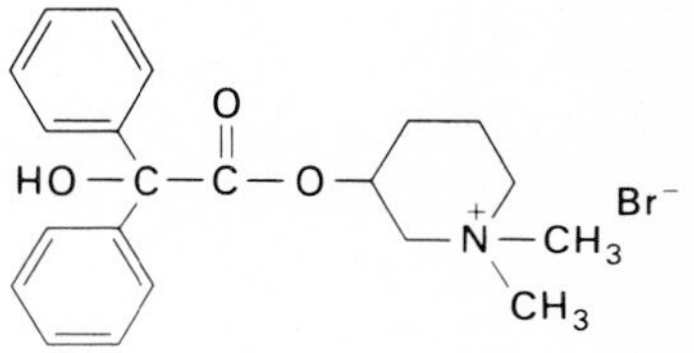

OXYPHENONIUM BROMIDE
(Antrenyl)

Dose: 5 mg every 4 hours by mouth.

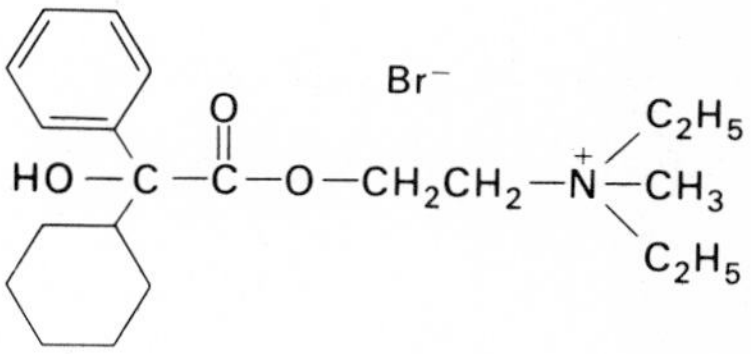

PENTHIENATE BROMIDE
(Monodral)

Dose: 5 mg every 4 to 8 hours by mouth.

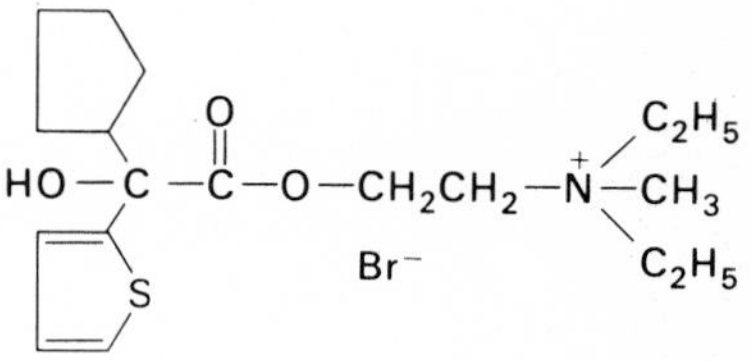

PIPENZOLATE METHYLBROMIDE
(Piptal)

Dose: 5 mg every 4 hours by mouth.

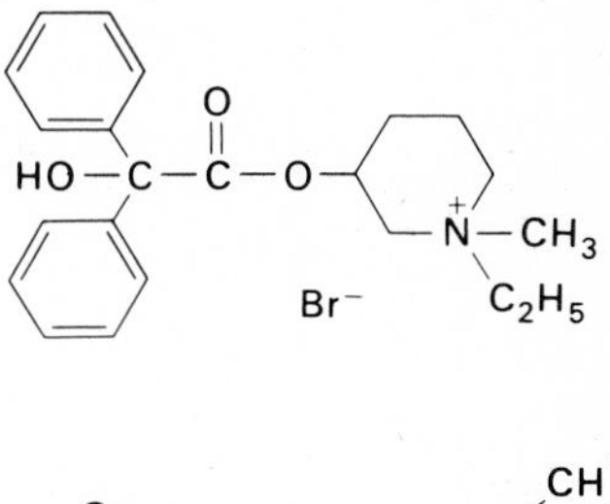

PROPANTHELINE BROMIDE
(Pro-Banthine)

Dose: 15 mg every 4 hours by mouth.

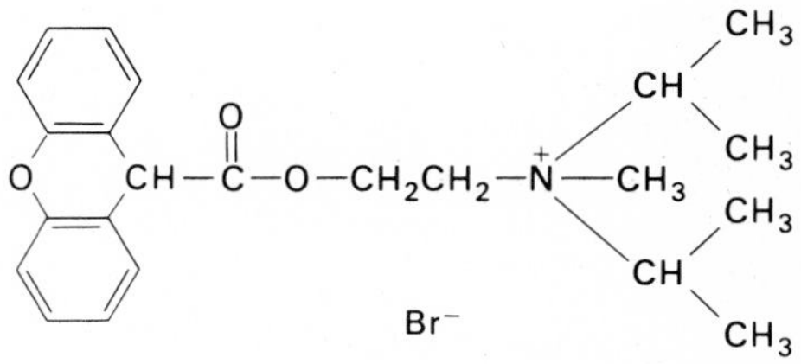

OTHERS

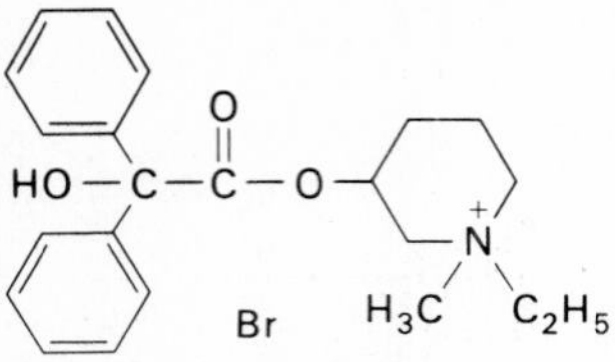

O
HO—C—C—O
N
Br H_3C C_2H_5

benzilonium Br (Portyn)

O CH_3 C_2H_5
HO—C—C—N—CH_2CH_2—N—CH_3
· Cl^- C_2H_5

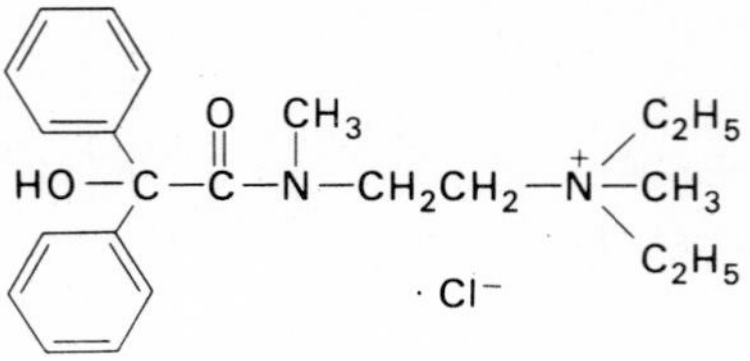

benzomethamine Cl (Contranul)

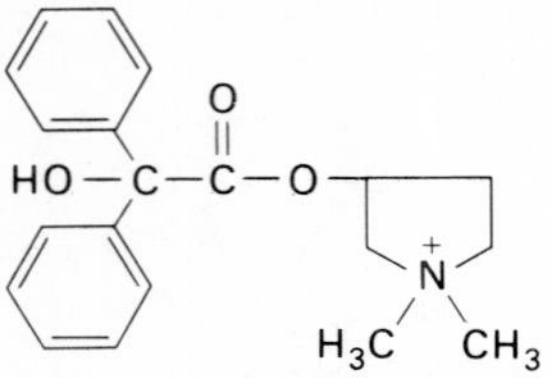

O
HO—C—C—O
N
H_3C CH_3

benzopyrrolate

O
CH—C—O
N · Br^-
H_3C CH_3

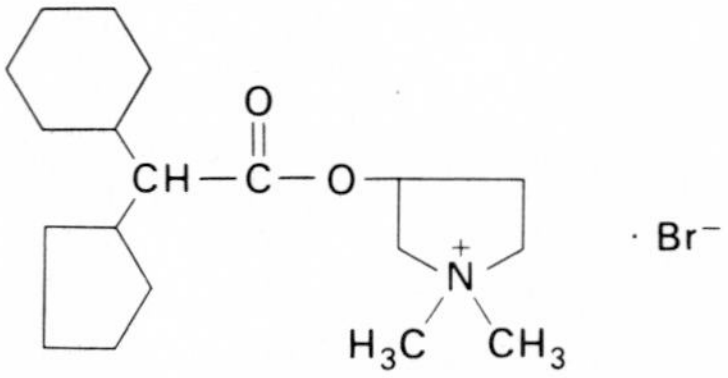

cyclopyrronium bromide

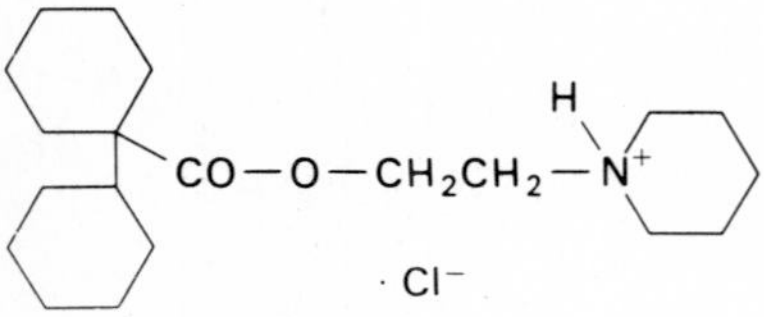

H
CO—O—CH_2CH_2—N^+
· Cl^-

dihexyverine Cl (Metaspas)

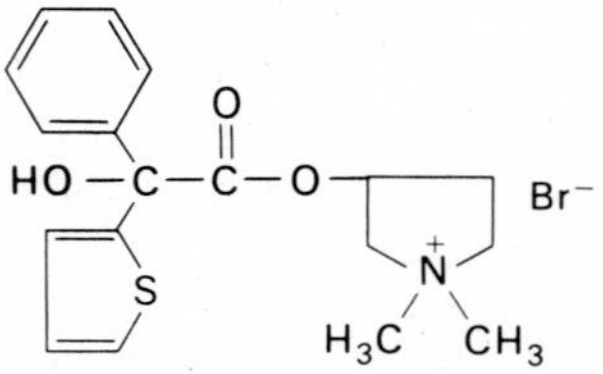

O
HO—C—C—O Br^-
S N
H_3C CH_3

heteronium Br (Hetrum)

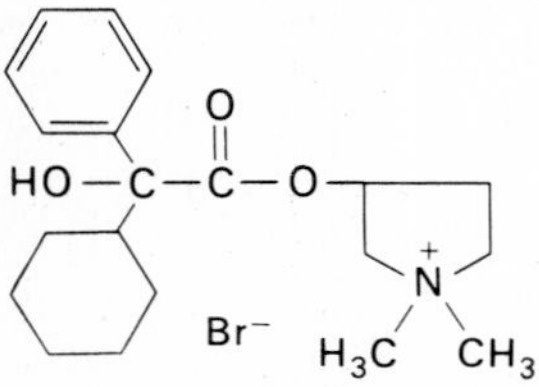

O
HO—C—C—O
N
Br^- H_3C CH_3

hexopyrronium Br

O C_2H_5
O CH—C—O—CH_2CH_2—N—CH_3
C_2H_5
Br^-

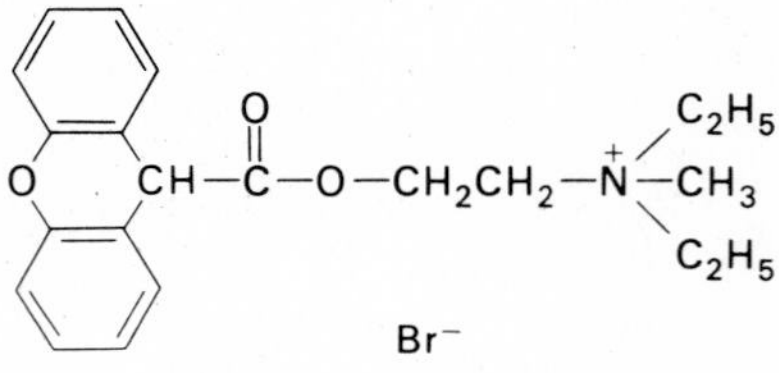

methantheline Br (Banthine)

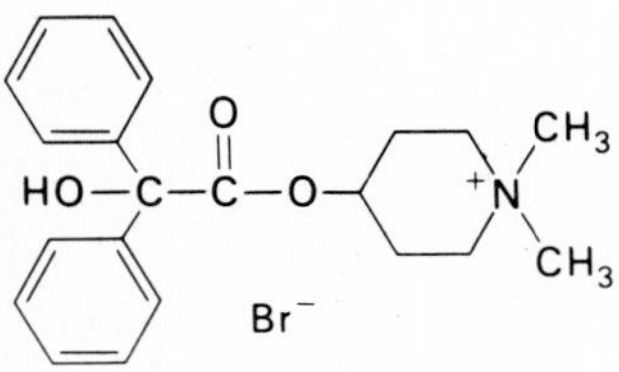

O CH_3
HO—C—C—O—$^+$N
CH_3
Br^-

parapenzolate Br

O
HO—C—C—O—CH_2 N
H_3C CH_3
$CH_3SO_3^-$

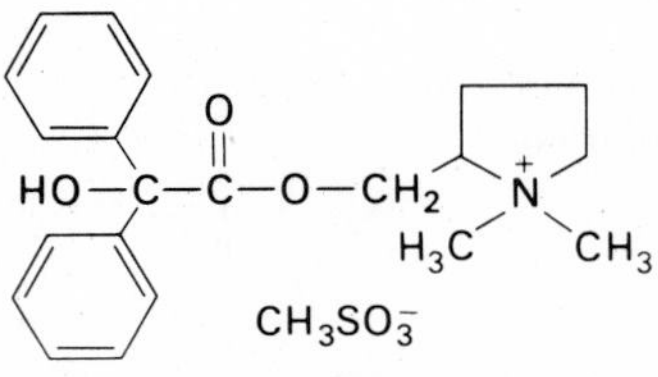

poldine mesylate (Nacton)

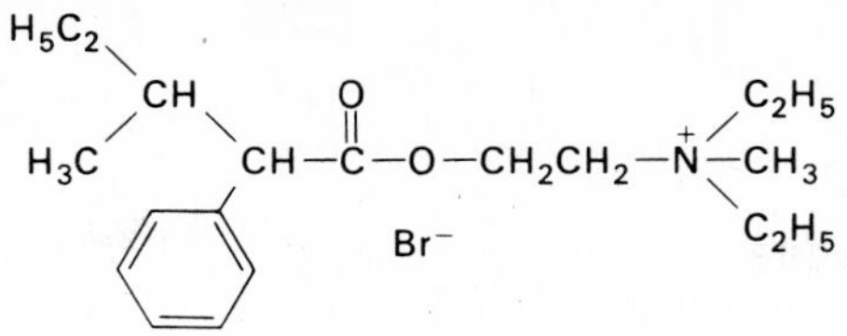

valethamate Br (Murel)

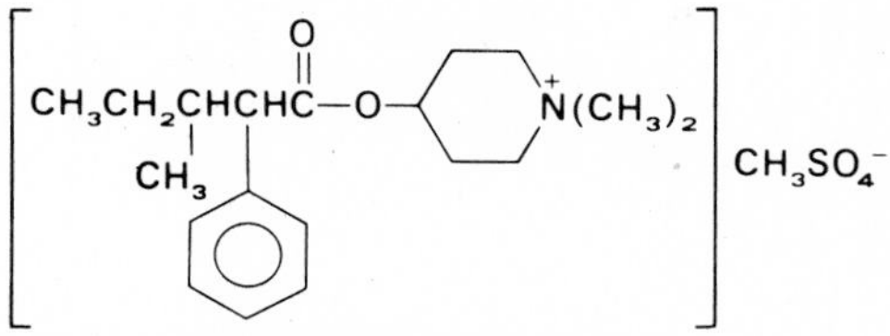

pentapiperium methylsulfate (Perium)

d. Carbamoyl esters

AMBUTONIUM BROMIDE

Dose: 10 mg every 4 hours.

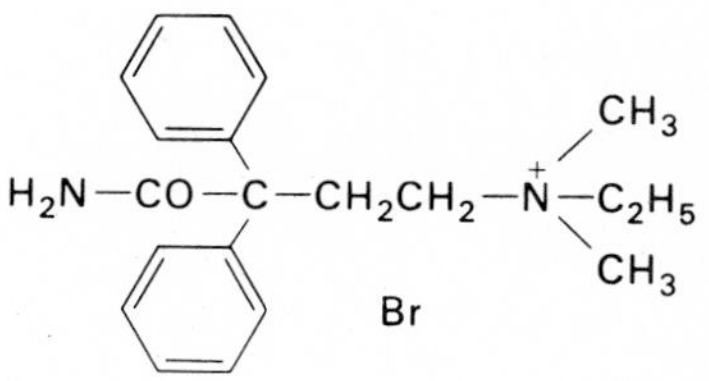

AMINOPENTAMIDE SULFATE (Centrine)

Long acting.

Dose: 0.5 mg every 4 hours by mouth.

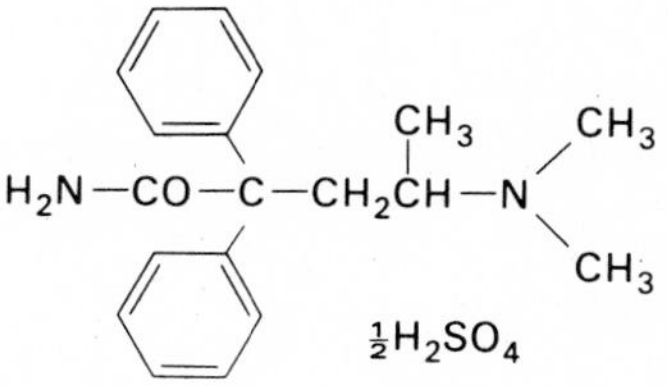

DIBUTOLINE SULFATE (Dibuline)

Dose: 25 mg subcutaneously.

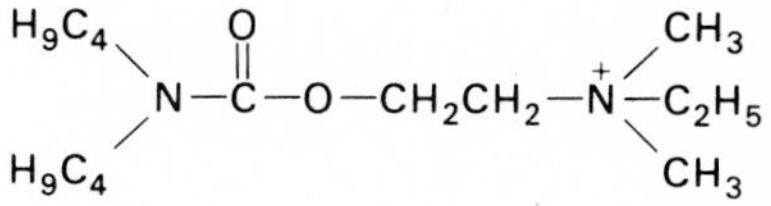

ISOPROPAMIDE IODIDE (Darbid)

Long acting.

Dose: 5 mg every 4 hours by mouth.

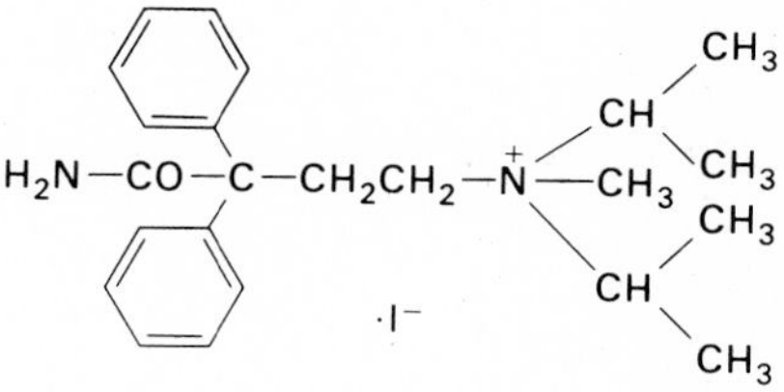

OTHERS

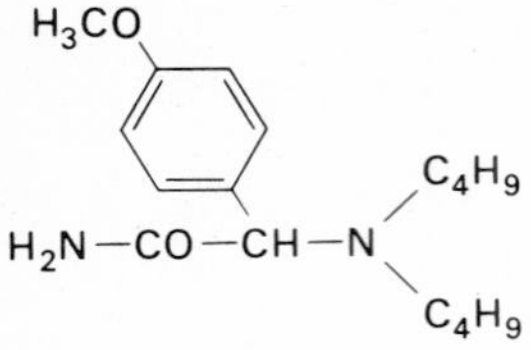

ambucetamide

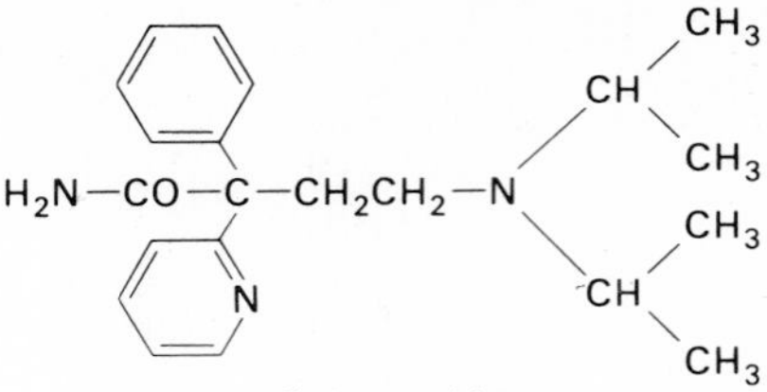

disopyramide

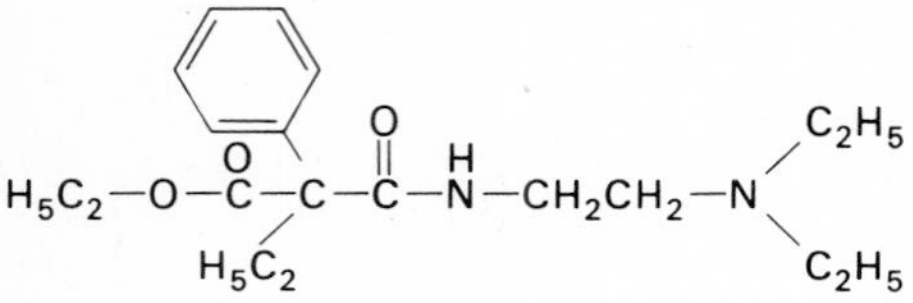

fenalamide (Spasmanide)

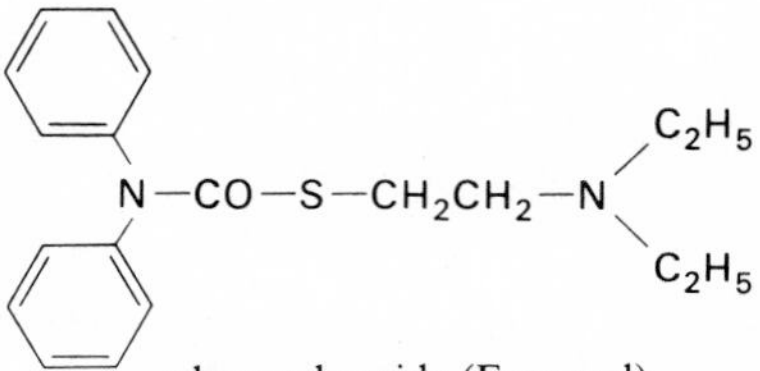

phencarbamide (Escorpal)

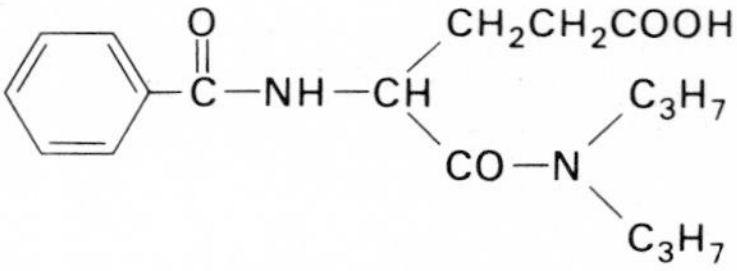

proglumide (Nulsa)

e. *Diphenyl methane derivatives* (effects primarily postganglionic unless quaternary, then ganglionic also)

DIPHEMANIL METHYLSULFATE (Prantal)
Dose: 100 mg every 3 hours by mouth.

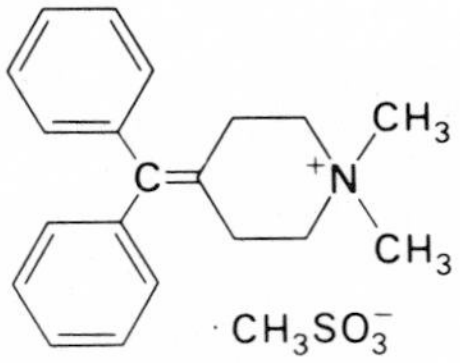

HEXOCYCLIUM METHYLSULFATE (Tral)
Dose: 50 mg every 3 hours by mouth.

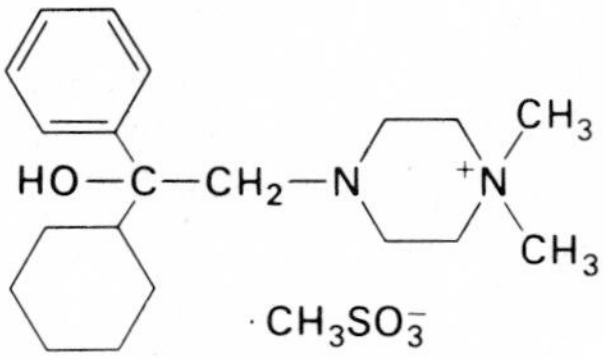

METHIXENE HYDROCHLORIDE (Trest)
Dose: 1 mg 3 times a day by mouth.

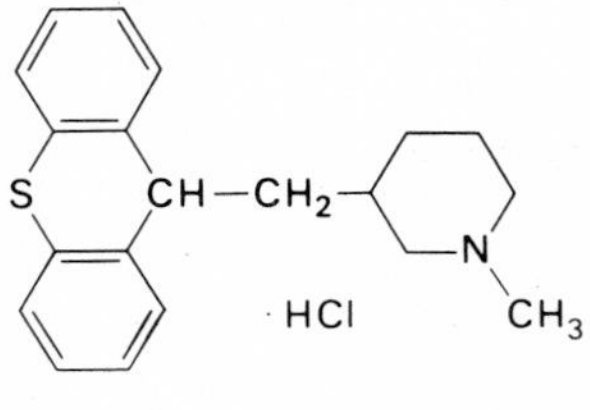

THIHEXINOL METHYLBROMIDE (Entoquel)

Produced dehydration in babies; withdrawn from market.

Dose: 15 mg 4 times a day by mouth.

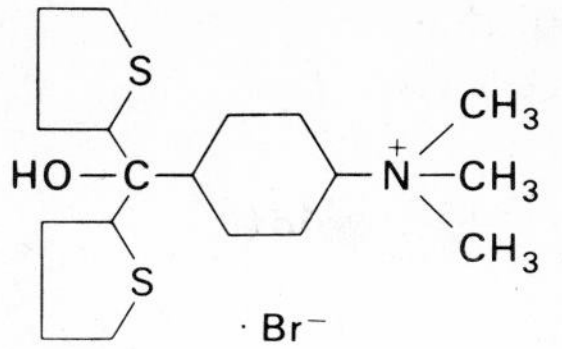

TRIDIHEXETHYL CHLORIDE (Pathilon)

Dose: 50 mg every 3 hours by mouth.

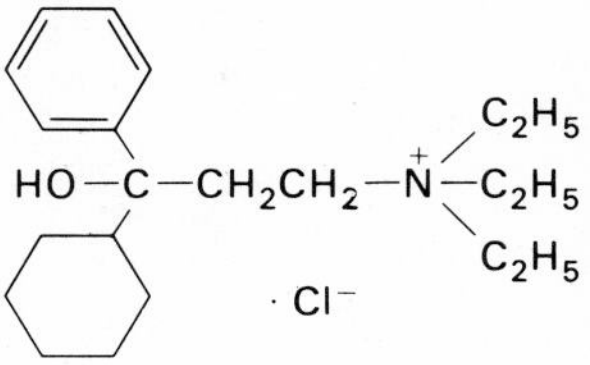

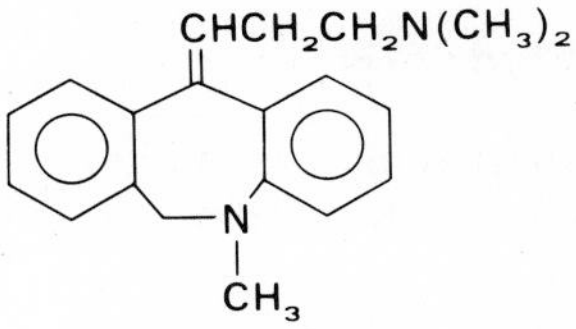

elantrine

OTHERS

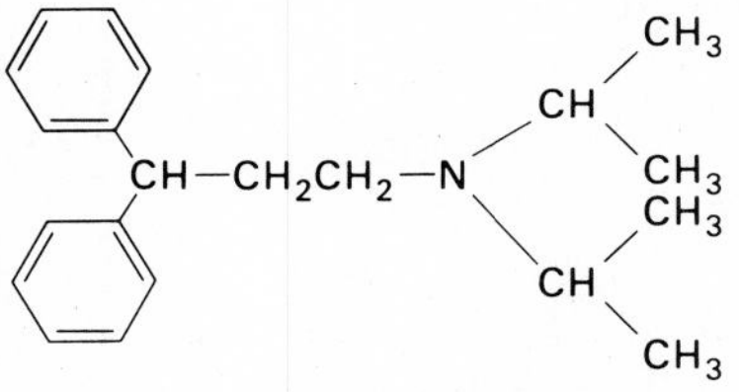

diisopromine

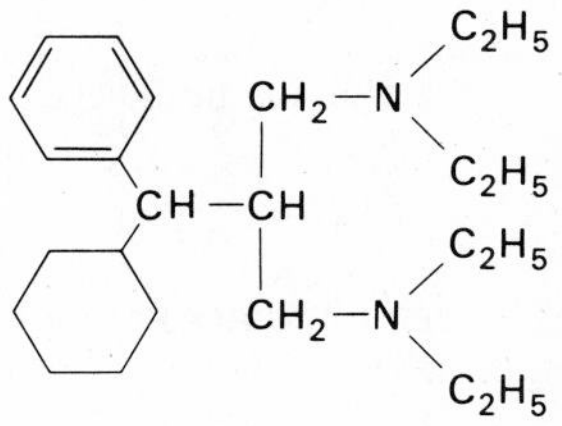

phenetamine

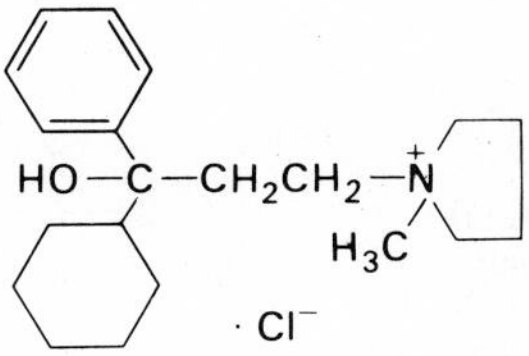

tricyclamol Cl (Elorine)

f. Others

METOQUIZINE

Under investigation.

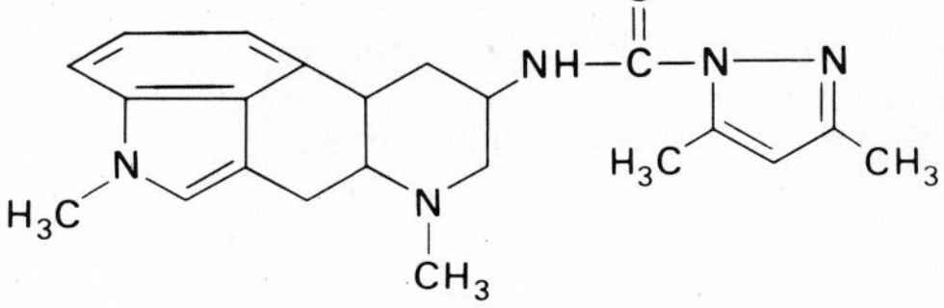

TOQUIZINE

Under investigation.

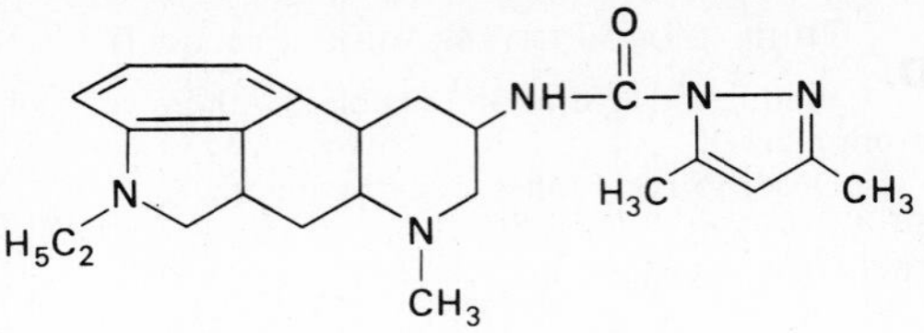

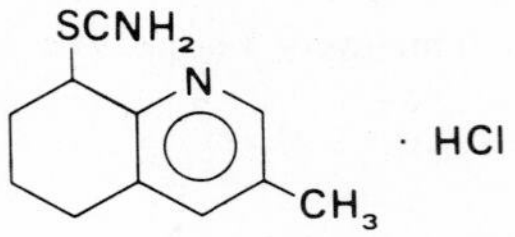

tiquinamide hydrochloride

C. Cycloplegics and Mydriatics

Anticholinergic drugs produce only local effects when applied to the conjunctiva and are useful in ophthalmology (general effects may be produced in babies).

1. Preparations

CYCLOPENTOLATE HYDROCHLORIDE (Cyclogyl)

Similar to homatropine; may be neutralized with pilocarpine.

Dose: 0.5% solution in the eye.

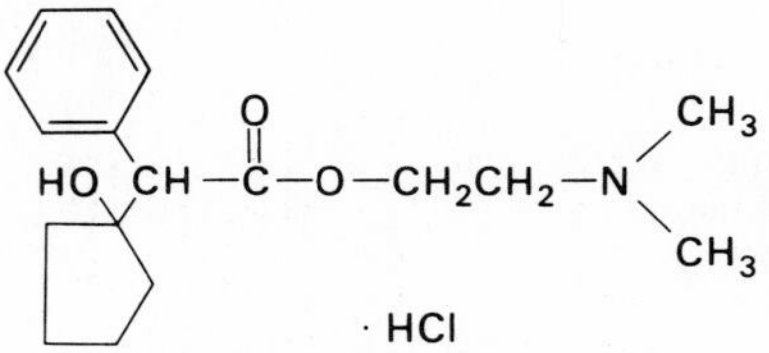

EUCATROPINE HYDROCHLORIDE (Euphthalmine)

Weaker and more transient; used as a mydriatic in eye examination.

Dose: 5% solution in the eye.

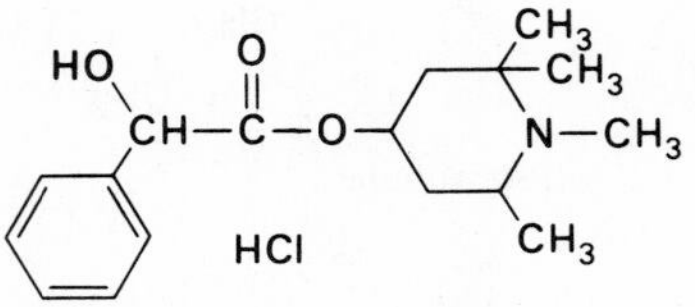

HOMATROPINE HYDROBROMIDE

In addition to its gastrointestinal uses, homatropine is useful as a cycloplegic and mydriatic when long action is desired: in iritis and corneal ulcers, as an anodyne, and in refraction.

Dose: 2% solution in the eye.

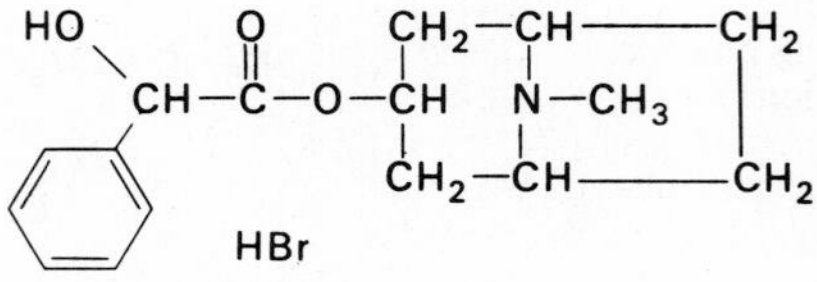

TROPICAMIDE (Mydriacyl)

Rapid and brief mydriasis for eye examination.

Dose: 0.5% to 1% solution in eye.

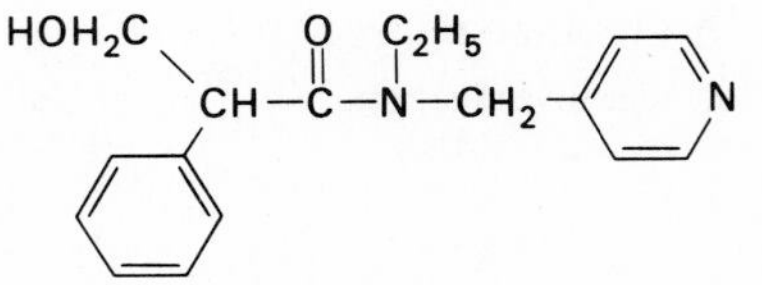

D. Centrally Acting Group

In addition to their anticholinergic effects, the atropine group of compounds produces sedation, and central actions on the basal ganglia; the latter have led to their use in parkinsonism.

1. Action. When used in parkinsonism the belladonna alkaloids may affect both tremor and rigidity beneficially but often produce uncomfortable side effects: dry mouth, blurred vision, dizziness, dysuria, hypotension, nocturnal confusion, memory loss, and even toxic psychosis and glaucoma.

2. Uses. a. Therapy in parkinsonism at best is less than good; about one-half the patients are substantially improved.

b. A large number of synthetic derivatives have come into use, but are not necessarily superior. Most resemble atropine, but some have strong antihistamine actions as well. In general, compounds with trivalent ("tertiary"; nonquaternary) N are preferred, presumably because of better penetration into the brain.

3. Preparations

a. Atropine group

TINCTURE OF BELLADONNA

Dose: 0.5 ml every 4 hours by mouth. Dose to be titrated to give maximum relief with tolerable side effects.

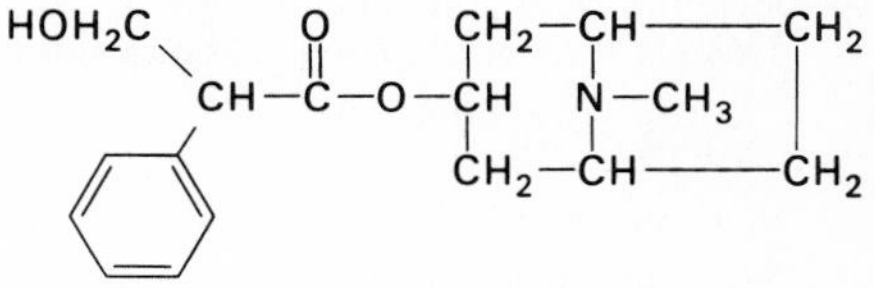

HOH$_2$C, O, CH$_2$—CH, CH$_2$, CH—C—O—CH, N—CH$_3$, CH$_2$—CH, CH$_2$

atropine sulfate

BENZTROPIN MESYLATE
(Cogentin)

Shows antihistaminic as well as atropine effects; is a rather good general purpose drug in parkinsonism. Long acting but does not produce central stimulation; also a local anesthetic. Some danger of the precipitation of glaucoma and urinary retention.

Dose: 1 to 2 mg daily by mouth.

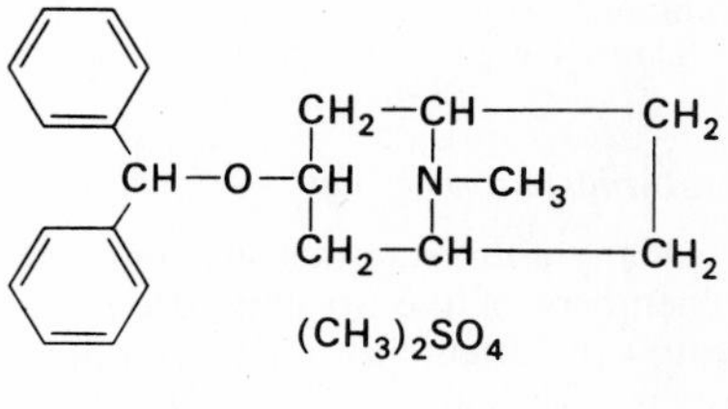

CH$_2$—CH, CH$_2$, CH—O—CH, N—CH$_3$, CH$_2$—CH, CH$_2$

$(CH_3)_2SO_4$

BIPERIDEN (Akineton)

Dose: 2 mg 1 to 4 times a day by mouth.

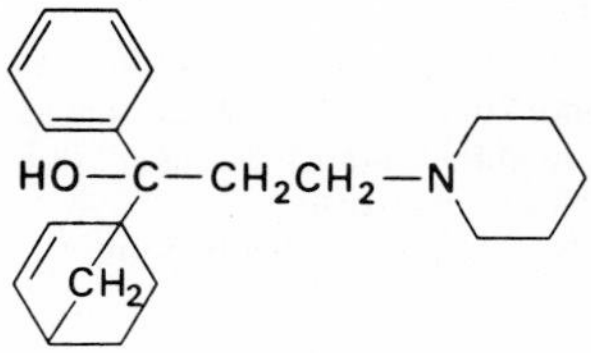

HO—C—CH$_2$CH$_2$—N, CH$_2$

CARAMIPHEN HYDROCHLORIDE
(Panparnit)

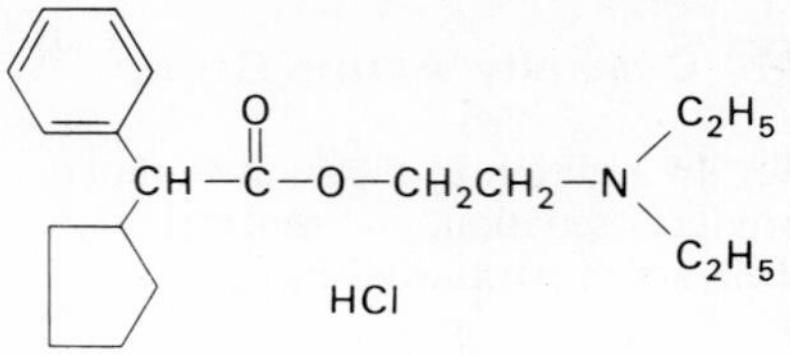

Side effects may be troublesome. Experimentally depresses decerebrate rigidity and spinal reflexes by a central action.

Dose: 12.5 mg or more 4 times a day by mouth.

CYCRIMINE HYDROCHLORIDE
(Pagitane)

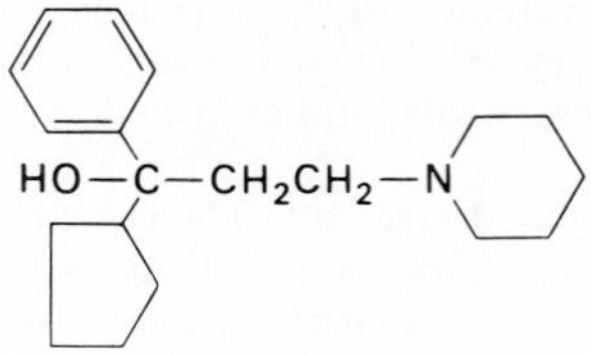

Dose: 5 mg 3 or more times a day by mouth.

ETHYBENZTROPIN (Ponalid)

Benztropin with methyl on N replaced by ethyl.
Dose: 5 mg by mouth 2 or 3 times a day.

PROCYCLIDINE HYDROCHLORIDE
(Kemadrin)

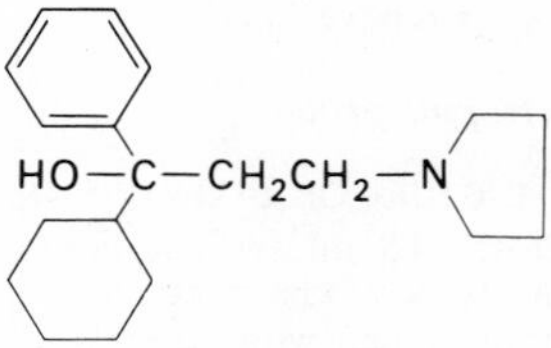

Relaxes voluntary muscles also, and therefore considered to be of especial advantage in rigidity.

Dose: 2.5 mg or more several times a day.

STRAMONIUM

Dose: 0.1 gm every 4 hours by mouth.

TRIHEXYPHENIDYL HYDROCHLORIDE
(Artane)

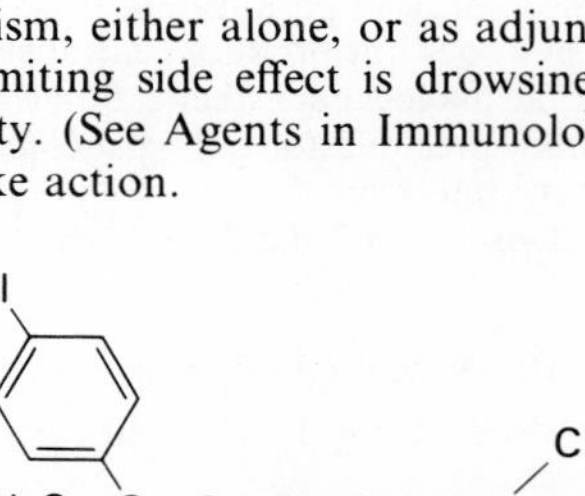

Potent; affects rigidity more than tremor; shows a minimum of side effects; a widely used agent.

Dose: 1 mg or more by mouth several times a day.

b. Antihistamine group

Many antihistamines are useful in parkinsonism, either alone, or as adjuncts to members of the atropine group. The most limiting side effect is drowsiness, because the attendant inactivity potentiates rigidity. (See Agents in Immunologic Disease.) Mechanism presumably their atropinelike action.

CHLORPHENOXAMINE HYDROCHLORIDE
(Phenoxene)

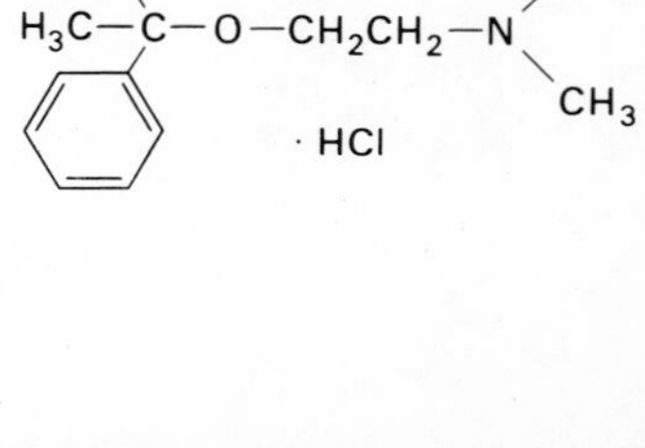

Lessens rigidity, fatigue, akinesia; has little effect on tremor; produces only minor dry mouth. Useful in coincident glaucoma as it does not produce pupillary changes.

Dose: 50 mg 3 times a day by mouth.

DIETHAZINE HYDROCHLORIDE
(Diparcol)

Dose: 0.1 gm 4 times a day, increased gradually to tolerance.

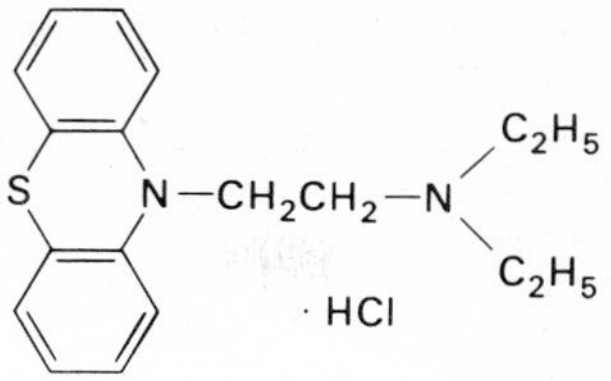

DIPHENHYDRAMINE HYDROCHLORIDE
(Benadryl)

Representative of general purpose antihistamines.

Dose: 25 mg 3 times a day by mouth.

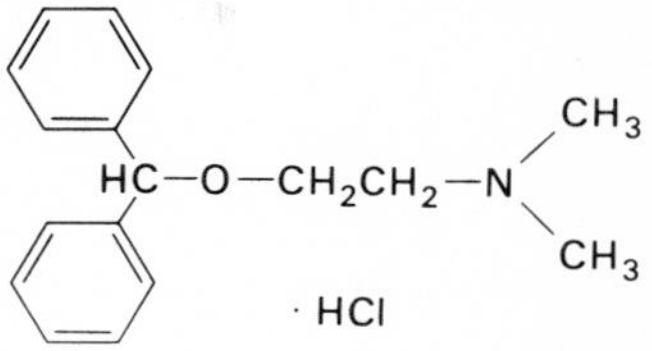

ETHOPROPAZINE HYDROCHLORIDE
(Parsidol)

Produces some ganglionic blockade as well as anticholinergic and antihistaminic effects. Said to be effective against both rigidity and tremor.

Dose: 100 mg 3 times a day by mouth.

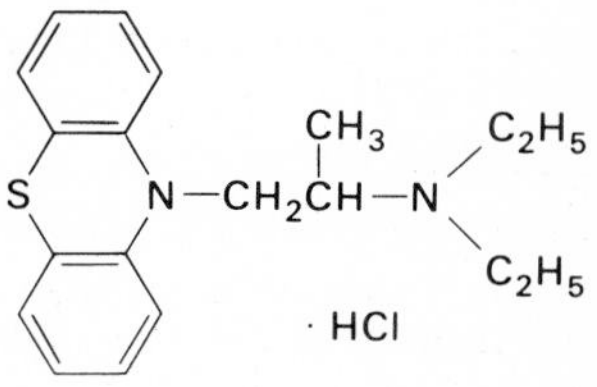

ORPHENADRINE (Norflex)

A rather weak antihistamine and muscle relaxant.

Dose: 20 mg 3 times a day by mouth.

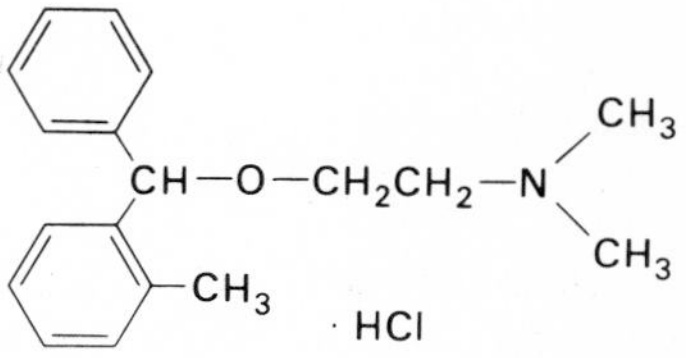

PHENINDAMINE TARTRATE (Thephorin)

Dose: 25 mg 4 times a day by mouth; usually not accompanied by sedation.

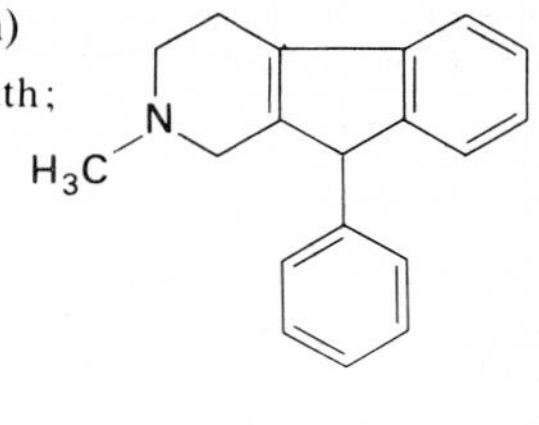

PHENYAPIN (Rigidyl)

Ethyl analogue of diphenhydramine.

TOFENACIN HYDROCHLORIDE

Dose: Under investigation.

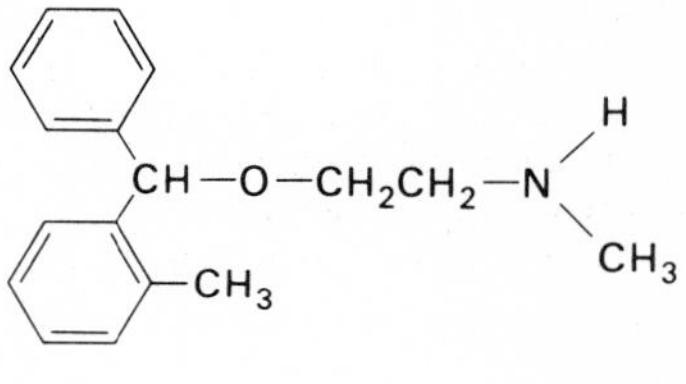

c. Other antiparkinsonian agents

LEVODOPA

See under Sympathetic Stimulants.

BENZETAMIDE

See under Sedatives.

AMANTADINE

See under Antiviral Agents.

E. Tremor Producing Agents

A number of tremor producing compounds have been used experimentally for the testing of antitremor compounds.

1. Preparations

TREMORINE (1,4-dipyrrolidino-2-butyne)

Produces tremors in mice; also is parasympathomimetic and causes salivation, diarrhea; antagonized by atropine.

Oxotremorine more potent and produces pure parasympathetic stimulation.

Dose: (in mice): 25 mg per kg (Trautner, Nature, 183:1462, 1959) (Csillik, Science, 146: 765, 1964).

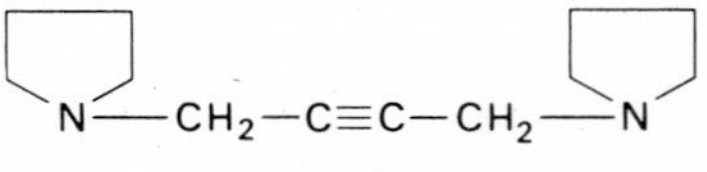

N—CH_2—C≡C—CH_2—N

tremorine

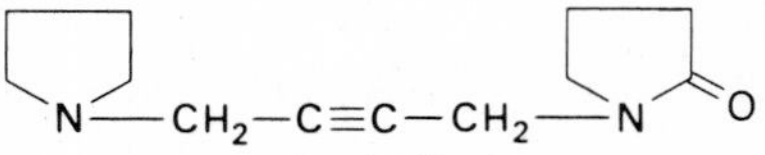

N—CH_2—C≡C—CH_2—N O

oxotremorine

3-AMINO-1,1,3-TRIPHENYLPROPAN-1-OL

More potent tremor producer. Resembles diphenylmethane anticholinergics. In doses of 30 mg per kg in mice produces tremor, restlessness, Straub tail, and other neurological effects (Ayton, J. Pharm. Pharmacol., 15:217, 1963).

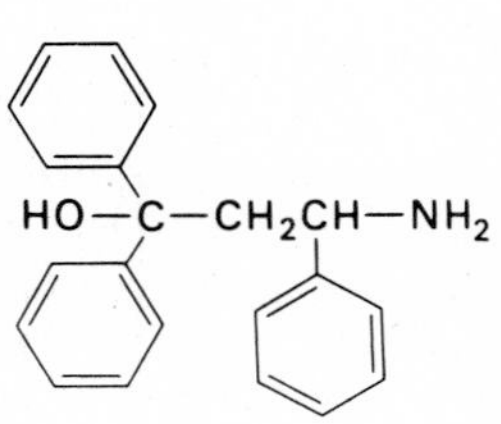

HO—C—CH_2CH—NH_2

II. POTENTIATING AGENTS

A number of compounds, some of which show chemical resemblances to the atropine or antihistamine groups, potentiate certain enzymatic reactions. These potentiating compounds exert minimal pharmacological effects when administered alone, but prolong the action, or enhance the intensity of action of other drugs. Although not used therapeutically they have great pharmacological interest.

1. **Chemistry**

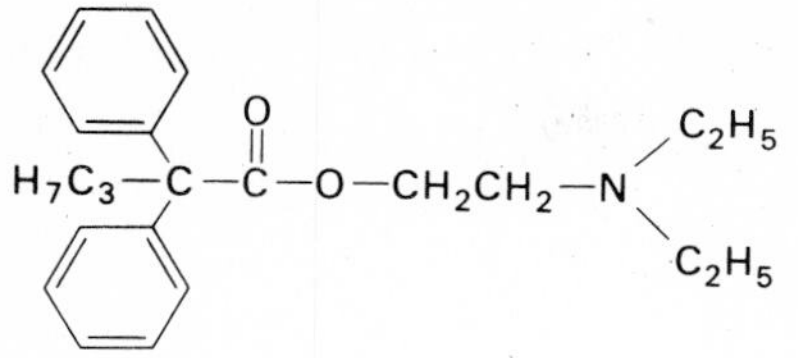

$$H_7C_3-C(C_6H_5)_2-C(=O)-O-CH_2CH_2-N(C_2H_5)_2$$

proadiphen hydrochloride
(SKF 525A)

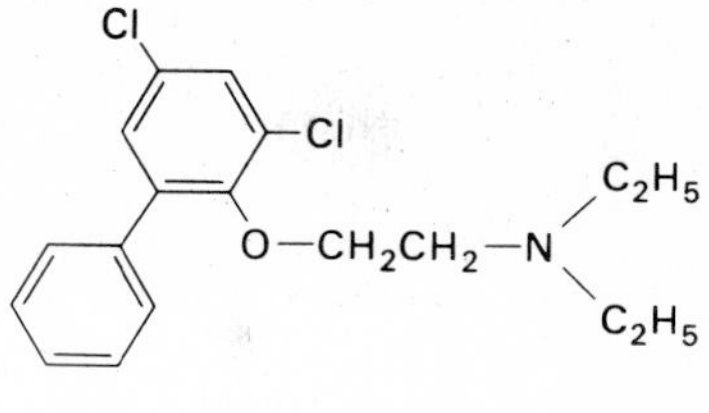

$$2,4\text{-}Cl_2\text{-}6\text{-}(C_6H_5)C_6H_2-O-CH_2CH_2-N(C_2H_5)_2$$

2,4-dichloro-6-phenylphenoxy-
diethylamine (Lilly 18947)

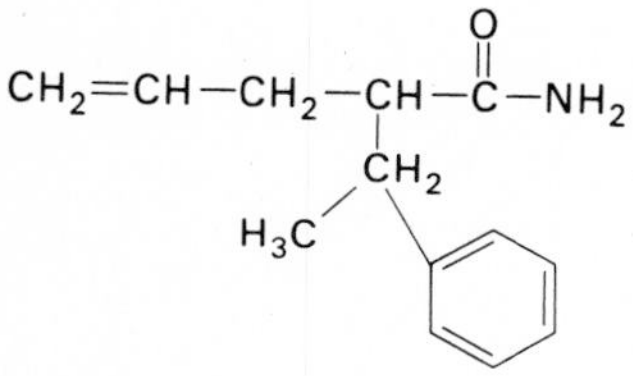

$$CH_2{=}CH-CH_2-CH(CH(CH_3)C_6H_5)-C(=O)-NH_2$$

2-(1-phenylethyl)-4-pentenamide
(NDR A-1358)

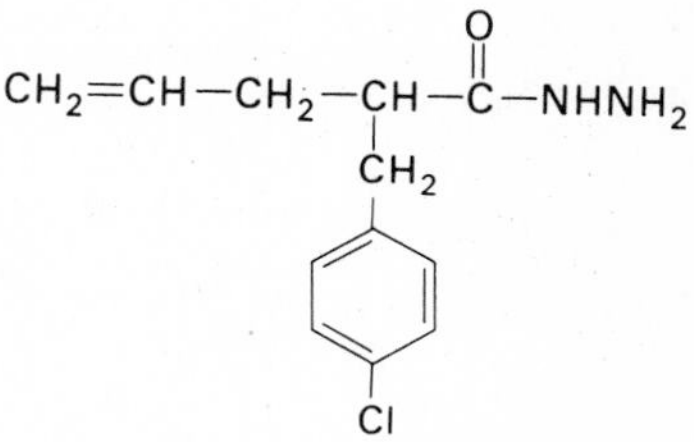

$$CH_2{=}CH-CH_2-CH(CH_2C_6H_4Cl)-C(=O)-NHNH_2$$

2-(*p*-chlorobenzyl)-4-pentenoic
acid hydrazide (NDR A-2435)

2. **Action.** Prolong the actions of hypnotics, analgesics, spinal cord depressants, sympathomimetic amines, hypotensives, and CNS stimulants.

3. **Mechanism.** a. Potentiation of the action of a drug could reasonably be expected from agents which would increase the responsiveness of receptors to drugs, which would block excretion of drugs, or which would block biotransformation (Brodie, J. Pharmacol. Exper. Ther., 119:197, 1957).

b. The potentiating agents utilize the third mechanism. The SKF and Lilly compounds enhance the activity of drugs by inhibiting enzyme systems in liver microsomes as follows (Throp, J. Med. Pharm. Chem., 2:15, 1960):

a′. Alkyl side chain oxidation: barbiturates
b′. Alkylamine dealkylation: meperidine, aminopyrine
c′. Sympathomimetic amine deamination: ephedrine
d′. Ether cleavage: codeine
e′. Phenol conjugation: morphine
f′. Aromatic hydroxylation

c. Each of the four compounds whose structure is given above potentiated the hypotensive effects in rats of reserpine, hydralazine, mecamylamine, a benzodioxane derivative, and a hexantrate (Goldstein, Amer. J. Pharm., 131:255, 1959).

SUMMARY: PARASYMPATHETIC DEPRESSANTS

TYPE	*ACTION AND MECHANISM*	*TOXICITY*	*USE*	*EXAMPLES*
Belladonna alkaloids	Parasympathetic inhibition by receptor block; mydriasis dry skin, mouth Alimentary and bronchial smooth muscle relaxation and diminished secretions	Dry mouth, difficulty in reading, difficulty in urination (older men)	Antispasmodic for alimentary bronchial, biliary, urinary tracts; mydriatic, central sedation	Atropine sulfate
Synthetic smooth muscle anti-spasmodics	Same, plus direct smooth muscle relaxation in some cases	Same	Same	Propantheline Br
Cycloplegics and mydriatics	Local dilation of pupil	Minor	Iritis, corneal ulcers, refraction	Cyclopentolate HCl
Antiparkinson group: atropine type	Decrease tremor and rigidity by central action on the basal ganglia	Dry mouth, etc., as for atropine	Parkinsonism	Trihexylphenidyl HCl
: anti-histamine type	Similar	Drowsiness	Same	Ethopropazine HCl

Reviews

Ingelfinger, F. Anticholinergic therapy of gastrointestinal disease. New Eng. J. Med., 268:1454, 1963.

Friend, D. Antiparkinsonism drug therapy. Clin. Pharmacol. Ther., 4:815, 1963.

45. Ganglionic and Myoneural Agents

I. GANGLIONIC AGENTS

In 1889 Langley showed that nicotine paralyzed autonomic ganglia and so started their pharmacological study.

Acetylcholine is the transmitter at the ganglionic synapse, whether sympathetic or parasympathetic. After its release by the preganglionic ending it crosses to the receptor of the postganglionic fiber and causes depolarization of the membrane. This depolarization initiates an action potential in the postganglionic cell, which is propagated down the fiber. Costa and co-workers have shown that acetylcholine also liberates catecholamines in sympathetic ganglia, which then reduce transmission, acting as a "modulator" (Science, 133:1822, 1961). It is likely that the modulator catecholamine is dopamine, which exerts its function through cyclic AMP (Greengard and Kebabjan, Fed. Proc., 33:1059, 1974).

Drugs may facilitate or hinder this crossing of the synapse; therapeutic interest is almost entirely in inhibitors. These inhibitors may block transmission by causing persistent depolarization, receptor competition, or by other mechanisms.

A. Agents Causing Persistent Depolarization (Nicotine)

NICOTINE

1. Chemistry. Alkaloid isolated in 1828 by Posselt and Reiman from *Nicotiana tobacum.*

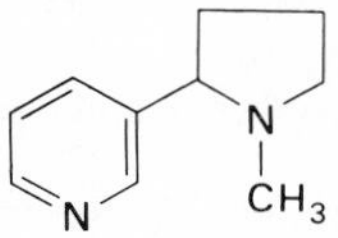

N

CH_3

N

2. Action and Mechanism. a. The action of nicotine on ganglia resembles that of acetylcholine in producing a strong initial stimulation of the receptor, but differs in that the resultant depolarization is greatly protracted. Thus paralysis of some duration is produced. During the brief stimulatory phase there may be nausea and increased intestinal activity, and a general constriction of arterioles and capillaries causing pallor, sweating, and increased blood pressure. During the paralytic phase the blood pressure falls.

b. Nicotine also liberates catechol amines from the adrenal medulla and peripheral stores with a resultant sharp vasoconstriction accentuating the ganglionic effect.

3. Pharmacodynamics. a. Readily absorbed from the mouth, lungs or intact skin.

b. A small amount (10 to 20%) is excreted unchanged in the urine, the rest is metabolized.

4. Toxicity. a. Acute poisoning causes respiratory paralysis.

b. Chronic poisoning may be responsible for tobacco amblyopia and thromboangitis obliterans.

5. Uses. a. Too unreliable for use in man as a therapeutic agent (excluding tobacco smoking).

b. Has enjoyed long use as a tool in the experimental laboratory, and as an insecticide.

c. Also, has recently been used in syringe bullets which are shot into wild animals, giving a "knockdown" of a minute or two during which they may be captured or treated.

6. Preparation

LOBELINE SULFATE (Nikoban)

Actions similar to nicotine but weaker; used as a tobacco deterrent. Its use as a respiratory stimulant is obsolete.

Dose: 0.5 mg by mouth.

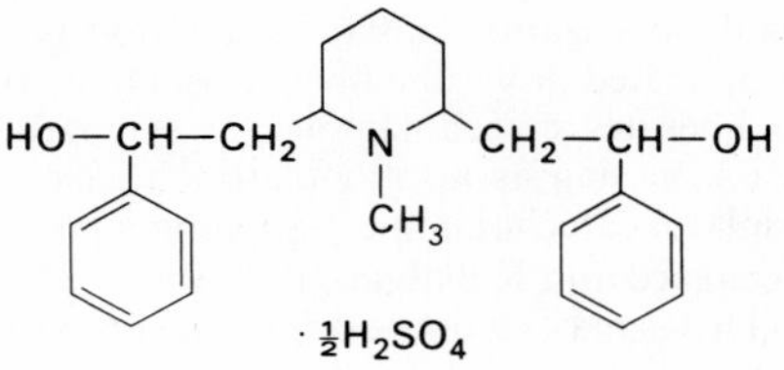

HO—CH—CH$_2$—[piperidine ring, N—CH$_3$]—CH$_2$—CH—OH (each CH bearing a phenyl ring) · $\frac{1}{2}H_2SO_4$

B. Agents Competing at Receptors (Tetraethylammonium)

A large number of agents inhibit ganglia by competing with acetylcholine at the receptor. These include such hypotensive agents as hexamethonium and mecamylamine (see Hypotensive Agents), and curare (see Myoneural Agents).

TETRAETHYLAMMONIUM

1. History. a. Marshall (1914) and Dale and Burn (1915) noted ganglionic blocking effects.

b. Acheson and Moe (1946) reintroduced as a therapeutic agent.

2. Chemistry. Resemblance to choline portion of acetylcholine:

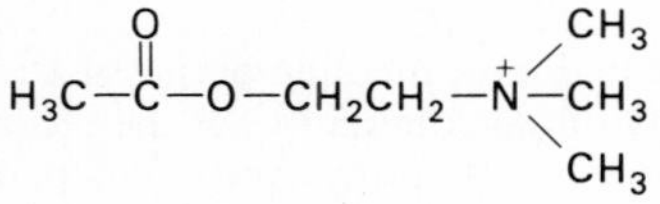

$$H_3C-\overset{O}{\overset{\|}{C}}-O-CH_2CH_2-\overset{+}{N}(CH_3)_3$$

acetylcholine

$$H_3C-CH_2-\overset{+}{N}(C_2H_5)_3$$

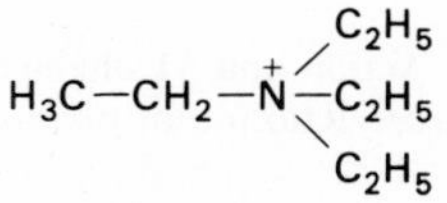

tetraethylammonium

3. Action and Mechanism. a. Produces a weak, transient ganglionic blockade by competing with acetylcholine for the receptors.

b. The main clinical result is peripheral arteriolar relaxation from the interruption of tonic sympathetic impulses, giving hypotension.

4. Pharmacodynamics and Toxicity. a. Poor oral absorption.

b. Fleeting action; tolerance develops rapidly.

c. Adequate therapeutic dosage causes postural hypotension which may be severe and impair cerebral circulation.

5. Uses. a. Formerly used to treat causalgia, peripheral vascular disease, and even hypertension.

b. Procedure difficult because of short action and need for intravenous injection.

6. Preparations

TETRAETHYLAMMONIUM CHLORIDE (TEA; Etamon)

Dose: 100 mg intravenously.
Obsolete.

MECAMYLAMINE HYDROCHLORIDE (Inversine)
Dose: 2.5 to 10 mg by mouth.

$NHCH_3$, CH_3, CH_2, CH_3, CH_3

C. Agents Inhibiting Ganglia by Other Mechanisms

Local anesthetics (and also calcium deficiency) may induce ganglionic blockade by interfering with the release of acetylcholine from the preganglionic nerve endings. These actions have no therapeutic importance.

II. MYONEURAL AGENTS

Myoneural agents affect the contraction of striated muscle at the neuromuscular junction. Either facilitation or inhibition is possible, and agents of either category are available for use.

The normal mechanism by which the impulse is carried from the tip of the motor nerve to the motor end plate on the muscle is comparable to that of autonomic ganglia and postganglionic parasympathetic nerve endings. Acetylcholine is the mediator.

Myoneural agents may alter the normal mechanism in at least three ways, i.e., by effects on or at the receptor (curare), by effects on the cholinesterase mechanism (neostigmine), or by effects on the formation or release of acetylcholine (botulinus toxin).

A. Inhibitors of Contraction by Maintenance of Polarization

CURARE

1. History. a. South American Indians have long used curare as an arrow poison.

b. Claude Bernard (1857) showed that the effect was on the "nerve ending," not on the nerve or muscle—application of curare to nerve trunk had no effect; muscle could still be stimulated directly after curare.

c. King (1935) isolated an active principle, *d*-tubocurarine.

d. Griffith (1943) initiated its use in therapeutics to provide surgical relaxation.

2. Chemistry. a. Various alkaloids from *Chondrodendron tomentosum;* crude preparations called tube, pot, or calabash from the native containers.

b. Active alkaloids, such as *d*-tubocurarine, possess 2 quaternary nitrogens, 10 carbon atoms, or 14 Å, apart, just twice the length of the critical moiety of acetylcholine. However, other active alkaloids may not have this configuration.

3. Action. a. Curare competes with and raises the threshold for acetylcholine at the myoneural receptors of all striated muscles, producing paralysis.

b. Highly innervated muscles such as the eye muscles are affected first, and the respiratory muscles, especially the diaphragm, are affected last.

c. Autonomic ganglia are also blocked.

4. Mechanism. Curare interferes with acetylcholine by occupying the receptors competitively; more acetylcholine can overcome the inhibition, but the threshold is raised.

5. Pharmacodynamics. a. Not well absorbed by mouth.

b. After injection part is bound in the liver and muscles and a smaller part excreted in the urine.

6. Toxicity. a. The principal danger of overdosage is respiratory paralysis. If this should occur, artificial respiration should be instituted and neostigmine plus atropine, or edrophonium, may be used after spontaneous diaphragmatic respiration has begun.

b. Histamine release may cause bronchospasm, hypotension, and excessive secretions.

7. Uses. a. To produce muscular relaxation during surgical anesthesia, and occasionally in tetanus or during electroshock therapy.

b. Not particularly useful in chronic spastic, ambulant states because parenteral administration is necessary.

8. Preparations

METOCURINE IODIDE
(Metubine iodide)

Dose: 2 to 5 mg intravenously.

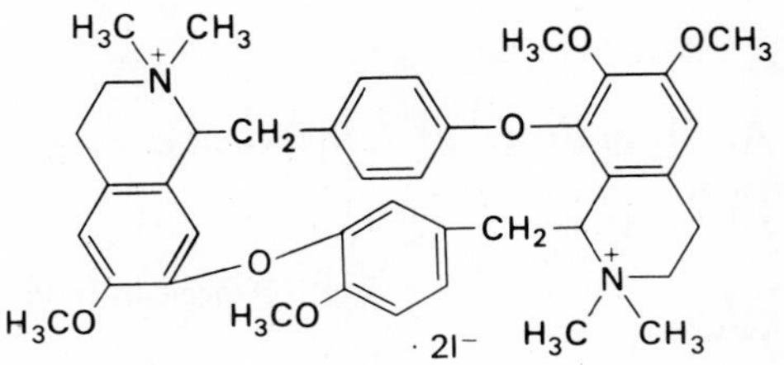

H_3C CH_3 $\overset{+}{N}$ CH_2 O H_3CO OCH_3 O CH_2 $\overset{+}{N}$ H_3CO H_3CO $\cdot 2I^-$ H_3C CH_3

TUBOCURARINE CHLORIDE
(Tubarine; and others)

Dose: 5 to 15 mg intravenously.

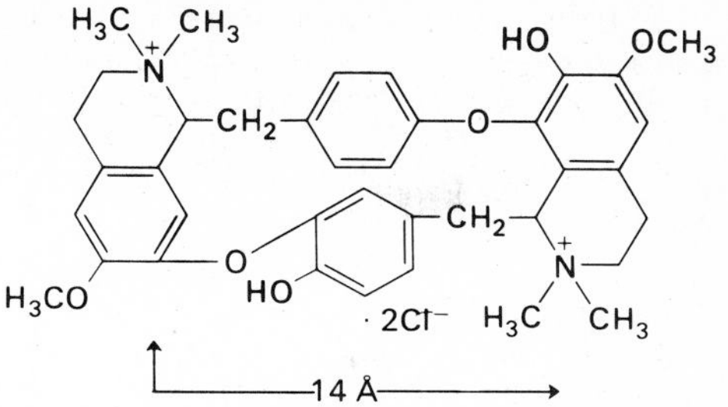

Chondodendron tomentosum extract (Intocostrin): Activity due principally to tubocurarine. Dose: 6 to 9 mg intravenously. Obsolete.

SYNTHETIC CURARE RELATIVES

1. Preparations

BENZOQUINONIUM CHLORIDE
(Mytolon)

Intermediate in mechanism between curare and decamethonium, but blocked by edrophonium. May cause bradycardia and excessive salivation.

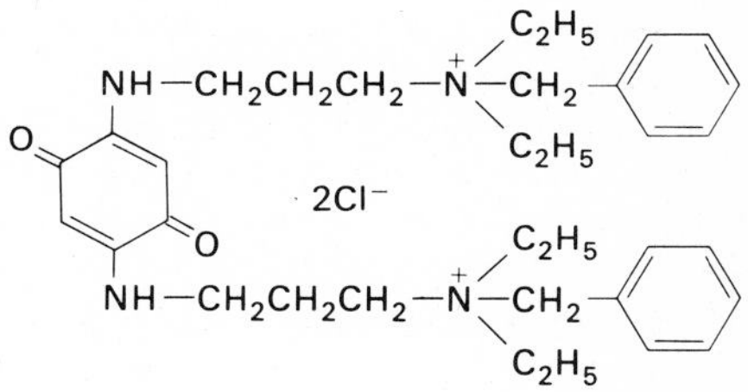

GALLAMINE TRIETHIODIDE (Flaxedil)

About one-third as potent as curare, shorter acting, and exhibits minimal side effects, but may cause tachycardia by blocking parasympathetic ganglia. Widely used as a muscle relaxant during surgical anesthesia. Edrophonium the preferred antidote.

Dose: 1 mg per kg body weight intravenously.

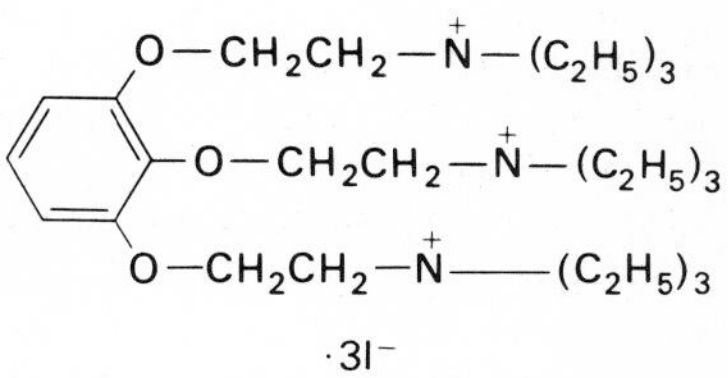

HEXAFLURENIUM BROMIDE (Mylaxen)

Produces mild nondepolarization and neuromuscular blockade; also inhibits plasma cholinesterase. Potentiates succinylcholine.

Dose: 400 mcg per kg intravenously, followed in 3 minutes by 300 mcg per kg succinylcholine.

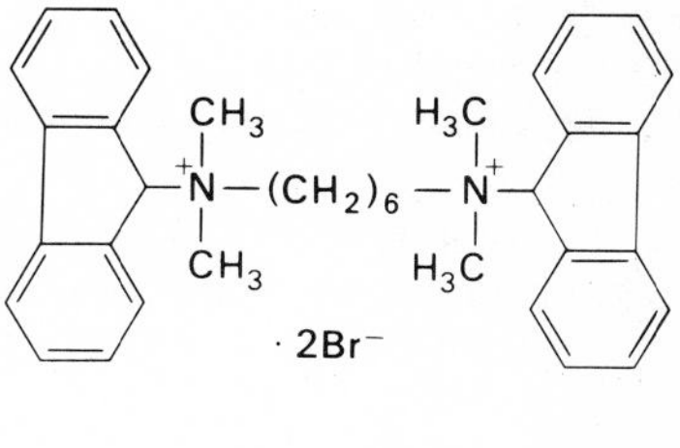

OTHERS

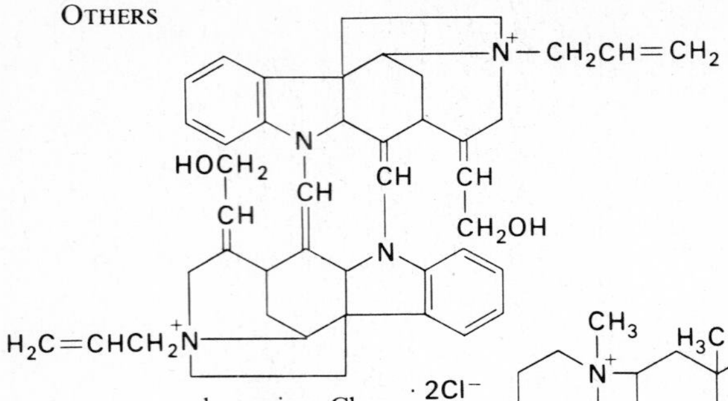

alcuronium Cl

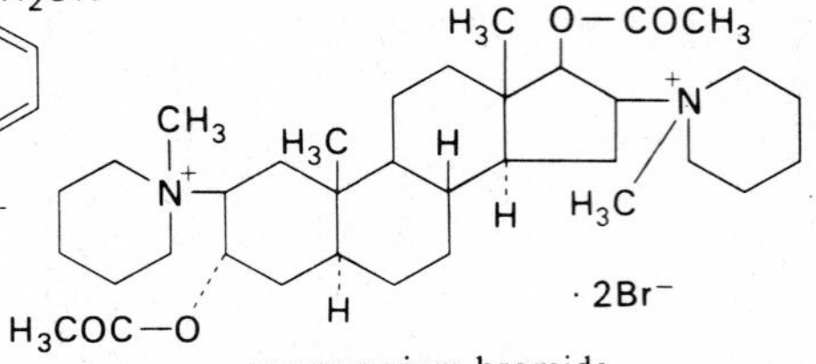

pancuronium bromide

B. Inhibitors of Contraction by Maintenance of Depolarization (Decamethonium)

DECAMETHONIUM GROUP

1. Chemistry. General similarly to curare, i.e., widely separated ammoniums, but in long thin molecules (leptocurares) in contrast to bulky molecule of curares (pachycurares).

2. Action. a. Decamethonium produces brief paralysis of striated muscle with about one-fifth the dose of curare and without ganglionic paralysis.

b. Succinylcholine (which is a diacetylcholine) gives a still more fleeting muscular paralysis.

3. Mechanism. a. Differ from curare in producing depolarization of the motor end plate, just as acetylcholine does (phase I block), but the depolarization lasts much longer than that from acetylcholine. Prolonged use results in a curarelike, nondepolarizing block (phase II block).

b. After the initial contraction the muscle remains relaxed for the duration of the action of the drugs. The action is a direct one on the end plate and does not depend upon the persistence of acetylcholine itself.

4. Pharmacodynamics. a. Decamethonium produces muscular relaxation for about 10 to 30 minutes after intravenous administration; succinylcholine is even more evanescent and must be given by continuous intravenous infusion.

b. Succinylcholine destroyed in the bloodstream by pseudocholinesterase; decamethonium excreted by the kidney.

5. Toxicity. a. Respiratory paralysis. Succinylcholine may produce prolonged apnea because of the absence of pseudocholinesterase, either on a genetic basis or from exposure to organic phosphate insecticides.

b. Should be treated with artificial respiration and not with neostigmine or edrophonium, in contrast to the curare group, because these agents would augment the effect of any acetylcholine present and further the depolarization with deepening of the paralysis. However, the antagonists may be used to differentiate degree of block.

6. Uses. a. To produce muscular relaxation during surgical anesthesia.

b. Agents given by intravenous drip may be used to give excellent moment to moment control.

7. Preparations

DECAMETHONIUM BROMIDE (Syncurine)

Dose: 0.5 to 3 mg intravenously. Repeat in 10 to 30 min as necessary.

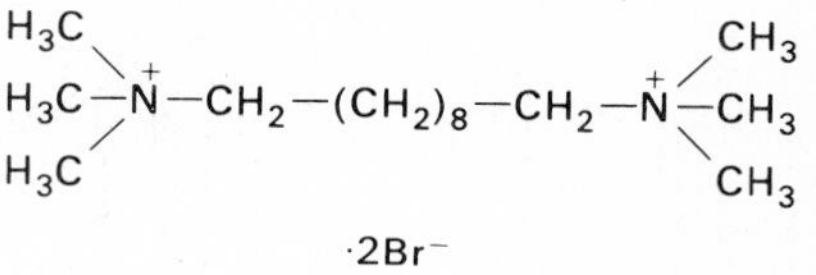

$$(H_3C)_3\overset{+}{N}-CH_2-(CH_2)_8-CH_2-\overset{+}{N}(CH_3)_3 \cdot 2Br^-$$

SUCCINYLCHOLINE CHLORIDE (Anectine; and others)

Dose: 20 to 60 mg for brief paralysis; 0.2% solution for continuous intravenous drip.

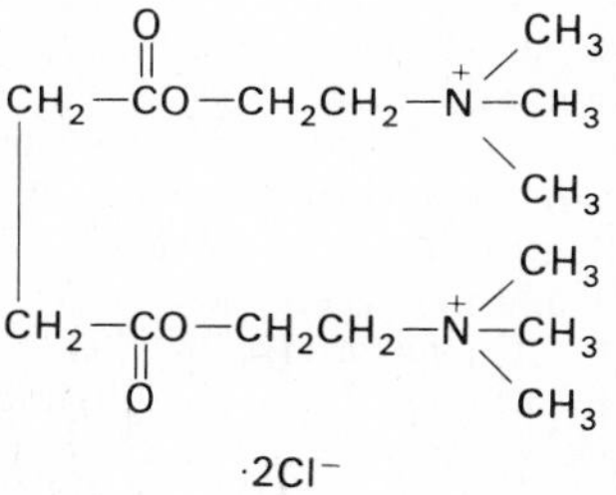

$$\begin{array}{l} CH_2-CO-CH_2CH_2-\overset{+}{N}(CH_3)_3 \\ | \\ CH_2-CO-CH_2CH_2-\overset{+}{N}(CH_3)_3 \end{array} \cdot 2Cl^-$$

(each CO is C=O)

C. Cholinesterases

1. Action. Cholinesterases, which hydrolyze choline esters, are of two general types:

a. Acetylcholinesterase (specific, or "true" cholinesterase): Primarily concerned with nervous transmission; occurs at motor end plates, in ganglia, and in the CNS gray substance (also in RBC). It splits acetylcholine most readily, propionylcholine less, and butyrylcholine least. It should be noted that butyrylcholine has been found in the brain and may serve some function as a transmitter there.

b. Butyrylcholinesterase (nonspecific, or "pseudo" cholinesterase): Primarily concerned with hydrolyzing choline esters in the tissues generally, and not with the transmission of nervous impulses. It may be involved in the effects of drugs on nervous transmission, however, by hydrolyzing the drugs in the blood stream before they can reach the synapses and end organs. Occurs in plasma, intestinal mucosa, pancreas, liver, CNS white matter. It hydrolyzes butyrylcholine most easily, propionylcholine less, and acetylcholine least.

2. Mechanism. a. Cholinesterases hydrolyze esters in two steps, first by attaching to them, and secondly by "pulling" them apart, as diagrammed:

acetylcholine

Attachment

van der Waal's forces

esteratic site (covalent bond)

$7 Å$

acetylcholinesterase

anionic site (ionic bond)

Splitting

acetyl

$HO{-}CH_2CH_2{-}N^+(CH_3)_3$

choline

a′. Attachment: Acetylcholine is attracted to acetylcholinesterase at two main points, the esteratic and anionic sites, supplemented by weaker van der Waal's forces.

b′. Splitting: The ester linkage is then broken by the greater pull of the attachment sites, possibly explainable by assuming that they are slightly farther apart than the length of the acetylcholine. The choline moiety is then immediately released, and in a second step the acetyl moiety is released as acetic acid.

b. Cholinesterase may be temporarily inhibited by an ester which can attach to it (7 Å between the binding atoms); the ester is itself later split, freeing the enzyme (neostigmine type). Inhibition may occur by binding of only the anionic site (edrophonium).

c. Cholinesterase may be permanently inactivated by compounds which it cannot split and which therefore continue to occupy the enzyme (phosphorylation by organophosphorus compounds) at the esteratic site.

D. Agents That Facilitate Contraction by Reversible Inhibition

NEOSTIGMINE GROUP

1. Chemistry. Relatives of neostigmine (see also Parasympathetic Stimulants).

2. Action. Increase the strength of voluntary muscles in myasthenia gravis and curare poisoning.

3. Mechanism. a. Enhance the effect of acetylcholine by serving as alternate substrates for acetylcholinesterase. A cloud or flood of neostigmine may be imagined to intercept acetylcholinesterase, allowing acetylcholine longer access to the motor end plate.

b. However, the inhibition is only temporary as the agents are gradually hydrolyzed and the enzyme is gradually freed.

c. Also acetylcholinelike, direct stimulation of the receptor.

4. Pharmacodynamics and Toxicity. a. Absorbed poorly (quaternaries); but may be adequate by oral therapy.

b. Overdosage may cause muscular fasciculations, weakness, and paralysis.

c. Must be used cautiously in asthma because of postganglionic action to produce bronchial spasm.

d. Artificial respiration and atropine should be used in poisoning.

5. Uses. a. To control the muscular weakness of myasthenia gravis, the result of a fundamental inadequacy of acetylcholine at the neuromuscular junction. A number of explanations have been offered to explain the defect; it may be the result of a presynaptic biochemical defect impairing synthesis (Desmidt, Nature, 182:1673, 1958). There also seems to be an uncertain relationship with the thymus.

b. As curare antidotes with atropine to counteract muscarinic effects; should not be used as antidotes against decamethonium or succinylcholine where excess of acetylcholine already present.

6. Preparations

AMBENONIUM CHLORIDE
(Mytelase)

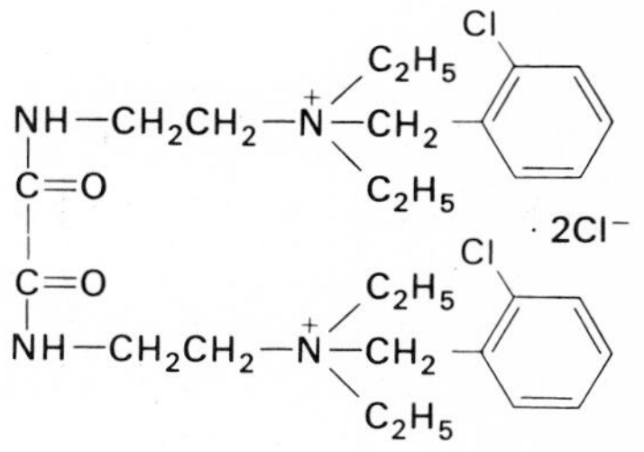

Somewhat more potent and longer acting than neostigmine. Reported to produce less gastrointestinal hyperactivity and salivation, possibly because its larger molecule limits its penetration to these receptors. However, lack of these warning signs in treating myasthenia gravis may allow inadvertent overdosage.

Dose: 5 to 25 mg several times a day by mouth.

BENZPYRINIUM BROMIDE
(Stigmonene)

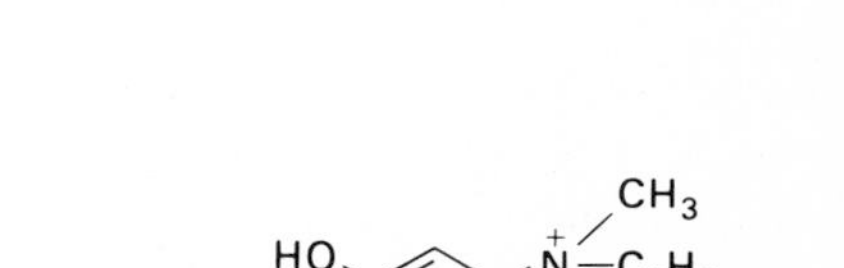

Similar to neostigmine; used in myasthenia gravis, and as a cholinergic agent to relieve postoperative distension, urinary retention, for pregnancy testing.

Dose: 2 mg intramuscularly.

EDROPHONIUM CHLORIDE
(Tensilon)

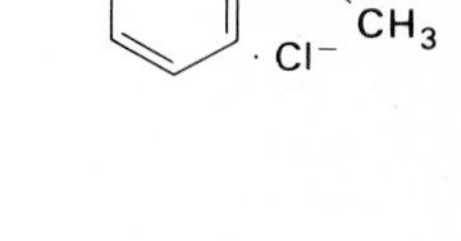

Brief action. Desirable antidote in curare poisoning. Minimal muscarinic effects. Also used in the diagnosis of myasthenia gravis in preference to neostigmine because its effect is briefer. Increase in muscle strength may occur within a minute in patients with the disease.

Dose: 10 mg intravenously.

NEOSTIGMINE BROMIDE
(Prostigmine)

Dose: 15 mg or more several times a day by mouth.

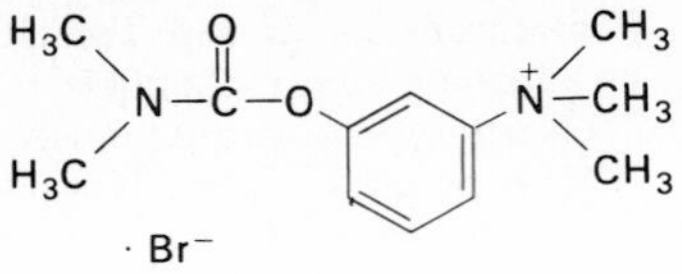

PYRIDOSTIGMINE BROMIDE
(Mestinon)

Resembles neostigmine but is less potent and correspondingly less toxic. Used in myasthenia gravis.

Dose: 60 mg or more several times a day by mouth.

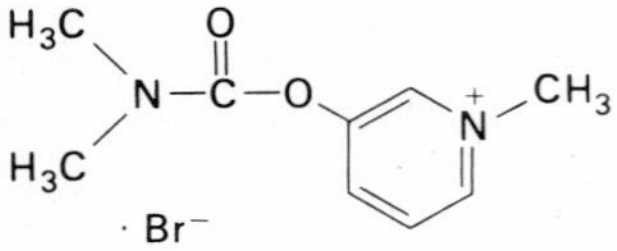

E. Agents That Facilitate Contraction by Persistent Inhibition

ORGANOPHOSPHORUS COMPOUNDS

1. History. a. Tetraethylpyrophosphate (TEPP) known since 1854.

b. Schrader (in the 1930's) synthesized paraoxon, parathion, and other members as possible nerve gases for military purposes.

2. Chemistry. Organic phosphates. Examples:

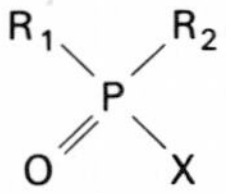

basic structure

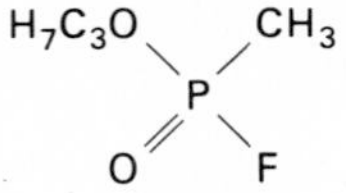

sarin

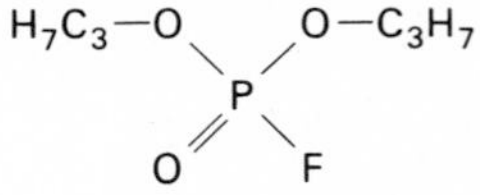

diisopropylfluorophosphate (DFP)

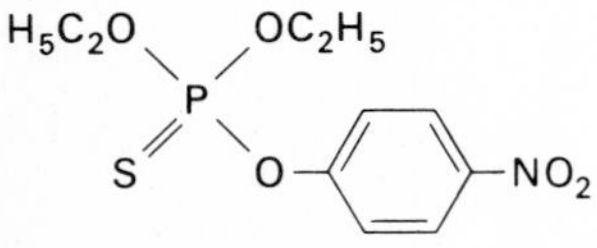

parathion

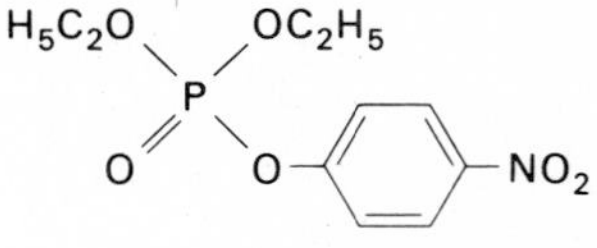

paraoxon

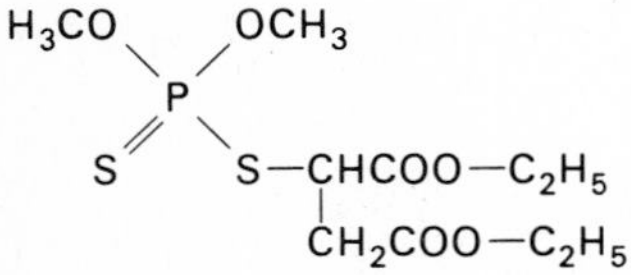

malathion

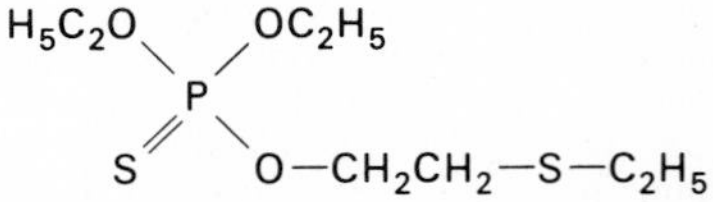

systox

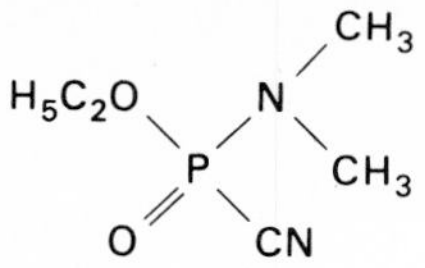

tabun

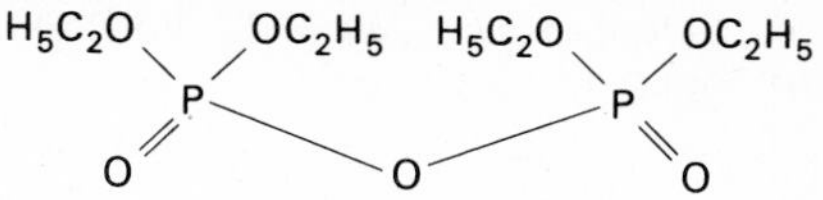

tetraethylpyrophosphate (TEPP)

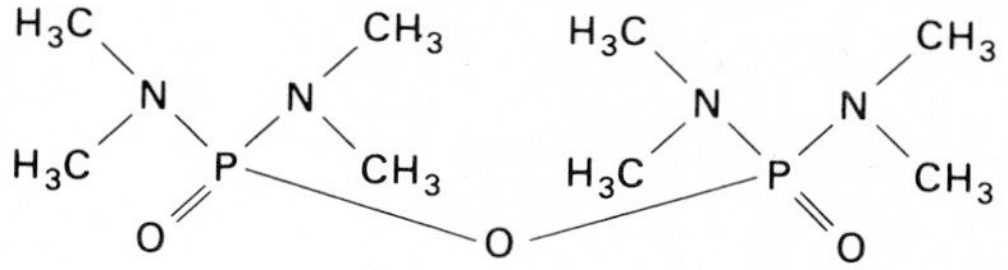

octamethylpyrophosphoramide (OMPA)

3. Action. Inhibit both types of cholinesterase; acetylcholine accumulates, producing the following effects:

a. Postganglionic: miosis, rhinorrhea, bronchial constriction, sweating, nausea, diarrhea, bradycardia.

b. Ganglionic: hypertension.

c. Neuromuscular: fasciculation, muscle cramps.

d. Central: anxiety, insomnia, headache, apathy, confusion, ataxia, coma, convulsions.

4. Mechanism. a. Organophosphorus cholinesterase inhibitors unite with the enzyme in a firm bond to the esteratic site which is not subject to hydrolysis. For example, the attachment of sarin may be represented as follows:

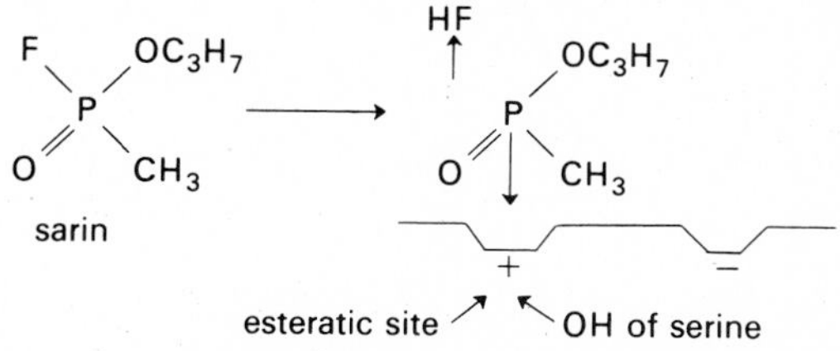

sarin

HF

esteratic site

OH of serine

b. Some of the compounds also possess a quaternary nitrogen (corresponding to that of choline) and hence may form a bond at the ionic site as well. Even if such a compound is hydrolyzed with the release of this portion, the phosphorus-esteratic site bond remains (see Holmstedt, Pharmacol. Rev., 11:567, 1959 for a general discussion).

c. It has been suggested that the thiophosphates may be changed in the liver to oxygen analogues before acting (DuBois, J. Pharmacol. Exp. Ther., 124:194, 1958).

5. Pharmacodynamics. Absorbed from various sites, including the skin.

6. Toxicity. a. Some members intensely poisonous.

b. Death may come from convulsions, paralysis of the respiratory and circulatory centers, increased bronchial secretion and bronchospasm, and paralysis of the respiratory muscles.

7. Uses. a. Widely used as insecticides but less satisfactory in medicine.

b. Isoflurophate and echothiophate are used in wide angle glaucoma (see Parasympathetic Stimulants), but trials in myasthenia gravis have been disappointing.

F. Reactivators of Cholinesterase

PRALIDOXIME GROUP

1. History. Jandorf (1951), Wilson (1951), and Wagner-Jauregg (1953) showed that hydroxylamine and hydroxamic acids could dislodge organophosphorus inhibitors from cholinesterase.

2. Chemistry. Non-, mono-, or bis-quaternary oximes.

3. Action and Mechanism. a. Reactivate cholinesterase and also depolarize receptors (Wills, Proc. Soc. Exp. Biol. Med., 101:196, 1959); thus antagonize the actions of organophosphates (and curare, but not succinylcholine).

b. The process of reactivation, in which the reactivator unites with the organophosphorus compound and "pulls" it away from the enzyme, may be diagrammed as follows:

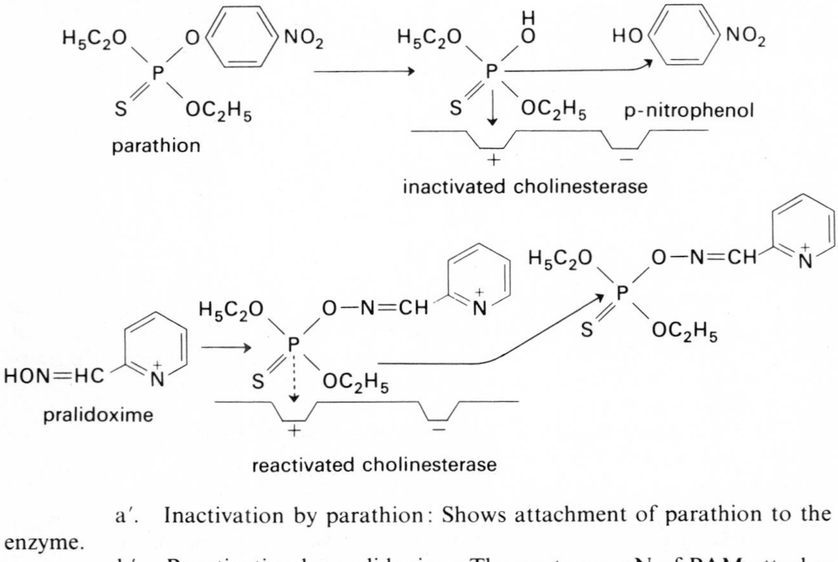

H_5C_2O O NO_2 P S OC_2H_5

parathion

H_5C_2O H O P S OC_2H_5 HO NO_2

p-nitrophenol

\+ −

inactivated cholinesterase

HON=HC N+

pralidoxime

H_5C_2O O—N=CH N+ P S OC_2H_5

\+ −

reactivated cholinesterase

H_5C_2O O—N=CH N+ P S OC_2H_5

a′. Inactivation by parathion: Shows attachment of parathion to the enzyme.

b′. Reactivation by pralidoxime: The quaternary N of PAM attaches at the anionic site on the enzyme long enough to "pull" the anion free; it is then quickly released, freeing the new complex.

4. Pharmacodynamics and Toxicity. a. Pralidoxime requires parenteral administration. Pharmacological actions and toxicity under study.

b. High doses or rapid administration may result in neuromuscular blockade and atropinelike effects.

5. Uses. a. Pralidoxime is used as an antidote in poisoning by organophosphorus insecticides and warfare chemicals of this type.

b. It is also used in cholinergic crises arising during the treatment of myasthenia gravis, and to check the action of anticholinesterases in the eye.

c. Treatment of organophosphorus cholinesterase inhibitors should include:

a′. Removal of poison, intubation, aspiration of stomach and mouth, artificial respiration.

b′. Atropine, up to 100 mg or more per day.

c′. Reactivators, such as pralidoxime (see Namba and Hiraki, J.A.M.A., 166:1835, 1958).

6. Preparation

PRALIDOXIME CHLORIDE (PAM; Protopam chloride)

Monoquaternary oxime.

Dose: 10 to 50 mg per kg body weight in 100 ml of saline by slow intravenous infusion.

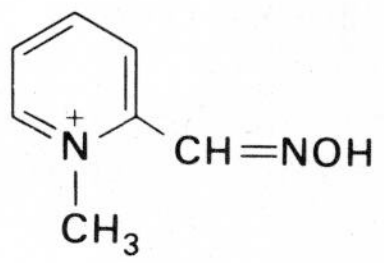

$\overset{+}{N}$ CH=NOH
CH_3

PRALIDOXIME MESYLATE

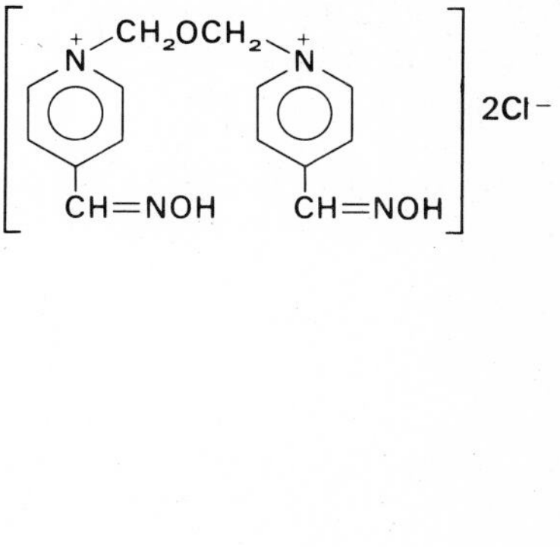

$[\overset{+}{N}$–CH_2OCH_2–$\overset{+}{N}]$ $2Cl^-$
CH=NOH CH=NOH

OBIDOXIME CHLORIDE

Dose: 3 to 6 mg per kg body weight by slow intravenous injection.

OTHERS

TRIMEDOXIME BROMIDE

DIACETYL MONOXIME (DAM)

G. Agents That Alter the Synthesis of Acetylcholine

Although the agents principally considered in this chapter act in the neighborhood of the receptor, or on the cholinesterase mechanism, three important toxins affect the release or synthesis of acetylcholine.

Guanidine reverses neuromuscular block and may be helpful in botulinus poisoning (15 to 35 mg per kg per day by mouth) (Cherington, New Eng. J. Med., 282:197, 1970).

BOTULINUS TOXIN

Considered to act just proximally to the site of acetylcholine release from the tip of the axone, either by impaired synthesis or impaired release.

DINOFLAGELLATE TOXIN and some snake toxins

Presumed to act similarly to botulinus toxin.

TICK TOXIN

The toxin causing tick paralysis is also thought to act just proximally to the site of acetylcholine release, by blocking passage and release.

HEMICHOLIUM (HC-3)

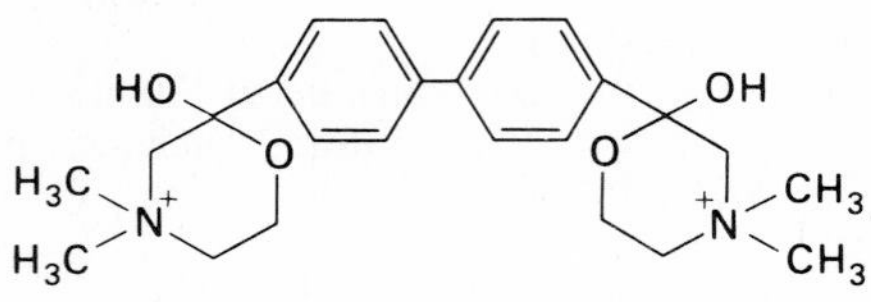

Presumed to inhibit formation of acetylcholine by preventing passage of choline through cellular membrane (Gardiner, Nature, 191:86, 1961).

Cyclized acetylcholine moieties may interfere with release of acetylcholine from nerve endings (Schueler, Fed. Proc., 20:561, 1961).

HO OH O O H_3C $\overset{+}{N}$ CH_3 H_3C $\overset{+}{N}$ CH_3

SUMMARY: GANGLIONIC AND MYONEURAL AGENTS

TYPE	*ACTION AND MECHANISM*	*TOXICITY*	*USE*	*EXAMPLES*
Ganglionic agents	Nausea, vasoconstriction, sweating; ganglionic stimulation, then paralysis with hypotension	Respiratory paralysis	Hypertension	Tetraethylammonium Cl
Myoneural inhibitors	Maintenance of polarization	Same	Relaxation during anesthesia	Tubocurarine Cl
Myoneural inhibitors	Maintenance of depolarization	Same	Same	Succinylcholine Cl
Myoneural facilitators	Inhibition of acetylcholinesterase	Muscular fasciculation, weakness, paralysis	Myasthenia gravis, curare antidotes	Neostigmine Br
Cholinesterase reactivators	Removal of organophosphate anticholinesterases from enzyme site	Neuromuscular blockade	Organophosphate poisoning	Pralidoxime

Reviews

Grob, D. Neuromuscular pharmacology. Ann. Rev. Pharmacol., 1:239, 1961.

D'Arcy, P., and Taylor, E. Quaternary ammonium compounds in medicinal chemistry. J. Pharm. Pharmacol., 14:193, 1962.

Silvette, H., Hoff, E., Larson, P., and Haag, H. Actions of nicotine on central nervous system functions. Pharmacol. Rev., 14:137, 1962.

Volle, R. Pharmacology of the autonomic nervous system. Ann. Rev. Pharmacol., 3:129, 1963.

Karczmar, A. Neuromuscular pharmacology. Ann. Rev. Pharmacol., 7:241, 1967.

46. Muscle Relaxants

Agents that relax skeletal muscle have been sought for use in various types of muscle spasticity. Success has been greatest with compounds that block internuncial synapses, especially in the spinal cord. Other compounds, such as curare, which block neuromuscular transmission, are not easily adaptable to chronic, ambulant therapy. Atropine and relatives which reduce the spasm in parkinsonism by central action are ineffective in other types of striated muscle spasm.

A. Propanediol Derivatives (Mephenesin)

A large group, some of which are also used as tranquilizers or hypnotics (see Sedatives and Hypnotics).

1. History. Mørch (1947) introduced mephenesin.

2. Chemistry. Propanediols, or derived compounds, most of which contain carbamate groups.

3. Action and Mechanism. a. Inhibit the synapses of internuncial neurones in the spinal cord, brain stem, and elsewhere to give an ascending muscular relaxation and paralysis. Complex reflexes tend to be abolished, simple reflexes to remain.

b. The mechanism of the action is unexplained at the chemical level.

c. Carisoprodol exhibits a mild atropinelike effect as well as muscle relaxation.

d. Meprobamate and derivatives show central muscle-relaxing effects of other sedatives.

4. Pharmacodynamics. Members of the group are well absorbed by mouth; little is known of their metabolic fate. Rapid metabolism of mephenesin group limits effectiveness.

5. Toxicity. a. Side effects include occasional sleepiness, weakness, vertigo, and lassitude.

b. Hemolysis and hemoglobinuria have been noted after intravenous administration.

6. Uses. a. To relieve muscle spasm in sprains, arthritis, bursitis, myositis, chorea, torticollis, spastic paraplegia, and the like.

b. Although the drugs are widely used, the results are usually short of spectacular.

c. Mephenesin is used as an antidote in strychnine poisoning, in which spinal reflexes are greatly heightened.

7. Preparations

CARISOPRODOL (Soma)
Dose: 350 mg 3 or 4 times a day by mouth.

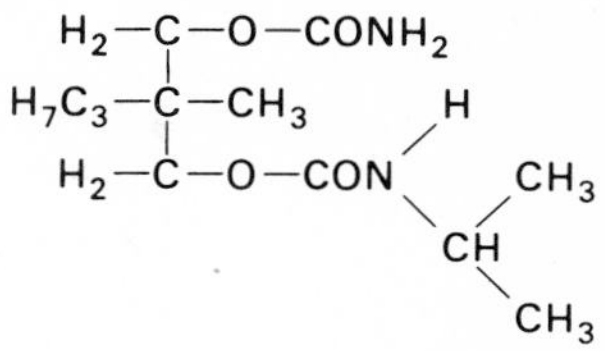

$H_2-C-O-CONH_2$
$H_7C_3-C-CH_3$ H
$H_2-C-O-CON$ CH_3
CH
CH_3

CHLORPHENESIN CARBAMATE (Maolate)
Dose: 0.3 gm 4 times a day by mouth.

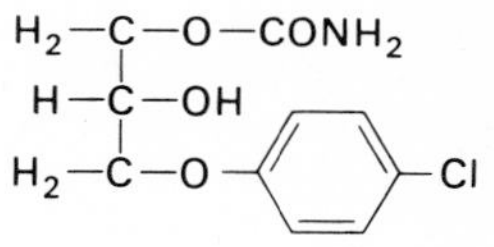

$H_2-C-O-CONH_2$
$H-C-OH$
H_2-C-O- Cl

MEPHENESIN (Tolserol; and many others)
Dose: 1 to 3 gm 3 to 5 times a day by mouth.

H_2-C-OH
$H-C-OH$
H_2-C-O-
H_3C

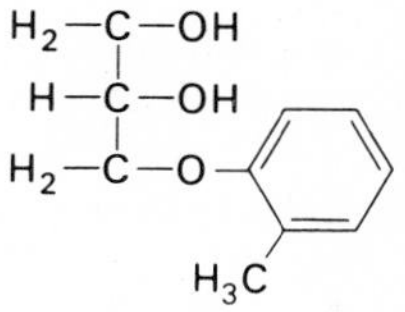

MEPHENESIN CARBAMATE (Tolseram)
Somewhat more slowly absorbed than mephenesin.
Dose: 1 to 3 gm 3 to 5 times a day by mouth.

$H_2-C-O-CONH_2$
$H-C-OH$
H_2-C-O-
H_3C

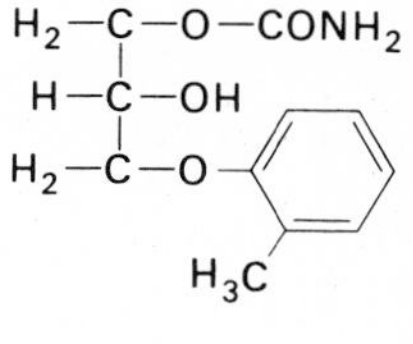

METHOCARBAMOL (Robaxin)
Reported to have a longer action than mephenesin.
Dose: 1 to 1.5 gm 3 times a day by mouth.

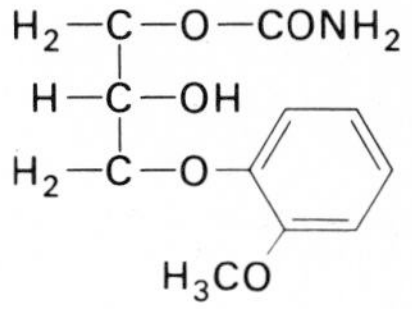

$H_2-C-O-CONH_2$
$H-C-OH$
H_2-C-O-
H_3CO

PROMOXOLANE (Dimethylane)
Dose: 0.5 gm 4 times a day by mouth.

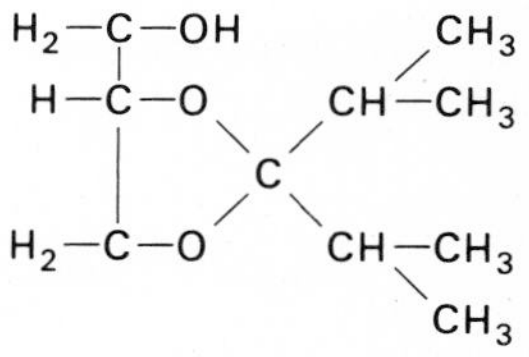

H_2-C-OH CH_3
$H-C-O$ $CH-CH_3$
C
H_2-C-O $CH-CH_3$
CH_3

STYRAMATE (Sinaxar)

Said to be devoid of any sedative effects.
Dose: 0.2 to 0.4 gm 3 times a day by mouth.

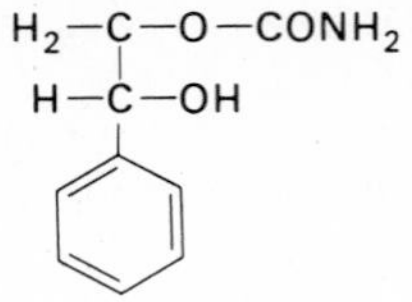

$H_2-C-O-CONH_2$
$H-C-OH$
(phenyl)

OTHERS

Emylcamate, meprobamate (see Sedatives).

B. Benzoxazole Derivatives

1. Chemistry. Benzimidazole and benzoxazole derivatives.

2. Action and Mechanism. a. Benzimidazole (not used clinically) and the benzoxazole derivatives interrupt nervous impulses in polysynaptic pathways in the cord and brain stem, much as mephenesin does. The result is an ascending paralysis, which may involve the intercostals.

b. The mechanism of action is unknown, though purine competition has been suggested.

c. Zoxazolamine, but not chlorozoxazone, also exerts a marked uricosuric effect through inhibition of tubular reabsorption of urate.

3. Pharmacodynamics and Toxicity. a. Well absorbed by mouth.

b. Side effects usually not severe but may include anorexia, headache, weakness, drowsiness, and skin rash; however, zoxazolamine may produce severe hepatitis and was marketed for only a short time.

4. Uses. As relaxants in muscle spasm and spasticity. Effects similar to those for mephenesin, but tend to be more potent and longer lasting.

5. Preparation

CHLORZOXAZONE (Paraflex)

Dose: 250 mg 3 times a day by mouth.

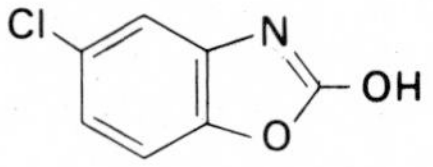

Cl N OH O

C. Thiazanone Derivatives (Chlormezanone)

1. Chemistry. Thiazanone derivatives.

2. Action and Mechanism. a. Skeletal muscle relaxant and anticonvulsant; resemble meprobamate in general effects.

b. Mechanism of action not determined; probably like other sedatives.

3. Pharmacodynamics and Toxicity. Absorbed by mouth; have a low order of toxicity.

4. Uses. a. In musculoskeletal disease and neurological muscle spasm.
b. Also as a mild tranquilizer.

5. Preparation

CHLORMEZANONE (Trancopal)

Dose: 0.1 to 0.3 gm or more 3 times a day by mouth.

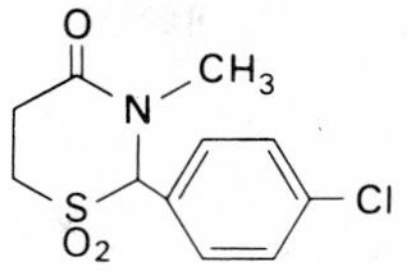

D. Oxazolidones

1. Chemistry. Oxazolidones, related to trimethadione type of anticonvulsant; also have been described as "cyclic carbamates."

2. Action and Toxicity. a. Mild sedatives; muscle relaxation may be only a part of sedation.
b. Question of hemolytic anemia and liver damage with metaxalone.

3. Uses. Relatively ineffective, but may be used as sedatives.

4. Preparations

MEPHENOXALONE (Trepidone)

Mild tranquilizer and muscle relaxant resembling meprobamate.

Dose: 400 mg 4 times a day by mouth.

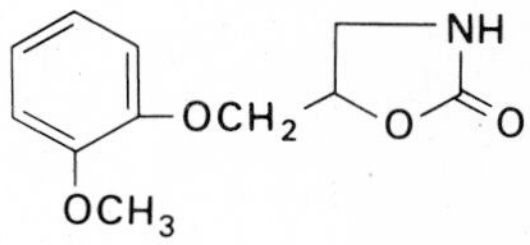

METAXALONE

Tranquilizer and muscle relaxer.
Under investigation.

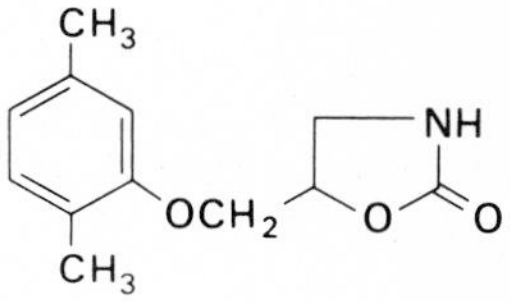

E. Other Muscle Relaxants

DIAZEPAM

See Tranquilizers.

FLETAZEPAM

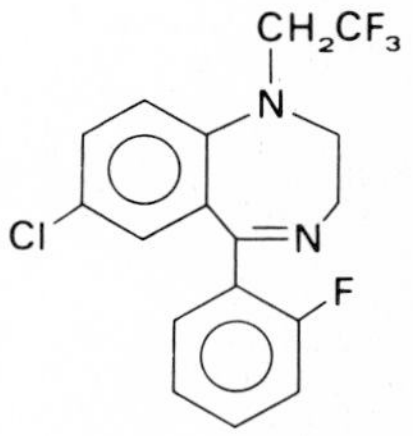

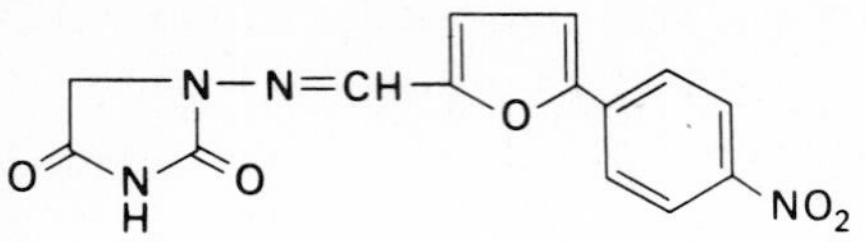

dantrolene

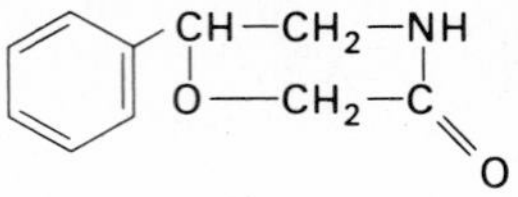

flumetramide

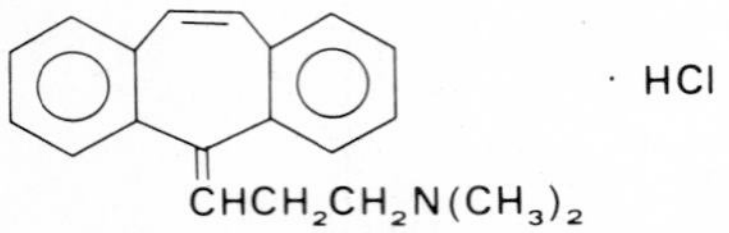

cyclobenzaprine hydrochloride

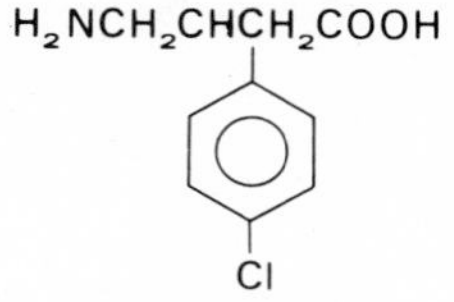

$H_2NCH_2CHCH_2COOH$

baclofen

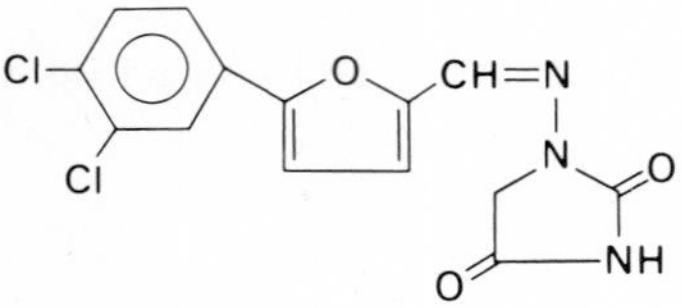

clodanolene

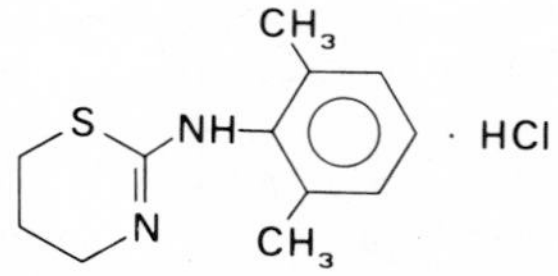

xylazine hydrochloride (Rompun)
(veterinary)

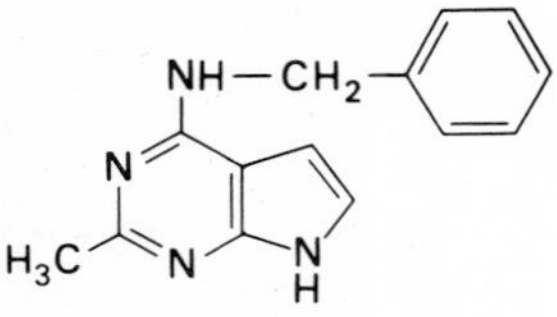

rolodine

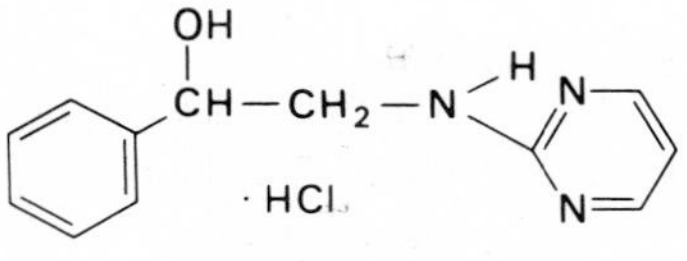

fenyripol HCl

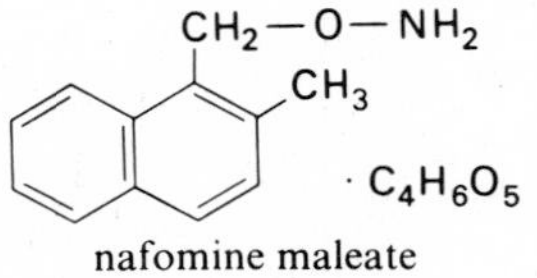

$\cdot C_4H_6O_5$

nafomine maleate

SUMMARY: MUSCLE RELAXANTS

TYPE	*ACTION AND MECHANISM*	*TOXICITY*	*USE*	*EXAMPLES*
Propanediol derivatives	Inhibit internuncial neurons in spinal cord	Sleepiness, weakness, vertigo, hemolysis	Muscle spasm, strychnine poisoning	Mephenesin
Benzoxazole derivatives	Similar	Anorexia, drowsiness, skin rash	Muscle spasm	Chlorzoxazone
Thiazanone derivatives	Not known	Minor	Same	Chlormezanone

47. General Anesthetics and Therapeutic Gases

I. GENERAL ANESTHETICS

General anesthetics are agents that depress the central nervous system reversibly, producing loss of consciousness, analgesia, and muscular relaxation with minimal depression of the vital functions. Under their influence surgical operations or other painful procedures may be done without recall by the patient.

A. Inhalation Anesthetics

1. History. a. Davy (1799) noted that nitrous oxide could produce unconsciousness; Faraday (1818) reported that ether could allay pain; Hickman (1824) used carbon dioxide as an anesthetic for animal surgery.

b. Long (1844) used ether as a surgical anesthetic; Wells (1845) attempted to use nitrous oxide; Morton (1846) demonstrated the anesthetic use of ether publicly; Simpson (1847) used chloroform successfully.

c. Luckhardt and Thompson (1918) introduced ethylene; Lucas and Henderson (1928) introduced, and Waters (1930) used, cyclopropane; Leake and Chen (1930) suggested the use of divinyl ether; Raventos (1956) introduced halothane.

2. Chemistry. Diverse, relatively simple molecules; mostly hydrocarbons and halogenated hydrocarbons.

3. Action. a. The variety of agents, with different potencies, induction times and character of action, make generalization difficult, but the actions of a complete anesthetic (one which can cause respiratory arrest without the aid of another agent), such as ether, may be somewhat arbitrarily divided into a series of stages and planes.

b. The action starts with a depression of the reticular activating system of the midbrain, producing analgesia and sleepiness. Cortical depression follows, and with the resulting release of lower centers the excited phase of induction is seen. Progressive depression of the midbrain and spinal cord follows, and is accompanied by surgical anesthesia and loss of reflexes. Depression of the medulla is minimal until the deeper planes are reached, but then becomes increasingly prominent until respiration and circulation fail.

c. The stages of anesthesia may be summarized as follows:

Stage I: Inebriation and analgesia in a still conscious patient, who may tolerate mildly painful procedures; the stage is terminated by loss of consciousness. "Ether analgesia" is return to deep Stage I from Stage III, and may in skillful hands allow surgery.

Stage II: Delirium, excitement, irregular breathing, motor activity, signs of general sympathetic discharge, susceptibility to external stimuli; the stage is terminated by relaxation.

Stage III: Surgical anesthesia, progressive loss of reflexes and depression of vital functions.

Plane 1: Relaxation, regular respiration, pupils smaller, eyelid reflexes disappear. Suitable for procedures not requiring marked muscular relaxation (thoracic, neurosurgical, thyroid, bladder, hernia operations).

Plane 2: Increased relaxation, decreased respiration, eyeball movements cease. Suitable for most procedures requiring moderate relaxation and inhibition of pharyngeal, peritoneal, and other reflexes (throat, joint, abdominal surgery).

Plane 3: Accentuation of the signs of plane 2. Required for some phases of upper abdominal surgery and for breech extraction.

Plane 4: Respiration entirely diaphragmatic and by accessory muscles, pupils widely dilated; danger of circulatory and respiratory collapse.

Stage IV: Breathing stops, but the medullary paralysis is usually reversible with artificial respiration and redistribution of the anesthetic in the body.

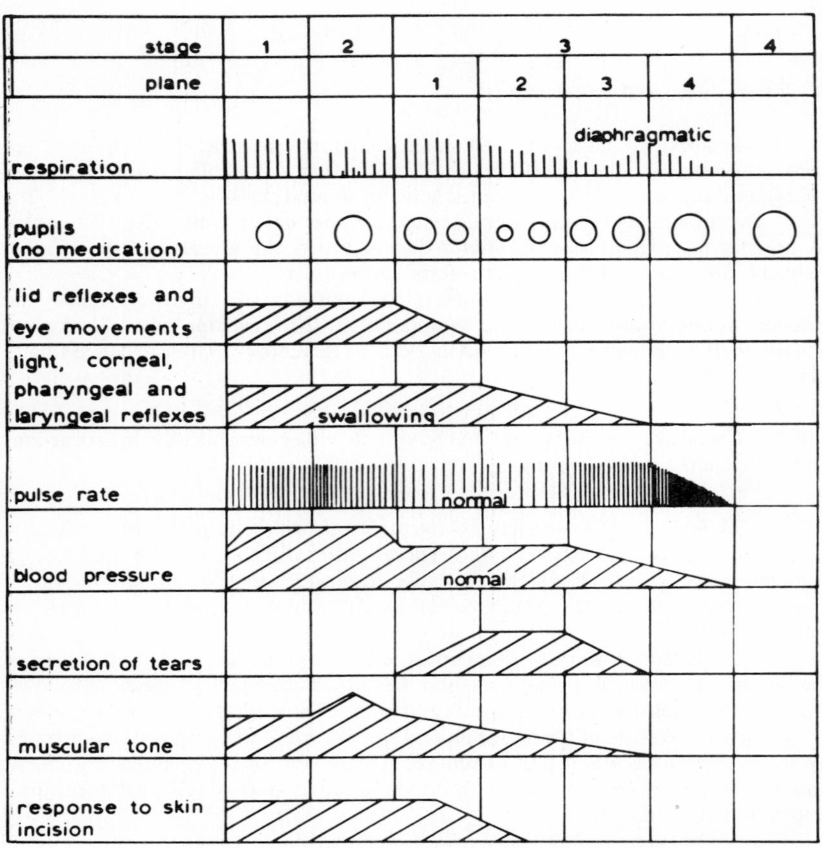

4. Mechanism. a. The fundamental mechanism appears to be an interference with energy production and utilization in the cell.

b. Concentrations of anesthetics effective in vivo inhibit the extra oxygen uptake which results from electrical or potassium stimulation of brain slices; slow the breakdown of immediate energy sources such as ATP and phosphocreatine.

c. Anesthetics also depress synaptic transmission in isolated ganglia.

d. Within a homologous series, high lipoid solubility favors anesthetic action. However, this factor, and others involving solubility, permeability and surface tension, are probably related to the problem of the transport of anesthetics to the site of action, rather than to the mechanism of action.

e. Alternative: Some anesthetics form microcrystals with tissue water which trap protein side chains and increase impedance to the point of anesthesia (Pauling, Science, 134:15, 1961).

NITROUS OXIDE

1. Chemistry. N_2O. Inert, colorless gas; nonflammable but supports combustion above 450°C. Stored in tanks as a liquid.

2. Action. a. CNS: Relatively weak anesthetic; at atmospheric pressure with full oxygenation will not depress below plane 1 of Stage III. To achieve surgical anesthesia some asphyxia is required, unless pressures greater than 1 atmosphere are used.

b. Other systems: Not depressant at nonasphyxial concentrations.

3. Pharmacodynamics. a. Inhaled and absorbed as a gas; unaltered in the body and excreted via the lungs.

b. Induction is easy and recovery rapid because of low blood:gas solubility ratio and lack of irritating properties.

4. Toxicity. Least toxic anesthetic gas at nonasphyxial levels; if higher concentrations are used intense asphyxia may raise BP dangerously in elderly persons. Does not cause liver or kidney damage.

Relative fatalities of common anesthetics:

Tribromethanol	1 in 1,000
Chloroform	1 in 2,000–3,000
Cyclopropane	1 in 3,000
Ether	1 in 5,000–15,000
Nitrous oxide	1 in 50,000–1,000,000

5. Uses. a. To induce anesthesia.

b. For brief anesthesia, as for tooth extraction.

c. As a principal agent in "balanced anesthesia." This consists of premedication with a basal anesthetic (barbiturate), a narcotic analgesic (meperidine), and a vagal inhibitor (atropine); induction by a short-acting barbiturate (thiopental); maintenance of unconsciousness, analgesia, and reflex inhibition by an anesthetic gas (75% to 80% N_2O) and an intravenous narcotic analgesic (meperidine); maintenance of muscle relaxation by a curare-type agent (gallamine). Such a procedure has the advantages of being highly versatile, nonexplosive, and well received by the patient. Disadvantages include the large doses of intravenous agents which may be poorly tolerated by debilitated patients and leave postoperative CNS depression and inadequate ventilation. Many other agents are used in variants of balanced anesthesia.

d. Advantages of N_2O include: nonexplosive, nonirritating, nontoxic, rapid induction and recovery. Disadvantages: weakness, poor muscular relaxation; asphyxia.

6. Preparation.

NITROUS OXIDE

Dose: up to 80% by nonrebreathing or semiclosed techniques.

ETHER

1. Chemistry. $(C_2H_5)_2O$. Relatively inert, colorless, unpleasant liquid; stored in cans (decomposition to aldehydes and peroxides retarded by copper). Boiling point: 35°C. Explosive in air (1.8% to 36%); in oxygen (2% to 82%).

2. Action. a. CNS: A potent, complete anesthetic; an inhaled concentration of 6% to 8% will maintain surgical anesthesia, and therefore anoxemia does not occur. Good margin of safety, as 12% to 15% required to produce respiratory arrest.

b. Respiratory system: Continuous depression; masked above plane 2 by reflex stimulation from irritation of bronchial tree. Copious secretions from bronchi may be reduced by parasympatholytics. Bronchodilatation occurs from sympathetic activity.

c. Cardiovascular system: Cardiovascular center usually depressed after respiratory center. Heart depressed and vessels dilated, but masked above plane 2 by sympathetic activity and epinephrine liberation. Ether does not sensitize the heart to epinephrine, nor are dangerous arrhythmias common.

d. Gastrointestinal system: Initial stimulation of smooth muscle, followed by relaxation. Hyperactivity may occur during recovery, with vomiting; or, if hypoxic or hypercarbic, postoperative ileus.

e. Other systems: Epinephrine induced glycogenolysis leads to elevated blood sugar; minimal depression of liver function; minimal irritation of kidneys with casts and RBC in the urine. Curarelike inhibition of neuromyal impulse provides excellent muscle relaxation; pregnant uterus inhibited and can be completely relaxed.

3. Pharmacodynamics. Inhaled and absorbed as a vapor; unaltered in the body; 85% to 90% eliminated by the lungs.

4. Toxicity. Irritation of respiratory tract; postoperative atelectasis and pneumonia. Collapse and respiratory depression from excessive administration should be treated by artificial respiration until the excess of ether has been washed out of the tissues.

5. Uses. a. Cheap; safe; satisfactory anesthetic for major, prolonged operations, especially in the elderly because of minimum cardiovascular effects.

b. Also used to quiet convulsions or tetanic seizures, and in labor.

c. Advantages include high therapeutic index, toleration by patients, excellent muscular relaxation without undue CNS depression, promotion of good ventilation.

d. Disadvantages include explosiveness, respiratory secretion, long induction and recovery time, unpleasant odor, depletion of liver glycogen, postoperative nausea and vomiting, decreased tolerance to hemorrhage.

6. Preparation

ETHER (Diethyl ether)

Dose: By open drop, or from vaporizers in nonrebreathing, semiclosed, or closed systems.

CHLOROFORM

1. Chemistry. $CHCl_3$. Thin, volatile liquid with a sweetish odor; boils at 61°C, enough higher than ether to make it more easily handled and stored in tropical climates. Nonflammable; forms phosgene if heated in an open flame.

2. Action. a. CNS: A potent, complete anesthetic; an inhaled concentration of 1.5% will maintain surgical anesthesia, but 2% will cause respiratory arrest, a low margin of safety. Cardiovascular and respiratory centers are simultaneously depressed.

b. Respiratory system: Nonirritating in concentration necessary for induction; hence depression of respiration is proportional to depth of anesthesia (different from ether where irritation stimulates respiration in early stages).

c. Cardiovascular system: Depression of vasomotor center and heart, and fall in blood pressure. Sensitizes to epinephrine, which predisposes to ventricular fibrillation; also stimulates vagus, which may cause vagal arrest, especially during induction.

d. Other systems: Effects on gastrointestinal tract similar to ether; glycogenolysis raises blood sugar; liver function is impaired, and permanent damage may follow administration for more than one-half hour, especially if hypoxia or hypercarbia occur; also renal tubular damage. Relaxes skeletal muscle, but without curarelike effect; activity of pregnant uterus inhibited only by deep anesthesia.

3. Pharmacodynamics. Inhaled and absorbed as vapor; unaltered in the body and excreted in the lungs.

4. Toxicity. Excessively dangerous because of the low therapeutic margin, and danger of cardiac arrhythmias and necrosis of liver and other parenchymatous organs.

5. Uses. a. No application if other, superior agents are available.

b. Advantages include nonexplosiveness and easy induction with simple apparatus.

c. Disadvantages include low margin of safety and danger of cardiac and liver toxicity.

6. Preparation

CHLOROFORM

Dose: By open drop, or from vaporizers in nonrebreathing or semiclosed systems.

ETHYLENE

1. Chemistry. $CH_2{=}CH_2$. An explosive gas with an unpleasant odor.

2. Action. Similar to N_2O; slightly more potent, but not enough to relieve anoxia.

3. Pharmacodynamics and Toxicity. Similar to N_2O.

4. Uses. Seldom used; no great advantage over N_2O in use and is explosive.

CYCLOPROPANE

1. Chemistry. Colorless, faintly unpleasant gas; stored in tanks as a liquid. Explosive in air (3% to 10%), in oxygen (2.5% to 50%).

2. Action. a. CNS: A complete anesthetic; an inhaled concentration of 20% to 25% will maintain surgical anesthesia; 40% is required to produce respiratory failure. Stimulates the parasympathetic system.

b. Respiratory system: Continuous depression without provoking secretions. Hypercarbia may be present without hypoxia. Bronchoconstriction may occur.

c. Cardiovascular system: Inhibition of heart, and degree of vasodilatation less than with ether. However, it sensitizes the myocardium to epinephrine, and ventricular arrhythmias may occur at deep levels of anesthesia, especially after hypoxia or hypercarbia.

d. Other systems: Minimal effects on gastrointestinal motility, but nausea and vomiting similar to ether; no serious hepatotoxicity or renal irritation; skeletal muscle relaxation incomplete except at deep levels of anesthesia.

3. Pharmacodynamics. Inhaled and absorbed as a vapor; eliminated unchanged by the lungs.

4. Toxicity. Danger of arrhythmias from sensitization to epinephrine. Hypoventilation and hypercarbia may result from lack of irritation.

5. Uses. a. Widely used, especially in poor risk and elderly patients.

b. Advantages include: easy, rapid induction, high therapeutic index, good toleration by patients, safety in the presence of shock or recent hemorrhage.

c. Disadvantages include: explosiveness, ventricular arrhythmias, postoperative nausea and vomiting.

6. Preparation

CYCLOPROPANE

Dose: By closed circuit (for economy).

$$H_2C\!\!<\!\!\underset{\textstyle \text{—}}{}\!\!>\!\!CH_2 \quad (\text{ring: } CH_2\text{–}CH_2\text{–}CH_2)$$

ETHYL CHLORIDE

1. Chemistry. C_2H_5Cl. A colorless, volatile liquid; boils at 13°C, which necessitates keeping it in glass or metal bottles under slight pressure; flammable.

2. Action. a. A complete anesthetic.

b. Also, when sprayed on the skin, the rapid evaporation produces almost instantaneous freezing, with temporary local anesthesia.

3. Pharmacodynamics and Toxicity. a. Inhaled and absorbed as a vapor.

b. Danger of vagal arrest or ventricular arrhythmia; hepatotoxic.

4. Uses. a. For rapid induction, or brief procedures, such as opening an ear drum.

b. Also may be used to supplement N_2O anesthesia, but in this case must not be used in a rebreathing system because it is hydrolyzed by soda lime.

c. For local "refrigeration" anesthesia.

5. Preparation

ETHYL CHLORIDE

Dose: By the open drop or spray method.

VINYL ETHER

1. Chemistry. $(CH_2{=}CH)_2O$. Colorless, unpleasant liquid; boils at 28.3°C; explosive in air (1.7%–27%), in oxygen (1.8%–85%).

2. Action. a. A potent, complete anesthetic; an inhaled concentration of 4% will maintain surgical anesthesia; 10% to 12% will cause respiratory arrest.

b. Other systems: Continuous depression of respiration without provoking copious secretion; myocardium not sensitized to epinephrine, but arrhythmias may occur with deep anesthesia.

3. Pharmacodynamics. Inhaled and absorbed as a gas; eliminated unchanged by lungs.

4. Toxicity. Nausea and vomiting uncommon; hepatotoxic if used for more than 30 minutes, or repeatedly at short intervals.

5. Uses. a. Suitable for brief operations.

b. Advantages include rapid induction and recovery, simplicity of administration, minor level of respiratory and gastrointestinal irritation.

c. Disadvantages include explosiveness, hepatotoxicity.

6. Preparation

VINYL ETHER (Divinyl ether; Vinethene)

Dose: By open drop.

TRICHLOROETHYLENE

1. Chemistry. $ClCH{=}CCl_2$. A volatile liquid with an odor like chloroform; nonflammable.

2. Action. Resembles chloroform but is more rapid in effect; analgesic in subanesthetic concentrations (0.25 vol %).

3. Pharmacodynamics. Absorbed through the respiratory epithelium; probably excreted in part as metabolic products.

4. Toxicity. Tachypnea, bradycardia, ventricular extrasystoles, and rarely tachycardia; amnesia may outlast anesthesia.

5. Uses. a. Too dangerous as an anesthetic, except in a concentration of 0.25% supplementing N_2O.

b. Widely used as an analgesic, often by self administration, to control labor pains, trigeminal neuralgia, and the pain of brief surgical procedures where muscular relaxation is not needed.

c. Should not come in contact with soda lime (forms dichloroacetylene, toxic to cranial nerves).

6. Preparation

TRICHLOROETHYLENE (Trilene)

Dose: By mask, inhaler device, or semiclosed system.

HALOTHANE

1. Chemistry. Colorless liquid; boils at 50°C; nonexplosive in oxygen (0.5% to 50%). Stable in brown bottles, not decomposed by soda lime.

2. Action. a. CNS: A potent, complete anesthetic; an inhaled concentration of 1% to 2% will maintain surgical anesthesia; 3% causes respiratory arrest, but this concentration may be used for induction.

b. Respiratory system: Continuous respiratory depressant; not irritating; causes bronchodilatation.

c. Cardiovascular system: Myocardial and vasomotor depressant; heart is sensitized to epinephrine, and ventricular arrhythmias may occur. Bradycardia controllable by parasympatholytic agents.

d. Other systems: Postoperative nausea and vomiting not severe; only a moderate muscle relaxant. Obtunds throat reflexes and relaxes masseter muscles, facilitating tracheal intubation.

3. Pharmacodynamics. Inhaled and absorbed as a vapor; a substantial portion retained for hours; some dechlorination occurs (Van Dyke, Biochem. Pharmacol., 13:1239, 1964).

4. Toxicity. Respiratory and cardiovascular depression; hypotension; hepatic necrosis and cholestatic jaundice reported. A toxic halogenated butene may increase under conditions of use.

5. Uses. a. For a rapid, flexible anesthesia where complete muscular relaxation is not needed (or gallamine may be given to secure relaxation); widely used.

b. Advantages: nonexplosive; useful adjunct to N_2O, decreasing the need for intravenous administration of depressants and muscle relaxants.

c. Disadvantages: low margin of safety, strong respiratory and circulatory depression, incomplete muscle relaxation. Moderately slow induction and recovery because of high blood:gas solubility coefficient.

d. Should not be used in presence of liver or biliary disease, pregnancy or labor.

6. Preparation

HALOTHANE (Fluothane)

Dose: From a calibrated vaporizer in a semiclosed system.

```
F         Br
 \       /
F—C—CH
 /       \
F         Cl
```

OTHER FLUORINATED HYDROCARBONS

METHOXYFLURANE (Penthrane)

A nonexplosive, high boiling (101°C) ether resembling ethyl ether except that it does not cause bronchial irritation and resultant respiratory stimulation. A more profound circulatory depressant than ether. Used in obstetrics at analgesic level. Occasional nephrotoxicity with inability to conserve water.

```
           F   Cl
           |  /
H3C—O—C—CH
           |  \
           F   Cl
```

FLUOROXENE (Fluoromar)

Resembles ether but is less flammable, but is also less potent; not in common use.

```
F
 \
F—C—CH2—O—CH=CH2
 /
F
```

FLUROTHYL (Indoklon)

Powerful convulsant used as an alternative to electric shock. May produce prolonged apnea; local venous thrombosis after intravenous use.

Dose: Intravenously or by inhalation.

```
F                  F
 \                /
F—C—CH2—O—CH2—C—F
 /                \
F                  F
```

$F(Cl)C$–cyclopropane ring with F, F, F and OCH_3

aliflurane

$CHF_2—O—CF_2—CHFCl$

enflurane

$HCF_2—O—CHClCF_3$

isoflurane

$F—CH_2—CF_3$

norflurane

$H_3C—O—CF_2—CHFBr$

roflurane

$F—CH_2—O—CH(CF_3)_2$

sevoflurane

$F—CF_2—CHFBr$

teflurane

B. Nonvolatile Anesthetics

INTRAVENOUS BARBITURATES

1. History. Lundy (1934) introduced thiopental as an intravenous anesthetic.

2. Chemistry. Barbituric acid derivatives with long side chains, or equivalent, at 5; oxygen at 2 often replaced by S.

3. Action. a. Complete anesthetics which depress in the same sequence as the volatile anesthetics. Analgesia occurs only at deep levels, and hence margin of safety is narrow.

b. Respiratory system: Nonirritating; mildly bronchoconstricting.

c. Cardiovascular system: Myocardial depressants and vasodilators; rapid injection may result in severe, transient hypotension. Do not sensitize the heart to epinephrine; do not induce arrhythmias in the absence of hypercarbia.

d. Other systems: Transient decrease in intestinal motility and tone, incidence of nausea and vomiting low; liver and renal function satisfactory, blood sugar not elevated; relaxation of skeletal and uterine muscle poor except at deep levels of anesthesia.

4. Mechanism. As for barbiturates generally (see Sedatives and Hypnotics).

5. Pharmacodynamics. a. Blood-brain equilibrium achieved within a minute of intravenous injection, with correspondingly rapid induction of anesthesia.

b. Rapid recovery from original dose owing to redistribution in other tissues. Delayed recovery from large doses as desaturation of tissues, including fat, may take several hours. Metabolized fairly completely in the liver (thiopental at rate of 10% to 15% per hour, principally through oxidation of the methylbutyl side chain).

6. Toxicity. a. Laryngospasm may occur during light anesthesia.
b. Severe respiratory and circulatory depression with deep anesthesia.

7. Uses. a. Useful in minor and emergency surgery; for the induction of balanced anesthesia; for rapid deepening of depression during other anesthesia; to control convulsions.
b. Advantages include rapid, pleasant induction without a mask.
c. Disadvantages include delicate administration, respiratory and circulatory depression at levels providing muscular relaxation.

8. Preparations

BUTHALITAL (Transithal)

Dose: 0.4 to 0.8 gm as 10% solution intravenously.

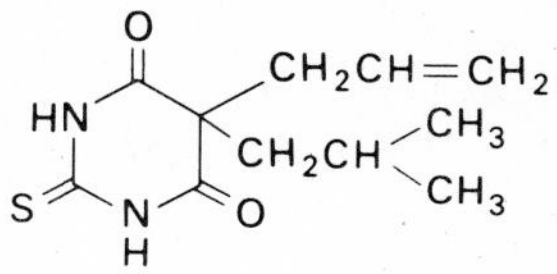

HEXOBARBITAL SODIUM (Evipal)

A nonthiobarbiturate similar in action to thiopental. No longer marketed as a general anesthetic, but used as a sedative.

Dose: 2 to 4 ml of 10% solution initially, supplemented by smaller doses as needed but not exceeding 10 ml.

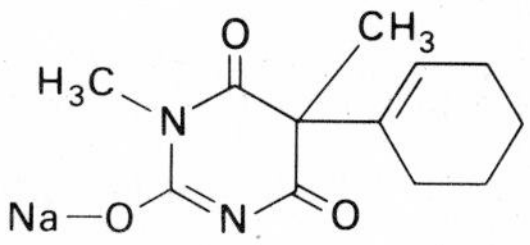

METHITURAL SODIUM (Neraval)

Similar to thiopental but half as potent.

Dose: 2 to 4 ml of a 5% solution initially, augmented as required.

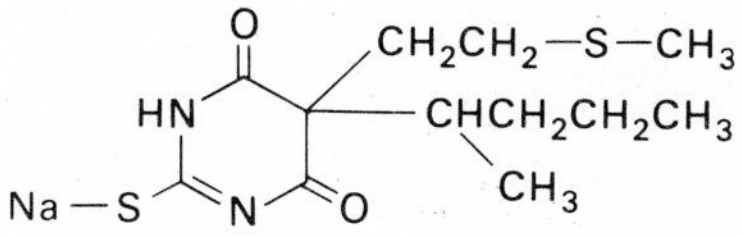

METHOHEXITAL SODIUM (Brevital)

Similar to thiopental but more potent and more briefly acting. Not used to stop convulsions as restlessness sometimes present.

Dose: 2.5 to 5 ml of a 1% solution initially, augmented as required.

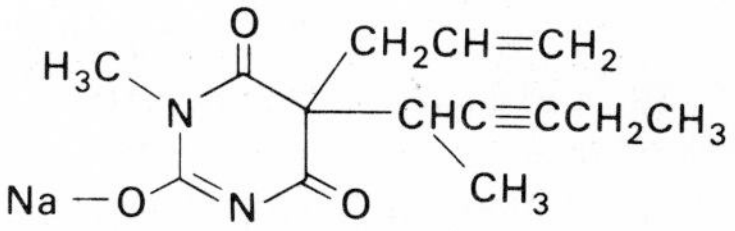

THIAMYLAL SODIUM (Surital)

Slightly more potent than thiopental but otherwise similar.

Dose: 4 to 8 ml of 2.5% solution initially, augmented as required.

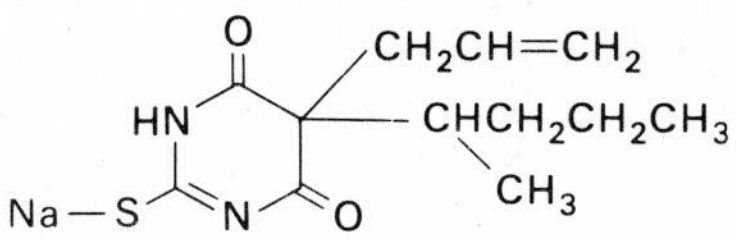

THIOPENTAL SODIUM (Pentothal)

Dose: 3 to 6 ml of 2.5% solution initially, followed by 2 to 3 ml at 30-second intervals as required (or corresponding doses of 5% solution).

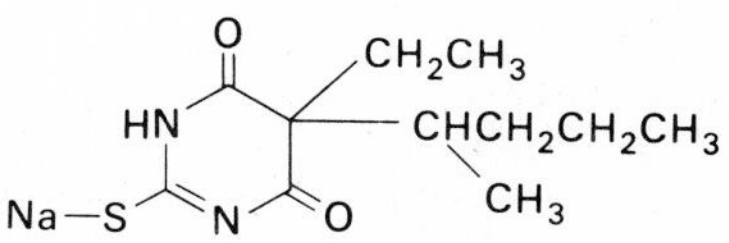

MAGNESIUM SALTS

1. Chemistry. a. Normal constituent of body. Serum magnesium about 85% ionized; balance bound to protein.

b. The adult requirement of Mg is about 0.2 to 0.6 mg per day.

2. Action and Mechanism. a. Magnesium functions as an intracellular electrolyte; as an essential metal for certain enzyme systems; and in the maintenance of normal neuromuscular irritability. Excess Mg decreases irritability; deficiency increases irritability. Ca and Mg are antagonistic on neuromuscular irritability.

b. Magnesium sulfate, or other magnesium salts, produce depression of the CNS when given parenterally. The action is rarely seen after oral administration because of minimal absorption and rapid excretion. The mechanism of action may be based on replacement of Ca on the surface of cells, which, when stimulated, admit Mg in place of Ca.

c. The grass tetany of cattle is related to an inadequate intake of Mg.

3. Pharmacodynamics and Toxicity. a. Brief tenure in body before excretion.

b. Principal hazard is excessive CNS depression; calcium (10 ml of 10% calcium gluconate) intravenously immediately abolishes the depression.

4. Uses. a. In producing strong sedation or basal anesthesia in tetanus and eclampsia.

b. Dangerous in adequate doses, and unreliable in safe doses.

5. Preparation

MAGNESIUM SULFATE
Dose: 20 ml of 20% solution intravenously.

CYCLOHEXANONE GROUP

1. Chemistry. Cyclohexanone or phencyclidine derivatives.

2. Action and Mechanism. a. Anesthesia and analgesia resembling that from ultrashort barbiturates. Produce sensory dissociation, especially for pain perception (Pender. J.A.M.A., 215:1126, 1971).

b. Do not produce vomiting, respiratory or circulatory depression, arrhythmias; do not produce muscle relaxation.

c. Mechanism unexplained.

3. Pharmacodynamics and Toxicity. a. Rapid onset and rapid recovery after parenteral administration.

b. Notably safe, but may produce transient hallucinations and a trancelike state.

4. Uses. a. Used for induction of anesthesia, short anesthesia, supplement to N_2O: minor surgery, cystoscopy, dressing changes, especially in children.

b. Trained personnel desirable; environment should be kept quiet.

5. Preparations

KETAMINE HYDROCHLORIDE (Ketalar; Ketaject)

Dose: 1 to 4.5 mg per kg intravenously (anesthesia in 1 minute, lasting 5 to 10 minutes); 6.5 to 13 mg per kg intramuscularly (anesthesia in 4 minutes, lasting 10 to 20 minutes).

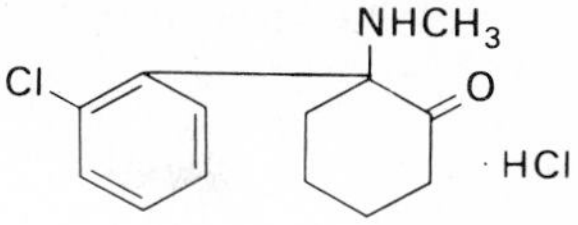

$NHCH_3$, Cl, O, · HCl

PHENCYCLIDINE HYDROCHLORIDE

Abandoned because of prolonged recovery time and psychotomimetic effects.

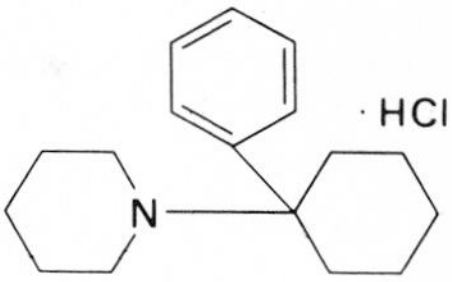

· HCl, N

TILETAMINE HYDROCHLORIDE

Under investigation.

$NH—C_2H_5$, O, S, · HCl

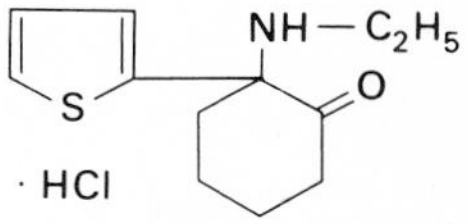

OTHER AGENTS

ETOXADROL HYDROCHLORIDE

Under investigation.

O, O, NH, C_2H_5, · HCl

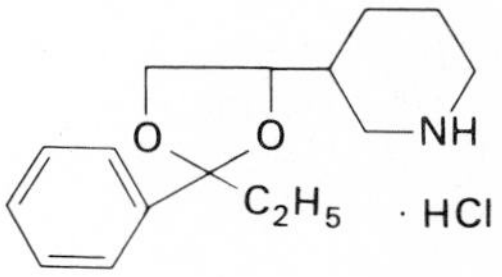

HYDROXYDIONE

Steroid formerly used as a basal or supplementary anesthesia.

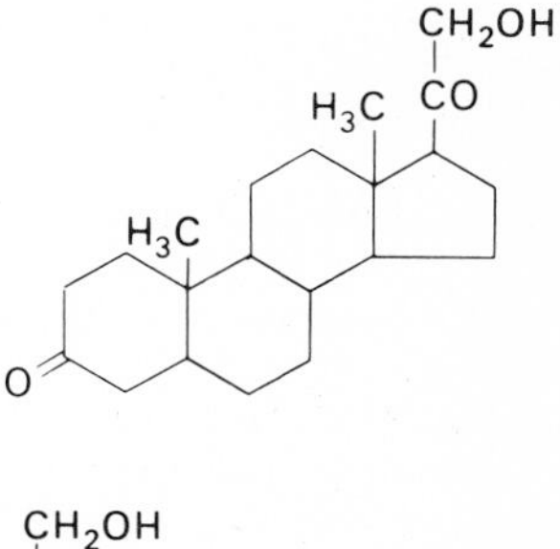

CH_2OH, H_3C CO, H_3C, O

OXYBATE SODIUM

Anesthetic supplement.
Under investigation.

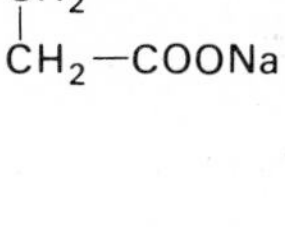

CH_2OH
CH_2
$CH_2—COONa$

PROPANIDID

Ultrashort intravenous anesthetic; nonbarbiturate. Rapidly broken down in the blood.

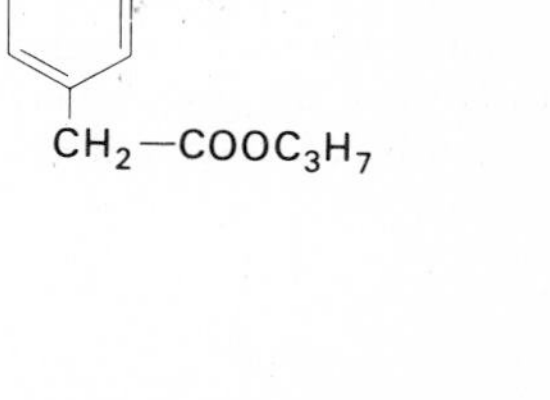

$O—CH_2—CO—N(C_2H_5)_2$, OCH_3, $CH_2—COOC_3H_7$

PROPOXATE

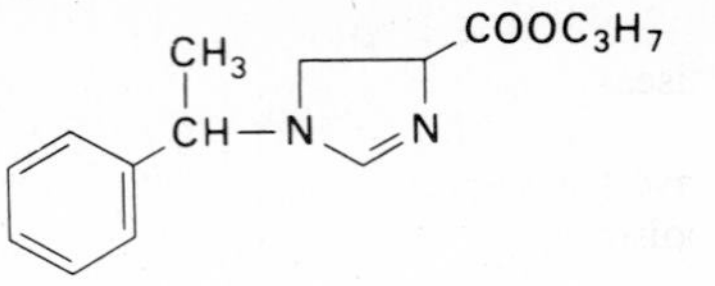

Potent, rapid anesthetic for coldblooded vertebrates.

Dose: 0.05 to 10 ppm in fresh or sea water.

TRIBROMETHANOL SOLUTION (tribromethanol in amylene hydrate; Avertin)

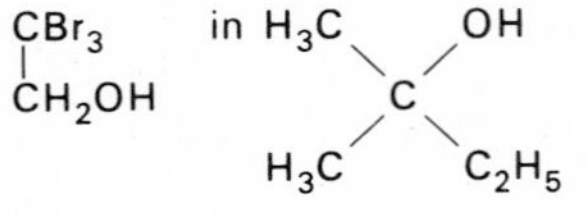

Formerly administered by rectum as a basal or preanesthetic agent.

CBr_3–CH_2OH in $(H_3C)_2C(OH)C_2H_5$

II. THERAPEUTIC GASES

OXYGEN

1. Chemistry. O_2. Colorless, odorless gas; supplied under pressure in steel cylinders.

2. Action and Mechanism. a. Relieves anoxia when mechanisms for oxygen absorption, conveyance, and utilization are not unduly impaired.

b. In the presence of impaired oxygen absorption from the lungs, as in pulmonary edema, absorption may be increased by a high concentration of inspired oxygen, and hemoglobin more completely saturated. Even in the absence of impaired absorption, an additional 2 volumes % can be dissolved in the blood with the administration of 100% oxygen.

c. Respiration is slightly depressed, followed in 6 to 8 minutes by stimulation, probably from irritant effects. Minimal vasoconstriction and bradycardia are produced, and definite (10% to 20%) decrease in cardiac output.

3. Pharmacodynamics. Absorbed from the lungs.

4. Toxicity. a. Breathing 100% oxygen for more than 12 hours causes substernal distress, decreased vital capacity, tracheobronchitis, and nonspecific symptoms such as fatigue, paresthesias, joint pain, anorexia, and nausea. Prolonged administration under positive pressure results in mood changes, loss of judgment, and eventually convulsions. Intermittent administration of concentrations above 70% for 1 to 3 weeks may lead to decreased erythrogenesis.

b. Administration to premature infants may cause retrolental fibroplasia.

c. "Oxygen apnea" may be produced in patients whose respiratory centers are depressed or damaged, with control of respiration via the carotid bodies; also in patients with chronic emphysema, with subsequent carbon dioxide narcosis.

5. Uses. a. Oxygen is a specific aid when alveoli are poorly ventilated (asthma, emphysema), or covered with fluid (pulmonary edema or pneumonia); when tissues are deprived of oxygen (shock, myocardial infarction, congestive failure, depressed respiratory center); and in carbon monoxide poisoning in which high oxygen tension aids in dissociation of carbon monoxide hemoglobin. In addition to the use of oxygen, the cause of the anoxia should be removed if possible.

b. Oxygen is also used for denitrogenation in the prevention of caisson disease, and to relieve distension of inflated hollow viscera.

c. Hyperbaric oxygen therapy using large pressure chambers is under investigation in circulatory and respiratory disturbances, anaerobic infections, CO poisoning, and to increase the sensitivity of tumors to radiation.

6. Preparation

OXYGEN

Dose: By inhalation in concentrations of 30% to 100% from nasal catheter, mask, tent, or chamber. By intermittent positive pressure in the prevention and treatment of atelectasis.

CARBON DIOXIDE

1. Chemistry. CO_2. Colorless, odorless gas; supplied under pressure in steel cylinders (with oxygen).

2. Action and Mechanism. a. Normal physiological roles: End product of cellular oxidation of carbon compounds; constituent of body buffer system; normal stimulant of the respiratory center and regulator of the cerebral circulation.

b. Pharmacological effects vary with the inhaled concentration: 1% produces a detectable increase in ventilation; 9% produces maximum increase in ventilation (tenfold; 60 to 70 liters per minute). Concentrations of 5% or more produce distressing symptoms including disorientation, apprehension, dyspnea, and headache. At concentrations of 10% or greater, narcotic effects appear; full anesthesia at an inhaled concentration of 30%. Convulsions may occur prior to anesthesia. At 40% ventilation is depressed below normal and fatalities appear; toxic effects begin at lower concentrations if the respiratory center is depressed.

3. Pharmacodynamics and Toxicity. a. Absorbed from the lungs and excreted via the lungs as carbon dioxide or via the kidneys as bicarbonate ion.

b. Toxic at concentrations above 5% in the inspired air, as noted under Action and Mechanism.

4. Uses. a. To prevent postoperative atelectasis by stimulation of ventilation.

b. Should not be used as a respiratory stimulant when hypoventilation and consequent hypercarbia are present.

5. Preparation

CARBON DIOXIDE

Dose: By inhalation of 5% to 10% concentrations in oxygen or air from a mask.

HELIUM

1. Chemistry. He. Inert, low density gas; a mixture of 80% helium and 20% oxygen has a specific gravity one-third that of air.

2. Action and Mechanism. a. Nontoxic gas which can replace nitrogen in inhaled air; because of its low density it may pass more easily than nitrogen through restricted passages in the bronchial tree.

b. About one-half the respiratory effort required to breathe an 80% helium mixture as an 80% nitrogen mixture.

3. Pharmacodynamics and Toxicity. Pharmacologically inactive and non-toxic.

4. Uses. a. To facilitate breathing in patients with acute or self-limiting obstruction of the respiratory tract, particularly in status asthmaticus.

b. Also, its low coefficient of solubility and high rate of diffusion as compared with nitrogen make it useful in the treatment of caisson disease or decompression sickness.

5. Preparation

HELIUM

Dose: By inhalation in 80% concentration with 20% oxygen from a mask.

SUMMARY: GENERAL ANESTHETICS AND THERAPEUTIC GASES

TYPE	*ACTION AND MECHANISM*	*TOXICITY*	*USE*	*EXAMPLES*
Inhalation anesthetics	Produce general anesthesia in stages Fundamental mechanisms not clear	Respiratory depression	General anesthesia	Nitrous oxide
Nonvolatile anesthetics	Same	Same	General or basal anesthesia by intravenous or intramuscular route	Thiopental sodium
Therapeutic	Oxygen to relieve anoxemia or CO_2 to stimulate respiratory center	Minor	Anoxemia, respiratory depression	Oxygen, CO_2

Reviews

Comroe, J., and Dripps, R. The physiological basis for oxygen therapy. Springfield, Ill., Charles C Thomas, Publishers, 1950.

Symposium on carbon dioxide. Anesthesiology, 21:585, 1960.

Hamilton, W. The limited clinical pharmacology of nitrous oxide. Clin. Pharmacol. Ther., 4:663, 1963.

Ngai, S., and Papper, E. Anesthesiology. New Eng. J. Med., 269:28, 1964.

Bunker, J., and Van Dam, L. Effects of anesthesia on metabolic and cellular functions. Pharmacol. Rev., 17:183, 1965.

Van Dam, L. Anesthesia. Ann. Rev. Pharmacol., 6:379, 1966.
Dobkin, A., and Su, G. Newer anesthetics and their uses. Clin. Pharmacol. Ther., 7:648, 1966.
Hedley-Whyte, J., and Winter, P. Oxygen therapy. Clin. Pharmacol. Ther., 8:696, 1967.
Cherkin, A. Mechanism of general anesthesia by nonhydrogen-bonding molecules. Ann. Rev. Pharmacol., 9:259, 1969.

48. Local Anesthetics

Local anesthesia may be defined as the reversible abolition of sensory perception, especially of pain, in a restricted area of the body. Qualities desirable in a local anesthetic include: low toxicity, minimal irritation, vasoconstriction, effectiveness topically and by injection, and reversibility. Local anesthetics are called topical when applied to the surface of the skin or a mucous membrane.

Local anesthetics may interrupt nervous conduction along an axone, at sensory endings, or elsewhere, by the following mechanisms:

a. Axone: Interference with the propagation of the nerve impulse by stabilizing the membrane potential. This has been explained on the basis of chemical combination of the anesthetic molecule with polar groups in the lipoprotein membrane, and perhaps also by interference with oxidative processes within the cell. They probably reach the site of action on the nerve membrane as free bases, then are converted to the cationic form at the tissue pH and exert their action as quaternary N compounds.

b. Sensory ending: The mechanism at sensory endings is presumably similar to that on axones.

c. Ganglionic and myoneural junctions: It has been proposed that in these areas those anesthetics which resemble acetylcholine, and therefore might compete with it, act by competitive interference, either at the receptor or as substrates for cholinesterase. Whether acetylcholine interference plays a part in the anesthesia at other areas is uncertain. May act by regulation of movements of ions in cells, especially by reducing availability of calcium, and not by a cholinergic mechanism (Feinstein, Nature, 214:151, 1967).

d. Motor nerves: Depression follows sensory depression, without a phase of stimulation. Small fibers (sensory) are blocked before large fibers (motor) because their large surface-to-volume ratio favors penetration quantitatively.

A. Cocaine

1. History. a. Niemann (1860) isolated cocaine and noticed that it numbed his tongue; von Anrep (1879) discovered that subcutaneous injection produced anesthesia.

b. Koller (1884), at the suggestion of Freud, used as anesthetic in the eye; Hall (1884) used in dentistry; Halsted (1885) began to study nerve block.

2. Chemistry. a. A benzoic acid ester of the base ecgonine; similarity to atropine.

b. Obtained from the leaves of *Erythroxylon coca;* or made semisynthetically.

3. Action. a. Depresses nerve endings and trunks, first sensory, then motor; anesthesia potent, topical or injected.

b. Vasoconstriction from "cocaine sensitization" of norepinephrine and epinephrine (see Sympathetic Stimulants). Probably prevents re-uptake of released amines.

c. Central stimulation, producing excitement and erratic behavior.

4. Mechanism. Elevates the threshold of nerve excitability by chemical combination with membrane; competes with acetylcholine (see introductory section).

5. Pharmacodynamics. Easily absorbed; partly altered in the body, probably by plasma cholinesterase, and excreted slowly over several days. Slow destruction favors toxicity.

6. Toxicity. a. Overdosage or systemic absorption produces central stimulation at first of a pleasurable nature, later with nausea, sweating, pupillary dilatation, hyperpyrexia, and convulsions. Finally, medullary depression, or cardiovascular collapse, may cause death.

b. Excited stage should be treated with intravenous barbiturate; later, depressed stage with artificial respiration.

c. Addicting (see Drug Addiction).

7. Uses. For topical anesthesia in the eye, nose, and throat; not used by injection as too toxic.

8. Preparation

COCAINE HYDROCHLORIDE

Dose: 2% to 4% solution (eye); 5% to 10% (nose or throat).

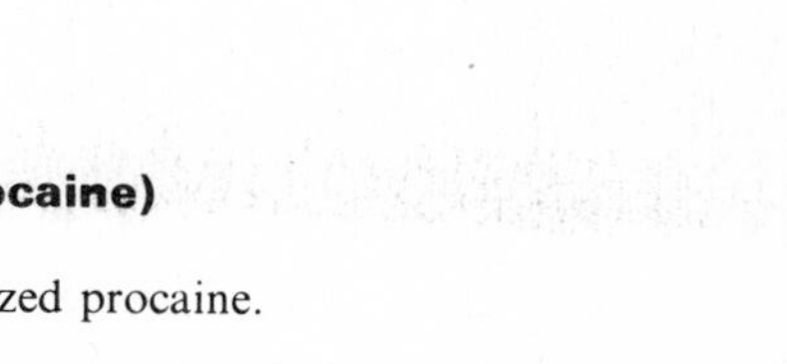

H_3COOC

CH—CH—CH_2

O

C—O—CH N—CH_3

CH_2—CH—CH_2

B. Synthetic Benzoic Esters (Procaine)

1. History. Einhorn (1905) synthesized procaine.

2. Chemistry. a. Esters of benzoic acid and diethylaminoethyl alcohols.

b. Structurally related to parasympathomimetic and parasympatholytic agents, and antihistamines.

3. Action and Mechanism. Procaine about one-half to one-third as potent as cocaine as an anesthetic, but only one-third to one-eighth as toxic when injected.

4. Pharmacology and Toxicity. a. Most poorly absorbed topically.

b. Hydrolyzed rapidly by esterases; *p*-aminobenzoic acid formed can interfere with sulfonamide therapy.

c. Overdosage gives excitement and convulsions, as with cocaine, but margin of safety greater and idiosyncrasy rarer. May depress medullary centers without prior stimulation.

5. Uses. Variously used for infiltration, intrathecal and topical anesthesia.

6. Preparations

AMOLANONE HYDROCHLORIDE (Amethone)

Dose: 0.33% for infiltration.

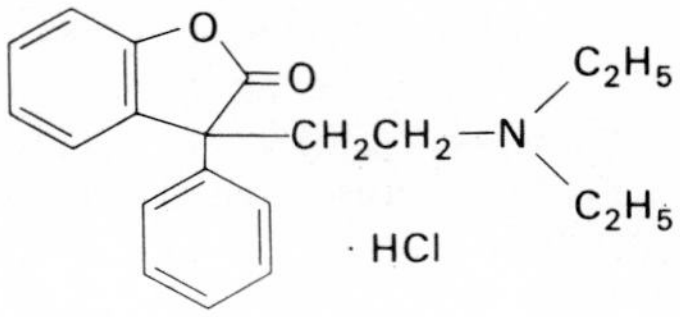

O, =O, $-CH_2CH_2-N(C_2H_5)_2$ · HCl

AMYDRICAINE HYDROCHLORIDE (Alypin)

Dose: 2% to 4% solution topically to mucous membranes.

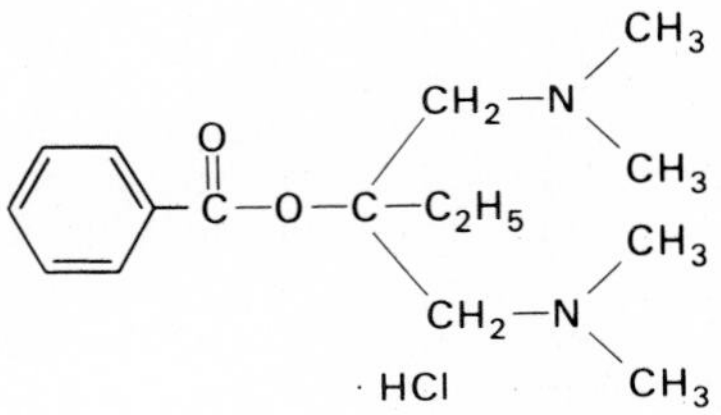

$C_6H_5-C(=O)-O-C(C_2H_5)(CH_2-N(CH_3)_2)(CH_2-N(CH_3)_2)$ · HCl

BENOXINATE HYDROCHLORIDE (Dorsacaine)

Used for eye examination and minor surgical procedures.

Dose: 0.4% topically in the eye.

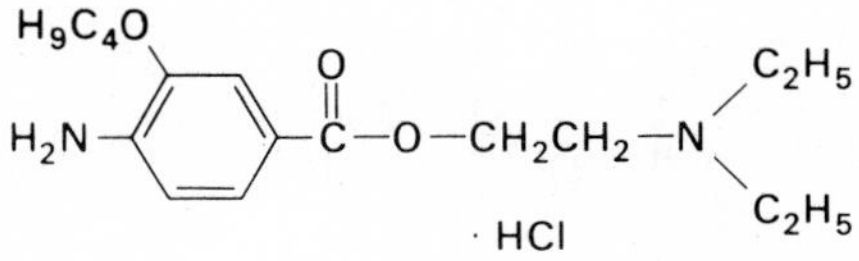

H_9C_4O, $H_2N-C_6H_3-C(=O)-O-CH_2CH_2-N(C_2H_5)_2$ · HCl

BENZOCAINE

Dose: 3% to 5% in dusting powders and ointments (insoluble).

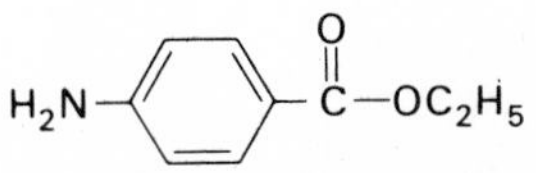

$H_2N-C_6H_4-C(=O)-OC_2H_5$

BUTACAINE SULFATE (Butyn)

More toxic and longer acting than cocaine.

Dose: 2% solution to eye, nose, throat, mouth; 1% to urethra.

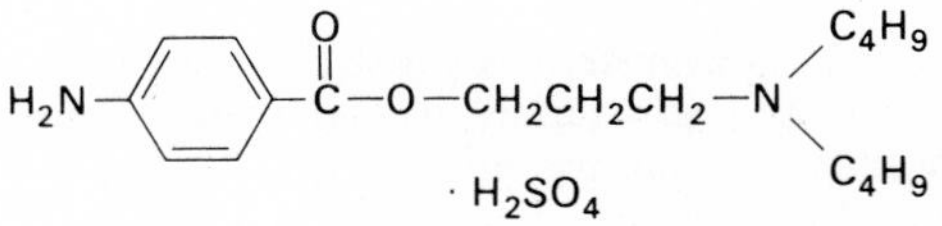

$H_2N-C_6H_4-C(=O)-O-CH_2CH_2CH_2-N(C_4H_9)_2$ · H_2SO_4

BUTETHAMINE HYDROCHLORIDE (Monocaine)

Slightly more potent and more toxic than procaine; used in dental and minor surgery.

Dose: 1% solution by infiltration.

$H_2N-C(=O)-O-CH_2CH_2-N(H)-CH_2CH(CH_3)_2 \cdot HCl$

BUTYL AMINOBENZOATE (Butesin)

Dose: As a dusting powder (insoluble).

$H_2N-C(=O)-OC_4H_9$

Butamben picrate (Butesin picrate)
Sensitizing.
Dose: 1% in ointments.

CHLOROPROCAINE HYDROCHLORIDE (Nesacaine)

Potency twice that of procaine; toxicity about the same.

Dose: 1% solution by infiltration.

$H_2N-C(=O)-O-CH_2CH_2-N(C_2H_5)_2 \cdot HCl$, Cl

CYCLOMETHYCAINE SULFATE (Surfacaine)

Used topically for surface anesthesia.

Dose: 0.5% to 1% in solutions or ointments.

$O-C(=O)-O-CH_2CH_2CH_2-N$, H_3C, $\cdot H_2SO_4$

HEXYLCAINE HYDROCHLORIDE (Cyclaine)

Dose: 1% solution for infiltration anesthesia; 15 to 20 mg in spinal anesthesia; 5% topically.

$C(=O)-O-CH(CH_3)CH_2-N(H) \cdot HCl$

LAROCAINE HYDROCHLORIDE

Dose: Locally, to eye and mucous membrane.

$H_2N-C(=O)-O-CH_2C(CH_3)_2CH_2-N(C_2H_5)_2 \cdot HCl$

MEPRYLCAINE HYDROCHLORIDE (Oracaine)

Dose: 2% by infiltration.

$C(=O)-O-CH_2-C(CH_3)_2-NH-C_3H_7 \cdot HCl$

NAEPAINE HYDROCHLORIDE (Amylsine)

Resembles cocaine but does not cause mydriasis; used as a corneal anesthetic.

Dose: 2% in the eye.

$H_2N-C(=O)-O-CH_2CH_2-N(H)-C_5H_{11} \cdot HCl$

ORTHOFORM

Dose: 10% to 20% in dusting powders (insoluble).

H_2N; $HO-$(ring)$-\overset{O}{\overset{\|}{C}}-OCH_3$

PARETHOXYCAINE (Intracaine)

Dose: 0.5% by infiltration.

H_5C_2O-(ring)$-\overset{O}{\overset{\|}{C}}-O-CH_2CH_2-N(C_2H_5)_2$

PIPEROCAINE HYDROCHLORIDE (Metycaine)

Similar to procaine but slightly more potent and longer lasting.

Dose: 0.75% solution for infiltration.

(ring)$-\overset{O}{\overset{\|}{C}}-O-CH_2CH_2CH_2-N$(ring, H_3C) $\cdot HCl$

PROCAINE HYDROCHLORIDE (Novocaine and others)

Dose: 1% solution by infiltration subcutaneously or intramuscularly (solutions contain epinephrine or other sympathomimetic to produce local vasoconstriction and retention of anesthetic); 100 to 150 mg intraspinally.

H_2N-(ring)$-\overset{O}{\overset{\|}{C}}-O-CH_2CH_2-N(C_2H_5)_2 \cdot HCl$

PROPARACAINE HYDROCHLORIDE (Ophthaine)

Dose: 0.5% solution topically in the eye.

H_2N; H_7C_3O-(ring)$-\overset{O}{\overset{\|}{C}}-O-CH_2CH_2-N(C_2H_5)_2 \cdot HCl$

PROPOXYCAINE HYDROCHLORIDE (Ravocaine)

Prolonged but toxic.

Dose: 0.5% by infiltration.

H_2N-(ring, OC_3H_7)$-\overset{O}{\overset{\|}{C}}-O-CH_2CH_2-N(C_2H_5)_2 \cdot HCl$

RISOCAINE

H_2N-(ring)$-\overset{O}{\overset{\|}{C}}-O-C_3H_7$

TETRACAINE HYDROCHLORIDE (Pontocaine)

Topical potency and toxicity equal cocaine; action prolonged as compared to procaine. Allergic sensitivity may appear, as with most local anesthetics used topically.

Dose: 1% to 2% solutions on surfaces; 6 to 20 mg intrathecally.

H_9C_4-HN-(ring)$-\overset{O}{\overset{\|}{C}}-O-CH_2CH_2-N(CH_3)_2 \cdot HCl$

C. Other Synthetics, Not Benzoic Esters (Dibucaine, Lidocaine)

1. Chemistry. Not esters of benzoic acid; contain —$NHCOCH_2$, or —$CONHCH_2$— groups.

2. Action and Mechanism. More potent than procaine; not inactivated by cholinesterases.

3. Pharmocodynamics and Toxicity. a. Act topically and by infiltration.
b. Dibucaine and lidocaine have opposite —NHCO— orientation; no cross sensitivity.

4. Uses. a. For infiltration and topical anesthesia.
b. Useful for patients sensitive to ester-type agents.

5. Preparations

BUPIVACAINE (Marcaine)
Long acting.
Dose: 0.25% to 0.75% solution for infiltration.

CH_3 / NH—CO / N / CH_3 / H_9C_4

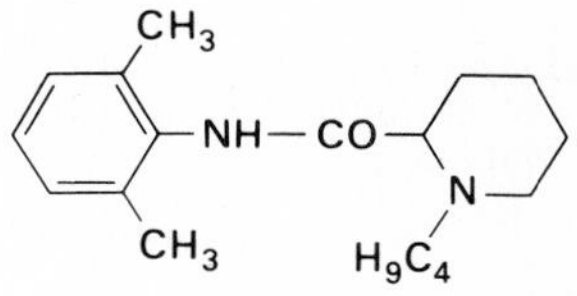

DIAMOCAINE CYCLAMATE
Under investigation.

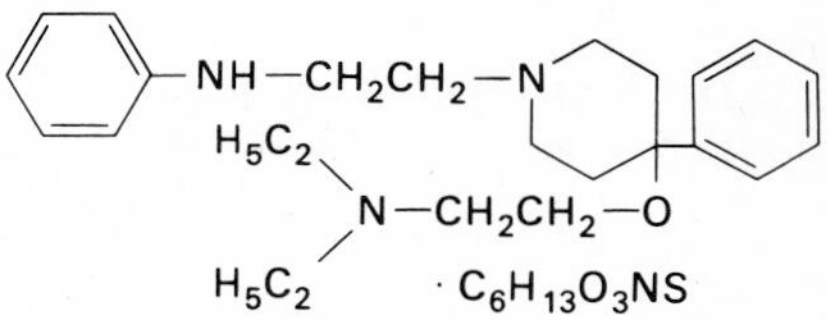

NH—CH_2CH_2—N / H_5C_2 / N—CH_2CH_2—O / H_5C_2 · $C_6H_{13}O_3NS$

DIBUCAINE HYDROCHLORIDE
(Nupercaine; Percaine)

Potency and toxicity 15 times procaine; dangerous.

Dose: 0.1% solution for infiltration and nerve block; locally in ointments (sensitizing).

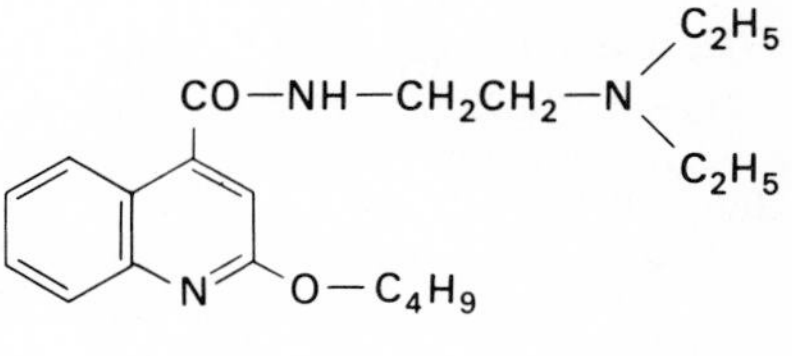

C_2H_5 / CO—NH—CH_2CH_2—N / C_2H_5 / N / O—C_4H_9

DIPERODON HYDROCHLORIDE
(Diothane)

Dose: 1% in solution or cream topically.

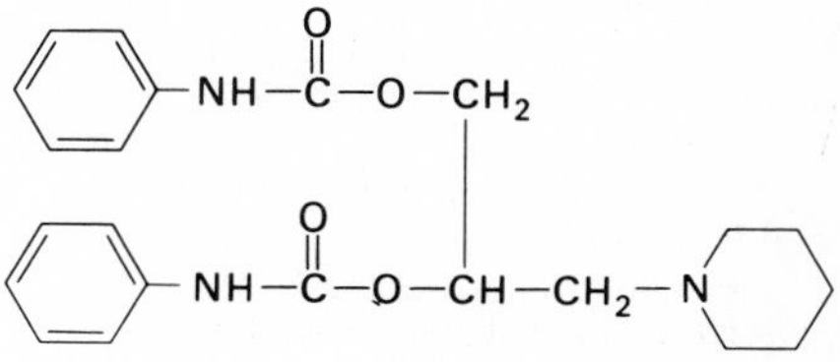

O / NH—C—O—CH_2 / O / NH—C—O—CH—CH_2—N

EUPROCIN HYDROCHLORIDE (in Otodyne)

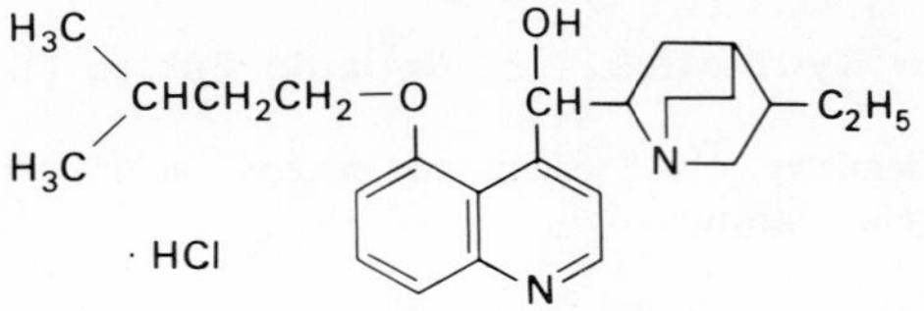

LIDOCAINE HYDROCHLORIDE (Xylocaine)

Potency five times procaine but no more toxic. Widely used.

Dose: 0.5% to 2% solution by infiltration or topically.

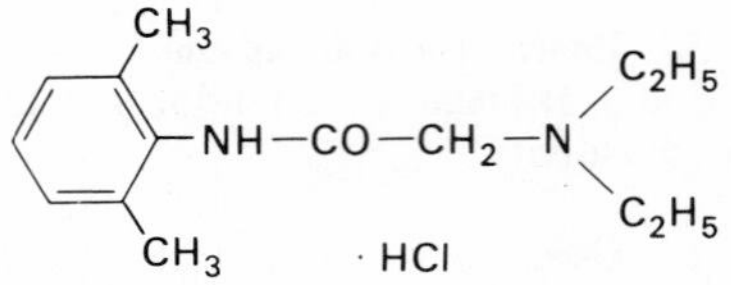

MEPIVACAINE (Carbocaine)

Similar to lidocaine, but possibly longer acting and less toxic.

Dose: 1% to 2% solution for infiltration.

Dexivacaine: Dextro isomer.

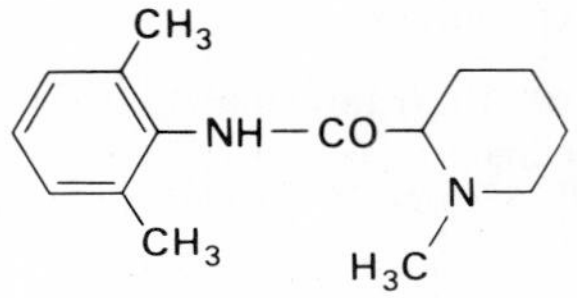

OXETHAZAINE (in Oxaine)

Topical; gives prolonged anesthesia to mucosa.

Dose: 10 to 20 mg by mouth; usually given in mixture with $Al(OH)_3$.

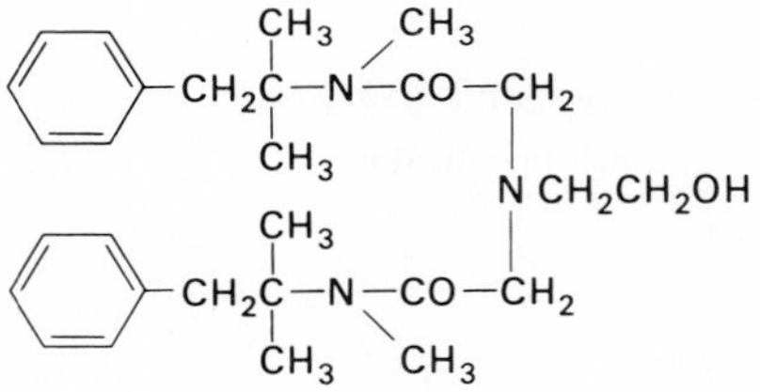

PHENACAINE HYDROCHLORIDE (Holocaine)

Dose: 1% solution used in the eye; promptly acting, slightly irritating.

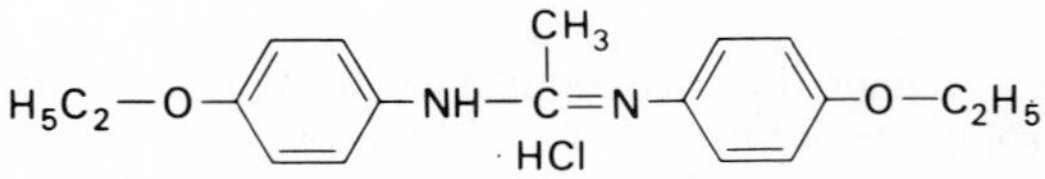

PRILOCAINE

Dose: 2% to 3% solution by infiltration or topically.

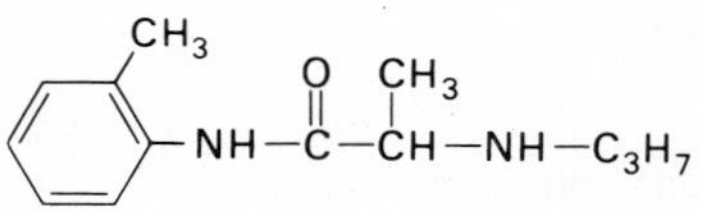

PYRROCAINE HYDROCHLORIDE (Endocaine)

For infiltration anesthesia.

Under investigation.

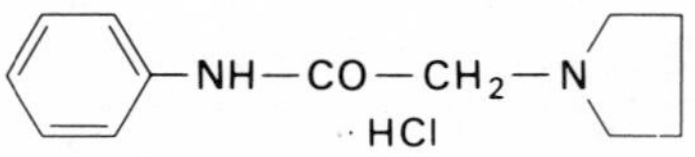

OTHERS

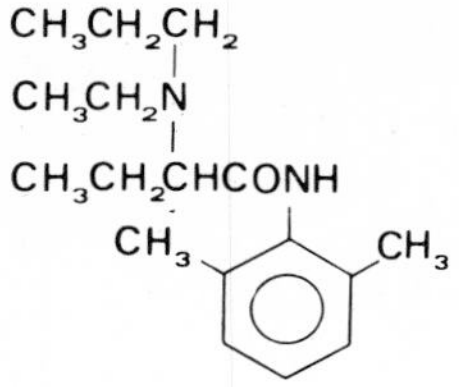

$CH_3CH_2CH_2$
CH_3CH_2N
$CH_3CH_2CHCONH$
CH_3 CH_3

etidocaine (Duranest)

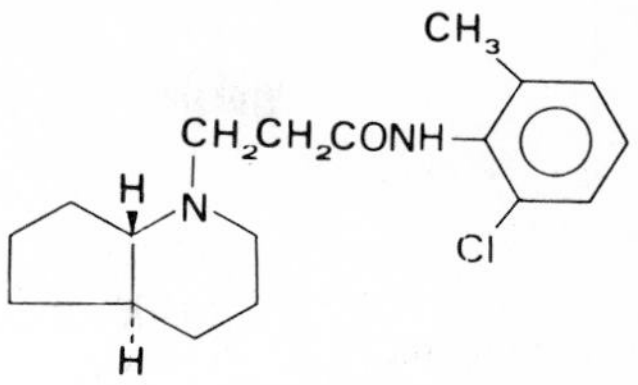

CH_3
CH_2CH_2CONH
H N
Cl
H

rodocaine

levoxadrol hydrochloride (Levoxan)
(See smooth muscle relaxants.)

D. Other Synthetic Types

a. Complex types

DIMETHISOQUIN HYDROCHLORIDE (Quotane)

Dose: 0.5% solution or cream locally for itching.

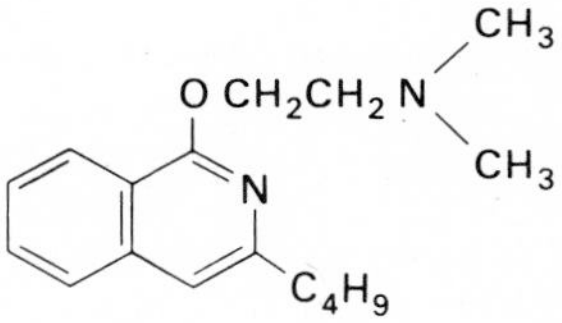

CH_3
O CH_2CH_2 N
N CH_3
C_4H_9

DYCLONINE HYDROCHLORIDE (Dyclone)

Dose: 0.5% to 1% topically.

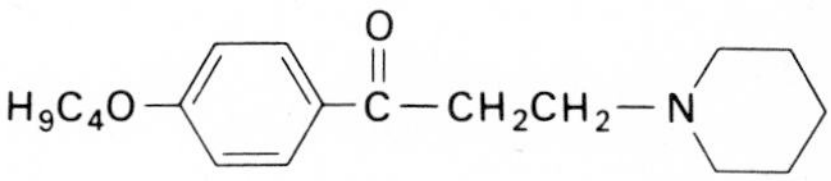

O
H_9C_4O—C—CH_2CH_2—N

PRAMOXINE HYDROCHLORIDE (Tronothane)

Dose: 1% topically for itching.

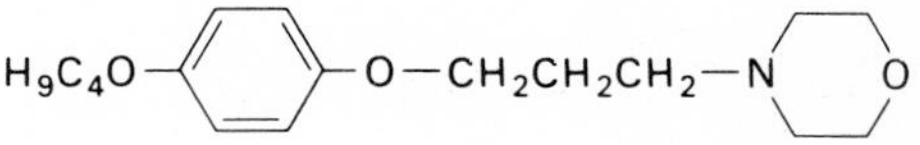

H_9C_4O—O—$CH_2CH_2CH_2$—N O

b. Aromatic alcohols

BENZYL ALCOHOL

Dose: 10% in ointments; as anesthetic in intramuscular injections; irritating.

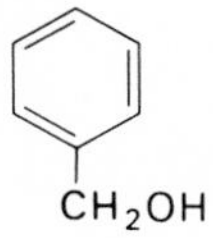

CH_2OH

EUGENOL

Feeble dental anesthetic.
Dose: Applied topically.

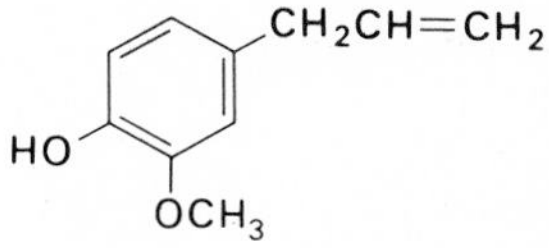

$CH_2CH{=}CH_2$
HO
OCH_3

SALIGENIN

Dose: 2 % as anesthetic in intramuscular preparations.

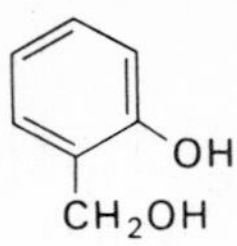

c. Others

FREEZING AGENTS: ETHYL CHLORIDE, CARBON DIOXIDE (solid), FREON

Used to anesthetize by freezing, Freon replacing ethyl chloride.

QUININE and UREA HYDROCHLORIDE

Pain, then anesthesia lasting several days; used as a sclerosing agent for hemorrhoids.

E. Spinal and Epidural Anesthesia

1. Spinal Anesthesia. a. Localized anesthesia by intrathecal administration of procaine, tetracaine, and other agents. Blocks sympathetic roots, then sensory, last motor. Relaxation excellent; blood pressure falls (sympathomimetic amine to sustain). Danger of shock and respiratory paralysis.

b. Former transverse myelitis not seen with better sterility and complete removal of detergents from syringes and equipment.

c. Administration: position of patient determines level of anesthesia; hypobaric and hyperbaric solutions (weighted with glucose).

d. Used for abdominal, pelvic, and lower extremity surgery.

2. Epidural Anesthesia. a. Localized anesthesia by extradural administration of procaine, tetracaine, piperocaine, lidocaine, and other agents. Subarachnoid space not entered, so headache and possible neurological complications of spinal anesthesia are prevented.

b. Dose of anesthetic large, so always potentially dangerous; small amount injected, then after observation the balance.

c. Caudal anesthesia, used especially in obstetrics.

SUMMARY: LOCAL ANESTHETICS

TYPE	*ACTION AND MECHANISM*	*TOXICITY*	*USE*	*EXAMPLES*
Benzoic acid ester: cocaine	Local anesthesia by membrane action on neuron	Central stimulation, convulsions	Topical anesthesia in ENT	Cocaine
Benzoic acid ester: synthetic	Same	Same	Local anesthesia by various routes	Procaine HCl
Nonbenzoic acid esters	Same	Same	Same	Lidocaine HCl

Reviews

Shanes, A. Drugs and nerve conduction. Ann. Rev. Pharmacol., 3:185, 1963.
Adriani, J., Zepernick, R., Arens, J., and Authement, E. Comparative potency and effectiveness of topical anesthetics in man. Clin. Pharmacol. Ther., 5:49, 1964.
Ritchie, J., and Greengard, P. On the mode of action of local anesthetics. Ann. Rev. Pharmacol., 6:405, 1966.

49. Nonnarcotic Analgesics

Analgesics alleviate pain or its appreciation without affecting consciousness.

In general the simple analgesics are most effective against pain of integumental origin, headache and muscle ache; the narcotics are more useful for deep or visceral pain. Narcotic analgesics of the morphine type produce more profound effects than simple analgesics like aspirin, and are potentially addicting with the development of tolerance and physical dependence.

At least four physiological mechanisms may be involved in analgesia:

a. Pain threshold: Morphine raises; aspirin does not.

b. Interpretation of pain: Altered by both morphine and aspirin. This function is difficult to assess; comparable to the ignoring of pain during joy, fear, euphoria, and other strong emotions.

c. Drowsiness: Morphine induces; aspirin does not. Often, but not always, a desirable accompaniment of analgesia.

d. Antiinflammatory effect: Absent with morphine; strong in many instances with aspirin and other simple analgesics.

Analgesics stand in partial contrast to hypnotics or sedatives, which produce calm, drowsiness, and sleep, but little or no analgesia. The simple, nonnarcotic analgesics are often antipyretics as well; this side effect is no longer considered to have much therapeutic merit.

A. The Salicylates

1. History. a. Rev. Edward Stone (1763) introduced salicylates (as willow bark) into medicine as analgesics.

b. Salicylic acid isolated from salicin (1838); acetylsalicylic acid synthesized (1853); used medically 1899 (Dreser).

2. Chemistry. Willow bark (*Salix*) contains salicin, a glycoside from which salicylate may be isolated; commercial salicylates synthetic.

3. Action. a. The pharmacological actions of salicylates are complex, and appear to be in part central and part peripheral.

b. Analgesia: Relief of pain; skeletal pain and headache better relieved than visceral pain. The analgesic, or antinociceptive, action has generally been assumed to be central, from an interference in the transmission of pain impulses between the hypothalamus and the sensory cortex, which alters the interpretation of the pain. However, it may also be in part peripheral, through a reduction of local edema (Smith, Ann. N.Y. Acad. Sci., 86:38, 1960).

c. Antipyresis: Probably the result of interference with the heat regulating centers in the hypothalamus, with a resulting dissipation of heat by cutaneous vasodilatation.

d. Antiinflammatory action: Similar to that characteristic of cortisone, aminopyrine, and certain cinchonic acid derivatives: hyaluronidase inhibited; circulating corticoid levels increased. Mechanism not understood.

e. Antiallergy: Some aspects of the antigen-antibody reaction are suppressed, as in rheumatic fever (may explain part of the antiinflammatory action); anaphylaxis and Arthus phenomenon not inhibited.

f. Metabolic and other actions: Respiration stimulated centrally; oxygen consumption increased; adrenal cortex stimulated; threshold for uric acid lowered; hypoglycemia by insulin mechanism (increased entry of glucose into muscle cells).

g. Keratolysis: Free acids are keratolytic and antiseptic (comparable to phenol).

4. Mechanism. a. Fundamental mechanism is inhibition of synthesis of prostaglandins, which produce fever, inflammation, and pain (Collier, Nature, 232:17, 1971).

b. It has been suggested (Winder, Nature, 184:494, 1959) that both the central antinociceptive and peripheral antipreinflammatory effects of aspirin are needed for maximal analgesia; that salicylamide is weaker than aspirin in the former, and therefore that the carboxyl is a sensitive group in the analgesic mechanism.

c. Salicylates inhibit mucosaccharide synthesis by limiting glucosamine-6-phosphate synthesis (Lee, J. Pharmaceut. Sci., 58:1152, 1969).

5. Pharmacodynamics. a. Salicylates are well absorbed from the gastrointestinal tract.

b. Widely distributed in the body; about 80% may be excreted in the urine, principally as salicyluric acid.

6. Toxicity. a. Systemic poisoning, or salicylism, first produces nausea, tinnitus and deafness, then diarrhea and hallucinations. In severe poisoning the respiratory center is directly stimulated by acidosis, producing hyperpnea (treat with alkali); later, alkalosis results from overbreathing, and death may result from respiratory paralysis.

b. Allergic reactions are infrequent.

c. Local irritation and gastrointestinal bleeding may be produced by most salicylates; minimized by ingestion of food or drink.

7. Uses. a. Aspirin and the analgesic salicylates are widely used to relieve headache, muscle and joint aches, and the malaise of minor infections.

b. They also produce gratifying relief of symptoms in rheumatic fever, and to a lesser extent in other kinds of arthritis.

c. Use as an antipyretic has been abandoned, as fever is recognized as only a symptom, and as sometimes beneficial; also because the drenching sweats produced as the fever falls may be uncomfortable.

d. Salicylic acid is used as a keratolytic for corns, often applied in collodion, and as an exfoliative agent in fungus infections, usually in ointments.

e. Methylsalicylate is used as a mild irritant in liniments.

8. Preparations

ACETYLSALICYLIC ACID (aspirin)

Combinations with antacids, buffers, and enteric coatings not advantageous.

Dose: 0.3 to 1 gm every 4 hours by mouth.

$O-COCH_3$

$COOH$

CARBASPIRIN CALCIUM (Calurin)

A complex salt with urea.

Slightly more soluble than aspirin and claimed to give less irritation; doubtful advantage.

Dose: 0.5 to 1 gm every 4 hours by mouth.

$O-COCH_3$ $O-COCH_3$.

$COO-Ca-OOC$

carbaspirin calcium

METHYLSALICYLATE (oil of wintergreen)

Absorption inadequate for systemic effect.

Dose: Locally as an ingredient in liniments.

OH

$COCH_3$ ($\|$ O)

SALICYLAMIDE (Salrin; and others)

Lacks full antiinflammatory and analgesic action of aspirin. Is not converted to salicylate and does not show cross sensitivity. Rapidly excreted and high levels difficult to maintain. Of doubtful advantage except in allergic sensitivity to aspirin.

Dose: 0.3 to 0.6 gm every 4 hours by mouth.

OH

$CONH_2$

SALICYLIC ACID

Dose: 6% locally in ointments.

OH

$COOH$

SODIUM SALICYLATE

Effects similar to aspirin but liberates free salicylic acid and is more irritating to the gastrointestinal tract; when administered with sodium bicarbonate, excretion is accelerated, reducing the effectivness.

Dose: 0.3 to 0.6 gm every 4 hours by mouth.

OH

$COONa$

OTHERS

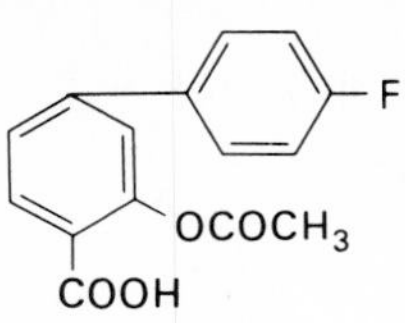

flufenisal

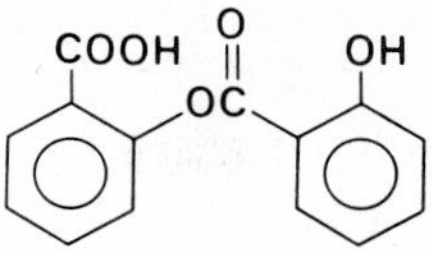

salsalate

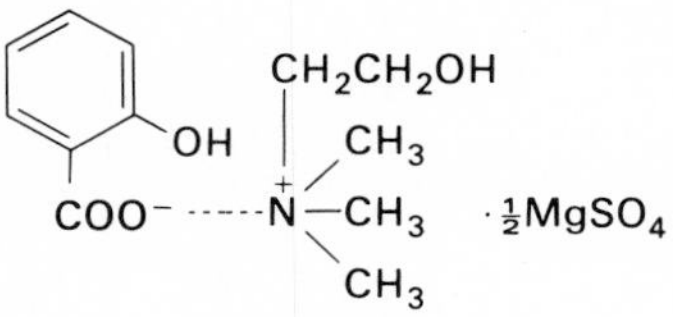

salcolex

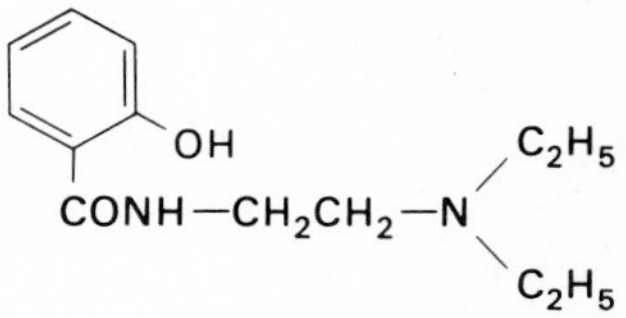

salethamide

B. Aniline Derivatives

1. Action and Mechanism. a. Acetanilid and phenacetin are comparable to aspirin as analgesics, but do not show antiinflammatory effects.

b. Both are probably changed into acetaminophen in the body, which may be the active form; the detailed mechanism of action is unknown.

2. Pharmacodynamics. Well absorbed by mouth; excreted as conjugated acetaminophen.

3. Toxicity. a. Rarely produce sensitization, but prolonged administration may cause sulfhemoglobinemia or methemoglobinemia, with cyanosis and anoxemia; also hemolytic anemia. Minimal gastric irritation.

b. Habituation may occur, but not physical dependence.

c. When taken in recommended or larger doses daily for months or years phenacetin apparently may cause interstitial nephritis and papillary necrosis, but the relationship is not clear-cut (Gilman, Amer. J. Med., 36:167, 1964; Milne, Ann. Rev. Pharmacol., 5:119, 1965).

4. Uses. Traditional use in analgesic (and antipyretic) mixtures; nevertheless, they are not as generally desirable as aspirin because of increased toxicity and dubious improvement in potency. Such mixtures commonly contain aspirin, phenacetin, and caffeine.

5. Preparations

ACETAMINOPHEN (Tempra, Tylenol)

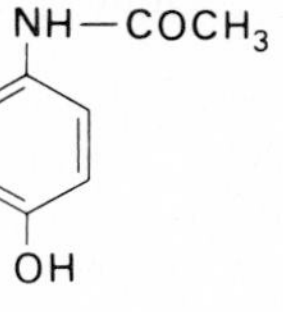

ACETANILID

Largely replaced by less toxic relatives.
Dose: 0.5 gm every 4 hours by mouth.

$NH-COCH_3$

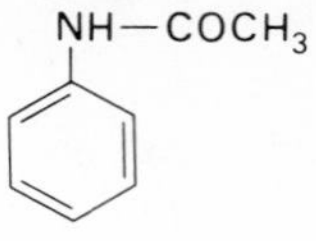

BUTACETIN (Tromal)

Under investigation.

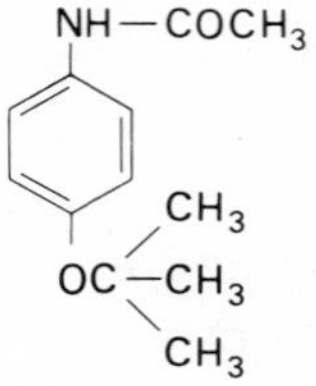

$NH-COCH_3$

$OC-(CH_3)_3$

PHENACETIN (acetophenetidin)

Dose: 0.3 to 0.6 gm every 4 hours by mouth.

$NH-COCH_3$

OC_2H_5

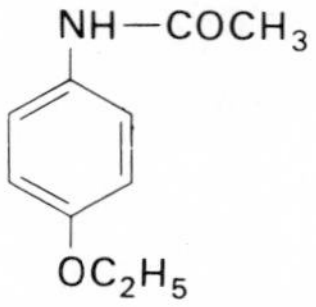

C. Pyrazolon Derivatives

1. History. a. Knorr (1883) prepared antipyrine, the first synthetic analgesic-antipyretic to come into clinical use.

b. Aminopyrine, introduced in 1893; recognized by Kracke (1938) as a cause of agranulocytosis.

2. Chemistry. Contain pyrazole nucleus.

3. Action and Mechanism. a. Potent analgesics and antiinflammatory agents.

b. Mechanism of action unknown.

4. Pharmacodynamics. Well absorbed; widely distributed; excreted in the urine in conjugated forms.

5. Toxicity. May produce nausea, anorexia, vertigo, rashes, water retention; induction of bleeding in peptic ulcers; agranulocytosis.

6. Uses. a. Aminopyrine and antipyrine have long been used as analgesics, but the danger of agranulocytosis has led to their near abandonment in the United States.

b. Phenylbutazone and oxyphenbutazone are used, preferably in short courses, in gout and rheumatoid arthritis.

c. Sulfinpyrazone is used in gout as an analgesic and uricosuric (see Inhibitors of Tubular Transport).

7. Preparations

AMINOPYRINE (Pyramidon)

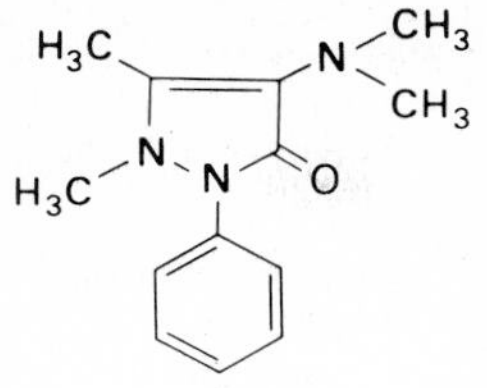

Potent analgesic.

Dose: 0.3 to 0.6 gm every 4 hours by mouth.

Dipyrone (Novaldin)

Sodium methanesulfonate derivative.

ANTIPYRINE

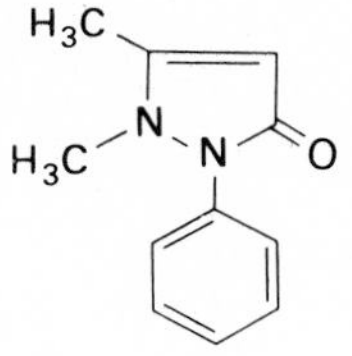

Resembles aminopyrine but is quicker acting and less potent.

Dose: 1 gm every 4 hours by mouth.

OXYPHENBUTAZONE (Tandearil)

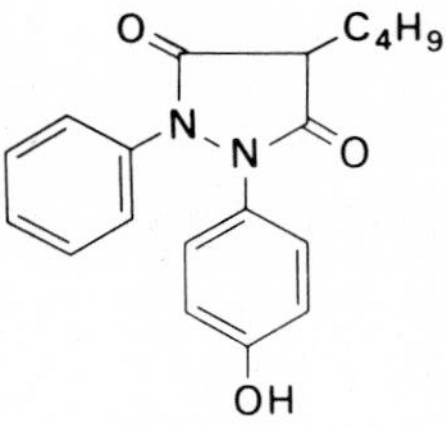

Metabolic product of phenylbutazone with similar effect and toxicity.

Dose: 100 mg 3 times a day by mouth for 10 days, then 2 times a day.

PHENYLBUTAZONE (Butazolidin)

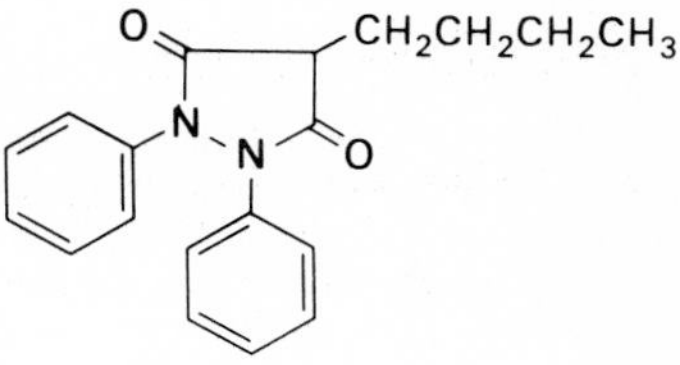

Dose: 0.3 to 0.6 gm 3 or 4 times a day by mouth.

Phenylbutazone sodium glycerate

OTHERS

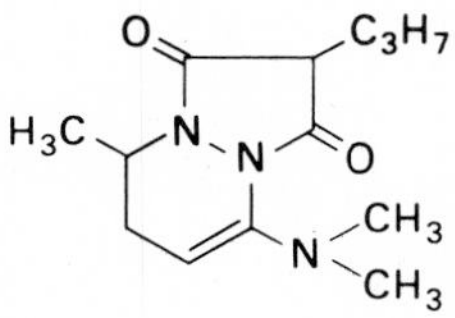

apazone

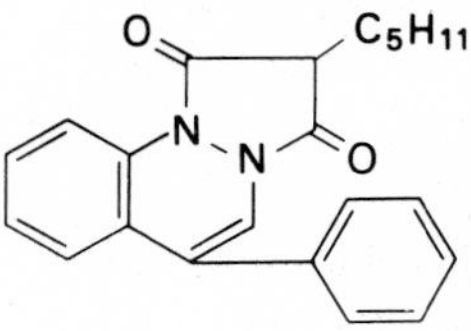

cintazone

D. The Colchicines

1. Chemistry. Colchicine is an alkaloid extracted from bulbs of the autumn crocus (*Colchicum autumnale*), which grows in Egypt. Used by von Störck for gout (1763). Demecolcine is semisynthetic.

2. Action and Mechanism. a. On uric acid metabolism: Potent agents in acute gout, but appear to act, not as analgesics, but in some way to reduce the inflammatory response to uric acid deposits. Pain is relieved after some hours, suddenly and with coincident nausea and diarrhea. Excretion of uric acid not altered; mechanism unknown.

b. Mitotic poison: Arrests mitosis in metaphase. Mechanism, and relationship to the effect in gout, undetermined.

c. Unifying mechanism may be binding to subunit protein of microtubules of cells, preventing polymerization; in gout, relief of pain may be from disruption of microtubules in leucocytes, preventing phagocytosis and resultant inflammation (Nature, 215:916, 1967).

3. Pharmacodyamics and Toxicity. a. Effective by mouth or injection.

b. Excessive dosage produces purging; extratherapeutic doses (experimental) produce cellular damage.

4. Uses. a. For the relief of acute gout.

b. Colchicine has been used for the visualization of chromosomes, for the induction of mutations (experimental), and for the treatment of cancer. For the latter purpose demecolcine may be superior, but is not curative.

5. Preparations

COLCHICINE

Replaced galenical Wine of Colchicum.

Dose: 0.5 mg by mouth every hour until symptoms are relieved or toxicity develops (about 8 doses) in gout; has also been given intravenously; 0.2 mg daily with probenecid 10 mg as maintenance therapy.

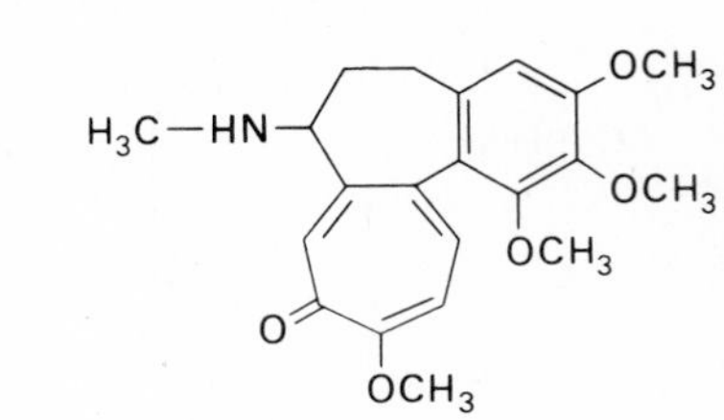

O
$H_3C-C-HN$
OCH_3
OCH_3
OCH_3
O
OCH_3

DEMECOLCINE (Colcemid)

Fewer gastrointestinal symptoms than colchicine, but this may encourage larger doses and increased marrow damage.

Dose: 2 mg intravenously in gout.

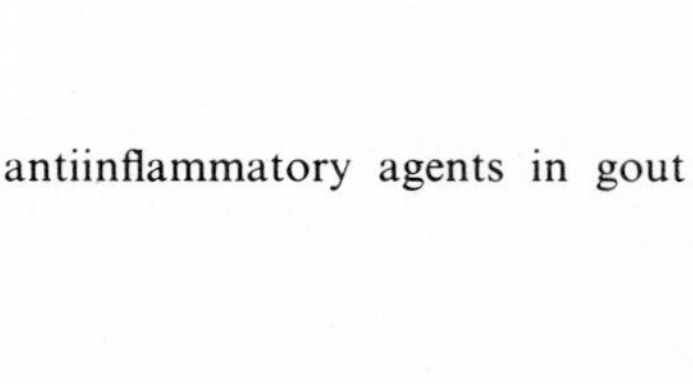

H_3C-HN
OCH_3
OCH_3
OCH_3
O
OCH_3

E. Purinols

See allopurinol and oxypurinol also for antiinflammatory agents in gout (Inhibitors of Tubular Transport).

F. Phenyramidol Group

1. Chemistry. Structural resemblances to sympathomimetics and phenampromide group.

2. Action and Mechanism. a. Phenyramidol is an analgesic, comparable in potency to aspirin; it is also a moderately potent skeletal muscle relaxant; does not show cardiovascular, local anesthetic, antiinflammatory, anticonvulsant, smooth muscle relaxing or metabolic effects, and is not addicting. The mechanism of action is unknown.

b. Phenampromide group addicting (see Narcotic Analgesics).

3. Pharmacology and Toxicity. a. Cause infrequent gastrointestinal distress and pruritis.

b. No euphoria; not habituating.

4. Uses. Phenyramidol is used for musculoskeletal pain, headache, premenstrual tension, and in peptic ulcer and dysmenorrhea. Preparations withdrawn from market.

5. Preparations

FENTANYL CITRATE (Sublimaze)

(See relationship to meperidine)

Dose: 25 to 100 mcg intramuscularly or intravenously.

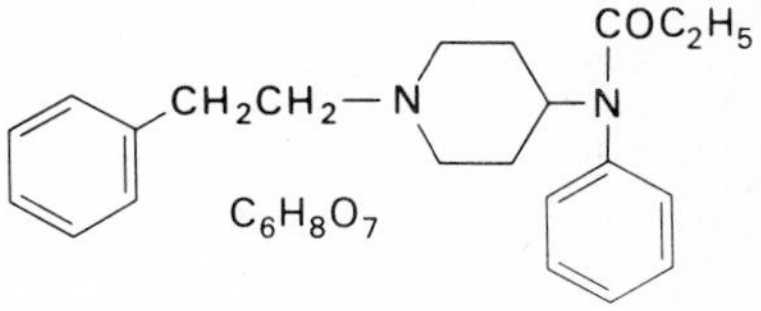

COC_2H_5

CH_2CH_2—N ... N

$C_6H_8O_7$

PHENYRAMIDOL HYDROCHLORIDE (Analexin)

Dose: 100 to 200 mg.

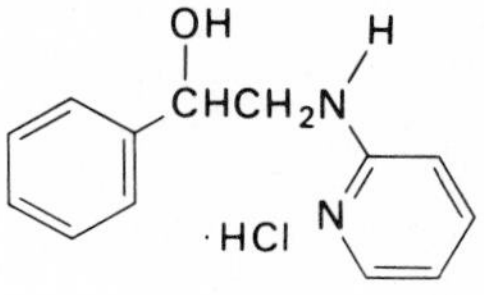

OH H

$CHCH_2N$

·HCl N

OTHERS

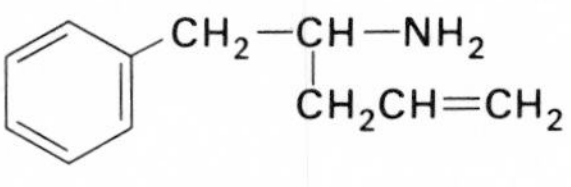

CH_2—CH—NH_2

$CH_2CH{=}CH_2$

alethamine

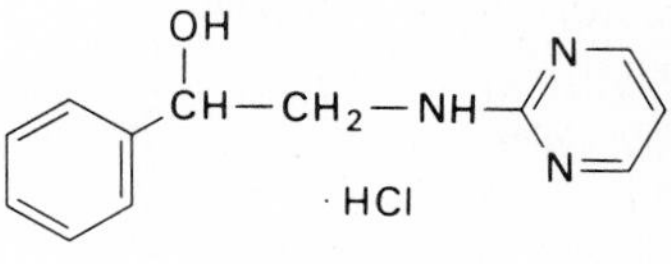

OH

CH—CH_2—NH— N N

·HCl

fenyripol HCl

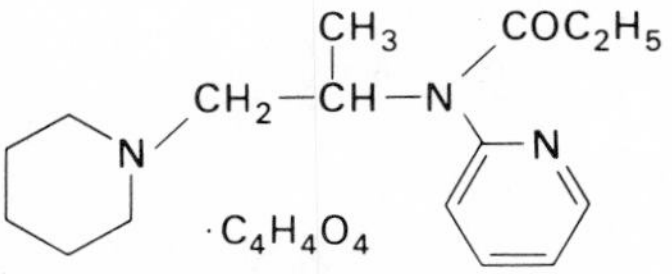

CH_3 COC_2H_5

CH_2—CH—N

N N

$\cdot C_4H_4O_4$

propiram fumarate

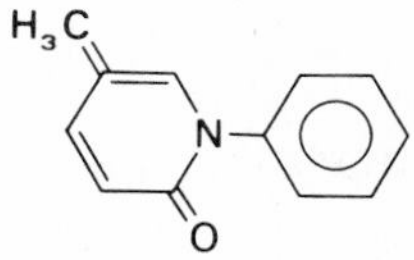

H_3C

N

O

pirfenidone

G. Fenamic Acid Derivatives

1. Action. Antiinflammatory and antipyretic of same order of effectiveness as aspirin.

2. Pharmacodynamics. a. Fair absorption, with peak in 2 to 4 hours after oral administration; unequal distribution in tissues.

b. Oxidation products excreted in urine.

3. Toxicity. May cause diarrhea, exacerbation of asthma; possible renal and marrow damage.

4. Uses. Alternative to, but less safe than, aspirin.

5. Preparations

FLUFENAMIC ACID (Arlef)

Strongly antiinflammatory but not antinociceptive; slower acting than aspirin; few side effects (Winder, Arch. Rheum., 6:36, 1963).

Dose: 300 mg by mouth daily.

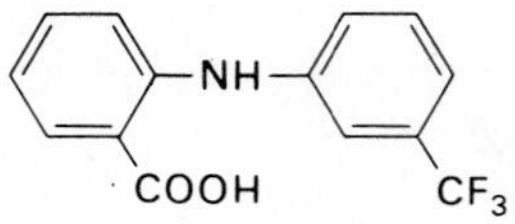

NH COOH CF_3

MEFENAMIC ACID (Ponstel)

Dose: 250 mg by mouth.

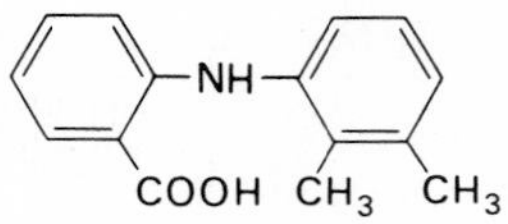

NH COOH CH_3 CH_3

OTHERS

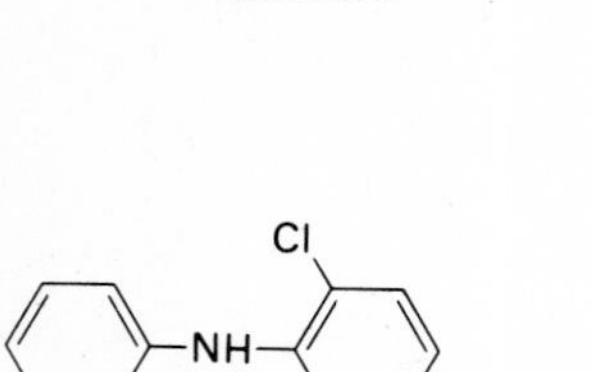

N NH CH_3 Cl $COOCH_2CH-CH_2OH$ OH

clonixeril

N NH COOH CH_3 Cl

clonixin

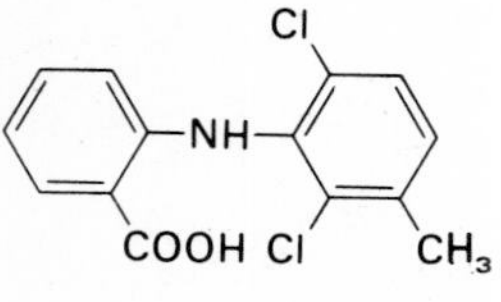

Cl NH COOH Cl CH_3

meclofenamic acid

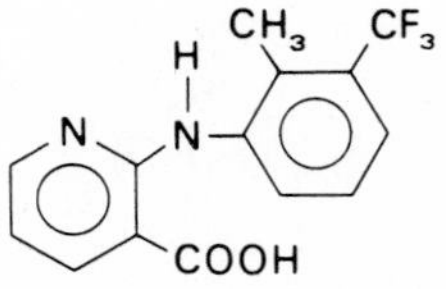

CH_3 CF_3 H N N COOH

flunixin

H. Indene and Related Derivatives

INDOMETHACIN (Indocin)

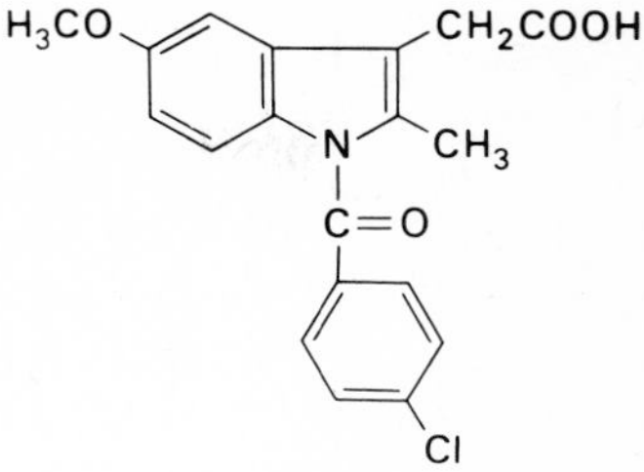

Strongly antiinflammatory; comparable in effectiveness to phenylbutazone in arthritis (Katz, Arth. Rheum., 6:281, 1963), but may be ulcerogenic (Lovgren, Brit. Med. J., 1:118, 1964). May produce drowsiness, tinnitus, psychic and gastrointestinal disturbances, skin rashes.

Dose: 25 mg 4 times a day by mouth.

H_3CO — CH_2COOH — CH_3 — N — C=O — Cl

OTHERS

$O-CH_2CH_2CH_2-N(CH_3)_2$ · HCl

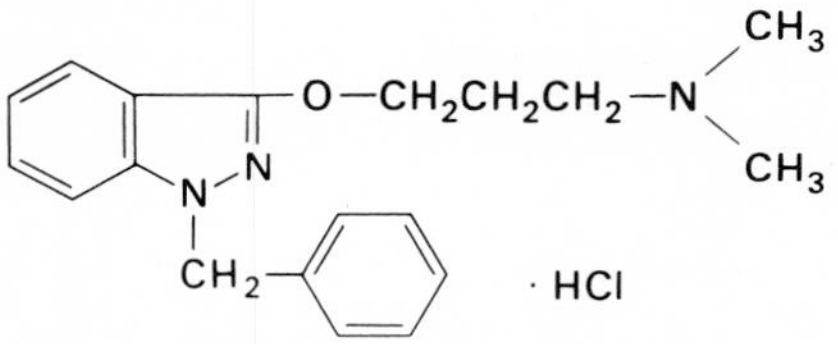

benzydamine HCl (Tantum)

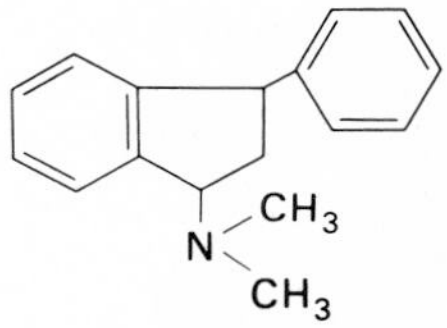

$N(CH_3)_2$

dimefadane

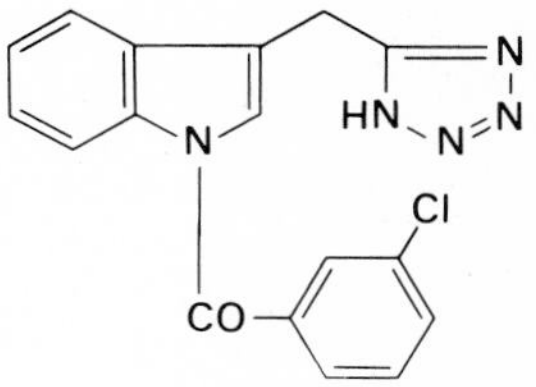

OCH_3 OCH_3

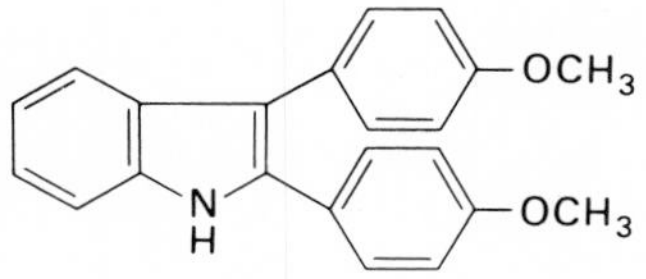

indoxole

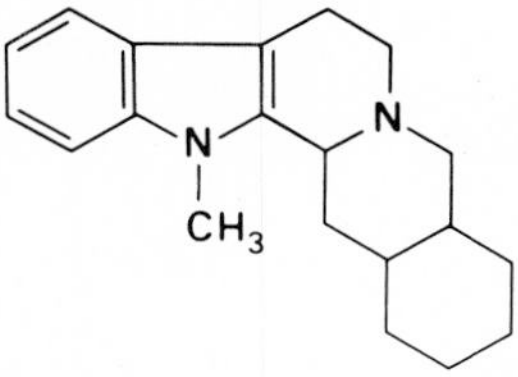

HN N N N — CO — Cl

intrazole

CH_3

mimbane HCl

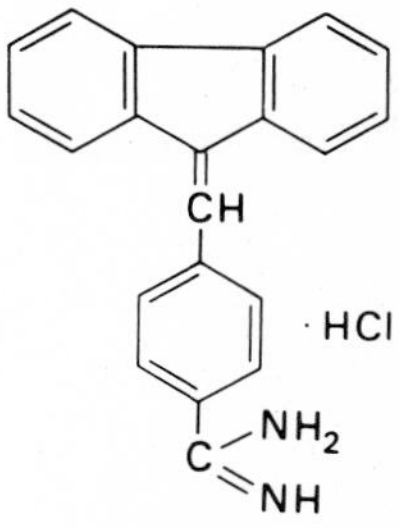

CH · HCl $C(NH_2)=NH$

paranylene HCl

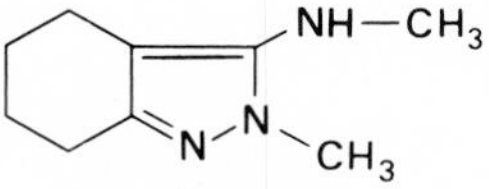

$NH-CH_3$ CH_3

tetrydamine

CH_2 N CH_2CH_2 N · HCl

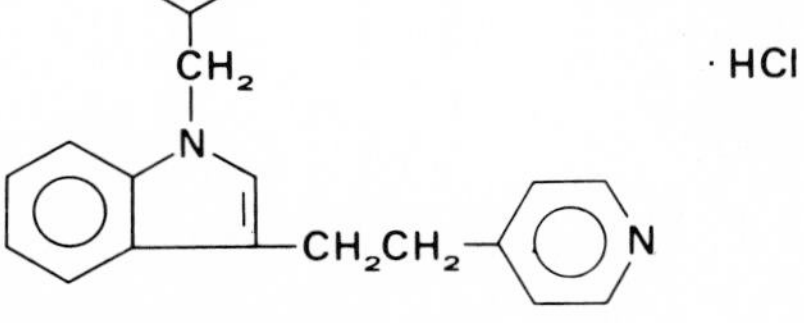

benzindopyrine hydrochloride

I. Ibufenac Group

alcolfenac

fenoprofen

fluprofen

ibufenac

ibuprofen

naproxen

ketoprofen

naproxol

fenbufen

J. Other Analgesic or Antiinflammatory Agents

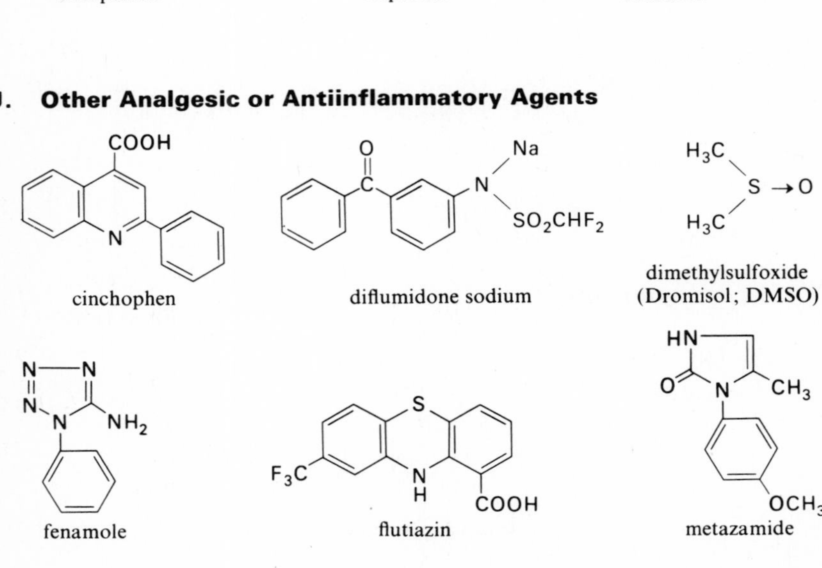

cinchophen

diflumidone sodium

dimethylsulfoxide (Dromisol; DMSO)

fenamole

flutiazin

metazamide

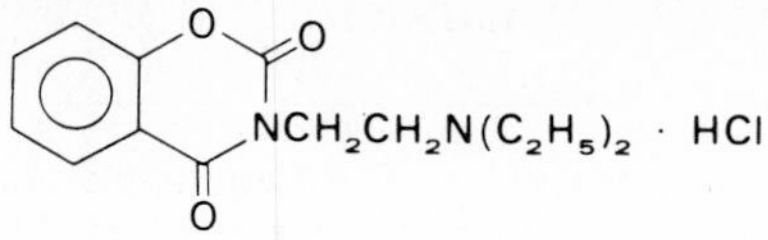

$NCH_2CH_2N(C_2H_5)_2 \cdot HCl$

letimide hydrochloride

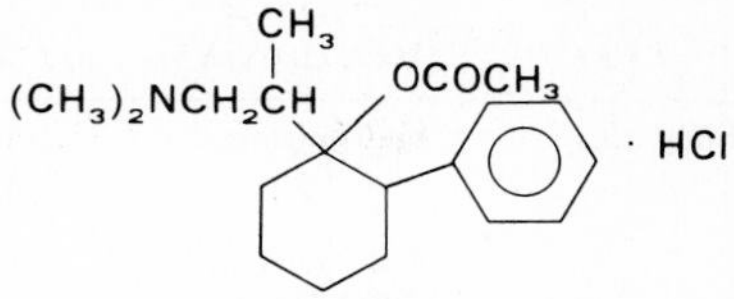

$(CH_3)_2NCH_2CH(CH_3)$ $OCOCH_3$ $\cdot HCl$

nexeridine hydrochloride

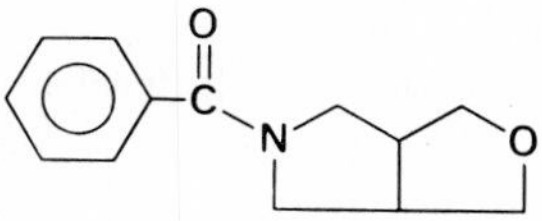

octazamide

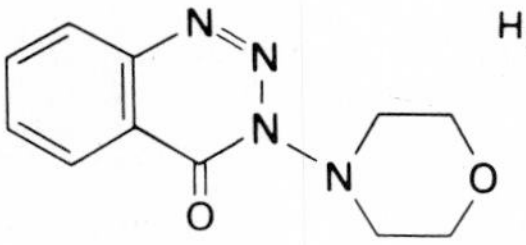

molinazone

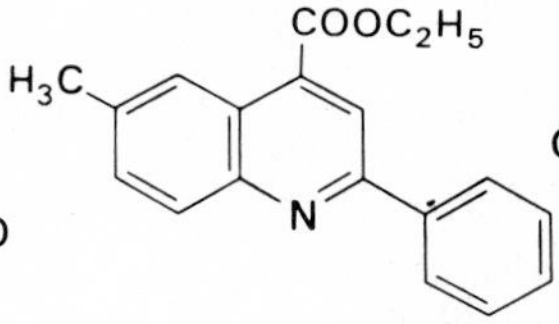

$COOC_2H_5$ H_3C

neocinchophen

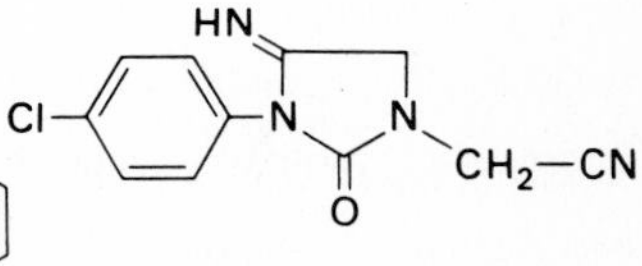

HN Cl $CH_2—CN$

nimazone

$CH_2CH_2—N(C_2H_5)_2$ $CH—C_2H_5$ $C_6H_8O_7$

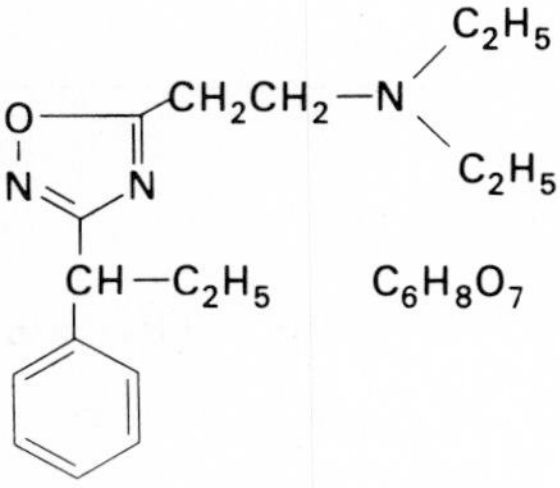

proxazole citrate (Toness)

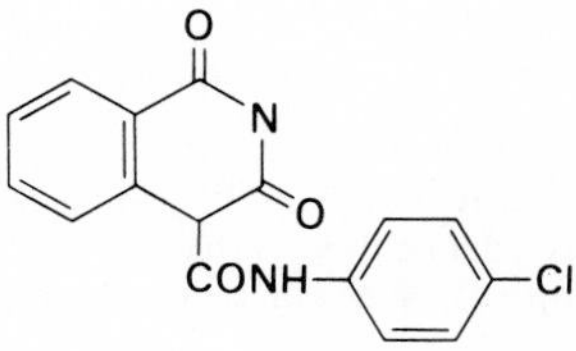

CONH— —Cl

tesicam

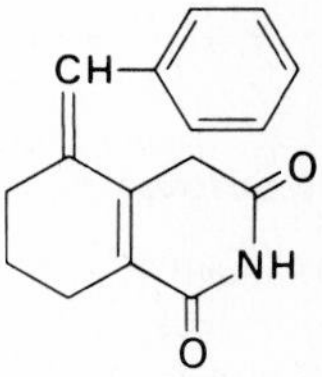

CH— NH

tesimide

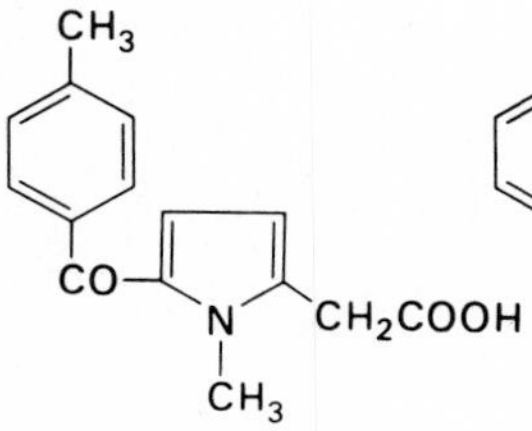

CH_3 CO— CH_2COOH CH_3

tolmetin

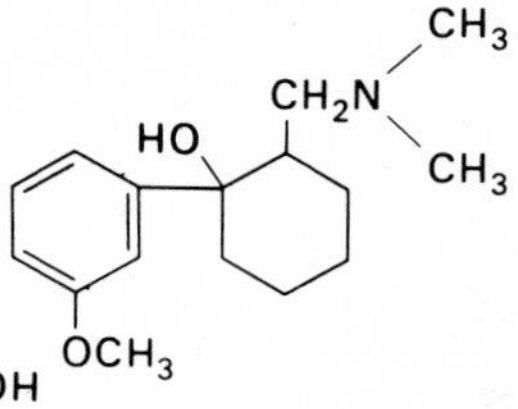

HO $CH_2N(CH_3)_2$ OCH_3

tramadol

$COOC_2H_5$ SO_2CF_3

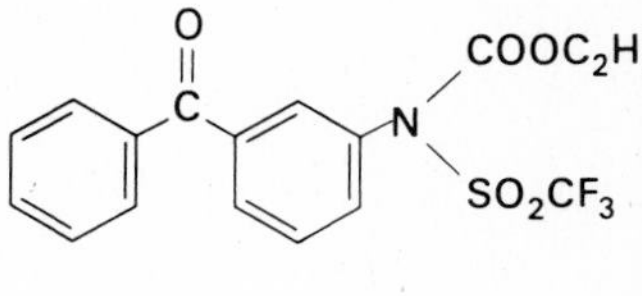

triflumidate

SUMMARY: NONNARCOTIC ANALGESICS

TYPE	*ACTION AND MECHANISM*	*TOXICITY*	*USE*	*EXAMPLES*
Salicylates	Analgesic and antiinflammatory Mechanism not understood	Tinnitus, acidosis	Analgesic, antiinflammatory	Aspirin
Aniline derivatives	Analgesic Mechanism not understood	Methemoglobin, hemolytic anemia	Analgesic	Acetanilid
Pyrazolon derivatives	Analgesic and antiinflammatory Mechanism not understood	Agranulocytosis, bleeding in peptic ulcer	Analgesic, antiinflammatory	Phenylbutazone
Colchicines	Antiinflammatory in gout Mitotic inhibitor	Purging	Acute gout	Colchicine
Phenyramidol group	Analgesic Mechanism not understood	Gastrointestinal distress	Analgesic	Phenyramidol
Indene derivatives	Analgesic and antiinflammatory Mechanism not understood	Same, plus drowsiness, tinnitus	Analgesic	Indomethacin

Reviews

Randall, L. Non-narcotic analgesics, in Physiological Pharmacology. Foot and Hoffman (eds.). New York, Academic Press, 1963.

Murray, W. Evaluation of aspirin in treatment of headache. Clin. Pharmacol. Ther., 5:21, 1964.

Shen, T. Anti-inflammatory agents. Topics Med. Chem., 1:29, 1967.

Kuzell, W. Nonsteroid anti-inflammatory agents. Ann. Rev. Pharmacol., 8:357, 1968.

Murray, W., and Piliero, S. Non-steroid anti-inflammatory agents. Ann. Rev. Pharmacol., 10:171, 1970.

50. Narcotic Analgesics

A. Opium

1. History. a. Opium may be the oldest drug on record. The poppy was known to the Sumerians before 4000 B.C., then to the Assyrians and to the Egyptians; the Ebers papyrus, dating from about 1500 B.C., includes prescriptions containing opium. Homer presumably mentions it, and Theophrastus used it in the third century B.C.

b. Paracelsus (1521) brought opium from Constantinople to Germany and from it made a tincture which also contained powdered pearls and gold salts; he called the mixture laudanum.

c. Sertürner (1803) isolated morphine from opium, the first isolation of a pure alkaloid; Gates and Tschudi (1952) achieved the first total synthesis of morphine.

2. Chemistry. Opium, the dried juice of the unripe capsule of *Papaver somniferum*, contains alkaloids of two types:

a. Phenanthrene derivatives: morphine (9%), codeine (0.5%), thebaine (0.2%), and others.

b. Benzylisoquinoline derivatives: noscapine (narcotine) (6%), papaverine (1%), and others (considered under Smooth Muscle Relaxants, and Antitussives).

3. Action and Mechanism. a. Opium has the actions of the alkaloids it contains, primarily morphine (considered in detail in the next sections).

b. In general, the actions are analgesic, sedative, and constipating; relatively more constipation may be produced than by preparations of pure alkaloids.

4. Pharmacodynamics and Toxicity. a. Galenical preparations of opium differ from preparations of pure alkaloids in not being unpleasantly bitter, and thus are adapted to oral use.

b. General pharmacological and toxicological characteristics are those of morphine.

5. Uses. Less used than formerly, but desirable constipating agents in diarrhea.

6. Preparations

PAREGORIC

Large noncritical dose makes this a preferred preparation especially for children.
Dose: 4 ml every 1 to 4 hours as needed (to control diarrhea) by mouth.

POWDER OF IPECAC AND OPIUM (Dover's Powder)

An example of the old, mostly discarded, complex preparations containing opium and used for colds and other minor ills. Another was Compound Mixture of Opium and Glycyrrhiza (Brown Mixture), 4 ml by mouth.
Dose: 0.6 gm by mouth.

TINCTURE OF OPIUM (laudanum)

Largely replaced by paregoric.
Dose: 0.6 ml as needed by mouth.

B. Morphine and Relatives

MORPHINE

1. Chemistry. a. Analgesic activity appears to depend upon a γ-phenyl-N-methyl piperidine grouping (Gero, Science, 119:12, 1954) in which the piperidine ring has a chair shape, and is not in the plane of the phenyl ring.

b. This grouping is common to all the morphine, methadone, and meperidine derivatives.

c. Receptor attachment related to this grouping (Beckett and Casy, J. Pharm. Pharmacol., 6:986, 1954) was proposed, but is now considered an incomplete explanation (Dole, Ann. Rev. Biochem., 39:821, 1970).

2. Action. a. Morphine exhibits a combination of depression and stimulation in the CNS and the gut.

b. Analgesia and hypnosis: Pain and anxiety are relieved by central effects which raise the pain threshold and produce euphoria and sedation. These effects combine to dull the appreciation and interpretation of unpleasant stimuli. Pain is much more depressed than other sensory stimuli, and there is little motor depression. The area or areas in the brain most involved in the analgesic action are not known; probably the fundamental depression is widespread.

c. Respiratory depression: Probably from a combination of depression of the respiratory center in the medulla and of the respiratory reflex; parallels analgesic potency. The cough reflex is similarly depressed.

d. Smooth muscle spasm: Morphine increases the tone, but decreases the rhythmic contractions, in many types of smooth muscle, primarily by stimulation of the motor side of the myenteric plexus, although drugs which stimulate the smooth muscle directly may be antagonized, suggesting the possibility of a direct effect as well (Lewis, Brit. J. Pharmacol., 15:425, 1960). In the gastrointestinal tract this produces colic and constipation, which may be troublesome in ordinary analgesic therapy (and in addicts, who do not become tolerant to this effect), or useful in the treatment of diarrhea. Ureteral or biliary tract spasm is increased by morphine, but the analgesia may outweigh this undesirable effect, especially when a painful stone is present.

Bronchial constriction is always an undesirable action, but is ordinarily minor; however, it may be lethal when combined with respiratory depression in asthma.

e. Nausea and vomiting: These result from stimulation of the emetic chemoreceptor trigger zone in the medulla; more common in ambulatory than in recumbent patients.

f. Circulatory and other effects: The vasomotor center is depressed; some vessels, including the coronary arteries, may be dilated; on the whole, circulatory effects are not outstanding and probably result from a combination of central actions and peripheral histamine release. Miosis is characteristic (effect on the oculomotor nerve), and other signs of vagal stimulation can be seen.

3. Mechanism. a. The mechanism of action of morphine is not clearly understood.

b. Elements of sympathetic and parasympathetic stimulation may be identified within the picture of morphine activity, but the principal effect appears to be in the CNS. Anticholinesterase activity is present, but probably is not critical.

4. Pharmacodynamics. a. Morphine is absorbed well by injection, but capriciously by mouth or mucous surface. Penetration into the spinal fluid is poor.

b. Metabolism and excretion are rapid; partly conjugated in the liver, and appears in the urine as the glucuronide. Most of a single dose can be identified in the urine in 24 hours.

5. Toxicity. a. Acute poisoning is characterized by increasing depression, slowed respiration, pinpoint pupils, flushing, and then cyanosis. Death occurs in 5 to 10 hours from doses in the neighborhood of 200 mg. Treatment is by the use of nalorphine.

b. Chronic toxicity (see Drug Addiction).

6. Uses. a. The principal use of morphine in man is to relieve pain; as an analgesic it is potent and effective in almost all types of pain; the effect is often improved by the accompanying sedation and decrease in anxiety.

b. It is also of use in the dyspnea of heart failure, in pulmonary edema and cough, and as a preanesthetic sedative.

7. Preparation

MORPHINE SULFATE

Dose: 5 to 15 mg subcutaneously or intramuscularly, or less often intravenously or by mouth.

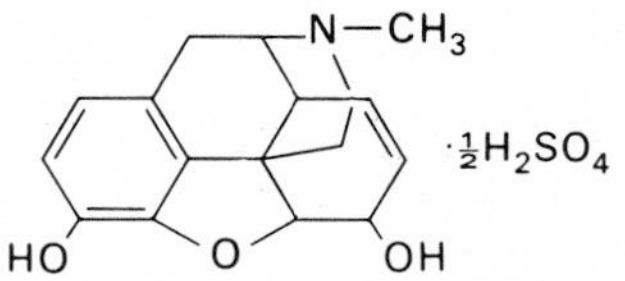

$N{-}CH_3$

$\cdot\frac{1}{2}H_2SO_4$

HO O OH

MORPHINE DERIVATIVES

1. Chemistry. a. The morphine molecule is subject to a variety of chemical alterations, and related compounds may also be synthesized.

b. In the morphine series the phenolic OH is usually retained; in the codeine group it is replaced with an OCH_3 group or equivalent.

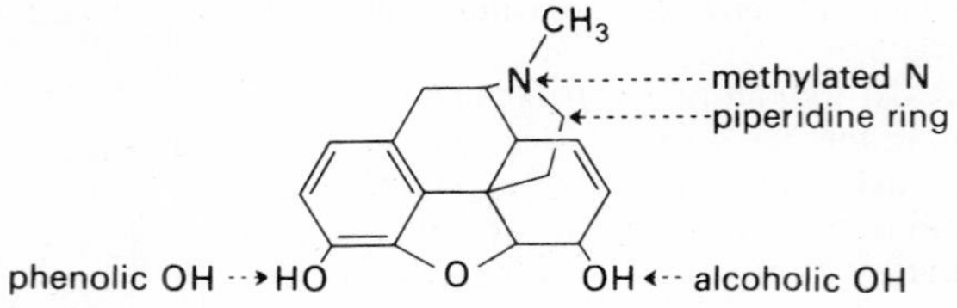

CH_3
N ← methylated N
← piperidine ring
phenolic OH → HO O OH ← alcoholic OH

morphine

c. Masking the phenolic OH usually decreases activity (heroin is an exception, but the acetyl group may improve penetration, and then be hydrolyzed). Alteration of the alcoholic OH is compatible with increased potency.

d. Replacement of the methyl on the nitrogen usually results in an antagonist; variations in saturation or substitution of the right hand ring may affect potency.

2. Preparations

a. Morphine series: As a group, the morphine series are strong analgesics, strong respiratory depressants, and strong smooth muscle stimulants; they are also strongly addicting.

APOMORPHINE HYDROCHLORIDE

Powerful emetic and depressant. May be used to empty the stomach in poisoning but ordinarily a stomach tube is safer; will subdue wildly excited patients.

Dose: 5 mg subcutaneously.

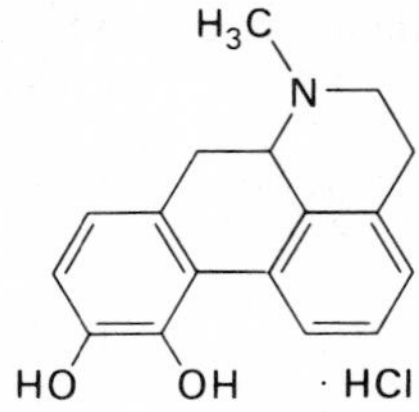

H_3C N HO OH · HCl

HEROIN (diacetylmorphine)

More potent than morphine and would be highly satisfactory if it were not also more addicting; not permitted in the United States.

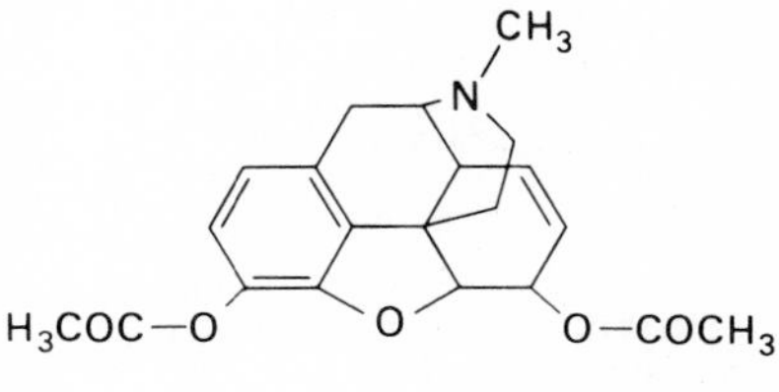

CH_3 N H_3COC-O O $O-COCH_3$

HYDROMORPHONE HYDROCHLORIDE (Dilaudid)

An oxidation product of morphine; similar in action but effective in a smaller dose. Popularly assumed to produce less nausea and vomiting.

Dose: 3 mg subcutaneously.

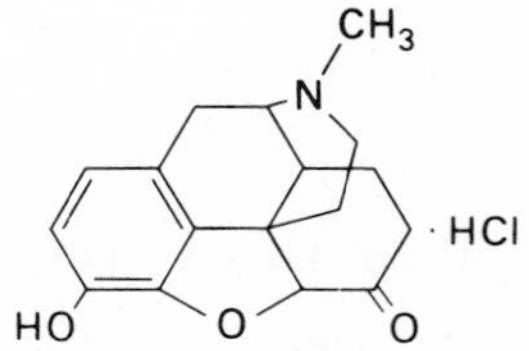

CH_3 N · HCl HO O O

LEVORPHANOL TARTRATE (Levo-Dromoran)

Potent and long lasting, but of doubtful advantage over morphine except more effective orally and is synthetic.

Dose: 1.5 to 3 mg by mouth or subcutaneously.

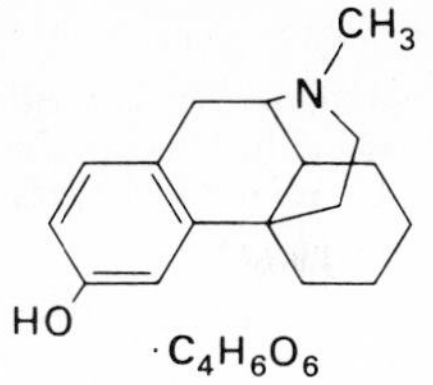

$\cdot C_4H_6O_6$

METOPON HYDROCHLORIDE (Methyldilaudid)

Introduced with hopes of reliable oral absorption, but proved to be unsatisfactory.

Dose: 4 mg by mouth.

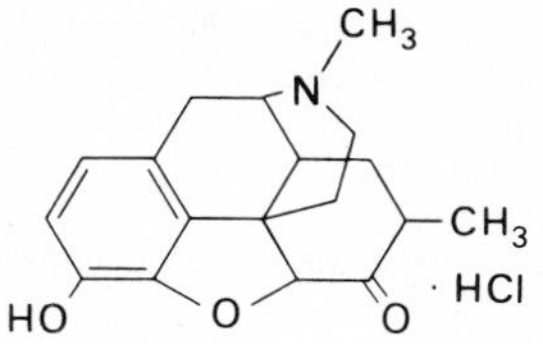

OXYMORPHONE HYDROCHLORIDE (Numorphan)

More potent than morphine but tolerance may develop more rapidly. Actual therapeutic advantage over morphine doubtful.

Dose: 1.5 mg subcutaneously.

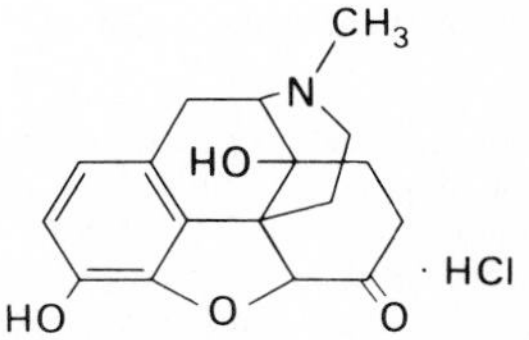

b. *Benzomorphan series:* Newer members of this series combine the benzomorphan nucleus with narcotic antagonist side chains on the piperidine N. Minimal addiction liability is the principal potential advantage over morphine.

BUPRENORPHINE HYDROCHLORIDE

Under investigation.

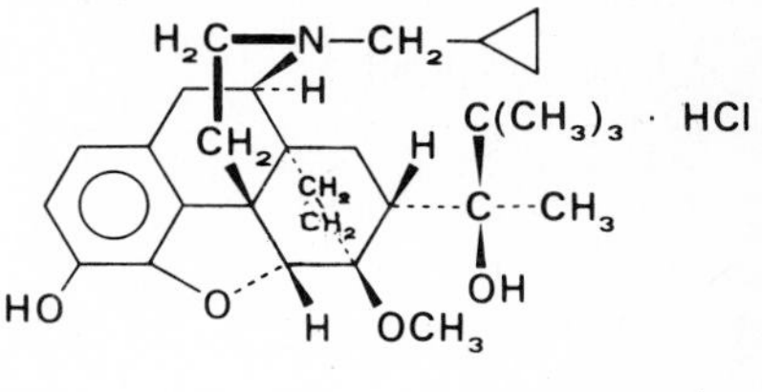

BUTORPHANOL

Dose: 2 mg by injection.

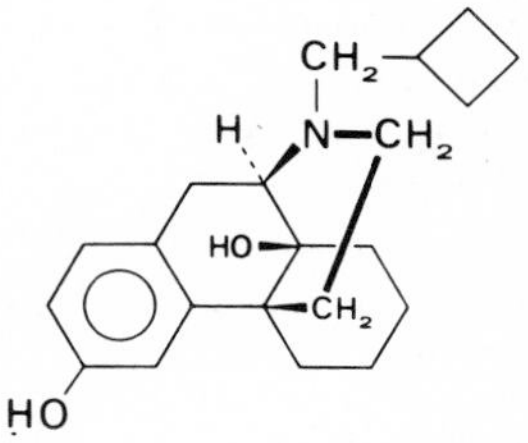

CARBAZOCINE

Under investigation.

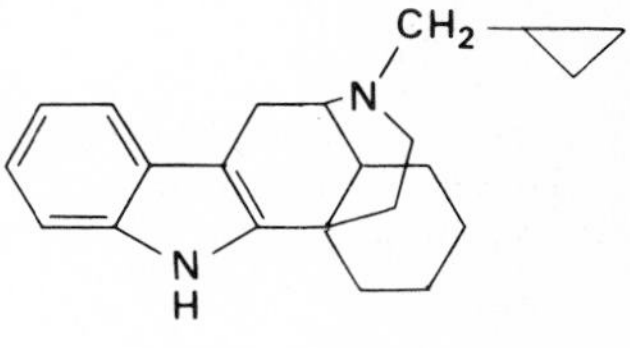

CYCLAZOCINE

Sedative and analgesic; side effects include euphoria and confusion. Long acting.
Dose: 2 mg by mouth or subcutaneously.

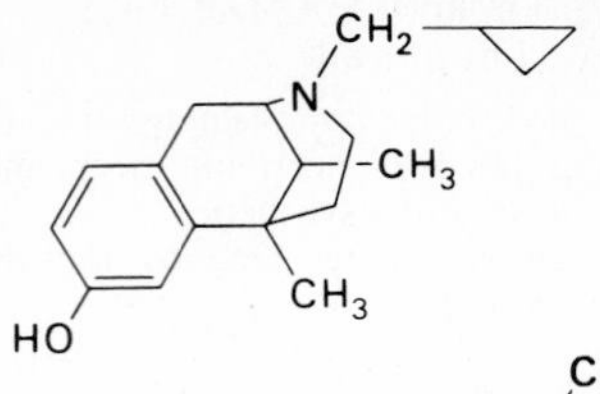

PENTAZOCINE (Talwin)

Promising alternative to morphine. Analgesic, soporific, respiratory, depressant, nauseant about equal to morphine. Minimum addiction liability; unsatisfactory in abstinence syndrome. Weak narcotic antagonist. May produce pain at site of injection.

Dose: 20 to 40 mg subcutaneously or intramuscularly.

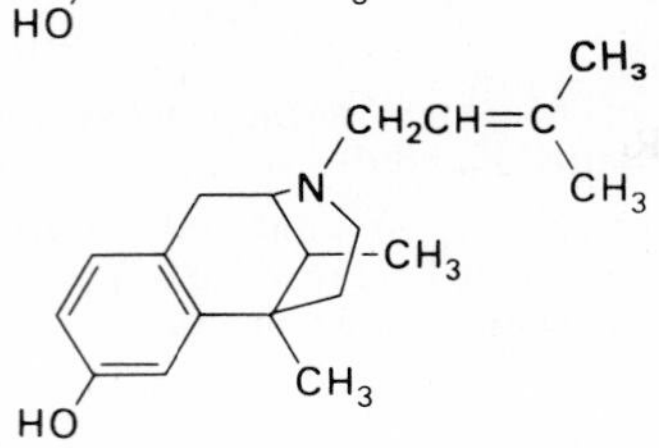

PHENAZOCINE HYDROBROMIDE (Prinadol)

Synthetic molecule. Four times as potent as morphine but generally similar and advantages over morphine questioned (DeKornfeld, Anesthesia, 21:159, 1960). May be less sedative and less hypotensive, but constipating. Oral use may be possible.

Dose: 3 mg intramuscularly.

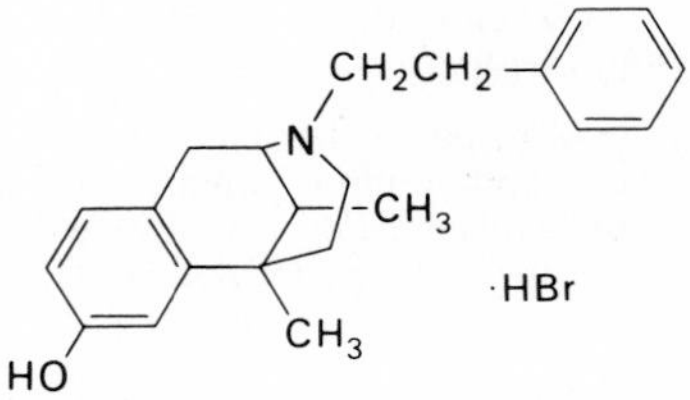

$\cdot HBr$

VOLAZOCINE

Under investigation.

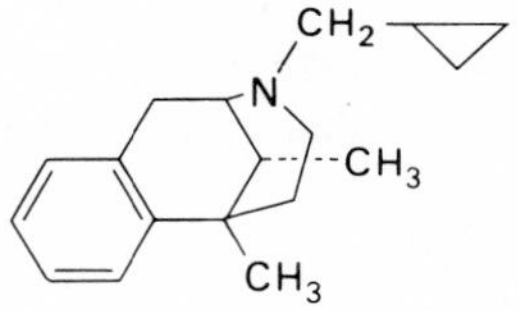

c. *Codeine series:* Characteristically weaker than morphine as analgesics, respiratory depressants, smooth muscle stimulants, and in producing addiction; however, the antitussive effect is not correspondingly reduced. They are therefore used as less potent analgesics and as cough suppressants. Codeine is convulsant in extratherapeutic doses, and this action is amplified in some of the series.

CODEINE SULFATE (or phosphate)

Narcotic action one-twentieth that of morphine; respiratory and cough depression one-third. Valuable for the control of mild pain and cough.

Dose: 30 to 60 mg orally or subcutaneously.

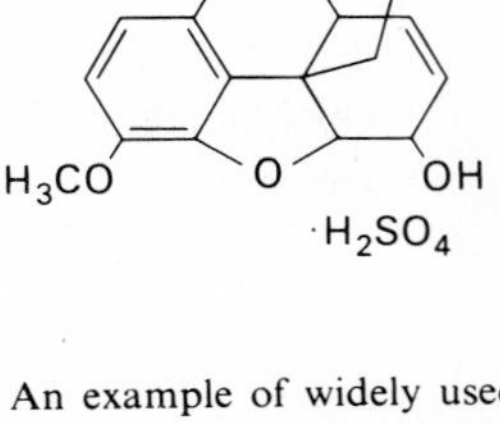

$\cdot H_2SO_4$

Elixir Terpin Hydrate and Codeine

Dose: 4 ml (contains 8 mg codeine) or more by mouth. An example of widely used cough syrups containing codeine.

CODOXIME

Antitussive.

Dose: Under investigation.

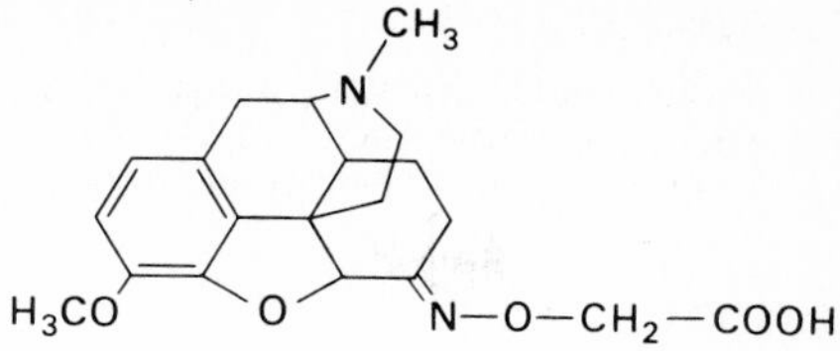

DEXTROMETHORPHAN HYDROBROMIDE (Romilar)

Used exclusively as an antitussive; not analgesic.

Dose: 10 to 20 mg by mouth.

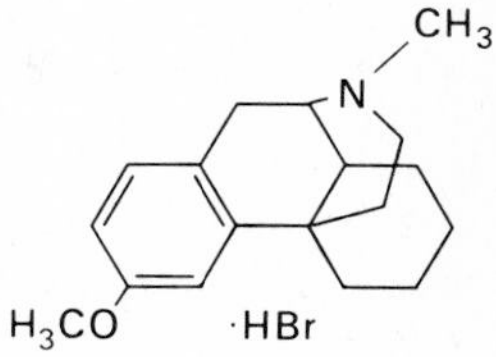

Elixir Terpin Hydrate and Dextromethorphan Hydrobromide

Dose: 5 ml (contains 10 mg dextromethorphan) by mouth.

DROCODE (Rapocodin)

A dihydrocodeine similar in action to codeine.

Dose: 10 to 60 mg by mouth.

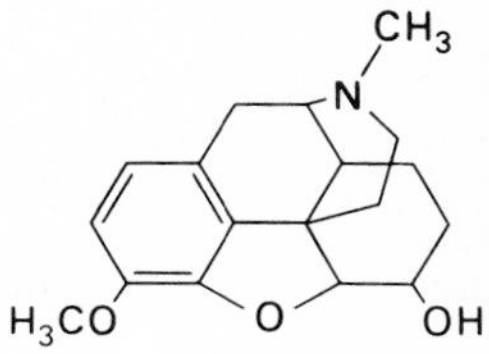

HYDROCODONE BITARTRATE (Dicodid)

A dihydrocodeinone, similar to codeine with no particular advantage. Stated to be more addicting than codeine; in the mixture, Hycodan.

Dose: 5 to 10 mg by mouth.

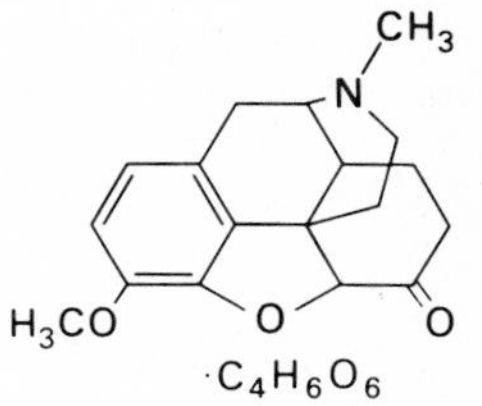

OXYCODONE HYDROCHLORIDE

More potent than codeine, and addicting. Used as an analgesic and cough suppressant; in the mixture, Percodan.

Dose: 10 to 20 mg orally or subcutaneously.

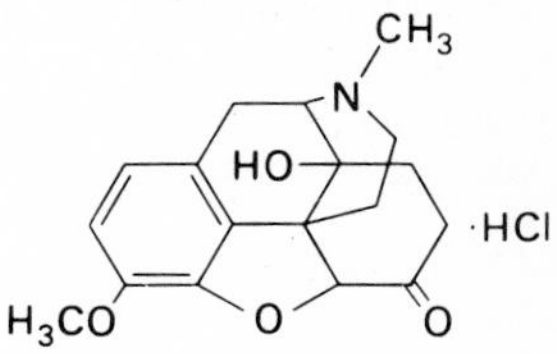

PHOLCODINE (Ethnine)

More antitussive than codeine, but not analgesic. Low toxicity; anticonvulsant in animals; not addicting.

Dose: 10 to 15 mg intramuscularly.

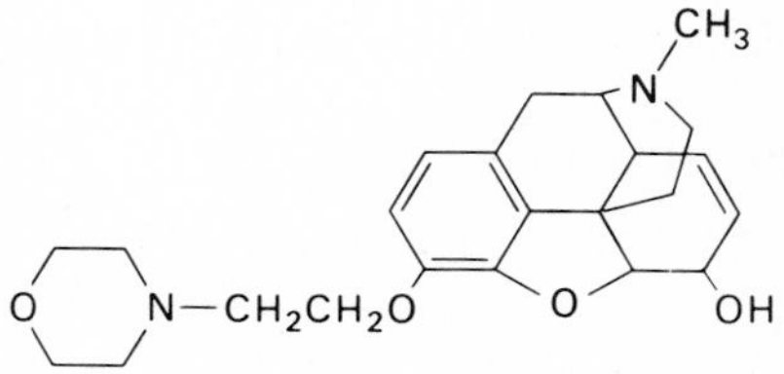

THEBAINE

Natural opium alkaloid with heightened convulsant action; not used clinically.

An intermediate in synthesis of morphine analogues.

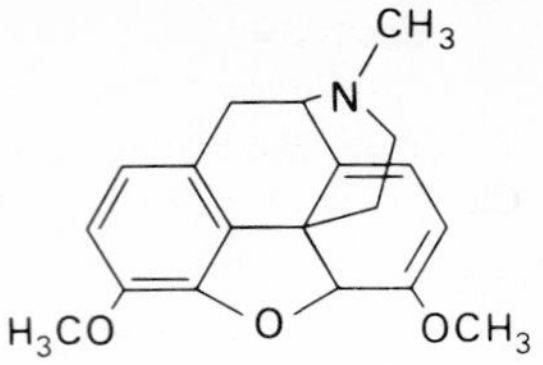

CH_3 N H_3CO O OCH_3

MORPHINE ANTAGONISTS

1. Chemistry. Morphine analogues in which the methyl on the N is replaced by a larger alkyl chain.

2. Action. a. Some (Naloxone) are pure antagonists, others have both anergesic and morphine-antagonizing action but are not used to relieve pain because of unpleasant psychic effects.

b. When given during the action of morphinelike narcotics, neutralize all their depressant effects within minutes (including respiratory depression and analgesia).

c. When given to addicts will precipitate a severe withdrawal reaction.

3. Mechanism. May act on two hypothetical morphine receptors having agonistic action on one and antagonistic action on the other.

4. Pharmacodynamics and Toxicity. Similar to morphine. Withdrawal symptoms in addicts may be seriously augmented.

5. Uses. a. Principal use as antidotes in overdosage with any narcotic analgesic.

b. Have also been given to mothers in labor who have received narcotics, in order to reduce postnatal respiratory depression in their babies.

c. May be used in suspected addicts in the nalorphine test: nalorphine, 3 mg, is given subcutaneously; a diagnostic dilatation of the pupils follows within 20 minutes in the presence of narcotic analgesics.

6. Preparations

LEVALLORPHAN TARTRATE (Lorfan)

Similar effect to nalorphine (smaller dose).

Dose: 0.5 to 2.0 mg subcutaneously, intramuscularly, or intravenously.

$CH_2CH{=}CH_2$ N $\cdot C_4H_6O_6$ HO

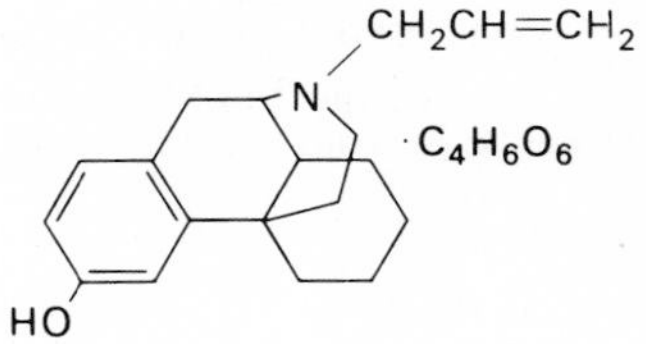

NALORPHINE HYDROCHLORIDE (Nalline)

Dose: 5 to 15 mg subcutaneously, intramuscularly, or intravenously.

$CH_2CH{=}CH_2$ N $\cdot HCl$ HO O OH

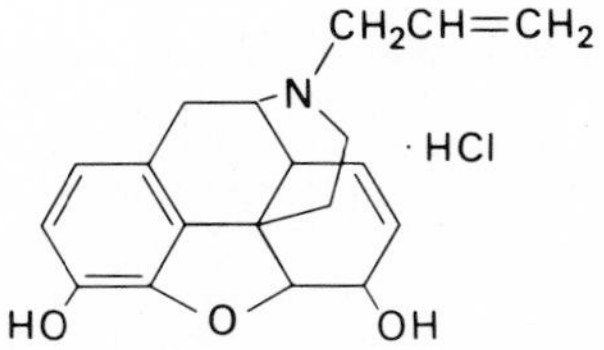

NALOXONE HYDROCHLORIDE (Narcan)
Pure antagonist.

Dose: 0.4 mg intramuscularly or intravenously. Can be repeated 2 to 3 times.

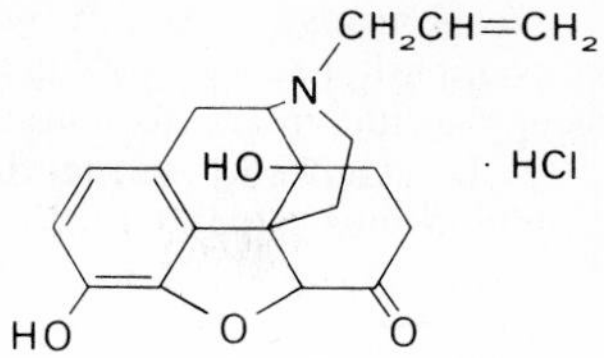

$CH_2CH{=}CH_2$ · HCl

OTHERS

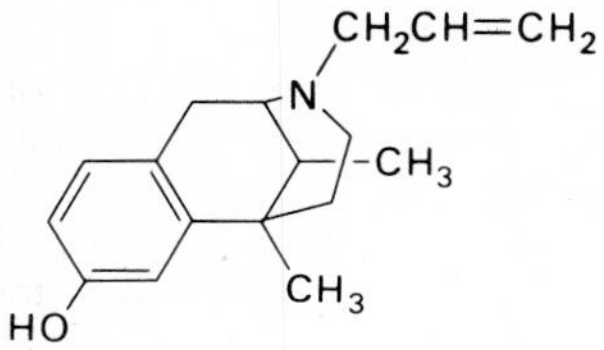

alazocine

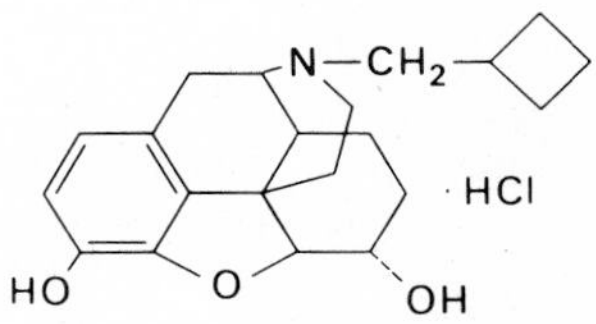

nalbufine HCl

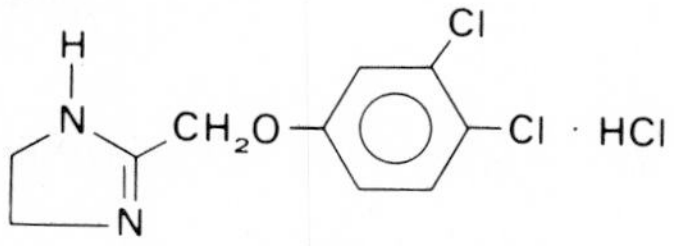

fenmetozole hydrochloride

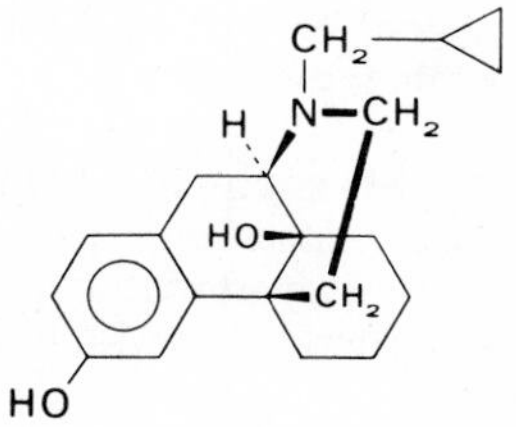

oxilorphan

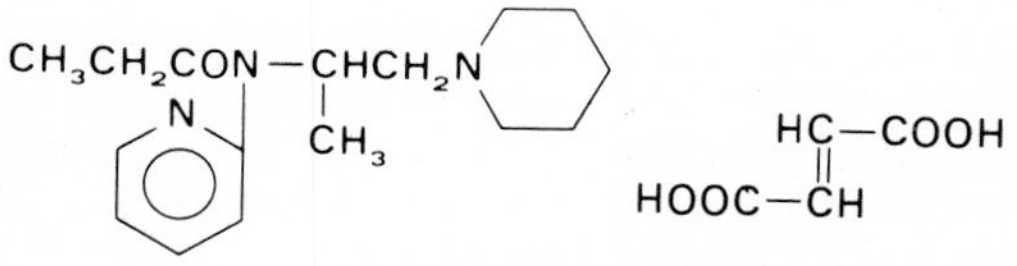

propiram fumarate

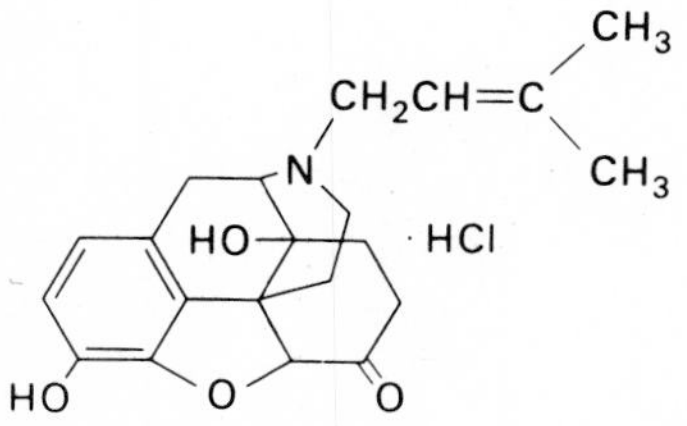

nalmexone HCl

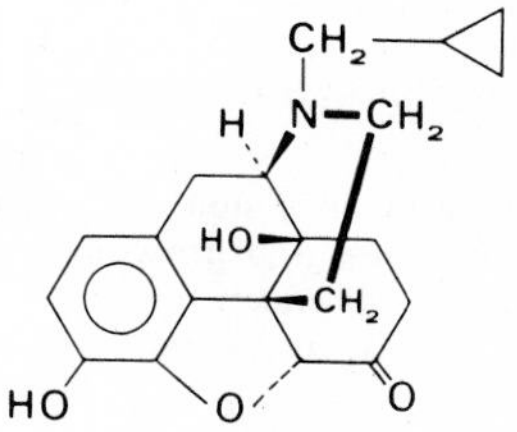

naltrexone

C. Methadone and Related Compounds

1. **History.** Methadone introduced by Bockmuhl and Schaumann (1941).

2. Chemistry. a. Although apparently resembling the diphenylmethane parasympatholytics or antihistamines, the strong analgesic effects suggest that they occupy a different conformation in the body.

b. Gero showed that they could assume a near γ-phenyl-N-methyl-piperidyl form, and thus explained their similarity to morphine (Science, 119:112, 1954).

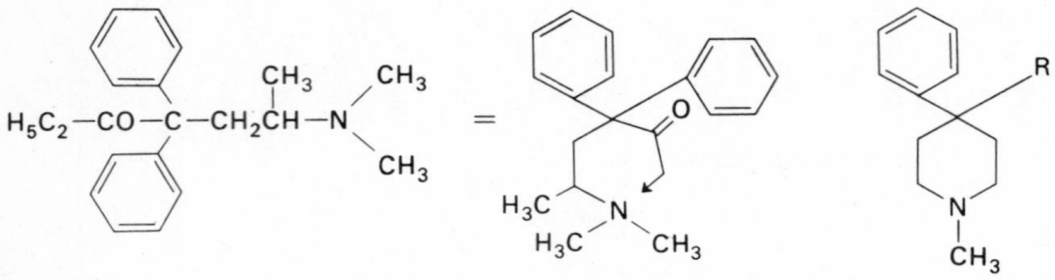

H_5C_2—CO—C—CH_2CH—N(CH_3)$_2$ = methadone (cyclic conformation)

methadone | methadone | γ-phenyl-N-methyl piperidine moiety

3. Action. General resemblance to the actions of morphine: produce strong analgesia, addiction, miosis, sedation, smooth muscle spasm, and respiratory depression. Withdrawal symptoms in addicted subjects developed more slowly than in morphine addicts.

4. Mechanism. a. Fundamental mechanism not understood, but probably acts by the same means as morphine.

b. Reported to impair the production of energy from carbohydrate in the CNS by interference with hexokinase.

5. Pharmacodynamics. Well absorbed orally. Rapidly metabolized by N-demethylation.

6. Uses. a. Useful alternatives to morphine for the relief of pain.

b. Also used during withdrawal treatment of morphinism.

c. Replacement for morphine and heroin in addiction.

7. Preparations

DEXTROMORAMIDE TARTRATE
(Dimorlin)

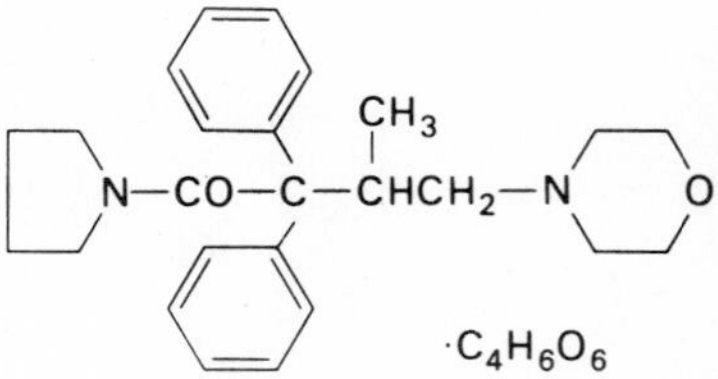

Analgesic potency similar to that of morphine; dizziness and drowsiness may be troublesome side effects.

Dose: 5 to 10 mg by mouth or subcutaneously.

N—CO—C—CHCH$_2$—N O (with CH_3) $\cdot C_4H_6O_6$

METHADONE HYDROCHLORIDE
(Adanon; Dolophine; and others)

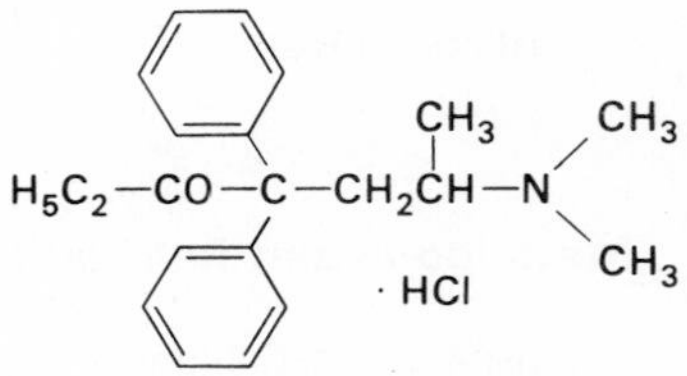

Dose: 2.5 to 10 mg subcutaneously or orally (never intravenously).

H_5C_2—CO—C—CH_2CH—N (with CH_3, CH_3, CH_3) $\cdot$ HCl

METHADYL ACETATE

LEVOMETHADYL ACETATE

Longer acting than methadone.

Dose: 50 mg every third day by mouth.

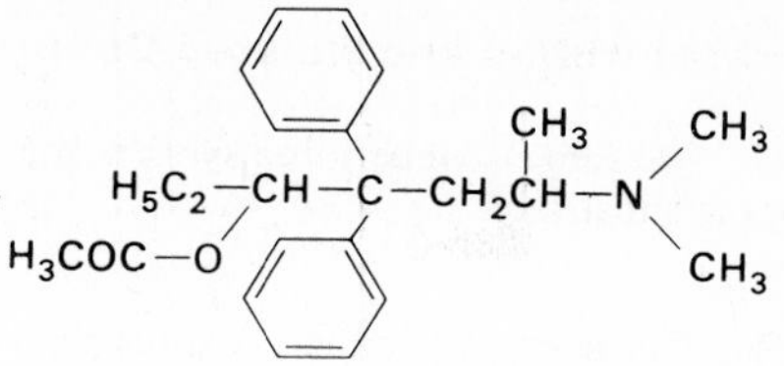

NORACYMETHADOL HYDROCHLORIDE

About the potency of morphine but with more nausea, drowsiness, and itching.
Dose: 30 mg by mouth; 5 to 15 mg intramuscularly.

PROPOXYPHENE HYDROCHLORIDE (Darvon)

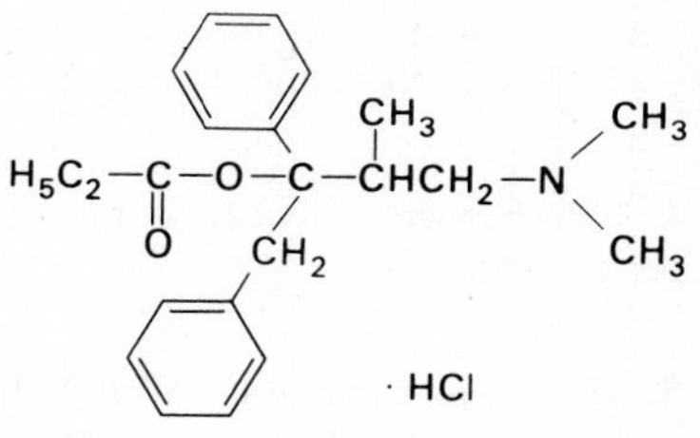

· HCl

Analgesic somewhat less potent than codeine; 65 mg equivalent to 0.6 gm aspirin; capable of relieving the symptoms of morphine abstinence, but itself unlikely to be used as an addicting agent because it is not euphorigenic, unless given intravenously, and is erosive when given subcutaneously. Nausea, vomiting, and skin rashes may be produced. Not under the Harrison Narcotic Act.

Dose: 50 mg up to 4 times daily by mouth.

Levopropoxyphene napsylate (Novrad).
Good antitussive; not analgesic.
Dose: 50 to 100 mg by mouth.

Propoxyphene napsylate

OTHERS

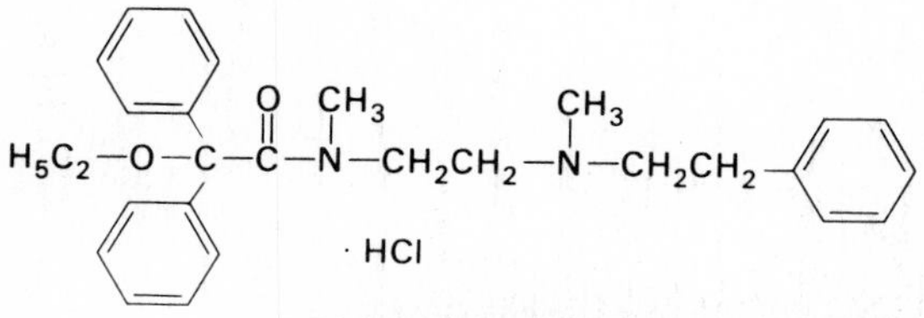

· HCl

carbiphene HCl (Bandol)

· HCl

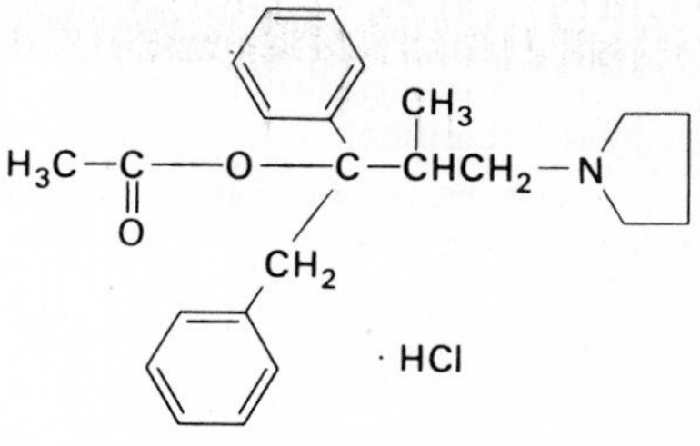

pyrroliphine HCl

D. Meperidine and Related Compounds

1. History. Meperidine synthesized by Eisleb and Schaumann (1939) as an atropine substitute.

2. Chemistry. Simplest expression of the γ-phenyl-N-methyl piperidine moiety.

3. Action. a. Meperidine intermediate between morphine and codeine as an analgesic; mildly sedative, and produces some peripheral vasodilatation; respiratory depression and nausea may be produced.

b. Related compounds generally similar; most somewhat less potent.

c. Some inhibit intestinal contractions effectively.

4. Mechanism. Probably similar to that of morphine; residing in the γ-phenyl-N-piperidine moiety.

5. Pharmacodynamics. Well absorbed orally. Rapidly metabolized by demethylation and hydrolysis to meperidinic acid.

6. Uses. a. Widely used as general purpose analgesics. Useful in anesthesia because of relatively short duration of action.

b. To control diarrhea.

7. Preparations

ALPHAPRODINE HYDROCHLORIDE (Nisentil)

Similar to meperidine, but slightly shorter acting.

Dose: 50 mg subcutaneously.

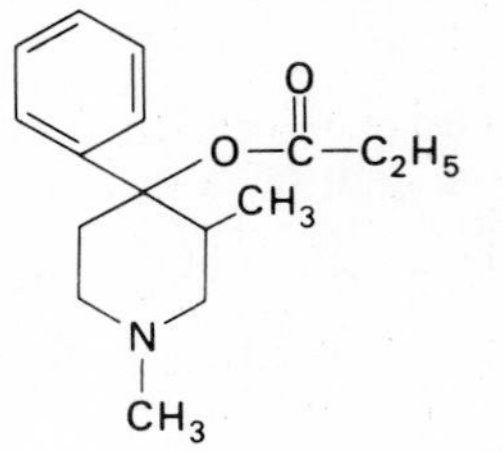

ANILERIDINE HYDROCHLORIDE (or phosphate) (Leritine)

Similar to meperidine, but twice as potent.

Dose: 25 mg by mouth or subcutaneously.

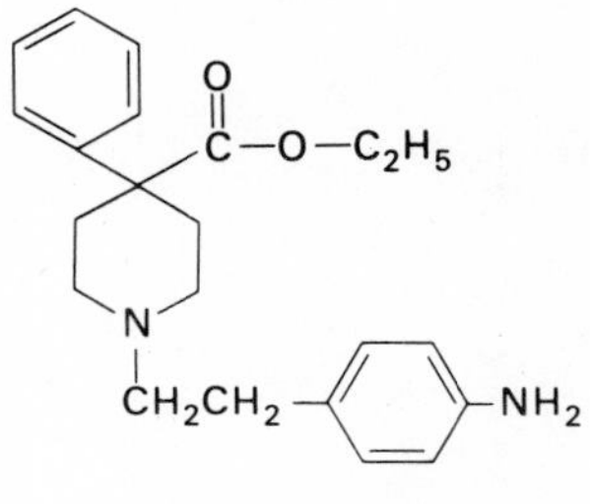

ETHOHEPTAZINE (Zactane)

Mild analgesic, comparable to aspirin; not reported to be addicting.

Dose: 50 to 100 mg by mouth.

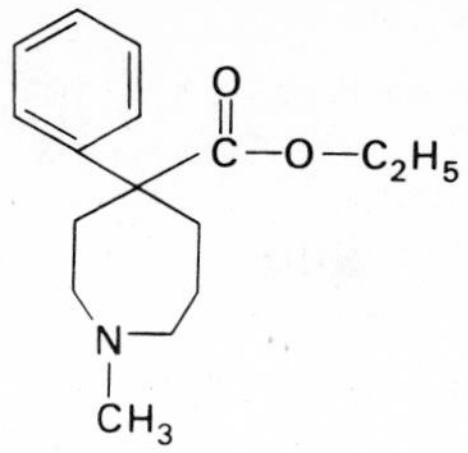

FENTANYL CITRATE (Sublimaze)

(See Phenyramidol group)

Potent; short acting.

Dose: 25 to 100 mcg intramuscularly or intravenously.

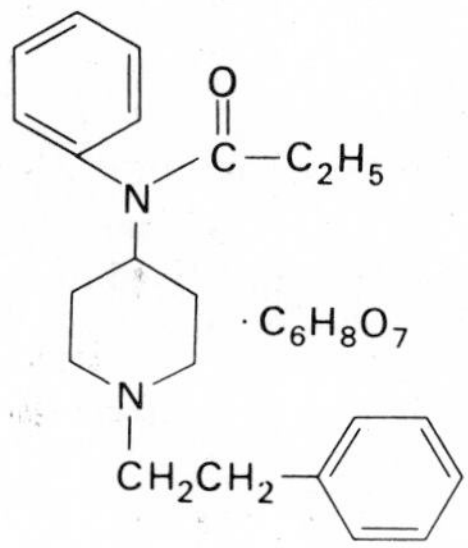

MEPERIDINE HYDROCHLORIDE (Demerol; Pethidine; and others)

Dose: 50 to 100 mg orally or intramuscularly.

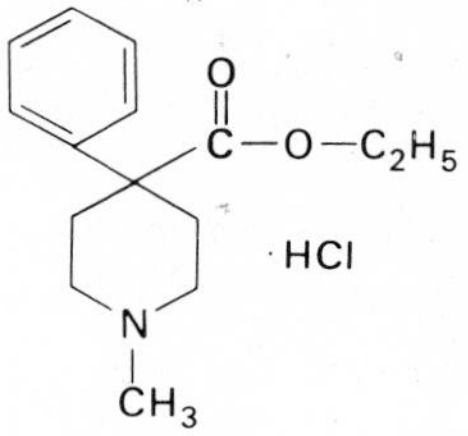

PIMINODINE ESYLATE (Alvodine)

Dose: 25 to 50 mg every 4 to 6 hours by mouth; 10 to 20 mg every 4 hours subcutaneously or intramuscularly.

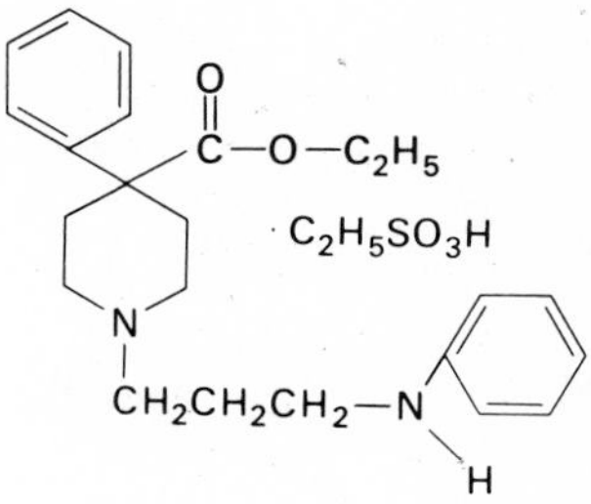

OTHERS

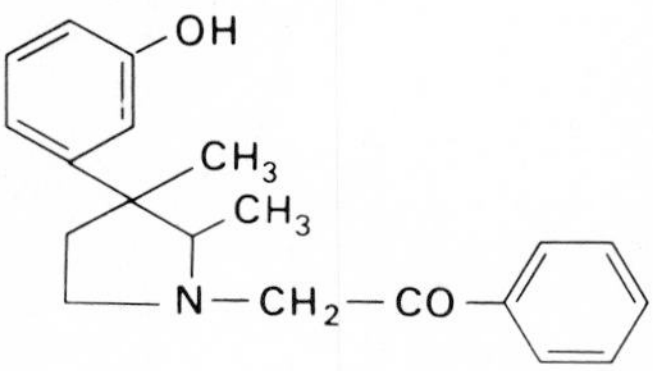

myfadol

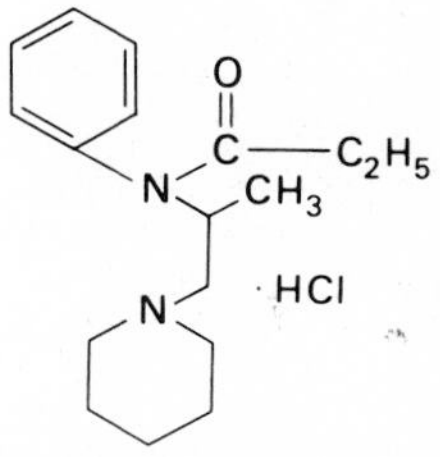

phenampromide HCl

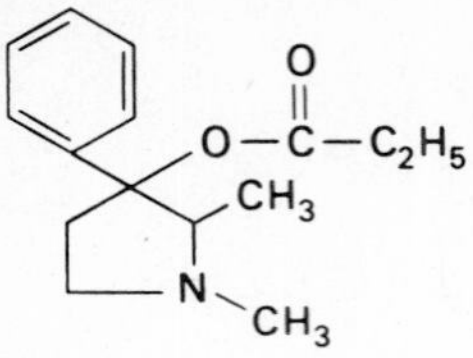

prodilidine (Cogesic)

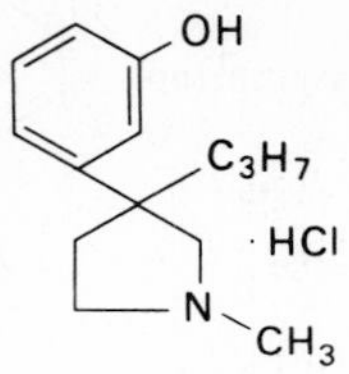

profadol HCl

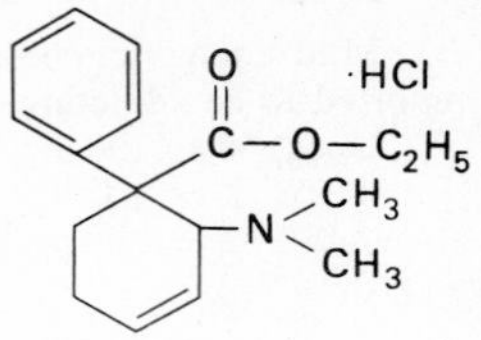

tilidine HCl

Antidiarrheal

DIPHENOXYLATE HYDROCHLORIDE (in Lomotil)

Strongly inhibitory of rhythmic contractions of smooth muscle; may be addicting. Used to control diarrhea: acute (as in food poisoning) or chronic (as in ulcerative colitis).

Dose: 5 mg 3 or 4 times a day by mouth. (Lomotil tablets contain 2.5 mg plus atropine 0.025 mg).

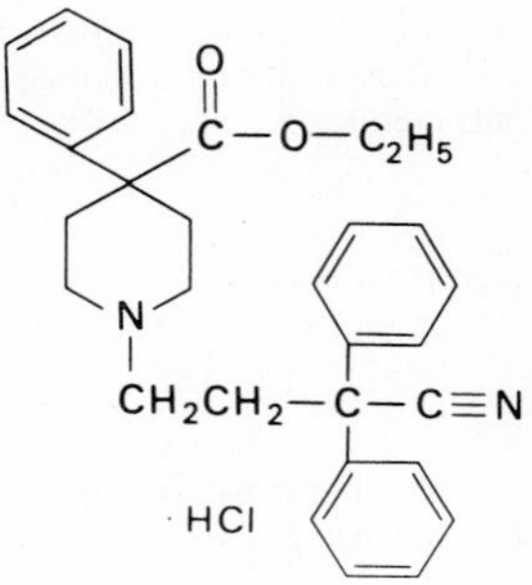

LOPERAMIDE HYDROCHLORIDE (Imodium)

Dose: 2.0 mg after each unformed stool.

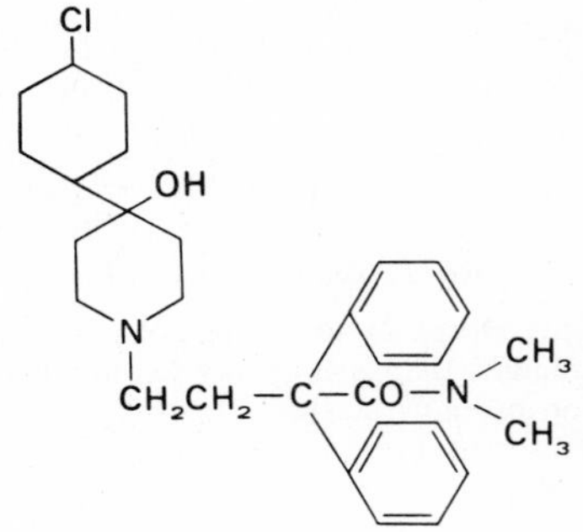

OTHERS

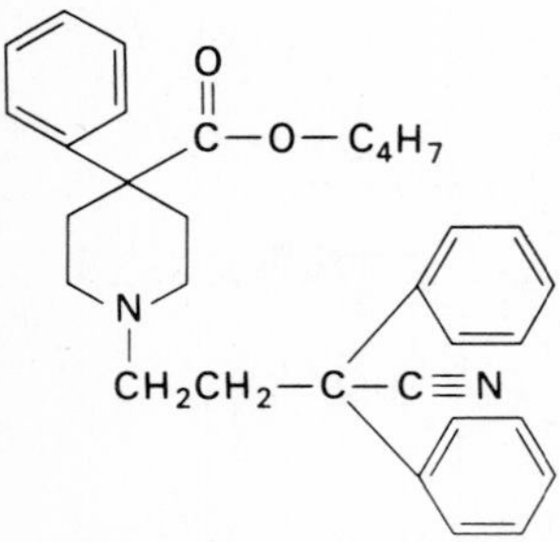

butoxylate HCl

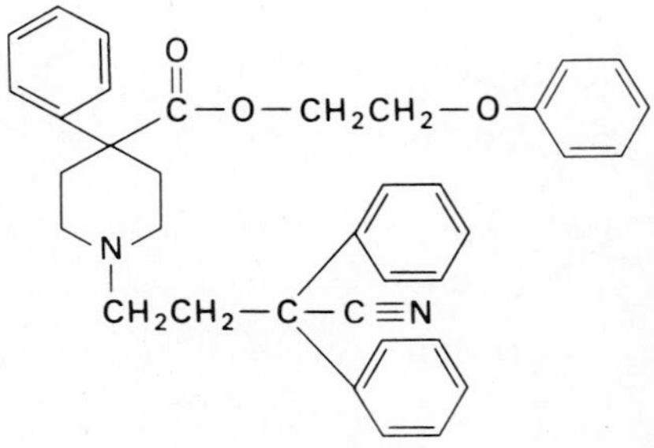

fetoxylate HCl

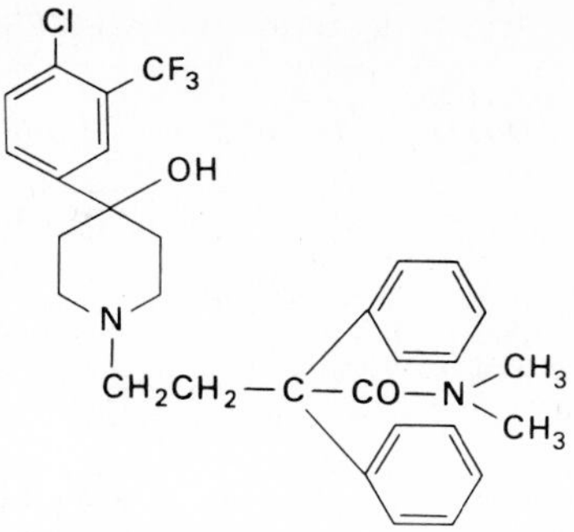

fluperamide

E. Others

METHOPHOLINE (Versidyne)

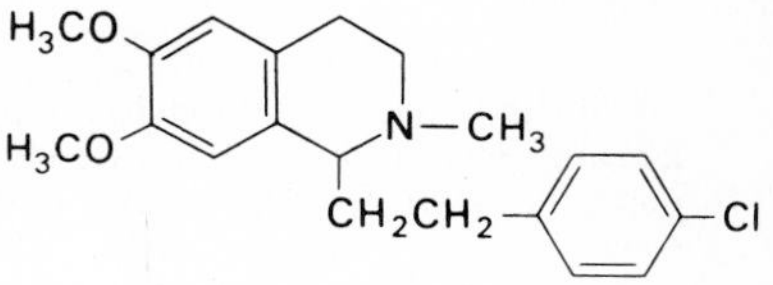

Benzoisoquinoline derivative. Analgesic parenterally (painful); weak antagonist of morphine abstinence.

Dose: 50 to 75 mg by mouth.

METHOTRIMEPRAZINE (Levoprome)

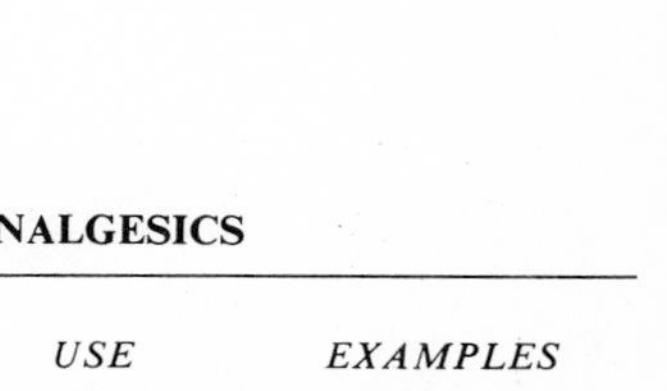

Phenothiazine analgesic comparable to morphine in potency, but producing less respiratory depression; not addicting; moderately sedative. Useful only in bed patients because of unpredictable orthostatic hypotension.

May cause drowsiness; nasal stuffiness, urinary retension.

Dose: 15 mg intramuscularly.

SUMMARY: NARCOTIC ANALGESICS

TYPE	*ACTION AND MECHANISM*	*TOXICITY*	*USE*	*EXAMPLES*
Opium	Quiet bowel Mechanism unknown	Sedation, addiction	Diarrhea	Paregoric
Morphine series	Analgesia sedation CNS and respiratory depression Smooth muscle contractions decreased Mechanism unknown	Respiratory depression, vomiting, addiction	Pain, cough, dyspnea	Morphine sulfate

(cont.)

SUMMARY: NARCOTIC ANALGESICS (cont.)

TYPE	*ACTION AND MECHANISM*	*TOXICITY*	*USE*	*EXAMPLES*
Codeine series	Same	Same	Same	Codeine sulfate
Antagonists	Same, but reverse effects of other morphine-type drugs	Worsening of morphine withdrawal	Opiate overdosage	Nalorphine
Methadone series	Similar to morphine	Similar to morphine	Pain, in morphine withdrawal	Methadone
Meperidine series	Same	Same	Pain, diarrhea	Meperidine

Reviews

Carroll, M., and Lim, R. Observations on neuropharmacology of morphine and morphine-like analgesia. Arch. Int. Pharmacodyn., 125:383, 1960.

Murphree, H. Clinical pharmacology of potent analgesics. Clin. Pharmacol. Ther., 3:473, 1962.

Grundfest, H. Effects of drugs on the central nervous system. Ann. Rev. Pharmacol., 4:341, 1964.

Lasagna, L. Clinical evaluation of morphine and its substitutes as analgesics. Pharmacol. Rev., 16:47, 1964.

Fraser, H., and Harris, L. Narcotic and narcotic antagonist analgesics. Ann. Rev. Pharmacol., 7:277, 1967.

Martin, W. Opioid antagonists. Pharmacol. Rev., 19:463, 1967.

51. Antitussives

Cough may be nonproductive or productive of sputum, this often being the sequence in disease. When nonproductive, suppression of the cough may be restful; when productive, suppression is still beneficially restful, but must be intermittent in order to allow periodic drainage of the sputum. Agents such as expectorants which make coughing easier by thinning the sputum may then also be of help.

A. Expectorants

1. Action and Mechanism. a. Expectorants are agents which facilitate coughing in productive coughs.

b. The mechanisms by which they act are diverse and not well understood, but physical changes in the character of the sputum in the direction of making it thinner and more profuse seem important.

2. Preparations

AMMONIUM CHLORIDE (NH_4Cl)

Thought to augment the sputum reflexly from irritation of the stomach.
Dose: 0.5 gm 3 times a day by mouth in liquid prescriptions.

SODIUM IODIDE (NaI, or other iodides)

Also considered to act through a gastric reflex, but locally as well, by osmotic effects as iodide is being secreted into the sputum.

Dose: 0.3 gm 3 times a day by mouth, usually in liquid prescriptions, saturated Solution of Sodium Iodide; Syrup Hydriodic Acid.

IPECAC (as syrup of ipecac)

Also thought to act through the gastric reflex.
Dose: 1 to 2 ml every 3 hours by mouth.

GLYCERYL GUAIACOLATE (guaiphenesin; Guaianesin)

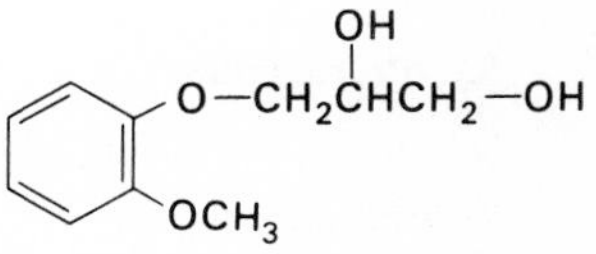

OH
O—CH_2CHCH_2—OH
OCH_3

Reduces viscosity of tenacious sputum; said to have value in dry, unproductive cough. Ingredient in proprietaries.

Dose: 100 to 200 mg every 2 to 4 hours by mouth.

TERPIN HYDRATE

Dose: 5 ml every 4 hours.

ACETYLCYSTEINE

Mucolytic.

CARBON DIOXIDE (CO_2)

Inhalation stimulates bronchial peristalsis and liquefies sputum.

STEAM

As inhalation, facilitates movement of sputum by moistening and lubricating; especially valuable in croup.

DETERGENTS

Loosen secretions and "roll them up" by surface action; they can then be coughed up more easily. Used in bronchial asthma, bronchitis, bronchiectasis. Example is "Alevaire" (contains Superinone, a detergent, plus sodium bicarbonate and glycerin) which is administered by aerosol produced in a special air compressor and nebulizer and delivered to a tent, face mask, or mouth or nose adapter; used an hour or more daily. Value uncertain (See Topical Agents).

B. Nonnarcotic Suppressives

1. Chemistry. The nonnarcotic suppressives are synthetics, most of which exhibit a combination of autonomic, antihistaminic, and local anesthetic action.

2. Action. Inhibit cough by various combinations of local anesthetic action, which anesthetizes the stretch receptors in the lungs; central suppression of the cough reflex at the vagal nuclei or other medullary centers; local drying of the respiratory tract; sedation. Most have not been studied adequately against pathological cough.

3. Pharmacodynamics and Toxicity. a. Most appear to be adequately absorbed and to act over 3 or 4 hours.

b. Members with local anesthetic action may numb the mouth; those with antihistaminic action may induce drowsiness, dizziness, excitation, depression; autonomics may produce dry mouth.

4. Uses. a. Most useful in mild, acute coughs, as in colds or bronchitis.

b. Simple coughs which result from irritation in the throat may often be suppressed by distraction of attention. Any thick, sweet, strongly flavored syrup or lozenge may suffice.

c. Coughing originating from irritation in the bronchi is less likely to respond to simple measures, and suppressives, both nonnarcotic and narcotic, may be useful.

5. Preparations

BENZONATATE (Tessalon)

Related to tetracaine.

Dose: 100 mg 3 times a day by mouth.

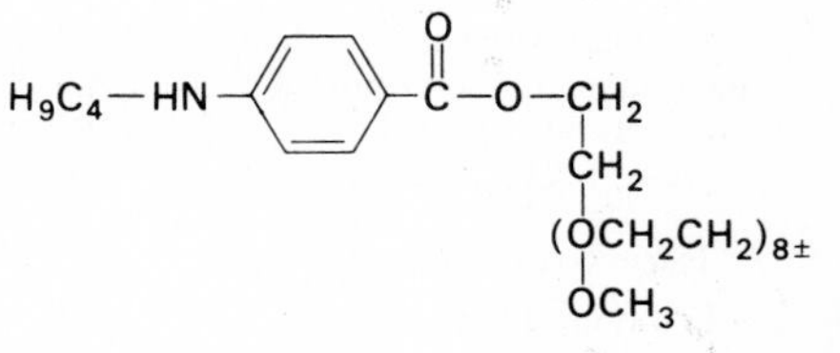

$H_9C_4{-}HN{-}C_6H_4{-}C(=O){-}O{-}CH_2{-}CH_2{-}(OCH_2CH_2)_{8\pm}{-}OCH_3$

CARBETAPENTANE CITRATE (Toclase)

Resembles antihistamines.

Dose: 15 to 30 mg 3 times a day by mouth.

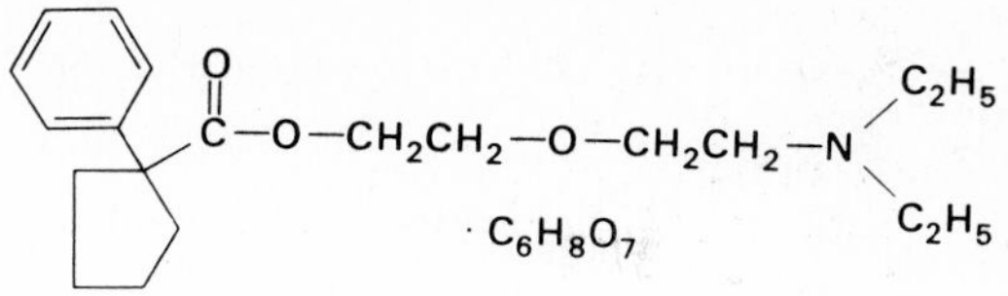

CHLOPHEDIANOL HYDROCHLORIDE (Detigon; ULO)

Slow action; peak in 3 hours, effect brief (2 hours).

Dose: 10 to 20 mg 3 times a day by mouth; usually given in a syrup.

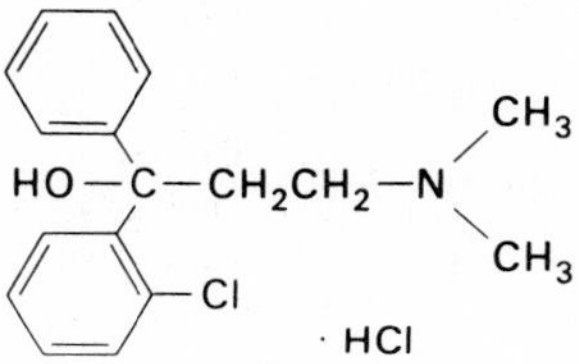

NOSCAPINE (narcotine; Nectadon)

Nonnarcotic, nonaddicting alkaloid from opium; mild antitussive.

Dose: 15 to 30 mg 3 times a day by mouth.

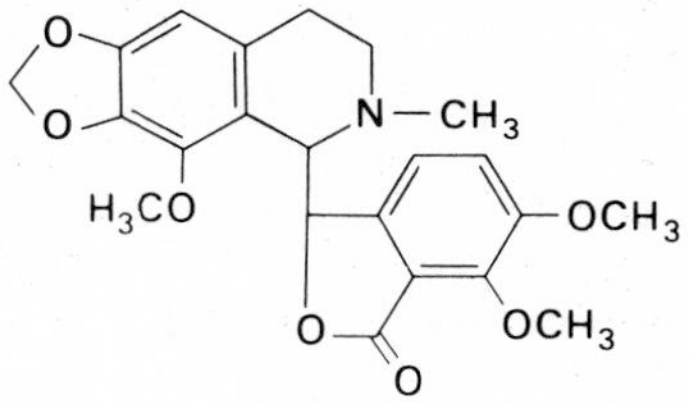

PIPAZETHATE HYDROCHLORIDE (Theratuss)

About one-half as antitussive as codeine. May cause bitter taste, nausea, tachycardia; little sedation.

Dose: 25 to 50 mg orally or by rectal suppository.

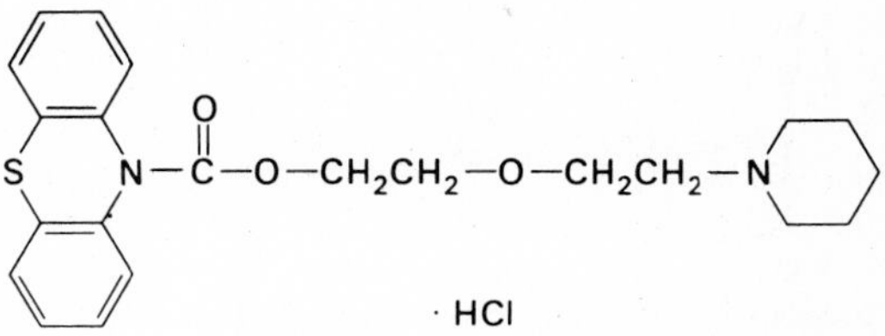

OTHERS

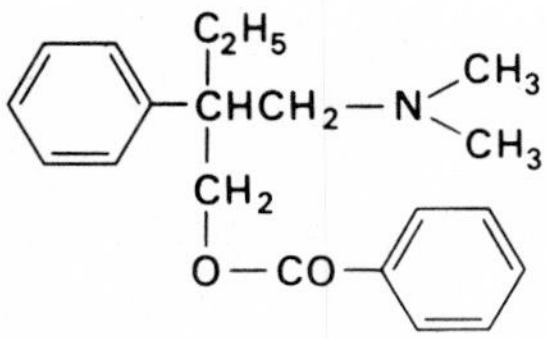

benzobutamine

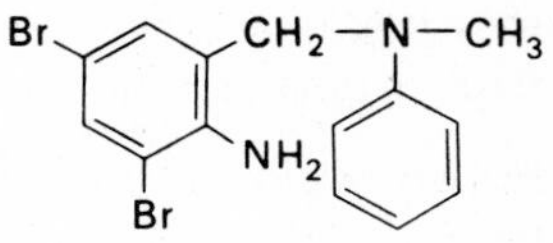

bromhexine HCl (Bisolvon)

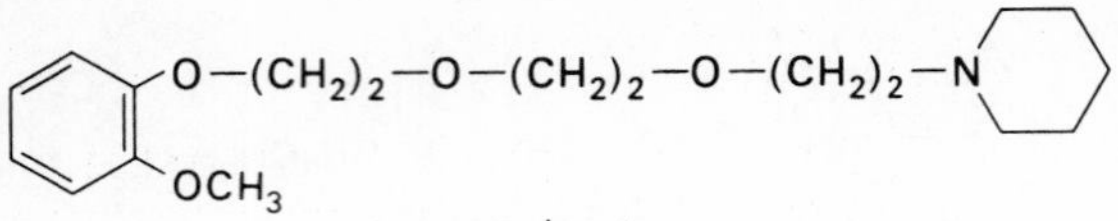

guaiapate

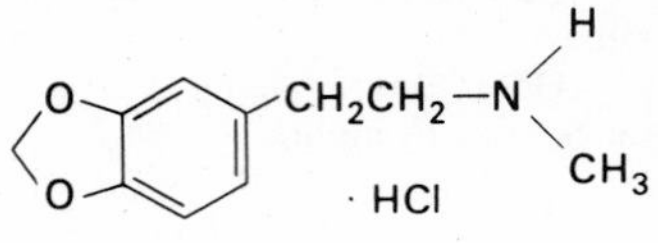

homarylamine HCl

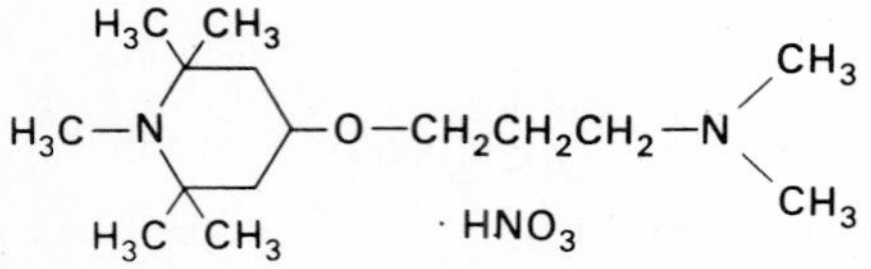

pemerid nitrate

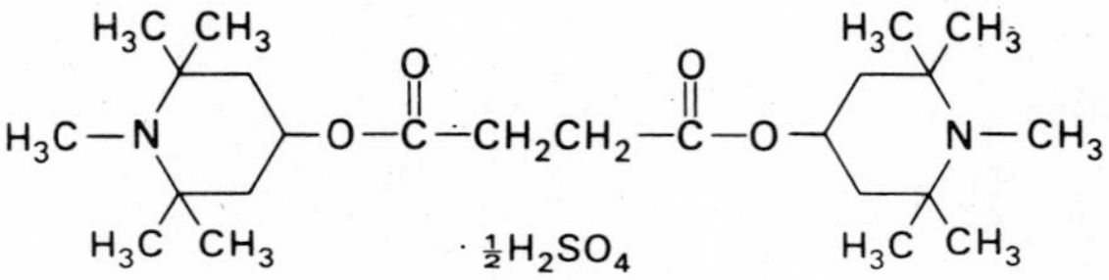

suxemerid sulfate

C. Narcotic Analgesics

CODEINE AND RELATIVES

The effects of codeine and numerous derivatives which depress cough by central medullary effects were considered in the previous chapter (see Narcotic Analgesics).

1. Preparations

CODEINE SULFATE

Should not be administered oftener than about every 4 hours in a productive cough in order to allow periodic escape from the suppressant.

Dose: 30 mg by mouth, or less.

Elexir terpin hydrate and codeine

Dose: 4 ml by mouth (contains 8 mg codeine).

DEXTROMETHORPHAN HYDROBROMIDE (Romilar)

Dose: 10 to 20 mg by mouth.

DROCODE BITARTRATE (Didrate)

Dose: 10 to 60 mg by mouth.

HYDROCODONE BITARTRATE (Dicodid)

Dose: 5 mg by mouth.

OXYCODONE HYDROCHLORIDE (in mixture, Percodan)

Dose: 10 mg orally.

SUMMARY: ANTITUSSIVES

TYPE	*ACTION AND MECHANISM*	*TOXICITY*	*USE*	*EXAMPLES*
Expectorant	Thin and increase sputum by osmotic or gastric reflex effect	Minor	To facilitate coughing	Ammonium Cl
Nonnarcotic suppressives	Inhibit coughing Mechanism not clear	Minor	To reduce coughing	Carbetapentane citrate
Narcotic suppressives	Inhibit coughing by depression of coughing center	Sedation, respiratory depression, addiction	Same	Codeine sulfate

Reviews

Bickerman, H. Clinical pharmacology of antitussive agents. Clin. Pharmacol. Ther., 3:353, 1962.
Doyle, F., and Mehta, M. Antitussives. Advances Drug Res., 1:107, 1964.
Salem, H., and Aviado, D. Antitussive Agents. London, Pergamon Press, 1970.
Boyd, E. Review of studies on the pharmacology of the expectorants and inhalants. Int. Z. Klin. Pharmakol. Toxik. 3:55, 1970.

52.
Sedatives and Hypnotics

Sedatives and hypnotics are agents conducive to calm or sleep. Sleep is a periodic state of rest and repair, in part a conditioned reflex; like appetite, the desire for sleep becomes acute, and then wanes. Insomnia, although sometimes associated with pain, is largely the result of the carry-over of unsolved problems from the day.

Drugs which allay apprehension, and drugs which assist sleep, are among the most useful in medicine, but are often gravely abused to avoid more direct, and ultimately more satisfactory, solutions to problems.

A. Halogenated Hydrocarbons

1. History. Chloral hydrate was synthesized by Liebig (1832) and introduced by Liebrich (1869). It was the first sedative to supplant opium and alcohol (used in "Mickey Finns" since 1870).

2. Chemistry. Series of halogenated hydrocarbons; related to chloroform.

3. Action and Mechanism. a. Central depressants inducing calm, sleep, and even anesthesia, according to dose used.

b. Respiratory and cardiovascular depression not marked by therapeutic dosage.

c. Mechanism not known but probably similar to that of other anesthetics.

4. Pharmacodynamics. a. Chloral hydrate is absorbed quickly (20 minutes); effects last 4 to 8 hours.

b. It is transformed into trichloroethanol, the principal agent present during the sedation, and excreted largely in the form of glucuronide (urochloralic acid).

c. Related derivatives generally resemble chloral hydrate, but have less unpleasant smells.

5. Toxicity. Relatively safe, but overdosage of chloral hydrate may give cardiac depression; fatal dose of chloral hydrate about 10 gm.

6. Uses. Chloral hydrate is a desirable hypnotic, especially in the elderly, because it gives a quick, relatively short sedation, without sequelae such as follow barbiturates. However, it is less convenient than the barbiturates and much less widely used; it may be useful in patients sensitive to barbiturates.

7. Preparations

CHLORAL HYDRATE

Dose: 0.5 to 2 gm by mouth, administered in solution, syrup, or capsules.

Chloral betaine (Beta-chlor)

Dose: 870 mg (500 mg chloral hydrate).

$(HO)_2CH{-}CCl_3$

CHLORHEXADOL (Lora)

Hydrolyzes to chloral hydrate in stomach.

Dose: 1.6 gm (1 gm chloral hydrate).

$H_3C{-}C(CH_3)(OH){-}CH_2{-}CH(CH_3){-}O{-}CH(OH){-}CCl_3$

CHLOROBUTANOL (Chloretone)

Used as a preservative for drugs and as an anesthetic for animals. Obsolete in human therapy.

$H_3C{-}C(OH)(CH_3){-}CCl_3$

PETRICHLORAL (Perichlor)

Slowly hydrolyzed to chloral hydrate and pentaerythritol in stomach.

Dose: 0.3 to 0.6 gm by mouth.

$C[CH_2{-}O{-}CH(OH){-}CCl_3]_4$

TRICLOFOS SODIUM

Breaks down to trichloroethanol.

Dose: 750 mg.

$NaO{-}P(=O)(OH){-}O{-}CH_2{-}CCl_3$

OTHERS

$HO{-}CH(NH{-}C(=O){-}C_2H_5){-}CCl_3$

carbochloral

$Cl_3C{-}CH_2OCOCH_2{-}CCl_3$

clorethate

B. Bromides

1. **History.** a. Glover (1842) showed depression in animals from bromide.
   b. Locock (1857) used in epilepsy; Behrend (1864) used as a clinical sedative.

2. Chemistry. Cation indifferent; KBr and NaBr common salts. Organic compounds not sedative.

3. Action and Mechanism. a. Produce both motor and sensory depression.

b. Mechanism not known, but probably a specific of the Br ions, and not the result of massive displacement of chloride (Goodwin, Nature, 221:556, 1969).

4. Pharmacology. a. Well absorbed.

b. Distribution wide with gradual replacement of chloride; excretion slow, by the chloride mechanism. At 1 gm per day, an effective level is not reached for one week; in one month this accumulates to a toxic level.

5. Toxicity. a. Bromism begins as confusion and may proceed to psychosis; after a period of excitement resembling delirium tremens, depression and apathy appear.

b. Particularly in persons with seborrhea, dermatitis also is produced.

c. Therapeutic blood levels are below 50 mg%; in poisoning they may reach 150 to 200 mg%.

d. Treatment is by the administration of chloride to replace the bromide; recovery may not be complete for 2 or 3 weeks.

6. Uses. Bromides have almost no use in modern medicine, having been replaced by less toxic drugs. However, they may still be found in proprietary sedatives and analgesics, and represent potential toxicity.

7. Preparation

SODIUM OR POTASSIUM BROMIDE (NaBr, KBr)

Practically obsolete.
Dose: 1 gm 3 times a day by mouth.

C. Paraldehyde

1. History. Cervello (1882) introduced into medicine.

2. Chemistry. Pungent, disagreeable polymer of acetaldehyde.

3. Action and Mechanism. a. Powerful CNS depressant, resembling alcohol in effects.

b. Produces moderately prolonged sleep (8 to 12 hours) with little or no motor or medullary depression.

4. Pharmacodynamics and Toxicity. a. Rapidly absorbed by mouth, but offensive smell makes administration difficult by this route except in alcoholics; fairly well absorbed from the rectum.

b. About one fourth of the administered drug is exhaled; most of the balance is metabolized.

c. It has a wide margin of safety, but 30 ml has been fatal.

d. Tolerance and dependence develop upon chronic usage.

5. Uses. An excellent sedative, but the offensive odor limits its use for the most part to alcoholics and psychotics. Should not be given with disulfiram as effects similar to those of disulfiram and alcohol may be produced.

6. Preparation

PARALDEHYDE

Dose: 4 to 20 ml by mouth or by rectum; 1 ml intramuscularly or intravenously.

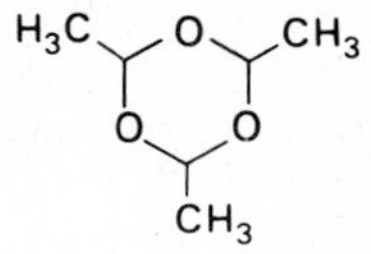

D. Carbamates, Ureides, and Higher Alcohols

The recent interest in tranquilizing drugs has renewed the use of a number of rather mild sedatives, and new examples have been introduced. There are resemblances between several of these compounds and the muscle relaxants and tranquilizers.

1. Chemistry. Variously composed carbamates, ureides, and higher alcohols; some are related also to propanediol muscle relaxants (mephenesin).

2. Action and Mechanism. a. Mild to moderately strong sedatives and hypnotics; some, such as meprobamate, are often assumed to be specific tranquilizers or muscle relaxants, but the principal effect is very similar to that of phenobarbital.

b. The mechanism of the sedation is unknown; any element of specific muscle relaxation would be due to internuncial neuron block in the spinal cord.

3. Pharmacodynamics and Toxicity. a. Satisfactorily absorbed by mouth; excreted largely as derivative substances.

b. In general of low toxicity, but serious toxicity has been noted from some of the drugs, as indicated individually.

4. Uses. As mild hypnotics and tranquilizers; in anxiety, tension headaches.

5. Preparations

a. Carbamates

BURAMATE

Sedative and anticonvulsant.
Under investigation.

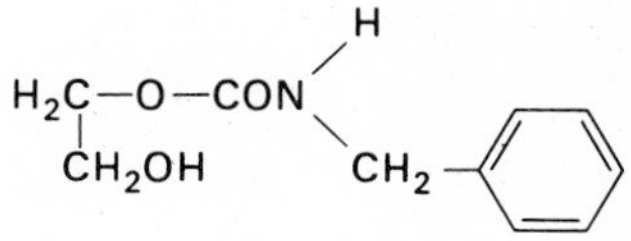

CINTRIAMIDE

Under investigation.

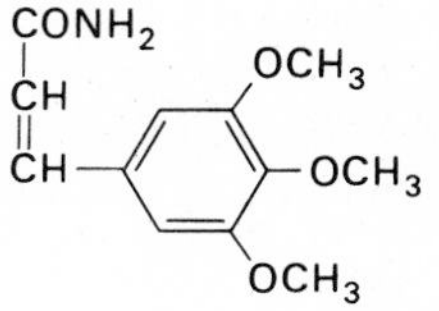

EMYLCAMATE (Nuncital; Striatran)

Has muscle relaxing properties as well as mild sedation.

Dose: 0.2 gm 3 or 4 times a day by mouth.

CH_3
$H_5C_2-C-O-CONH_2$
C_2H_5

ETHINAMATE (Valmid)

Dose: 0.5 gm 3 times a day by mouth.

$O-CONH_2$
$C\equiv CH$

HYDROXYPHENAMATE (Listica)

Dose: 200 mg 4 times a day by mouth.

$H_2-C-O-CONH_2$
H_5C_2-C-OH

MEBUTAMATE (Capla)

Sold as a central hypotensive (vasomotor center).

Dose: 300 mg 4 times a day by mouth.

$O-CONH_2$
H_3C-C
$O-CONH_2$
$H_3C-C-CH_3$
C_2H_5

MEPROBAMATE (Equanil, Miltown)

Meprobamate may produce tremulousness, nausea, depression; allergic symptoms (urticaria. petechiae, anaphylactoid phenomena, rash); thrombocytopenia; intolerance to alcohol; convulsions and other withdrawal symptoms of addiction reported after high, continued administration.

Dose: 400 mg 3 times a day by mouth.

$H_2-C-O-CONH_2$
$H_7C_3-C-CH_3$
$H_2-C-O-CONH_2$

OXANAMIDE (Quiactin)

Mild sedative.

Dose: 400 mg 3 times a day by mouth.

$CONH_2$
H_5C_2-C
O
H_7C_3-C
H

TYBAMATE (Solacen)

Dose: 250 to 500 mg 3 to 4 times a day by mouth.

$H_2-C-O-CONH-C_4H_9$
$H_7C_3-C-CH_3$
$H_2-C-O-CONH_2$

URETHAN

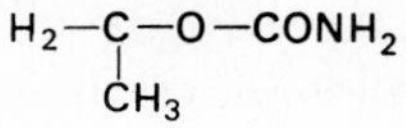

$H_2—C—O—CONH_2$
$\quad\;\; CH_3$

Used as an anesthetic in animals; also used in man for its antineoplastic actions (see Cancer Chemotherapy).

OTHERS

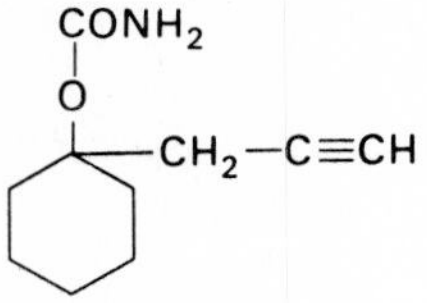

$CONH_2$
O
$—CH_2—C{\equiv}CH$

hexapropymate

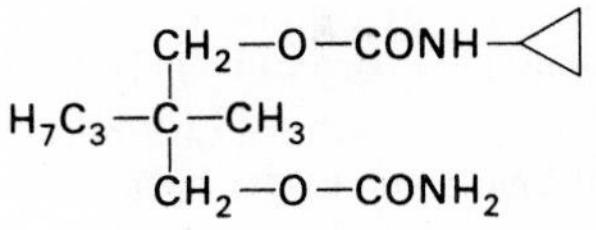

$CH_2—O—CONH—◁$
$H_7C_3—C—CH_3$
$CH_2—O—CONH_2$

lorbamate

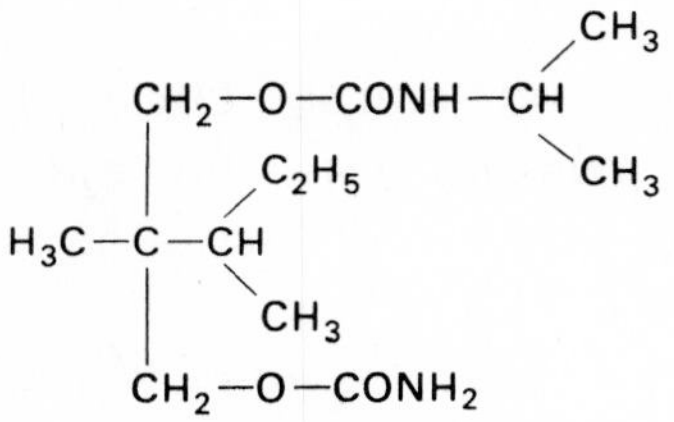

$CH_2—O—CONH—CH(CH_3)_2$
$H_3C—C—CH(C_2H_5)(CH_3)$
$CH_2—O—CONH_2$

nisobamate

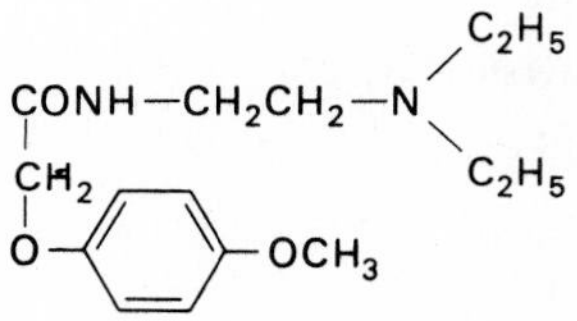

$CONH—CH_2CH_2—N(C_2H_5)_2$
CH_2
$O—C_6H_4—OCH_3$

mefexamide

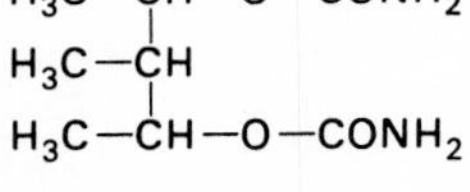

$H_3C—CH—O—CONH_2$
$H_3C—CH$
$H_3C—CH—O—CONH_2$

pentabamate

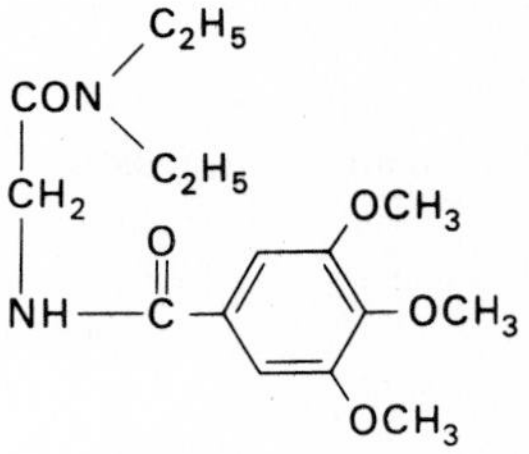

$CON(C_2H_5)_2$
CH_2
$NH—C(=O)—C_6H_2(OCH_3)_3$

tricetamide

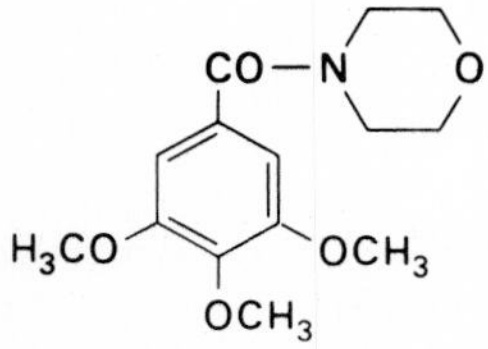

$CO—N(morpholine)O$
$H_3CO \quad OCH_3$
OCH_3

trimetozine

CH_3
$H_5C_2—C—O—CONH_2$
$C{\equiv}CH$

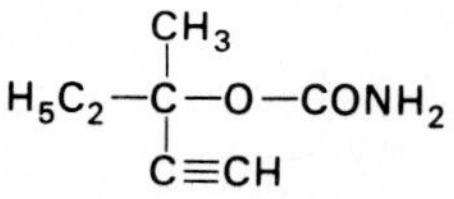

methylpentenylcarbamate

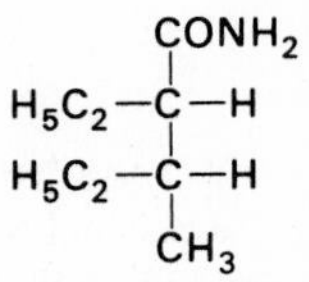

$CONH_2$
$H_5C_2—C—H$
$H_5C_2—C—H$
CH_3

valnoctamide

b. Ureides

ALLYLISOPROPYLACETYLCARBAMIDE (Sedormid)

Little used in the United States because of thrombocytopenia, but still used in Europe.

$$\begin{array}{l} NH{-}CO{-}CH(CH(CH_3)_2)(CH_2CH{=}CH_2) \\ \; | \\ C{=}O \\ \; | \\ NH_2 \end{array}$$

BROMISOVALUM (Bromural)

Slightly longer acting than carbromal.
Dose: 0.3 gm 3 times a day by mouth.

$$\begin{array}{l} NH{-}CO{-}CH(Br){-}CH(CH_3)_2 \\ \; | \\ C{=}O \\ \; | \\ NH_2 \end{array}$$

CAPURIDE

Under investigation.

$$\begin{array}{l} NH_2 \\ \; | \\ C{=}O \\ \; | \\ NH{-}CO{-}CH(C_2H_5){-}CH(CH_3){-}C_2H_5 \end{array}$$

CARBROMAL (Adalin; and others)

Feeble, short acting hypnotic; little used.
Dose: 0.3 gm 3 times a day by mouth.

$$\begin{array}{l} NH{-}CO{-}C(C_2H_5)_2{-}Br \\ \; | \\ C{=}O \\ \; | \\ NH_2 \end{array}$$

ECTYLUREA (Nostyn)

Dose: 150 to 300 mg 3 times a day by mouth.

$$\begin{array}{l} NH{-}CO{-}C(C_2H_5){=}CHCH_3 \\ \; | \\ C{=}O \\ \; | \\ NH_2 \end{array}$$

c. Higher alcohols

ETHCHLORVYNOL (Placidyl)

Mild sedative; used for insomnia.
Dose: 0.1 to 0.5 gm 3 or 4 times a day by mouth.

$$\begin{array}{c} CH{=}CHCl \\ | \\ H_5C_2{-}C{-}OH \\ | \\ C{\equiv}CH \end{array}$$

MEPARAFYNOL (Dormison)

Weak but nontoxic in sedative doses; anticonvulsant in subtoxic doses (hepatic damage).

Dose: 250 mg 4 times a day by mouth.

$$\begin{array}{c} CH_3 \\ | \\ H_5C_2{-}C{-}OH \\ | \\ C{\equiv}CH \end{array}$$

PHENAGLYCODOL (Ultran)

Produces drowsiness; probably little more than a placebo.

Dose: 300 mg 3 times a day by mouth.

Metaglycodol (meta isomer).

CH_3
$H_3C-C-OH$
$H_3C-C-OH$
Cl

E. Sulfones

1. Chemistry

H_3C $SO_2-C_2H_5$
C
H_3C $SO_2-C_2H_5$

sulfonal

H_3C $SO_2-C_2H_5$
C
H_5C_2 $SO_2-C_2H_5$

trional

2. Actions and Uses. Obsolete sedatives; Excessive toxicity; slow absorption with cumulation, hangover, dermatitis, porphyria, methemoglobinemia.

F. Barbiturates

1. History. a. A. von Baeyer (1864) synthesized barbituric acid.

b. Fischer and von Mering (1903) introduced barbital (diethylbarbituric acid) as a hypnotic.

2. Chemistry. a. Hydropyrimidine derivatives (malonylureas) with over 1,200 possible substitutions at C5 of pento or less.

b. Duration of activity dependent primarily upon substitutions at C5.

3. Actions

a. CNS:

a′. Low doses: Depression of sensory functions; sedation without analgesia, drowsiness; anticonvulsant.

b′. High doses: Depression of motor functions, then depression of medullary centers (circulatory and respiratory); increasing sedation, sleep, anesthesia.

b. Other systems: Blood sugar elevated; smooth muscle depressed; metabolic rate not greatly affected.

4. Mechanism. a. In sedative and hypnotic doses barbiturates appear to act principally at the level of the thalamus and the ascending reticular formation, with interference with the transmission of impulses to the cortex.

b. Underlying mechanism has not been completely explained; inhibition of enzymatic conversion of pyruvate to acetate may be involved.

c. May increase microsomal enzymatic activity involved in detoxification of other compounds.

5. Pharmacodynamics. a. Absorption is good by any route; parenteral use requires soluble sodium salts, which are alkaline (and therefore irritating).

b. Most are altered and broken down in the liver, but barbital (100 %), and phenobarbital (20 %), excreted by the kidneys.

c. Barbiturates (and other drugs) may stimulate the enzymes responsible for their own metabolism. This may, in part, explain tolerance and barbiturate-induced porphyria.

6. Toxicity. a. Overdosage produces severe depression, proceeding to coma and respiratory cessation.

b. Treat with artificial respiration if needed; warmth, gastric lavage and purge, "universal antidote" (charcoal, tannin, magnesium oxide), supportive fluids, oxygen, alkalinization of the urine, diuretics; stimulants controversial (amphetamine, picrotoxin, nikethamide, and others; see Stimulants); artificial kidney (Hadden, J.A.M.A., 209:893, 1969).

c. Occasional idiosyncrasies, especially rash.

d. Chronic poisoning characterized by confusion, dermatitis, addiction, and withdrawal syndrome (see Drug Addiction).

7. Uses. a. Anesthesia, acute sedation, or chronic sedation, depending upon the type of compound:

ACTION	*ONSET*	*DURATION*	*USES*
ultrashort	seconds	minutes	intravenous anesthesia (see General Anesthetics)
short	minutes	4–8 hours	brief hypnosis; preoperative sedation; insomnia
intermediate	1 hour	6–8 hours	insomnia
long	1 + hour	10–12 hours	continuous sedation; hypertension, psychoneurosis, epilepsy

b. Bases used by mouth; sodium salts by mouth, or parenterally.

c. Commercially available preparations present extensive duplication. In practice (excluding anesthesia), a short or intermediate drug, such as secobarbital or pentobarbital, and a long acting type, such as phenobarbital, will suffice for all needs.

8. Preparations

a. Short-acting

BUTALBITAL (allylbarbituric acid; Sandoptal)

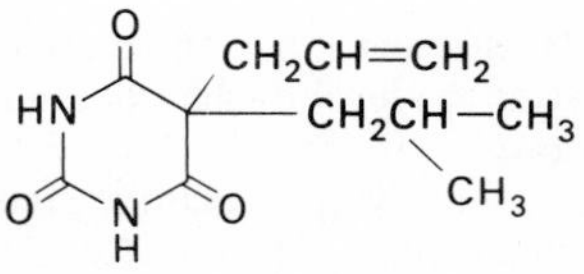

Dose: 0.2 to 0.4 gm by mouth.

O
HN
$CH_2CH{=}CH_2$
$CH_2CH{-}CH_3$
CH_3
O N O
H

CYCLOBARBITAL (Phanodorn)

Dose: 0.1 to 0.3 gm by mouth.

HEPTABARBITAL (Medomin)

Dose: 0.2 to 0.4 gm by mouth.

HEXOBARBITAL (Sombucaps)

Dose: 250 to 500 mg by mouth.

PENTOBARBITAL (Nembutal)

Dose: 0.1 to 0.2 gm by mouth; 0.1 to 0.5 gm intravenously (sodium salt).

SECOBARBITAL (Seconal)

Dose: 0.1 to 0.2 gm by mouth.

b. Intermediate-acting

ALLOBARBITAL

Dose: 0.1 to 0.3 gm by mouth.

AMOBARBITAL (Amytal)

Dose: 0.1 to 0.3 gm by mouth; 0.1 to 0.5 gm intravenously (sodium salt).

APROBARBITAL (Alurate)

Dose: 50 to 150 mg by mouth.

BUTABARBITAL (Butisol)

Dose: 50 to 200 mg by mouth.

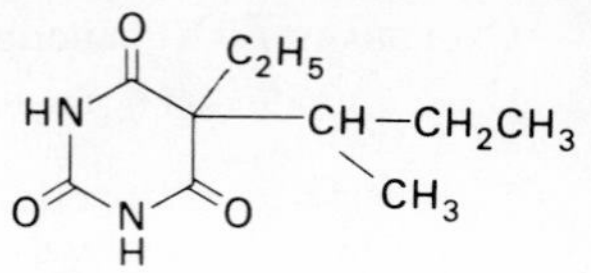

BUTALLYLONAL (Pernoston)

Dose: 0.2 gm by mouth.

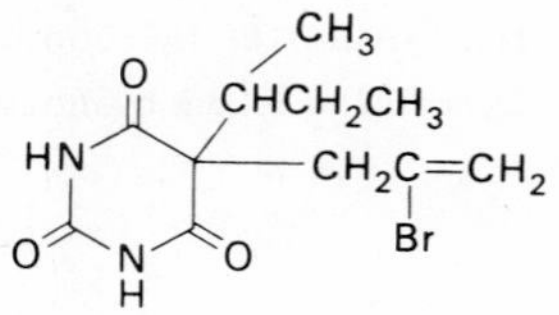

PROBARBITAL CALCIUM OR SODIUM (Ipral)

Dose: 0.2 to 0.4 gm by mouth

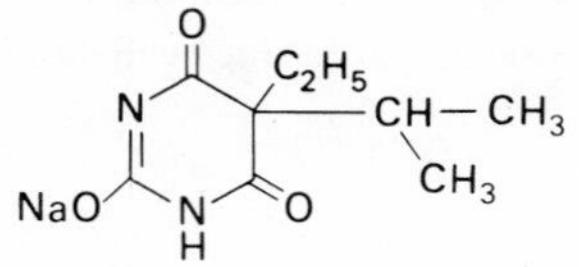

TALBUTAL (Lotusate)

Dose: 50 to 200 mg by mouth.

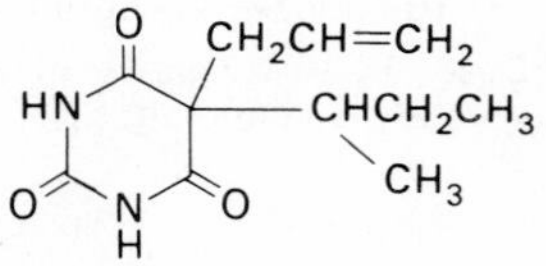

VINBARBITAL (Delvinal)

Dose: 0.1 to 0.4 gm by mouth.

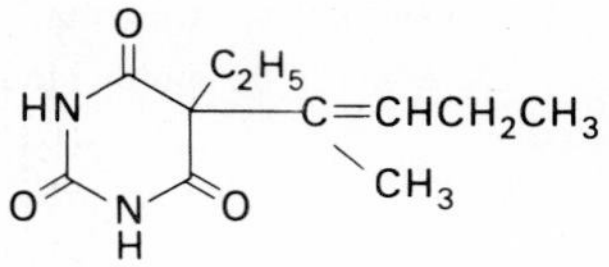

c. *Long-acting*

BARBITAL (Veronal)

Dose: 0.1 to 0.4 gm 3 times a day by mouth.

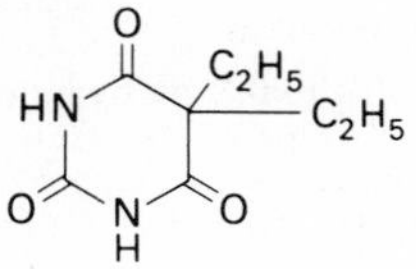

MEPHOBARBITAL (Mebaral)

Converted to phenobarbital in the body, and probably acts as such.

Dose: 30 to 60 mg 3 or 4 times a day by mouth.

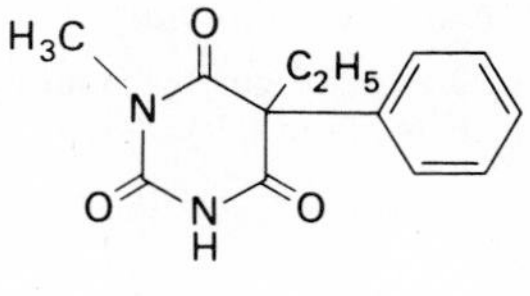

PHENOBARBITAL (Luminal)

Dose: 15 to 60 mg 1 to 4 times a day by mouth; 0.1 to 0.4 gm subcutaneously (sodium salt). Elixir of phenobarbital contains 4 mg per ml.

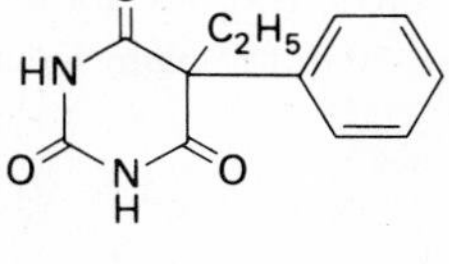

G. Glutarimide Derivatives and Related Groups

1. Chemistry. Piperidine derivatives; general resemblance to the barbiturates.

2. Action and Mechanism. a. Mild hypnotics, comparable to the short-acting barbiturates.

b. Mechanism of action not known.

3. Pharmacodynamics and Toxicity. a. Absorbed adequately by mouth.

b. Almost entirely metabolized by hydroxylation and conjugation.

c. Side effects relatively minor, but headache, nausea, and vertigo have been noted; rash common after glutethimide, and prolonged use has caused fever, psychosis, and addiction; addiction also reported after methyprylon.

4. Uses. Mild hypnotics for daytime sedation and for control of insomnia.

5. Preparations

GLUTETHIMIDE (Doriden)

Dose: 250 mg 3 times a day by mouth; 0.5 gm (to induce sleep).

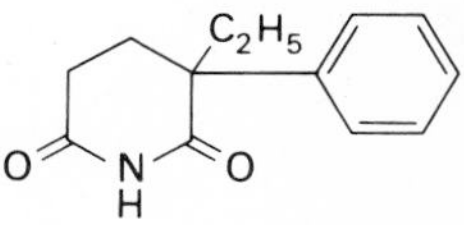

METHYPRYLON (Noludar)

Dose: 50 to 100 mg 3 times a day; 0.2 to 0.4 gm (to induce sleep).

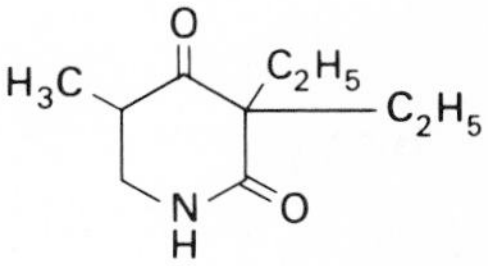

THALIDOMIDE (Kevadon)

Teratogenic when taken in early pregnancy (may cause monsters with phocomelia or other defects).

Action may be "antiimmune" and prevent rejection of fetus that had runt disease. Under trial against leprosy (inhibits lepra reaction that often follows sulfone treatment). Never marketed in the United States.

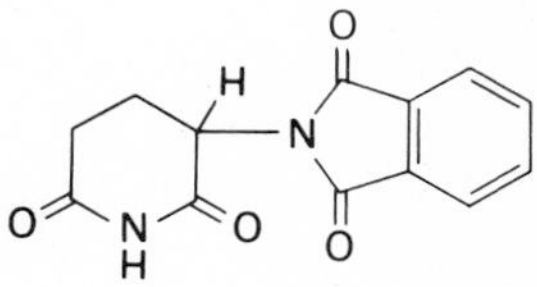

OTHERS

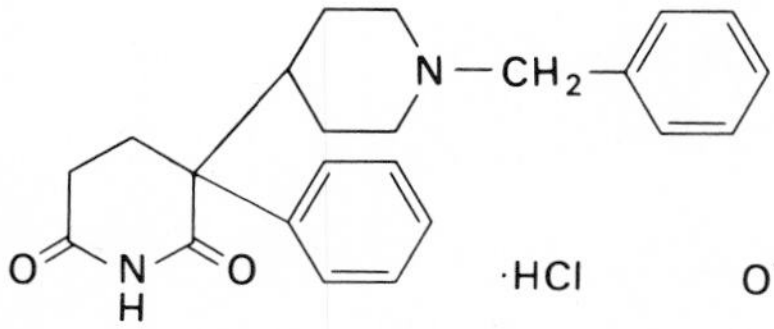

·HCl

benzetimide hydrochloride

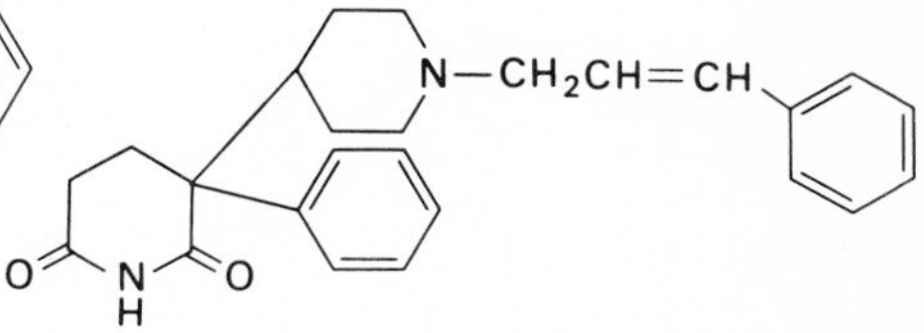

cinperene

dexetimide (dextroratatory isomer of benzetimide)

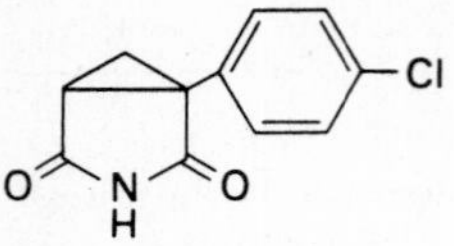

cyproximide

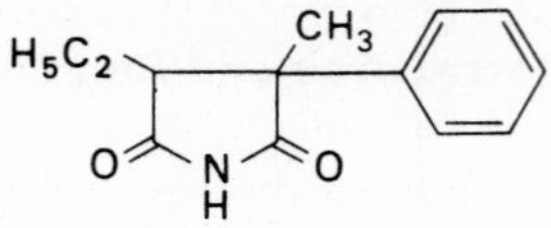

fenimide

H. Quinazolones

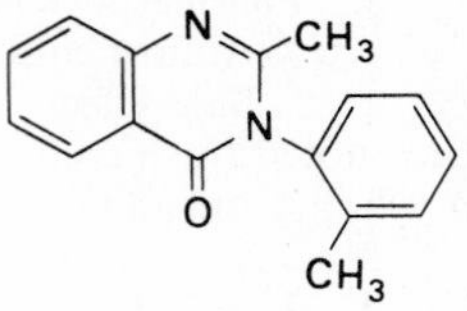

METHAQUALONE (Qualude)

Resembles short acting barbiturates.

Dose: 75 mg 4 times a day by mouth, or 150 to 300 mg at bedtime.

OTHERS

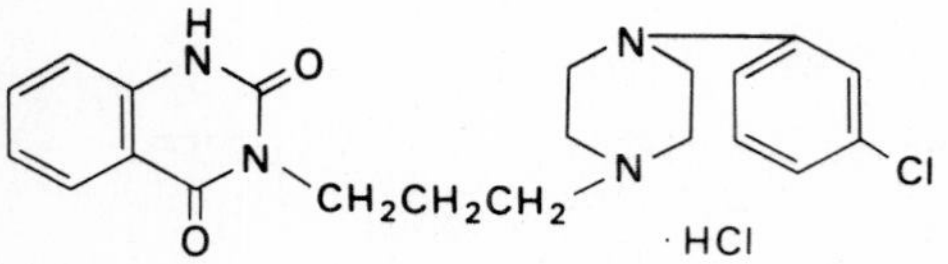

cloperidone HCl

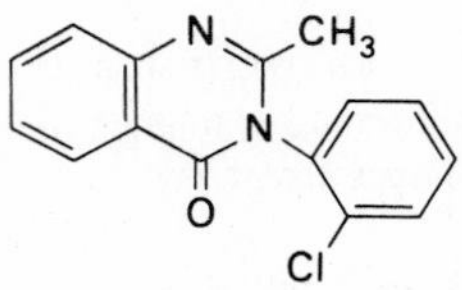

mecloqualone

I. Others

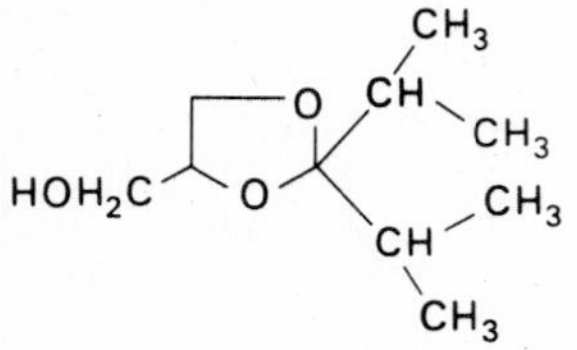

meproxarax

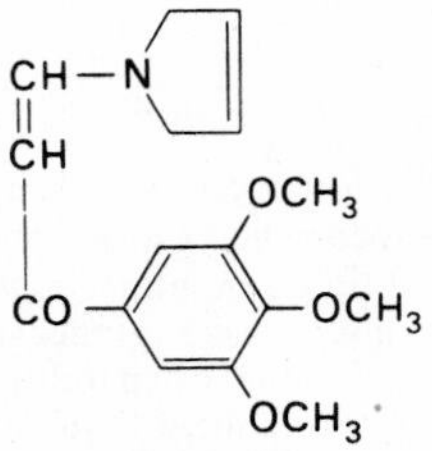

roletamide

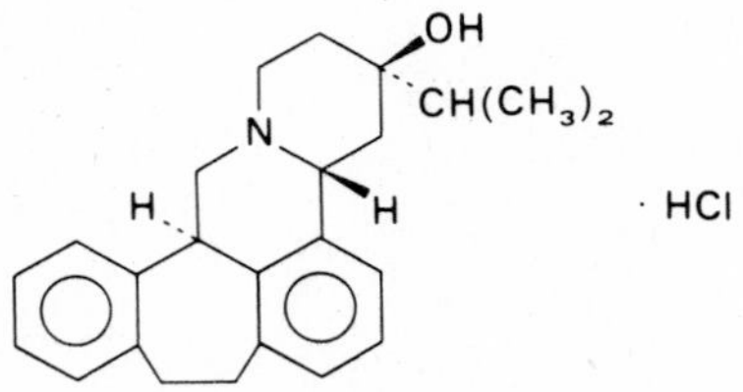

dexclamol hydrochloride

SUMMARY: SEDATIVES AND HYPNOTICS

TYPE	*ACTION AND MECHANISM*	*TOXICITY*	*USE*	*EXAMPLES*
Halogenated hydrocarbons	Central depression Mechanism unknown	Respiratory or cardiac depression	Insomnia	Choral
Bromides	Same	Confusion, dermatitis	Obsolete	Sodium bromide
Paraldehyde	Same	Respiratory depression, offensive smell	Sedative in alcoholics	Paraldehyde
Carbamates, ureides, and higher alcohols	Same	minimal, but addiction possible	Mild sedation	Meprobamate
Barbiturates	Same	Respiratory depression, Addiction possible	Sedation	Phenobarbital
Glutarimides	Same	Same	Same	Glutethimide

Reviews

Toman, J. Some aspects of central nervous system pharmacology. Ann. Rev. Pharmacol., 3:153, 1963.

Mark, L. Metabolism of barbiturates in man. Clin. Pharmacol. Ther., 4:504, 1963.

Grundfest, H. Effect of drugs on the central nervous system. Ann. Rev. Pharmacol., 4:341, 1964.

Burns, J. Implications of enzyme induction for drug therapy. Amer. J. Med., 37:327, 1964.

53. Anticonvulsants

Idiopathic epilepsy occurs as major convulsive seizures (grand mal), as momentary pauses of consciousness (petit mal), and as psychomotor attacks (epileptic equivalents), in which bizarre, autonomic actions replace actual convulsions, and in which consciousness is impaired rather than lost. In Jacksonian attacks only part of the body is involved and the cause may be a discernible local lesion in the brain rather than idiopathic. The incidence of epilepsy is about 1 in 200 of the population at large. Convulsions may also occur as symptoms in trauma, poisoning, and asphyxia.

Therapy of an acute convulsion, other than protective, is seldom possible, but continuing convulsions (status epilepticus) may be interrupted by intravenous diazepam, barbiturates, neuromuscular blocking agents, or general anesthesia. Historically, the bromides were the first widely used, effective drugs, but now have been almost entirely replaced by less toxic and more effective drugs.

A. The Barbiturate Group

The general qualities of the barbiturates are discussed in the preceding chapter (Sedatives and Hypnotics).

1. History. Hauptmann (1912) introduced phenobarbital as an antiepileptic drug, shortly after it was first used as a sedative; in the course of the next 15 years it had generally replaced bromides.

2. Chemistry. Barbiturates and closely allied compounds.

3. Action and Mechanism. a. Exert prophylactic influences against most types of epilepsy, as part of the general barbiturate action. Cortical arousal mechanisms suppressed.

b. Mechanism not known. Decreased sensitivity of neurones to abnormal electrical discharges.

c. Long-acting forms chosen because continuous suppression of epilepsy without excessive sedation more easily obtained with them, but sedation still a complication of barbiturate therapy.

4. Pharmacology and Toxicity. a. Methylated derivatives are probably slowly demethylated in the body and represent only a devious way of administering the basic compounds (Butler, Neurology, 8:106, 1958).

b. Mephobarbital may produce more skin rashes and febrile episodes than phenobarbital, but possibly less sedation.

5. Uses. a. Phenobarbital is effective in all types of epilepsy, but especially grand mal seizures.

b. In use, the accompanying sedation is usually a limiting factor, and may necessitate the simultaneous administration of another anticonvulsant as well.

c. Therapy should be continuous, without intermissions which might allow escape from control.

6. Preparations

PHENOBARBITAL (Luminal)

Dose: 15 to 100 mg 3 times a day by mouth.

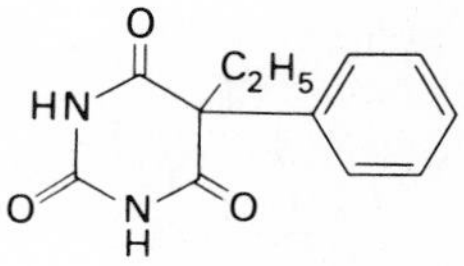

MEPHOBARBITAL (Mebaral)

Dose: 30 to 100 mg 3 times a day by mouth.

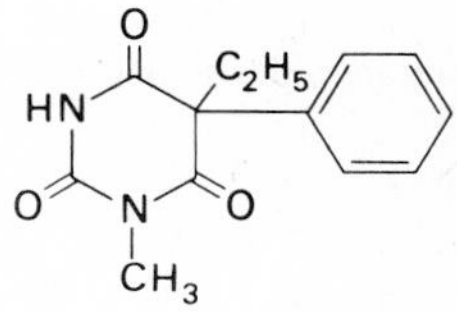

METHARBITAL (Gemonil)

Dose: 50 to 200 mg 3 times a day by mouth.

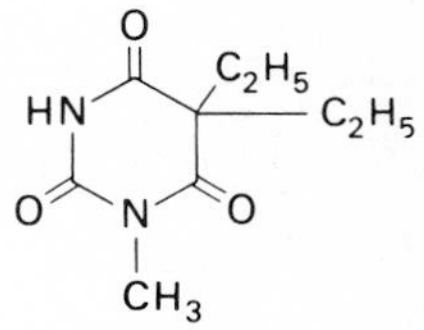

PRIMIDONE (Mysoline)

Not a complete barbiturate; reported to be most useful in grand mal and psychomotor epilepsy.

Dose: 125 mg daily by mouth, increased gradually as required to 250 mg 4 times a day.

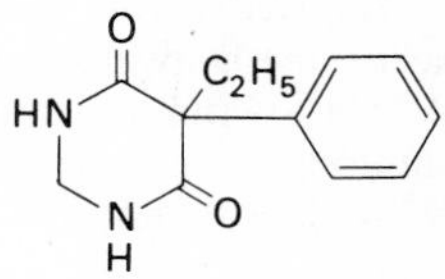

OTHERS

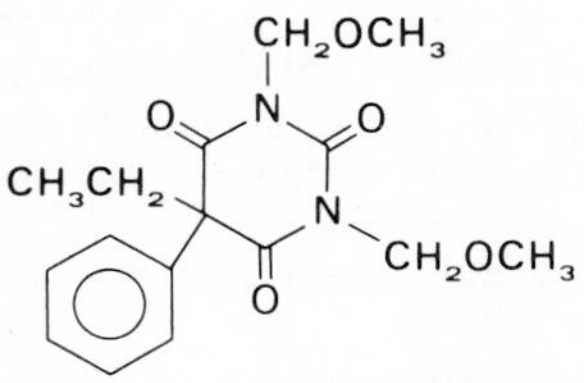

eterobarb (Antilon)

B. The Hydantoins

1. History. a. Phenylethylhydantoin (Nirvanol) (1916) used in chorea, but abandoned because of fever and rash.

b. Merritt and Putnam (1938) introduced diphenylhydantoin.

2. Chemistry. a. Hydantoins parallel barbiturates in structure, but with five-membered hydantoin ring.

b. Most other anticonvulsants also constructed on the "common denominator."

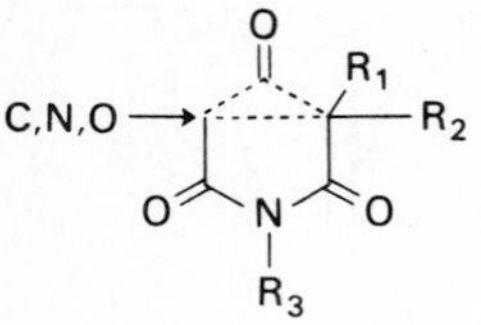

common denominator

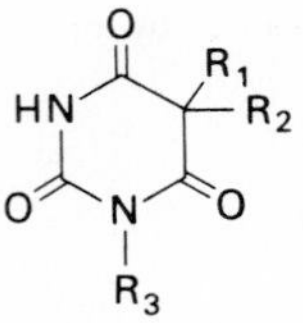

barbiturate

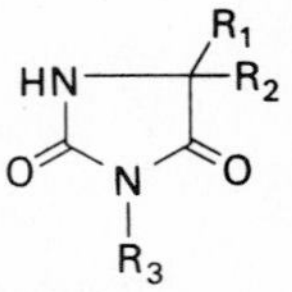

hydantoinate

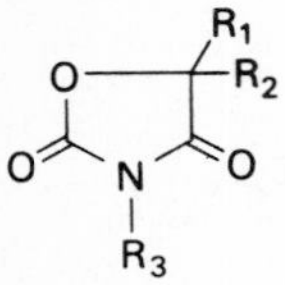

oxazolidone

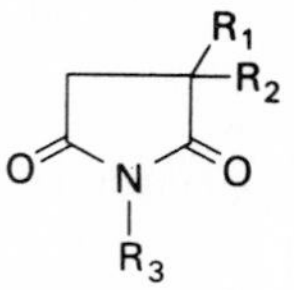

succinimide

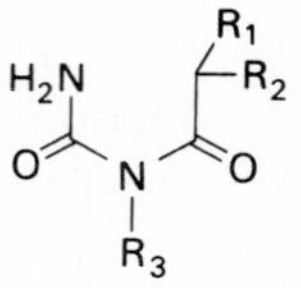

acetylurea

3. Action and Mechanism. a. Effective suppressants of grand mal attacks (except phethenylate vs. petit mal).

b. Primary action appears to be on motor cortex, where spread of impulse is inhibited; but, subcortical structures also inhibited; reduction of intracellular Na^+ reported. Peripheral nerves "stabilized."

c. Experimental suppression of electrically induced convulsions; but not pentylenetetrazol.

4. Pharmacodynamics and Toxicity. a. Well absorbed by mouth.

b. Partly excreted as a hydroxylated and conjugated form in the urine.

c. Produce less depression than barbiturates but may cause hyperplasia of the gums (not scurvy), nystagmus, tremor, dermatitis, lymphadenopathy.

5. Uses. a. Desirable and effective agents, alone or as supplements to phenobarbital, in grand mal epilepsy.

b. Also used in trigeminal neuralgia, probably because of effects on peripheral nerves.

6. Preparations

PHENYTOIN (Previous name: diphenylhydantoin) (Dilantin)

Dose: 30 to 100 mg 3 times a day by mouth.

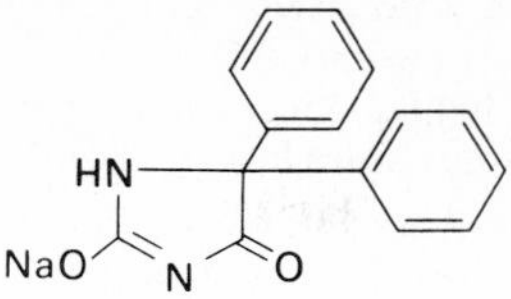

ETHOTOIN (Peganone)

Somewhat less effective than diphenylhydantoin.
Dose: 0.5 to 1 gm 3 to 6 times a day by mouth.

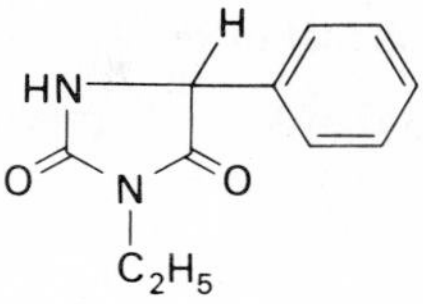

MEPHENYTOIN (Mesantoin)

More potent than diphenylhydantoin, but demethylated to phenylethylhydantoin in the body and may produce rash, fever, and aplastic anemia; little used.
Dose: 30 to 100 mg 3 times a day by mouth.

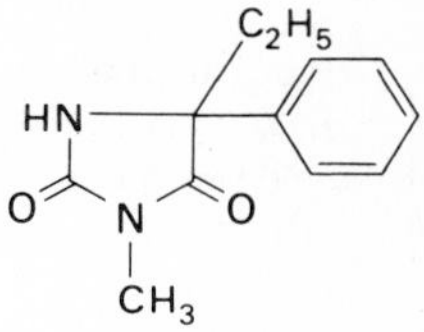

METHETOIN (Deltoin)

Dose: 30 increased to 100 mg in weekly steps by mouth.

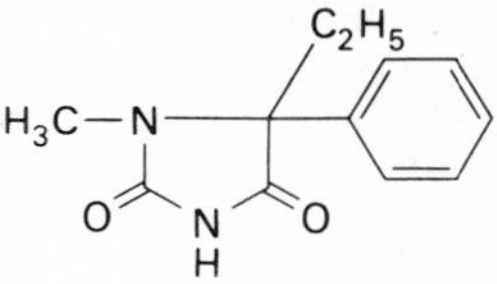

OTHERS

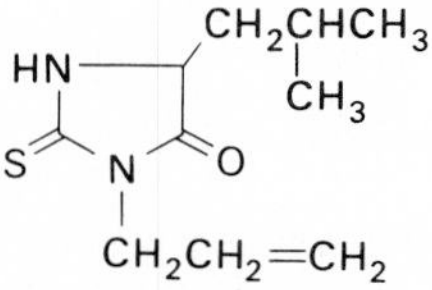

albutoin (CO-ORD)

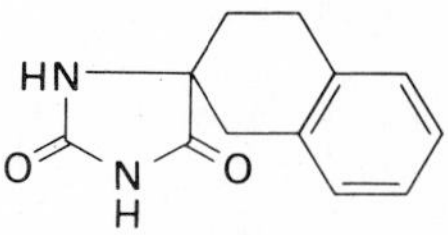

tetrantoin

C. Oxazolidones

1. Chemistry. Oxazolidone derivatives corresponding to hydantoin derivatives.

2. Action and Mechanism. a. Anticonvulsant, but effective against petit mal attacks, not grand mal; mildly sedative and analgesic.

b. Suppress primary focus and restrict spread to diencephalon.

c. Mechanism unknown.

3. **Pharmacodynamics and Toxicity.** a. Well absorbed.

b. Demethylated in the liver; demethylated product slowly excreted.

c. Toxicity unfortunately common; sedation, "glare" phenomenon (sensitivity to light), skin rashes, fever; accepted better by children than adults. Paramethadione causes less glare and rash than trimethadione.

4. **Uses.** To control petit mal epilepsy.

5. **Preparations**

DIMETHADIONE (Eupractone)

Under investigation.

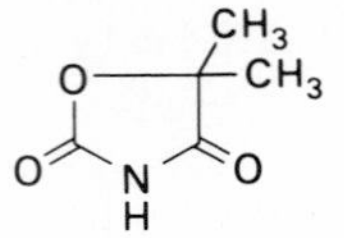

PARAMETHADIONE (Paradione)

Dose: 150 to 300 mg 3 times a day by mouth (children); 300 to 600 mg 3 times a day (adults).

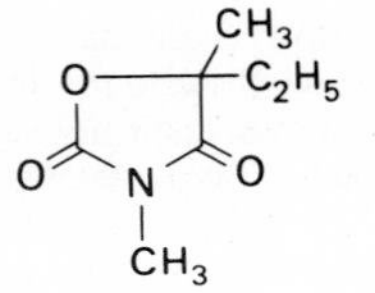

TRIMETHADIONE (Tridione)

Dose: 150 to 300 mg 3 times a day by mouth (children); 300 to 600 mg 3 times a day (adults).

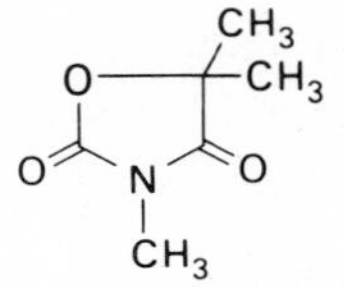

D. Succinimides

1. **Chemistry.** Like the oxazolidones, also correspond to hydantoin series.

2. **Action and Mechanism.** Effective against petit mal epilepsy, but less potent than trimethadione.

3. **Pharmacodynamics and Toxicity.** a. Well absorbed by mouth.

b. Toxicity: anorexia, diarrhea, drowsiness, ataxia, dermatitis, edema, albuminuria, and liver damage have been reported.

4. **Uses.** a. To control petit mal epilepsy.

b. Methsuximide said to be useful against psychomotor types.

5. **Preparations**

ETHOSUXIMIDE (Zarontin)

Has been reported to cause marrow damage and aplastic anemia.

Dose: 0.5 gm 2 to 4 times a day by mouth.

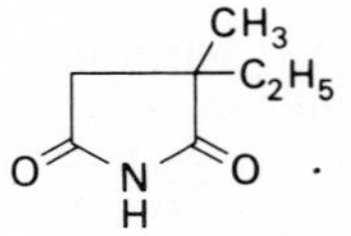

METHSUXIMIDE (Celontin)

Dose: 0.3 to 0.6 gm 2 or 3 times a day by mouth.

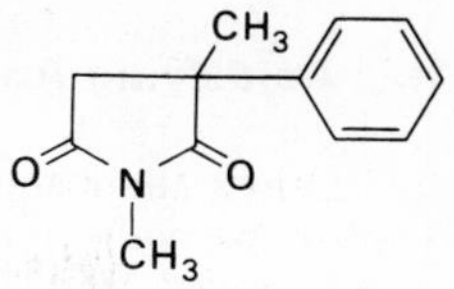

PHENSUXIMIDE (Milontin)

Dose: 0.5 to 1 gm 2 or 3 times a day.

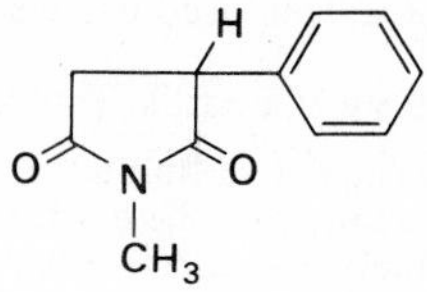

E. Glutarimide Group

AMINOGLUTETHIMIDE (Elipten)

May produce transient leukopenia; in higher doses, drowsiness, ataxia, nausea, and rashes; masculinization of young females.

Dose: 125 to 250 mg 1 to 3 times a day by mouth. Withdrawn from market.

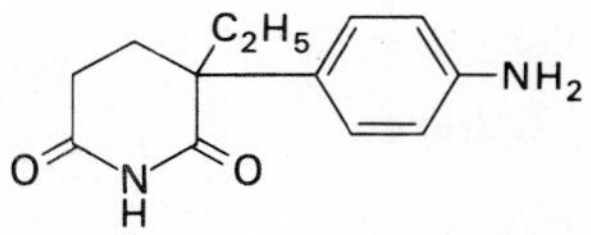

F. Acetylureas

1. Chemistry. Called "straight-chain" hydantoins.

2. Action and Mechanism. Potent agents, effective against psychic and psychomotor equivalents of epilepsy.

3. Pharmacodynamics and Toxicity. a. Well absorbed.

b. Completely metabolized, presumably in the liver.

c. Toxic; can produce hepatic damage, aplastic anemia, personality changes.

4. Uses. Only in severe equivalent epilepsy when other agents are ineffective: patients should be under close surveillance.

5. Preparation

PHENACEMIDE (Phenurone)

Dose: 250 mg 3 times a day by mouth.

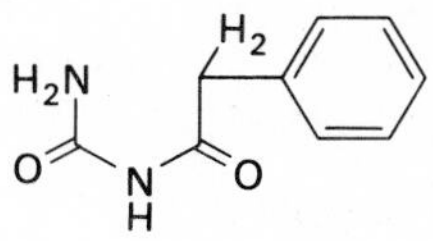

G. Benzodiazepines

(See under Tranquilizers.)

H. Acidifying Agents

Dehydration and the production of acidosis have been attempted in past years as partially effective measures in the control of epilepsy, but have not been well tolerated by patients, especially adults. More recently carbonic anhydrase inhibitors have been used more successfully (see Diuretics: ethoxzolamide).

SULTHIAME (Conadil, Trolone)

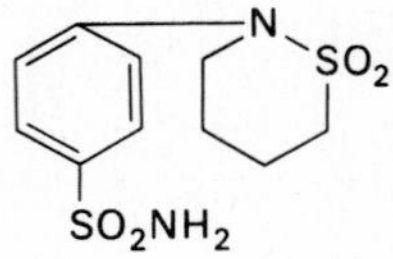

Carbonic anhydrase inhibitor.

Used in temporal lobe epilepsy and grand mal with psychomotor attacks, less effective in petit mal. Side effects include lethargy, anorexia, hyperpnea, ataxia, paresthesias, cold hands, colored visual illusions, psychotic episodes (Liske, J. New Drugs, 3:32, 1963).

Dose: 200 mg 3 times a day by mouth.

N SO_2

SO_2NH_2

I. Others

CARBAMAZEPINE (Tegretol)

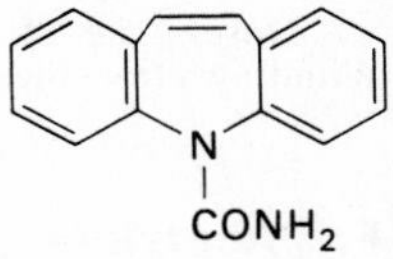

Reported to be active in all forms except petit mal (Theobald, Arzneimittel-Forsch., 13:122, 1963); used in trigeminal and other cranial nerve neuralgias. Side effects: drowsiness, dizziness, skin rashes.

Dose: 0.2 to 1.2 gm per day in divided doses by mouth.

N

$CONH_2$

SULTHIAME (Contravul)

OTHERS

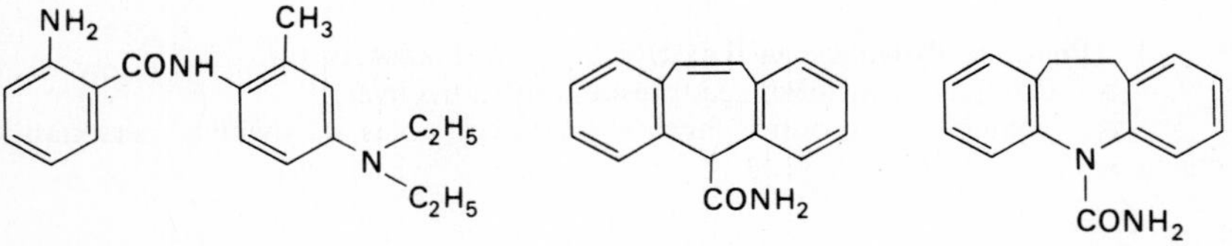

NH_2 CH_3 CONH N C_2H_5 C_2H_5

atolide

$CONH_2$

citenamide

N $CONH_2$

cyheptamide

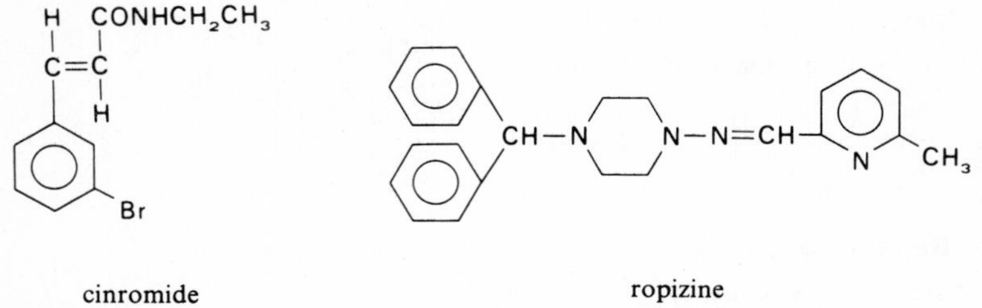

H $CONHCH_2CH_3$ C=C H Br

cinromide

CH—N N—N=CH— N CH_3

ropizine

$CH_3CH_2CH_2CHCOONa$
$CH_3CH_2CH_2$ (attached to CH)

valproate sodium (Depakene)

SUMMARY: ANTICONVULSANTS

TYPE	*ACTION AND MECHANISM*	*TOXICITY*	*USE*	*EXAMPLES*
Barbiturates	Anticonvulsant Mechanism unknown	Sedation	Epilepsy, all types	Phenobarbital
Hydantoins	Same	Hyperplasia of gums, dermatitis	Grand mal epilepsy	Phenytoin
Oxazolidones	Same	Glare phenomenon	Petit mal epilepsy	Trimethadione
Acetylureas	Same	Hepatic damage	Psychomotor epilepsy	Phenacemide

Review

Scholl, M. L. Treatment of seizure disorders. New Eng. J. Med., 269: 1304, 1963.

54. Tranquilizers

Tranquilizer is a somewhat idealized term, but carries the implication of mental calm without proportionate depression of mental activity or alertness.

Classical tranquilizers, like chlorpromazine and reserpine, differ from traditional sedatives in showing less dulling of sensorium, easier arousal, less ataxia, no anesthesia, more muscle tone, no excited stage, and less addiction; they potentiate barbiturates but lower the convulsive threshold.

Minor tranquilizers, such as the diphenylmethane group and the benzodiazepines, are similar to sedatives.

A. Phenothiazine Derivatives

1. History. Charpentier (1950) prepared chlorpromazine and other phenothiazine derivatives while searching for antihistamines and antiparkinsonian agents. They now overshadow all other tranquilizers and are widely used in the treatment of psychoses and for the relief of nausea and vomiting.

2. Chemistry. Phenothiazine nucleus plus a side chain of the dimethylaminoalkyl type; separation of the N atoms by two carbons characteristically yields antihistamines, by three carbons yields tranquilizers.

3. Action. a. Reduce motor activity, induce quietness, mild drowsiness, apathy.

b. Block conditioned, not unconditioned, reflexes.

c. Antiemetic; antiadrenergic; anticholinergic.

d. Differ from most sedatives in that actions mostly subcortical; depress the hypothalamus, reticular activating system, chemoreceptor trigger zone, and to some extent the vomiting center (sedation and antiemesis); stimulate the extrapyramidal system (parkinsonism).

4. Mechanism. a. Underlying mechanism not clear, but currently thought to be from a central adrenergic blocking action, probably the result of interference with access of norepinephrine to receptor and reentry into axone.

b. The following have been noted:

a′. Adrenolytic effects: Central block of norepinephrine and other amines, peripheral block of adrenergic receptors, prevention of uptake of amines and decreased storage, increased rate of epinephrine metabolism, and inhibition of deamination of serotonin.

b′. Membrane effects: Reduced permeability; may be mediated by donation of electron from drug to the inside of the organelle, polarizing the membrane and making it more stable (Gey, Nature, 194:387, 1962).

5. Pharmacodynamics. a. Absorbed well.

b. Distributed widely, including the hypothalamus; partly destroyed in the liver, and partly excreted as the sulfoxide.

6. Toxicity. a. General autonomic and metabolic effects: Weakness, chilliness, constipation, stuffy nose, blurred vision, dry mouth, hypotension, gain in weight, edema; lactation (hypothalamic effect); dermatitis including erythema, vesiculation and contact dermatitis; ignoring of pain of organic disease.

b. Organ damage: Intrahepatic obstructive hepatitis; marrow depression with agranulocytosis; most common with aliphatic side chain, less with piperazine, least with piperidine, but pigmentation of the retina may be produced by excessive dosage of the latter.

c. CNS effects: Following extrapyramidal syndromes, most pronounced with piperazine side chain:

a′. Akathisia: Inability to keep still; irresistible urge to be in motion; fright; may occur also with chlorpromazine or reserpine; control with antiparkinsonian agents and phenobarbital.

b′. Parkinsonism: Commonest in older patients and women; reversible but may take several months; treat with antiparkinsonian agents.

c. Dystonic syndrome: "Face, neck, tongue syndrome": Frequent (up to 10%); may also occur with reserpine, haloperidol, and others. Characterized by mandibular tics, protrusion of tongue, hypertonicity of muscles of neck impairing speech and swallowing, oculogyric spasms, torticollis, opisthotonos, tonic twitchings, and contractions of trunk muscles; rhythmical, intermittent, accompanied by anxiety, pallor, sweating, and rarely fever. Treat with intravenous caffeine sodiobenzoate 0.5 gm and antiparkinsonian drugs.

7. Uses

a. Aliphatic side chain group

a′. Potent tranquilizing agents; often preferable for home use as agranulocytosis is not a great danger, and CNS side effects may be controlled by antiparkinsonian drugs.

b′. Antiemetic.

b. Piperazine side chain group

a′. Valuable tranquilizers, especially in excited psychoses; have considerably altered the degree of detention and restraint of patients in psychiatric hospitals.

b′. Also used, but with more limited application, in psychoneuroses.

c′. As antiemetics; in acute porphyria; to potentiate analgesia.

c. Piperidine side chain group

a′. Adapted to use in ambulatory patients and neurotics; most effective in patients with excitement, hypermotility, tension, high drive, agitation, and hostility.

b′. Mepazine is also used as an antiemetic.

8. Preparations

a. Aliphatic side chain group

CHLORPROMAZINE HYDROCHLORIDE (Thorazine)

Dose: 10 to 200 mg 2 or 3 times a day by mouth; largest doses only in hospitalized patients.

S · HCl

N Cl

$CH_2CH_2CH_2-N(CH_3)_2$

PROMAZINE HYDROCHLORIDE (Sparine)

Less lipoid soluble (lacks Cl) and generally weaker than chlorpromazine, and produces less jaundice but more agranulocytosis.

Dose: 50 to 100 mg 3 times a day by mouth.

S · HCl

N

$CH_2CH_2CH_2-N(CH_3)_2$

TRIFLUPROMAZINE HYDROCHLORIDE (Vesprin)

Dose: 10 mg 2 or 3 times a day.

S · HCl

N CF_3

$CH_2CH_2CH_2-N(CH_3)_2$

PROPIOMAZINE

CH_3

$CH_2CH-N(CH_3)_2$

N $COCH_2CH_3$

S

ACEPROMAZINE MALEATE (Atravet, Plegicil)

For veterinary use only.

$CH_2CH_2CH_2N(CH_3)_2$

N $C(=O)-CH_3$ · $HC-COOH$ / $HC-COOH$

S

b. Piperazine side chain group

ACETOPHENAZINE MALEATE (Tindal)

Dose: 20 mg 3 times a day by mouth.

S

N $COCH_3$ $C_4H_4O_5$

$CH_2CH_2CH_2-N$ N$-CH_2CH_2OH$

BUTAPERAZINE MALEATE (Repoise)

Dose: 5 to 10 mg 3 times a day by mouth.

S

N COC_3H_7 $C_4H_4O_5$

$CH_2CH_2CH_2$—N N—CH_3

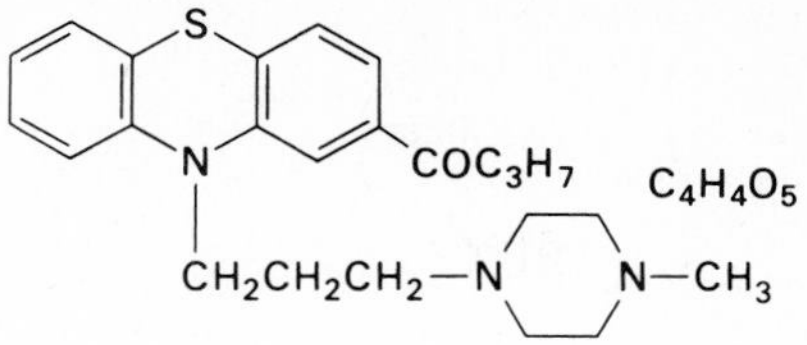

CARPHENAZINE MALEATE (Proketazine)

Dose: 25 to 50 mg 3 times a day by mouth.

S

N COC_2H_5 $C_4H_4O_5$

$CH_2CH_2CH_2$—N N—CH_2CH_2OH

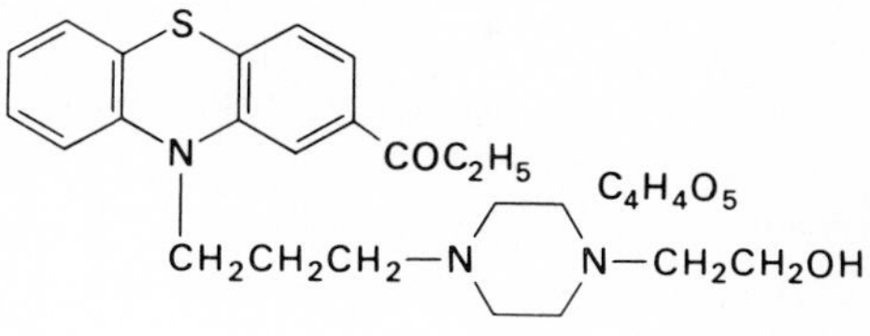

FLUPHENAZINE HYDROCHLORIDE (Prolixin; Permitil)

Dose: 0.5 to 3.0 mg 3 times a day by mouth.

S

N CF_3 · HCl

$CH_2CH_2CH_2$—N N—CH_2CH_2OH

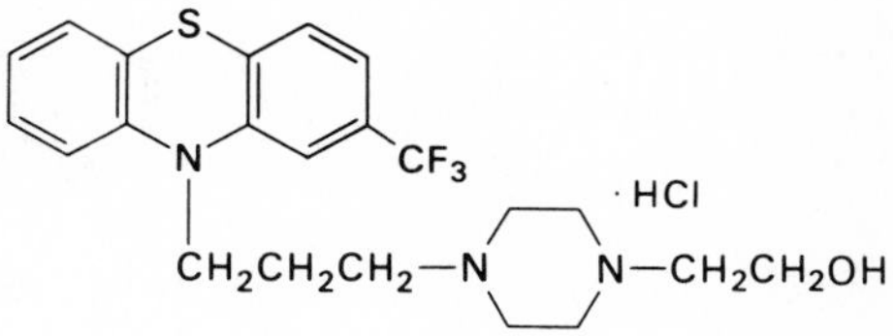

PERPHENAZINE (Trilafon)

Dose: 4 to 8 mg 3 times a day by mouth.

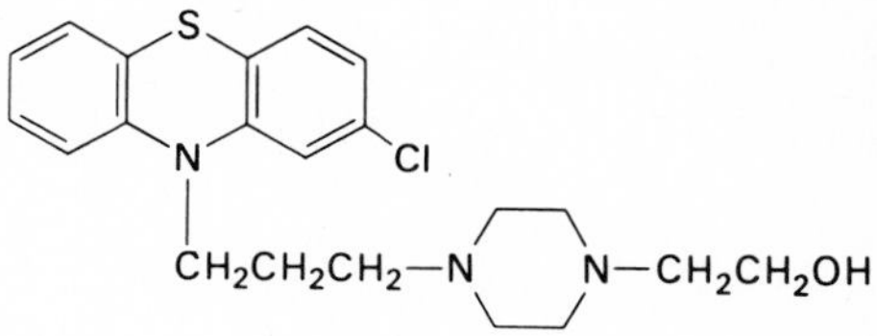

S

N Cl

$CH_2CH_2CH_2$—N N—CH_2CH_2OH

PROCHLORPERAZINE MALEATE (Compazine)

Dose: 10 to 30 mg 3 times a day by mouth.

S

N Cl $C_4H_4O_5$

$CH_2CH_2CH_2$—N N—CH_3

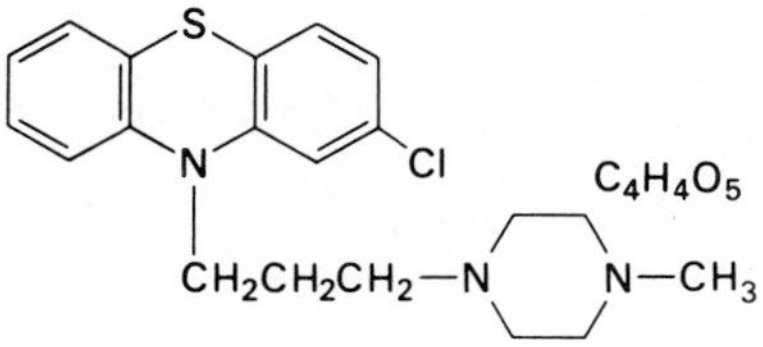

THIOPROPAZATE HYDROCHLORIDE (Dartal)

Stated to be hydrolyzed to perphenazine in the body.

Dose: 10 mg 3 times a day by mouth.

S

N Cl · HCl

$CH_2CH_2CH_2$—N N—CH_2CH_2

O—$COCH_3$

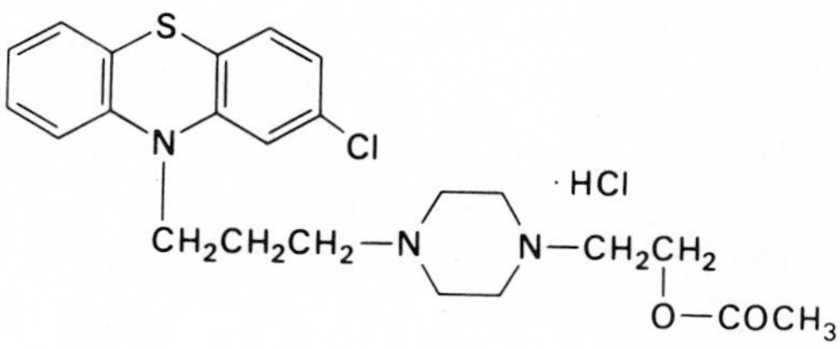

TRIFLUOPERAZINE HYDROCHLORIDE (Stelazine)

Dose: 2 to 5 mg 3 times a day by mouth.

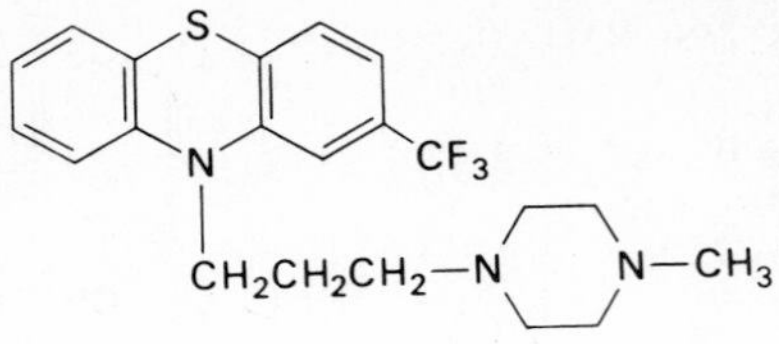

MESORIDAZINE (Serentil)

Dose: 25 mg twice a day to 75 mg 3 times a day by mouth.

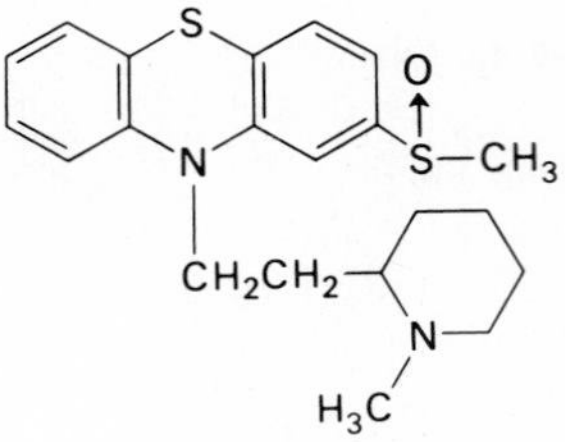

PIPERACETAZINE (Quide)

Dose: 10 to 30 mg 3 times a day by mouth.

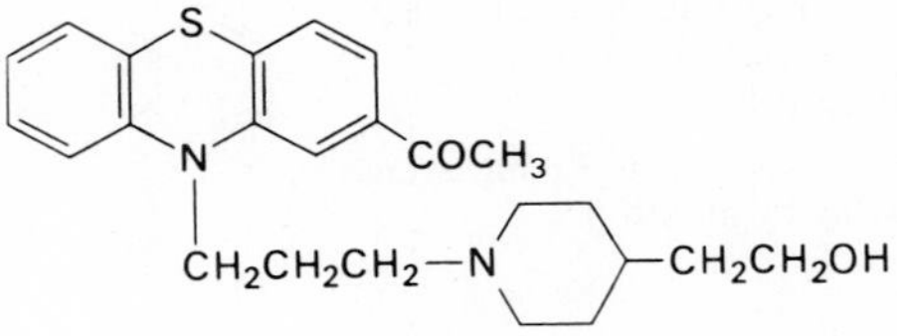

THIORIDAZINE (Mellaril)

Dose: 25 to 150 mg 3 times a day by mouth.

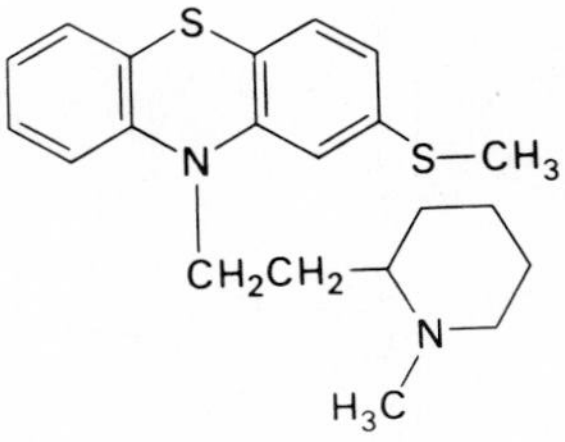

PIPOTIAZINE PALMITATE

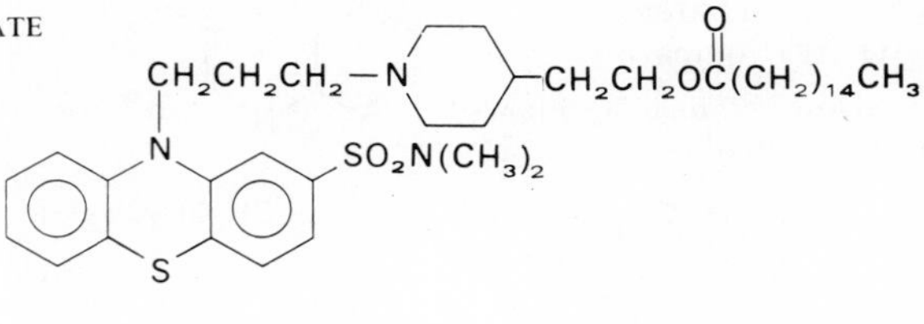

d. Thioxanthines and other analogues

CHLORPROTHIXINE (Taractan)

Calming agent only. May produce drowsiness; agranulocytosis.

Dose: 15 to 50 mg 3 or 4 times a day by mouth.

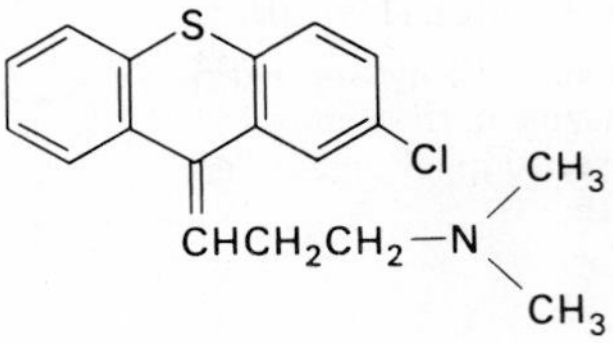

THIOTHIXINE HYDROCHLORIDE (Navane)

Said to be alerting; used in chronic withdrawn schizophrenics.

Dose: 2 mg 3 times a day by mouth, increased to 10 mg 3 times a day.

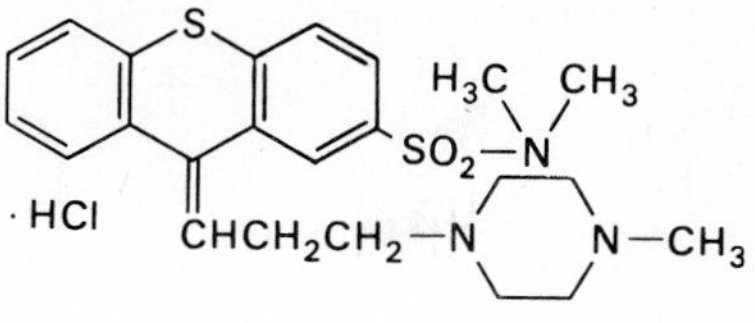

e. *Dibenzoxazepines*

LOXAPINE

LOXAPINE SUCCINATE (Daxolin, Loxitane)

Dose: 5 to 15 mg 3 times a day.

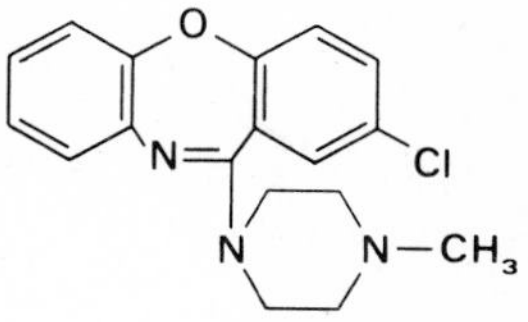

OTHERS

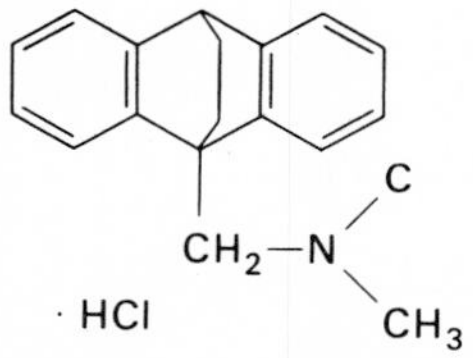

benzoctamine HCl (Tacitin)

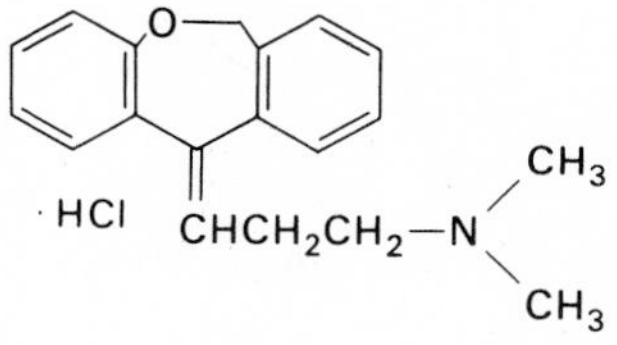

cidoxepin HCl

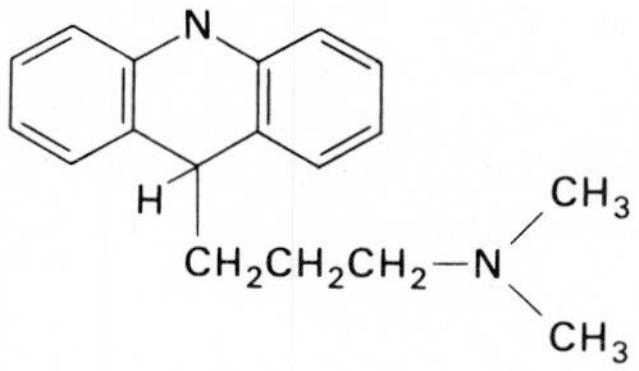

clomacran phosphate

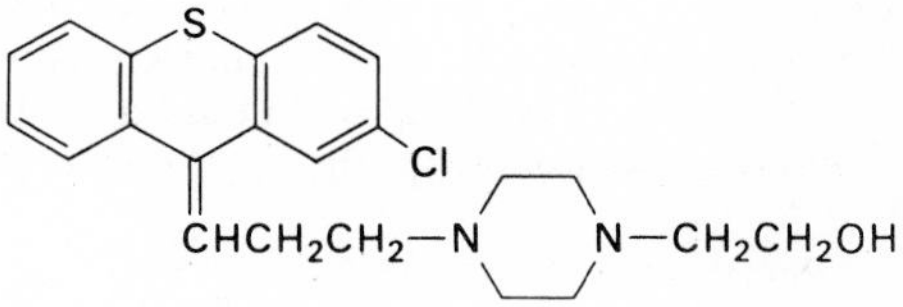

clopenthixol (Sordinol)

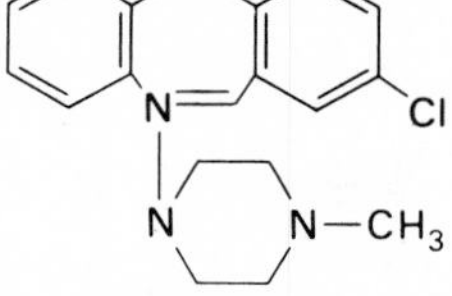

clothiapine

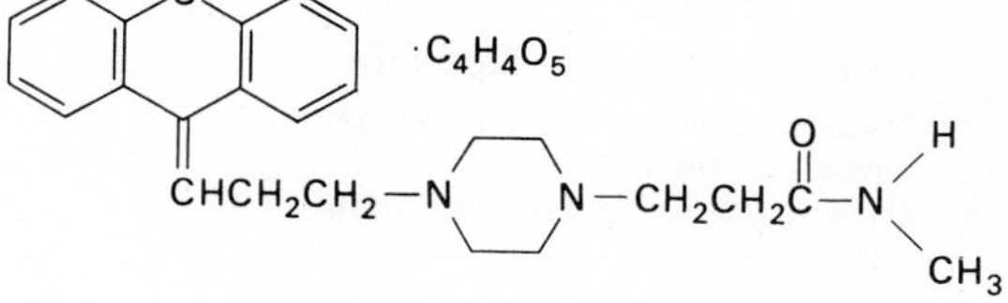

clothixamide maleate

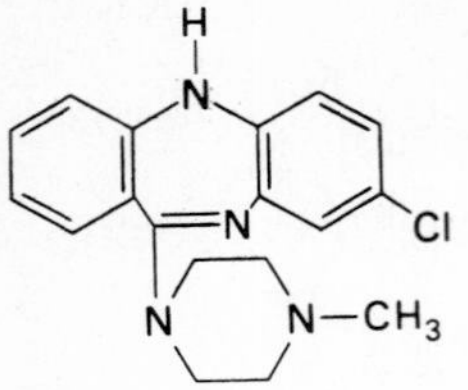

H N Cl N N—CH_3

clozapine

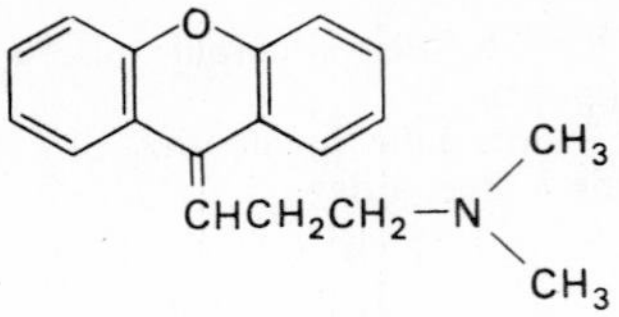

O $CHCH_2CH_2$—N(CH_3)(CH_3)

dimeprozan

O · HCl $CHCH_2CH_2$—N(CH_3)(CH_3)

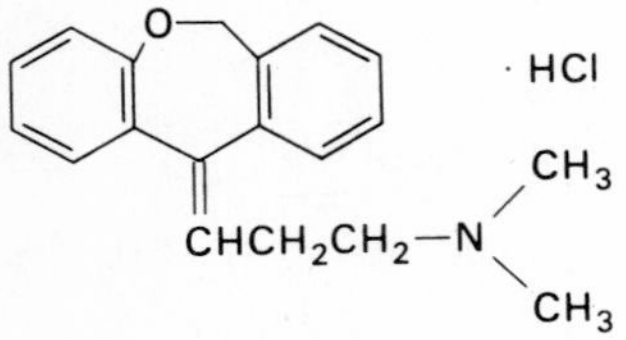

doxepin HCl
(Sinequan; Curatin)

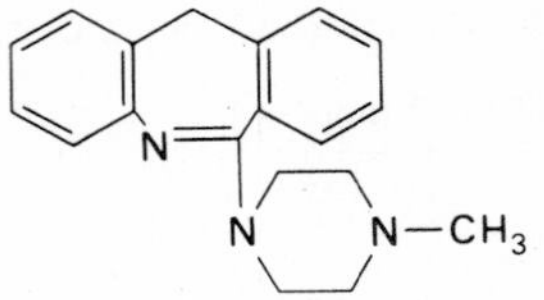

N N N—CH_3

perlapine

O · HCl $CHCH_2CH_2$—N —CH_2CH_2OH

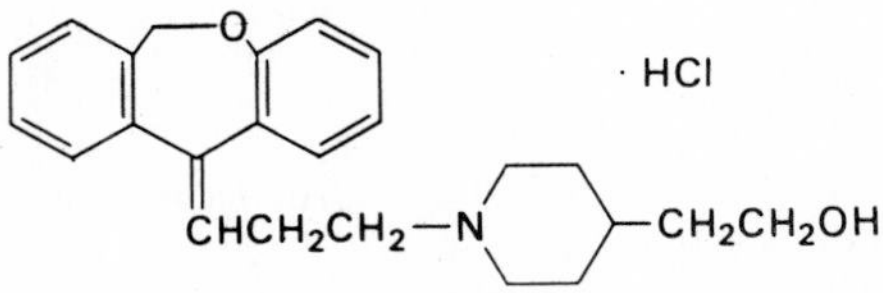

pinoxepin HCl

e. Antiemetics. Most of the phenothiazine tranquilizers have rather strong antiemetic or antinauseant actions; thus, chlorpromazine, prochlorperazine, and mepazine are used for this purpose. In others, listed below, the antinauseant is more prominent than the tranquilizer action. They may be effective in vomiting of psychic or organic cause, but are not particularly effective in motion sickness or Meniere's disease; for the latter the antihistamine group is more effective.

PIPAMAZINE (Mornidine)

Used especially in morning sickness.

Dose: 5 mg every 4 to 6 hours by mouth.

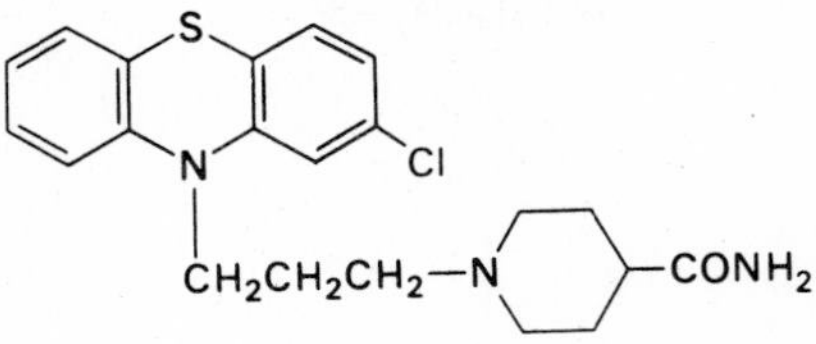

S N Cl $CH_2CH_2CH_2$—N —$CONH_2$

THIETHYLPERAZINE (Torecan)

Weak tranquilizer; minor drowsiness and dryness of the nose.

Dose: 20 to 30 mg daily by mouth.

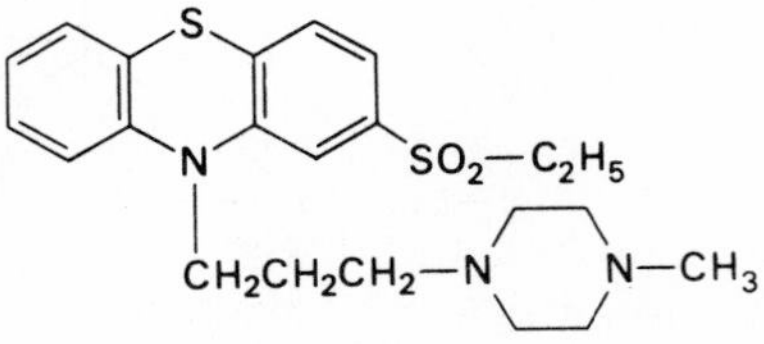

S N SO_2—C_2H_5 $CH_2CH_2CH_2$—N N—CH_3

TRIMETHOBENZAMIDE (Tigan)

(Not a phenothiazine derivative).

No sedative, hypotensive, or extrapyramidal effects.

Dose: 100 mg 4 times a day, orally or subcutaneously.

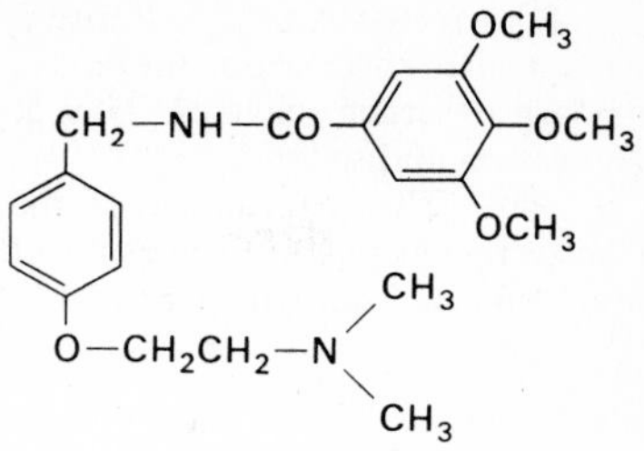

f. *Antipruritics.* May alleviate itching to some extent, of both allergic or nonallergic origin, but should be used hesitantly because of the danger of agranulocytosis.

METHDILAZINE HYDROCHLORIDE (Tacaryl)

Dose: 8 mg 2 to 4 times a day by mouth.

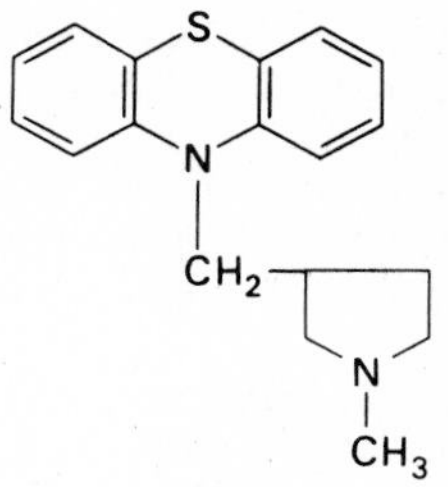

TRIMEPRAZINE (Temaril)

Dose: 2.5 mg 3 times a day by mouth.

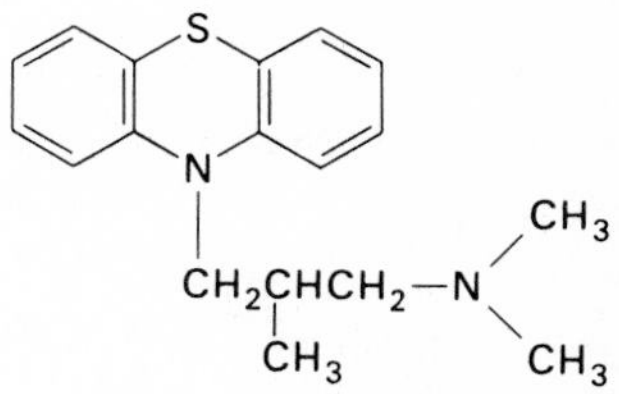

B. Rauwolfia Derivatives and Related Agents

RESERPINE GROUP

1. History. a. Centuries of use in India.

b. Mueller (1952) isolated, and Woodward (1956) synthesized reserpine.

2. Chemistry. Crude products and contained alkaloids from *Rauwolfia serpentina* and other species.

3. Action. a. Induce calm, sleep from which arousal is easy, and diminish aggressiveness.

b. Act subcortically, on the hypothalamus and reticular activating system (stimulate the latter, while chlorpromazine depresses).

c. Autonomic nervous system: Sympatholytic; hypotensive.

4. Mechanism. a. Cause a release of catechol amines and serotonin from storage sites throughout the body; the amines are then destroyed by monoamine oxidase or other enzymes. This depletion presumably is the cause of the central depression and sedation.

b. The mechanism of the release may actually be inhibition of active transport that pumps amines into the cells; passive leakage out is then uncompensated (Shore, Pharmacol. Rev., 14:531, 1962).

5. Pharmacodynamics. a. Absorption and distribution rather slow, but penetration into brain good.

b. Partial excretion of metabolic products in stool and urine.

6. Toxicity. a. CNS: Excessive sedation, nightmares, parkinsonism.

b. Sympatholytic: Nasal congestion, salivation, flushing, vomiting, diarrhea, bradycardia.

c. Other: Amenorrhea; increased gastric acid and volume and possibility of inducing bleeding from peptic ulcer.

7. Uses. a. Effective tranquilizers but less potent than phenothiazines; useful when the latter are not tolerated.

b. Used in excited psychoses, psychoneurosis, hypertension, thyrotoxicosis.

8. Preparations

DESERPIDINE
(Harmonyl)

Dose: 0.1 to 0.5 mg 1 to 3 or 4 times a day by mouth.

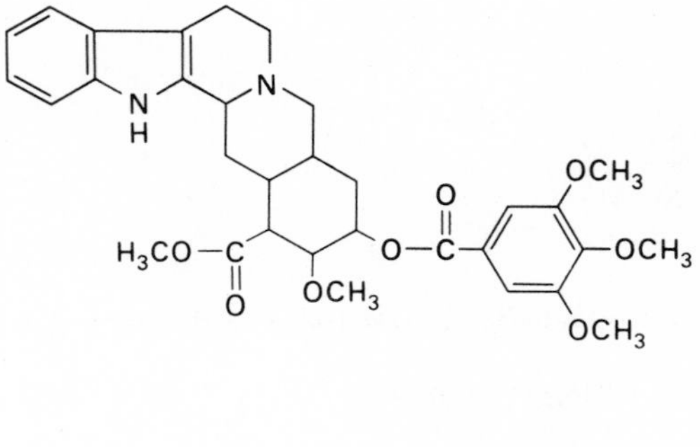

METOSERPATE HYDROCHLORIDE
(Pacitran)

Veterinary tranquilizer.

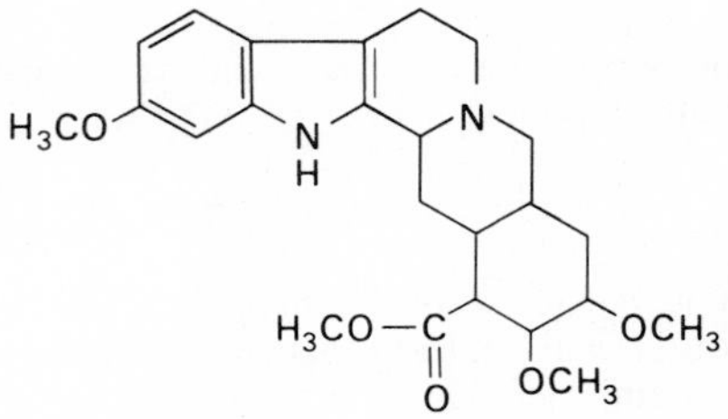

RESCINNAMINE
(Moderil)

Dose: 0.5 mg 2 times a day by mouth.

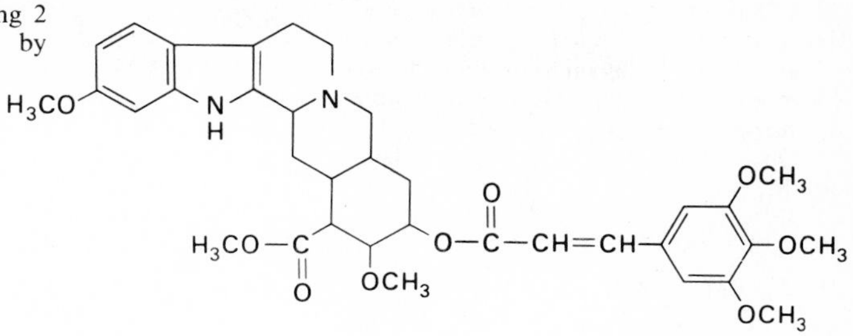

RESERPINE
(Serpasil; Rau-Sed; and many others)

Dose: 0.1 to 0.25 mg 1 to 3 or 4 times a day by mouth.

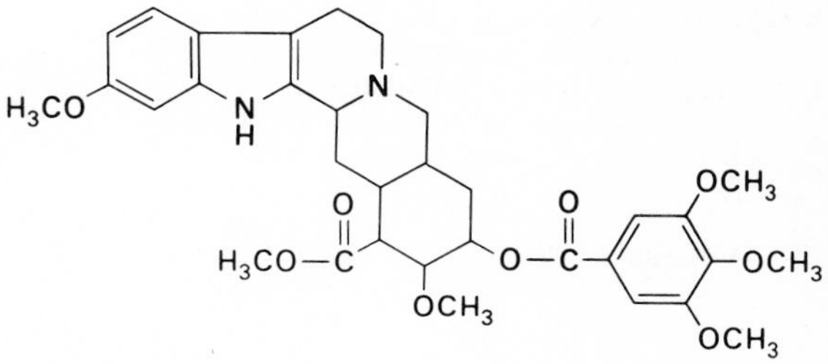

Alseroxylon (Rauwiloid)

Dose: 1 mg 2 to 4 times a day; extract of rauwolfia.

Rauwolfia (Raudixin; and others)

Powdered root of rauwolfia.
Dose: 100 mg 2 to 4 times a day by mouth.

OTHERS

A number of other agents are more or less distantly related to reserpine chemically, and resemble it in action.

BENZQUINAMIDE (Quantril)

Resembles reserpine in tranquilizing effects, and also shows antihistaminic, anticholinergic, antiemetic, and antiserotonin actions. However, mechanism may be different, as experimental animals do not show central or peripheral release of serotonin or norepinephrine. Side effects include little parkinsonism or sedation.

Dose: 200 mg 3 times a day or more by mouth.

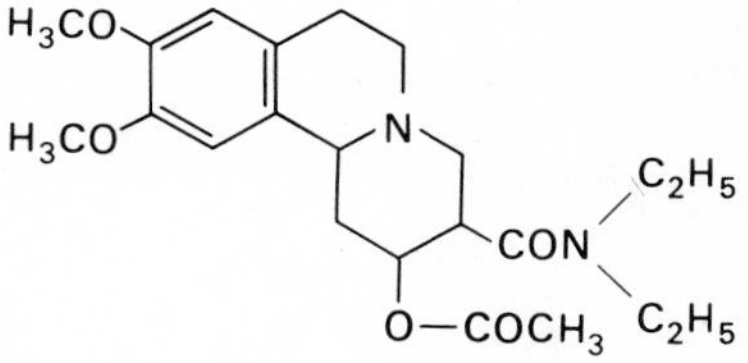

OXYPERTINE HYDROCHLORIDE

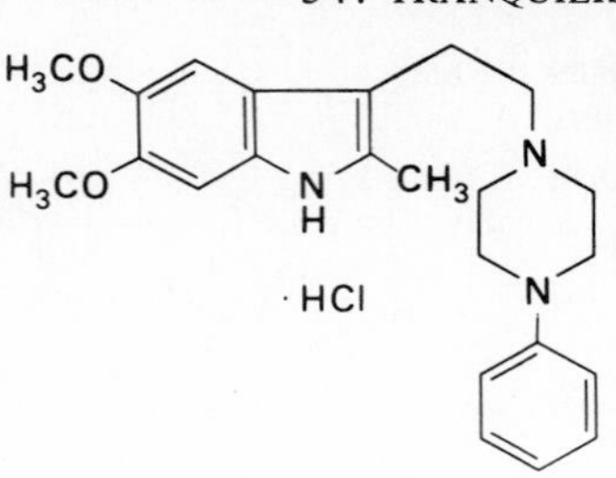

Resembles reserpine in mechanism and action. Side effects include anxiety, agitation, drowsiness, parkinsonism; possible disturbances in liver function (Hollister, J. New Drugs, 3:26, 1963). Useful as a tranquilizer in schizophrenics, except paranoids.

Dose: 10 to 40 mg 3 or 4 times a day by mouth.

TETRABENAZINE (Nitoman)

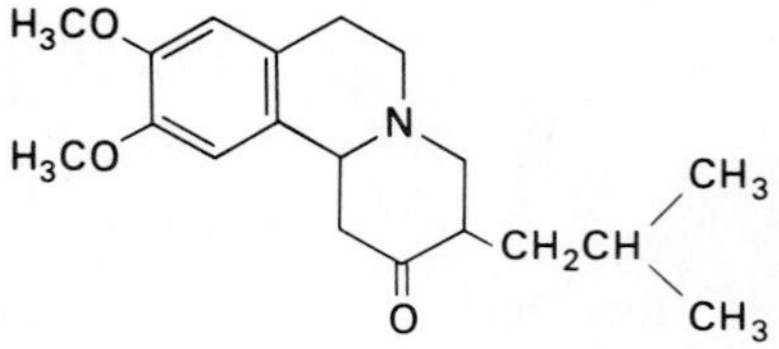

Less profound sedative than reserpine but resembles it in effect. It releases serotonin and norepinephrine in the brain but not peripherally. Previous administration of tetrabenazine before reserpine produces only tetrabenazine effects, suggesting competition at the same receptor. Side effects: excessive sedation, potentiation of barbiturates and anesthetics, depression of appetite, parkinsonism. Useful in patients with schizophrenia, especially during hallucinations.

Dose: 100 mg or more daily by mouth.

OTHERS

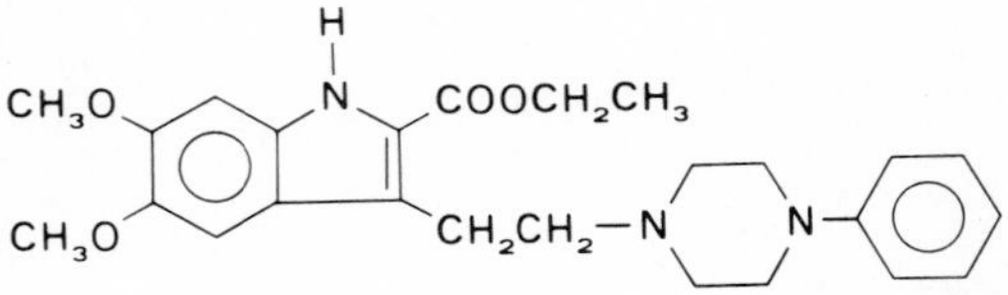

alpertine

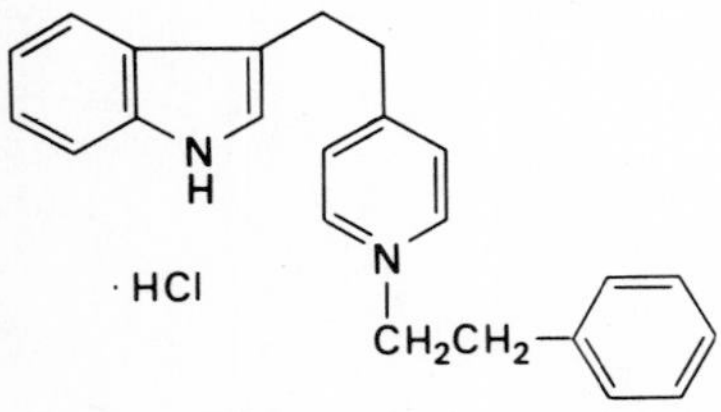

indopine HCl

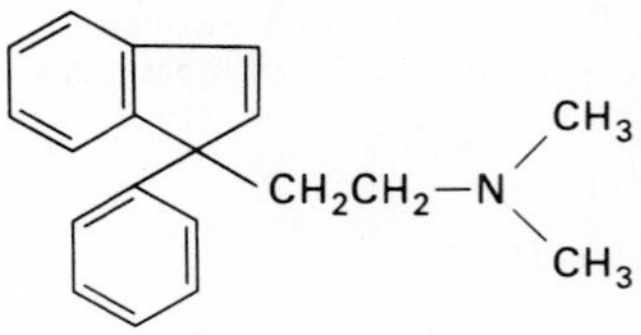

indriline HCl

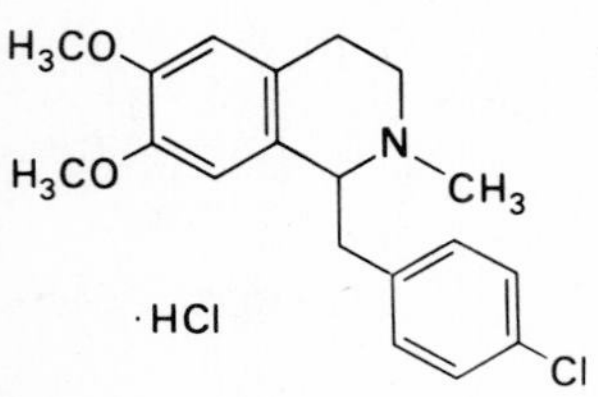

methopholine HCl

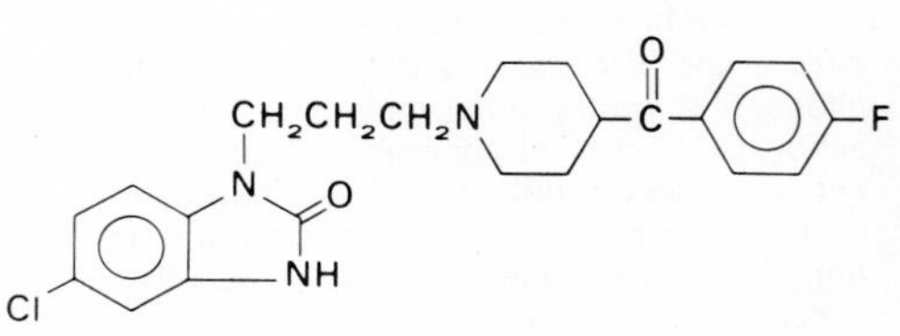

milenperone

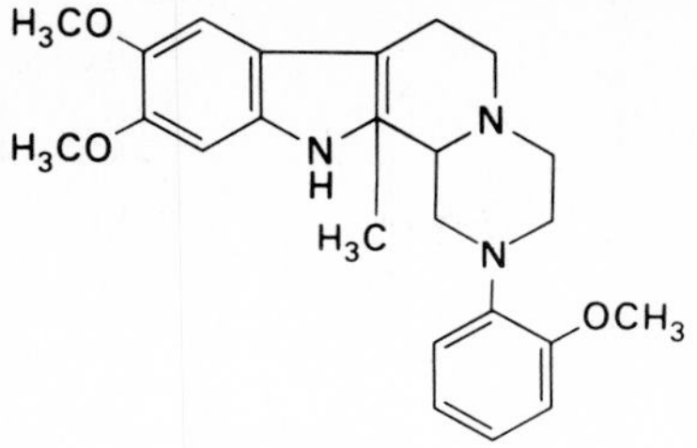

H_3CO H_3CO N H H_3C N N OCH_3

milipertine

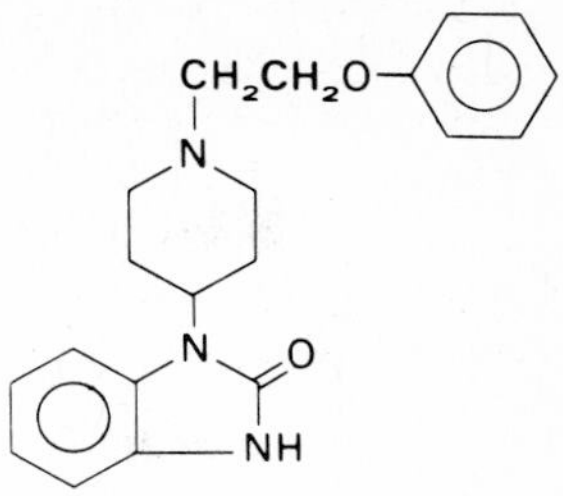

CH_2CH_2O N N O NH

oxiperomide

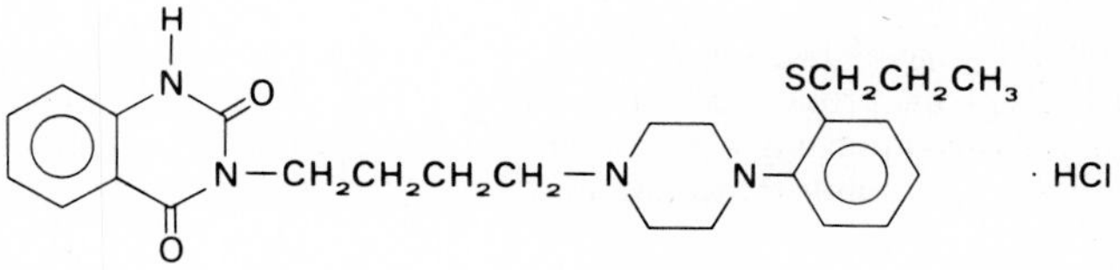

H N O N—$CH_2CH_2CH_2CH_2$—N N $SCH_2CH_2CH_3$ · HCl O

tioperidone hydrochloride

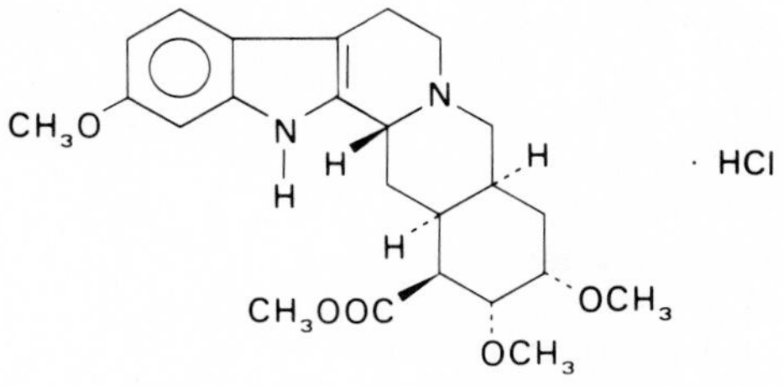

CH_3O N H H N H H CH_3OOC OCH_3 OCH_3 · HCl

metoserpate hydrochloride (Pacitran)
veterinary

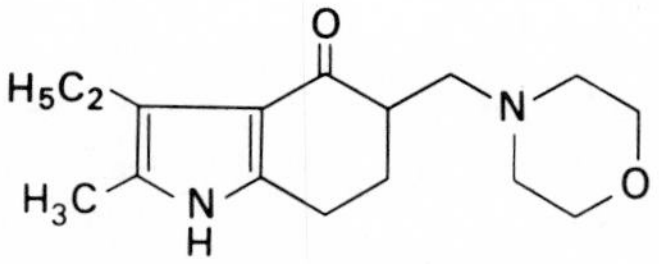

O H_5C_2 H_3C N H N O

molindone (Moban)

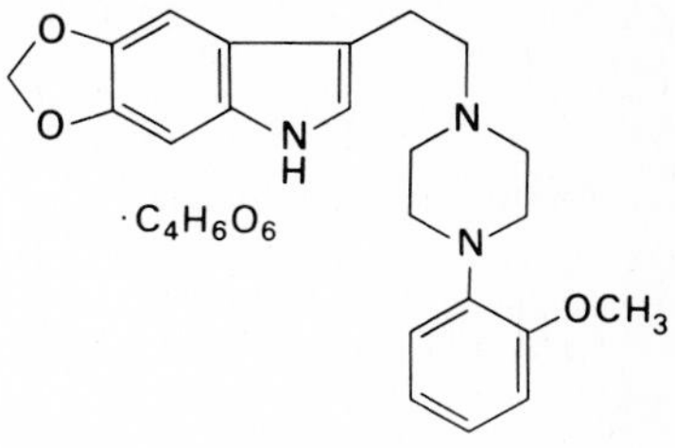

O O N H · $C_4H_6O_6$ N N OCH_3

solypertine tartrate

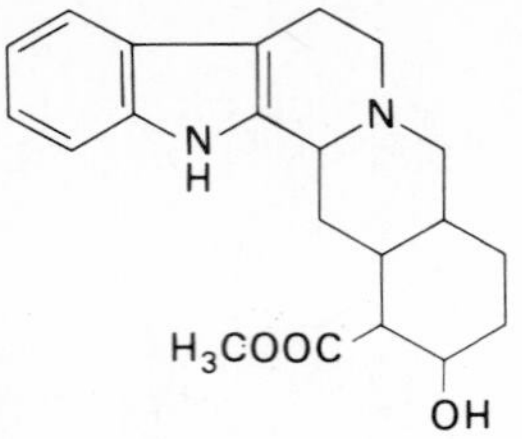

yohimbine

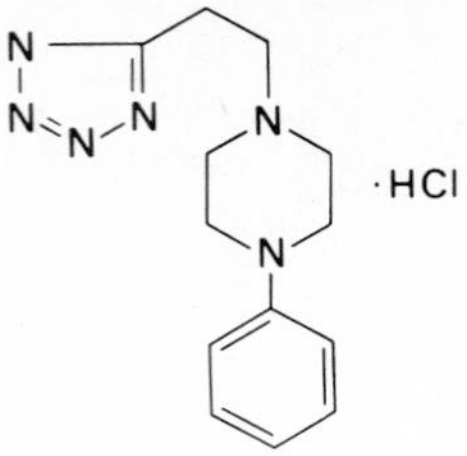

zolertine HCl

C. Diphenylmethane Derivatives (Benactyzine)

A number of agents bearing relationships to antihistamines and spasmolytics and usually showing pronounced autonomic effects have been found to have sedative or mild tranquilizing actions similar to those of the parent compounds. They are often called minor tranquilizers.

1. Chemistry. Diphenylmethane derivatives and related compounds.

2. Action and Mechanism. a. Mild sedatives and tranquilizers.
b. Most also possess autonomic effects, especially antispasmodic.

3. Uses. Tranquilizers, more used in neuroses than psychoses.

4. Preparations

a. Benzilic acid esters

BENACTYZINE HYDROCHLORIDE (Suavitil)

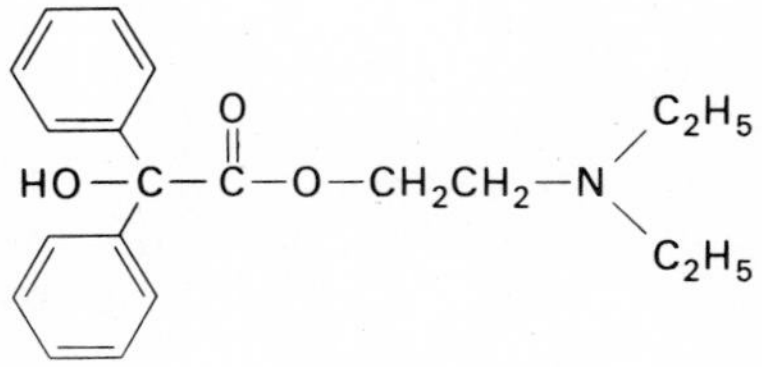

Questionable tranquilizer with one-fifth parasympatholytic action of atropine; inhibits conditioned reflexes, potentiates barbiturates and chloral, inhibits MAO; reduces bioelectric potentials of brain on EEG. Probably has no advantages as a tranquilizer to outweigh the atropine effects.

Dose: 1 mg or more 3 times a day.

PIPERILATE (pipethanate; Sycotrol)

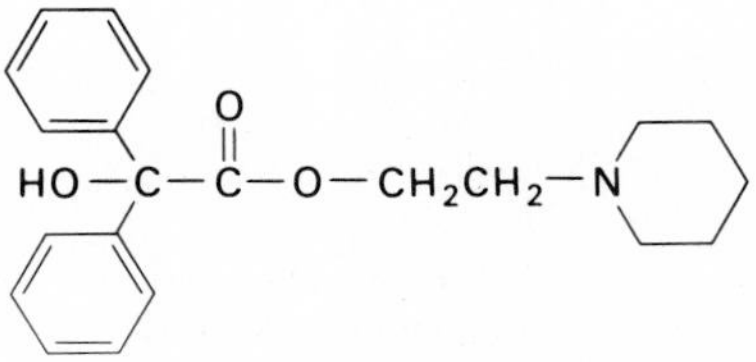

Said to relieve anxiety and tension.

Dose: 3 mg 3 or 4 times a day by mouth.

b. Diphenylmethane derivatives

AZACYCLONOL HYDROCHLORIDE (Frenquel)

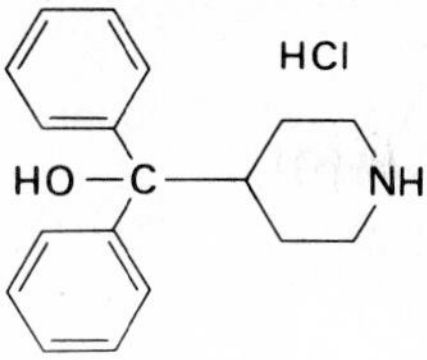

Antagonizes the stimulatory effects of the isomer pipradol; other action dubious but proposed for relief of hallucinations in schizophrenia; largely experimental. Preparations withdrawn from market.

Dose: 20 to 100 mg 3 times a day.

HO—C(C₆H₅)₂—(4-piperidyl) HCl

CAPTODIAMINE (Suvren)

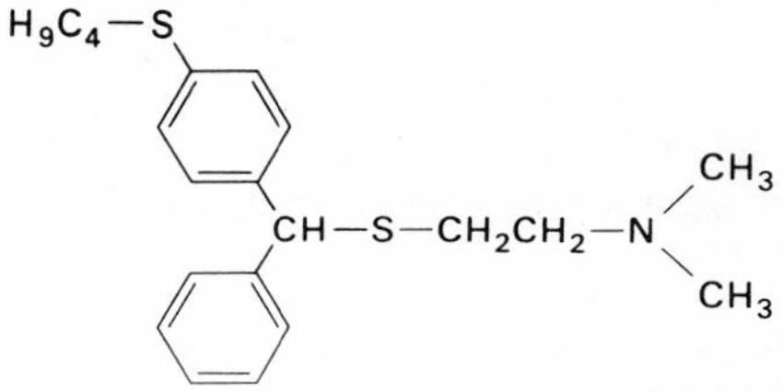

Said to calm without drowsiness, and to improve reaction time.

Dose: 100 mg 3 times a day by mouth.

$H_9C_4-S-C_6H_4-CH(C_6H_5)-S-CH_2CH_2-N(CH_3)_2$

HYDROXYZINE HYDROCHLORIDE OR PAMOATE (Atarax; Vistaril)

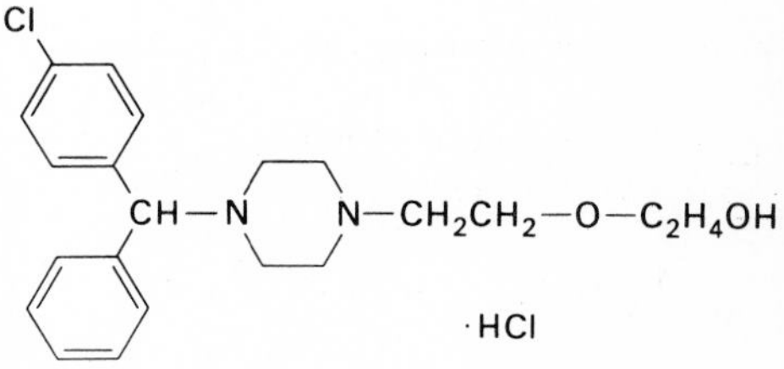

Rapidly acting mild sedative and tranquilizer, most useful in neuroses. Antihistaminic. May arrest ventricular arrhythmias.

Dose: 25 to 100 mg 3 times a day by mouth, or (hydrochloride) intramuscularly or intravenously.

$Cl-C_6H_4-CH(C_6H_5)-N(piperazine)N-CH_2CH_2-O-C_2H_4OH \cdot HCl$

OTHERS

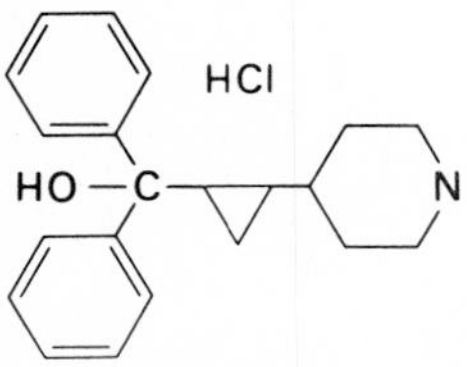

HO—C(C₆H₅)₂—(cyclopropyl)—(piperidyl N) HCl

cyprolidol HCl

$HO-C(C_6H_5)_2-CH(NH_2)(C_5H_{11})$

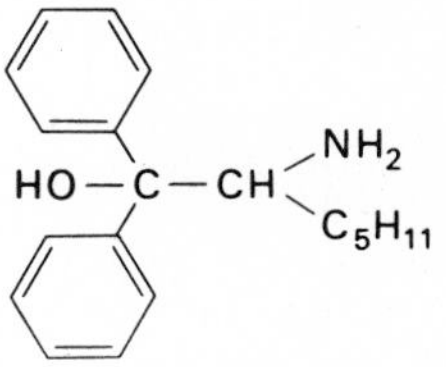

hexandrol

D. Butyrophenone Group (Haloperidol)

1. Chemistry. Butyrophenone derivatives.

2. Action and Mechanism. Similar in effect to chlorpromazine; depress subcortical brain, midbrain, and reticular formation.

3. Pharmacodynamics and Toxicity. Marked extrapyramidal effects, restlessness, autonomic actions, rashes.

4. Uses. Agitated schizophrenia, manic states, mental deficiency.

5. Preparations

HALOANISONE

Dose: 10 mg intramuscularly.

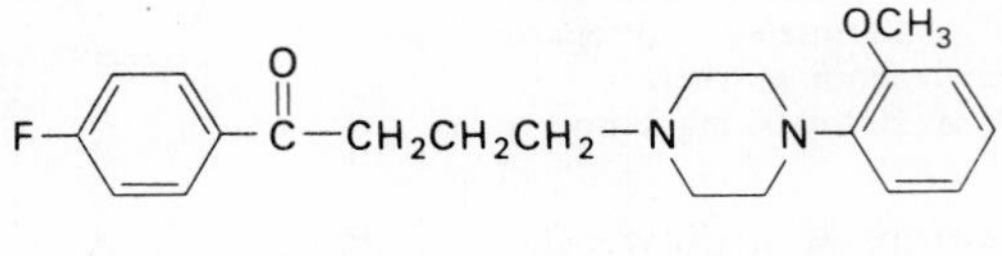

HALOPERIDOL
(Haldol; Serenase)

Dose: 1 to 2 mg 2 to 3 times a day.

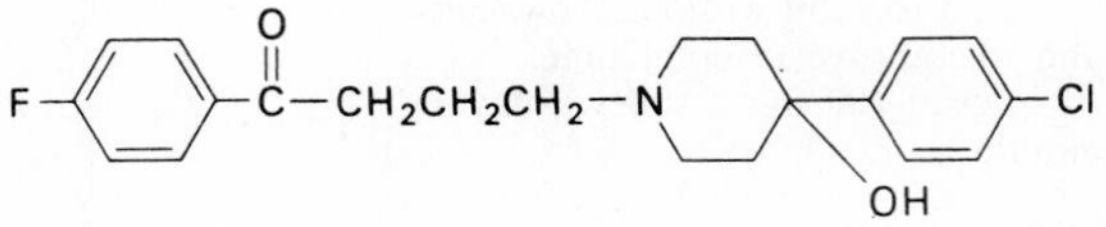

OTHERS

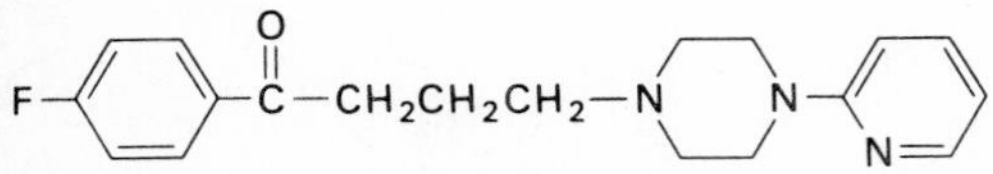

azaperone

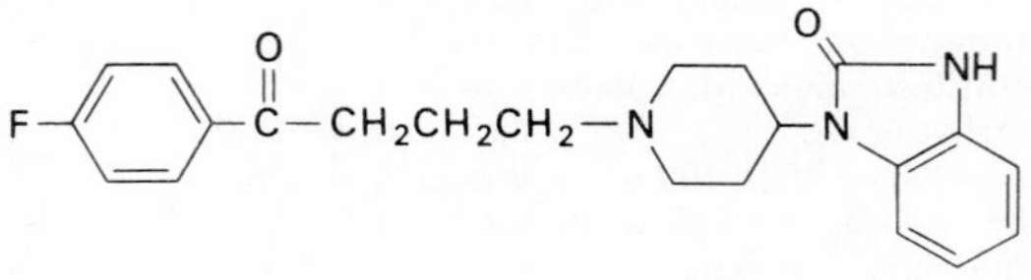

benperidol

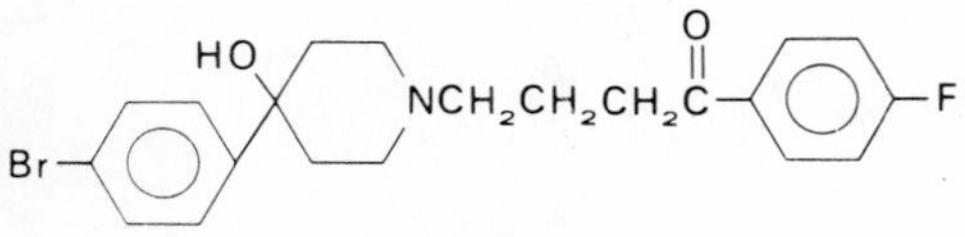

bromperidol

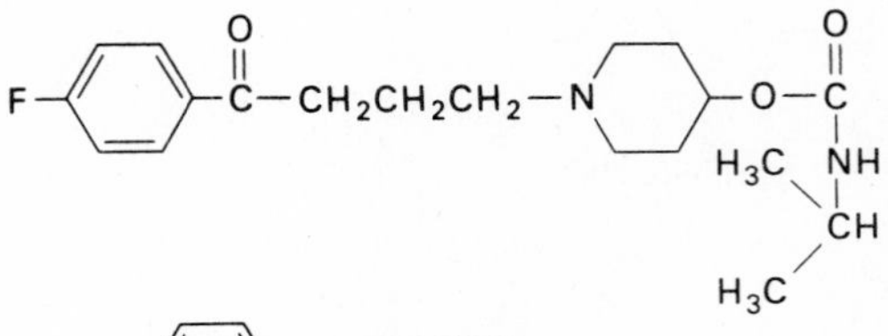

carperone

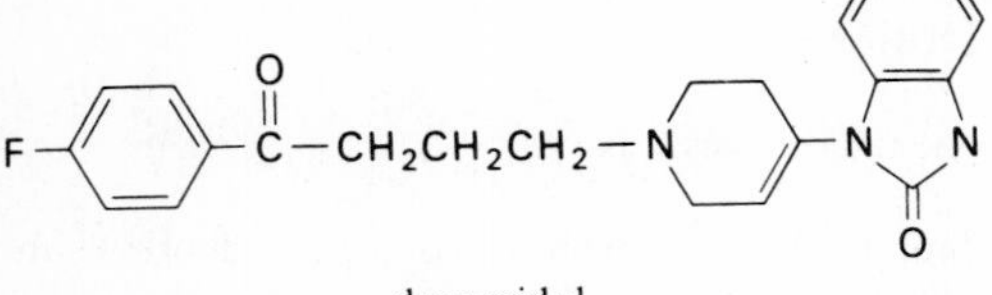

droperidol

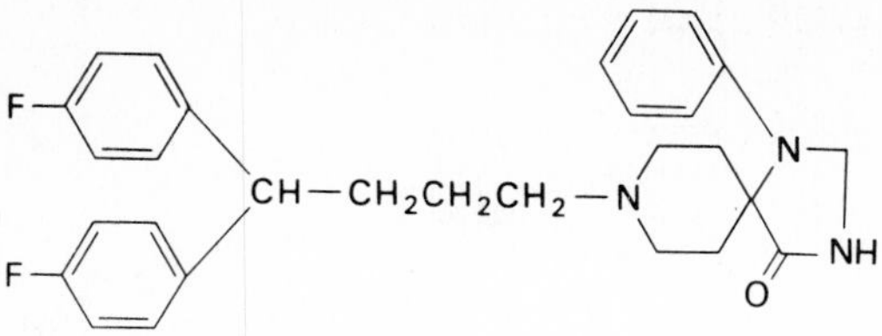

fluspirilene (Imap)

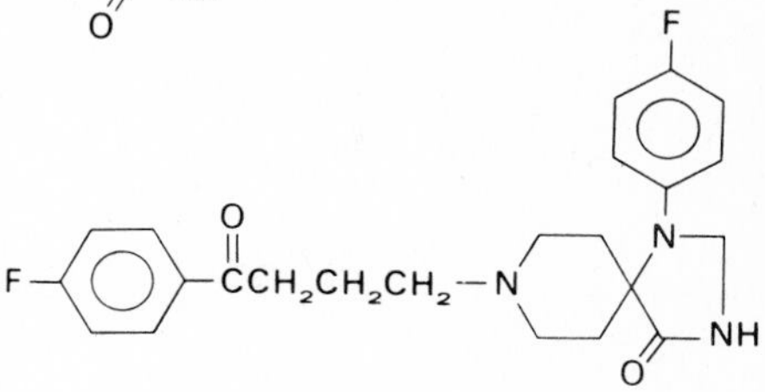

fluspiperone

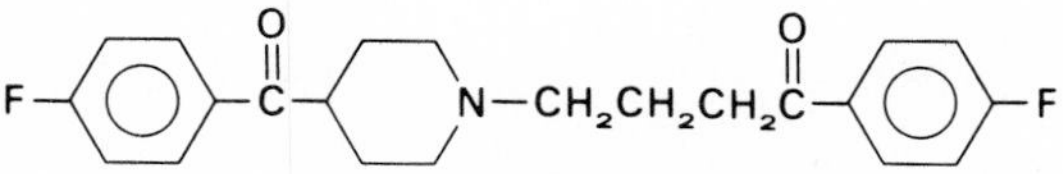

lenperone (Elanone)

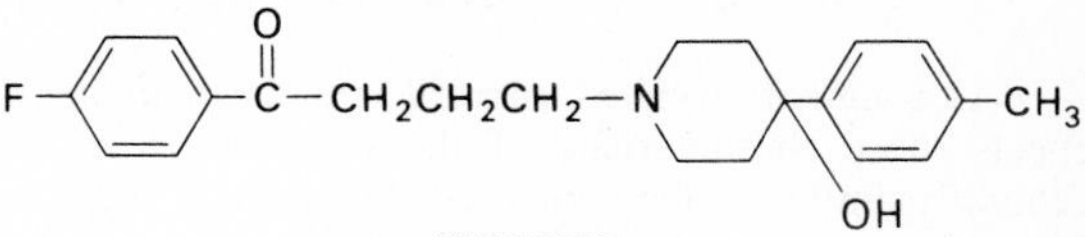

meperone

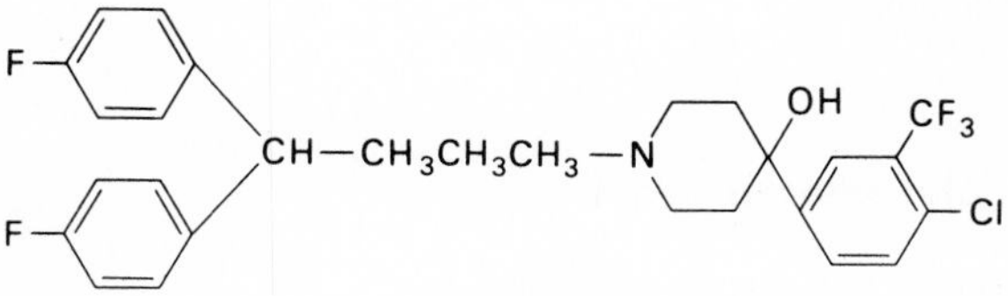

penfluridol

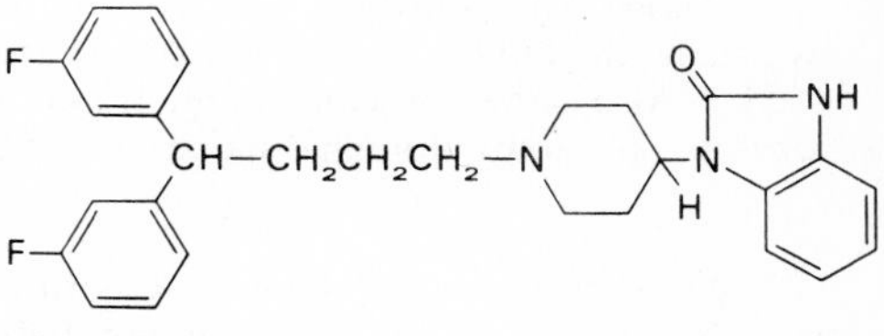

pimozide

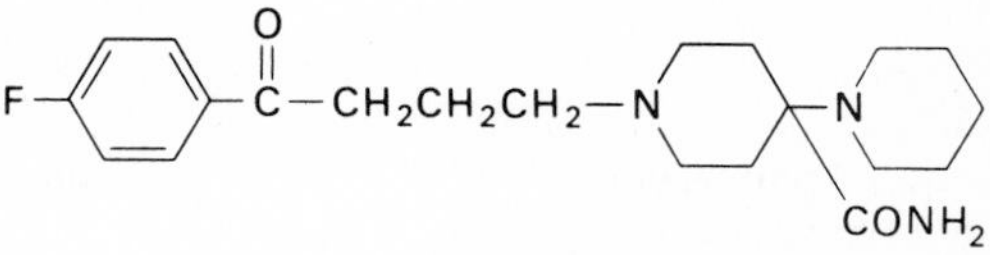

pipamperone

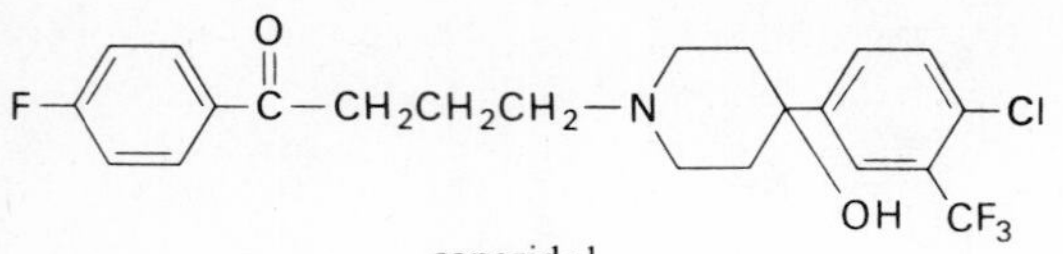

F—⟨C₆H₄⟩—C(=O)—CH₂CH₂CH₂—N⟨piperidine⟩(OH)—⟨C₆H₃(Cl)(CF₃)⟩

seperidol

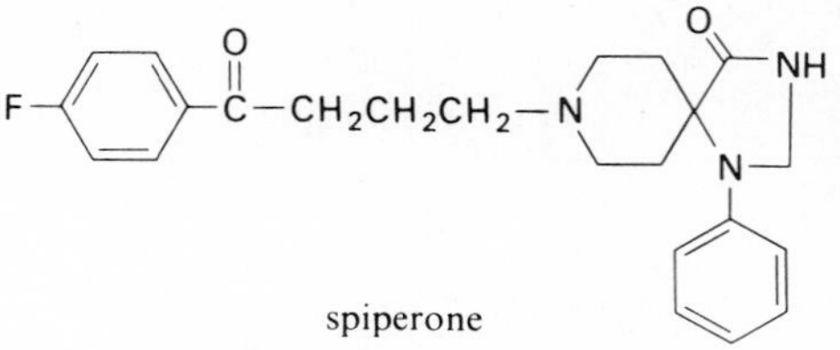

spiperone

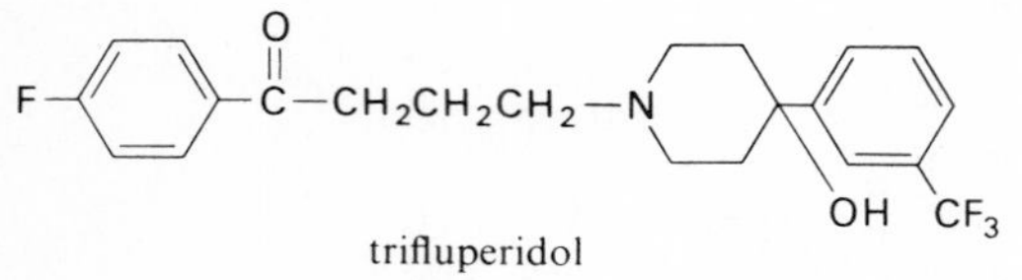

trifluperidol

E. Propanediol—Carbamate Series (Meprobamate)

Although often called tranquilizers, the propanediol-carbamate group produces effects more characteristic of the sedatives than of the tranquilizers. They are generally similar to phenobarbital in usefulness and have no application in psychoses. Meprobamate, the most used member, is helpful as a sedative in functional disorders (see Sedatives and Hypnotics).

F. Benzodiazepines (Chlordiazepoxide)

1. Chemistry. Benzodiazepine derivatives.

2. Action. a. Effective sedatives and muscle relaxants; do not appear to show specific tranquilizing or antipsychotic effects apart from sedative effects.

b. Also show anticonvulsant, appetite-stimulating, and weak analgesic actions; do not show autonomic actions or inhibition of conditional reflexes.

3. Mechanism. a. Unknown. Reported to inhibit respiratory function in mitochondria in vitro (Kadenbach, Nature, 192: 174, 1961).

b. Do not act by releasing serotonin or norepinephrine; do not affect MAO.

4. Pharmacodynamics. a. Absorbed slowly by mouth; effects develop over several hours.

b. Cumulation may occur; slow excretion, half-life 48 hours.

5. Toxicity. a. Ataxia, drowsiness, vertigo and syncope, itching, dermatitis, increased appetite, "rage reaction," impaired thinking.

b. Withdrawal symptoms, including seizures, have been seen 7 to 8 days following cessation of high doses.

6. Uses. a. Widely used as alternatives to phenobarbital or meprobamate in psychoneuroses, anxiety states, tension states; alcoholic intoxication; may have an advantage in that overdosage not fatal; undesirable in psychotics.

b. Diazepam is the drug of choice for the treatment of status epilepticus.

c. Also used as muscle relaxants.

7. Preparations

CHLORDIAZEPOXIDE HYDROCHLORIDE (Librium)

Dose: 25 to 100 mg daily by mouth.

NH—CH_3 N Cl N O

CLONAZEPAM (Clonopin)

Dose: 0.5 mg 3 times a day up to 20 mg/day.

H N O O_2N N Cl

CLORAZEPATE DIPOTASSIUM (Tranxilene, Tranxene)

Dose: 26 mg a day by mouth.

H OH N OH COOK · KOH Cl N

DIAZEPAM (Valium)

Similar to chlordiazepoxide but smaller dose.

Dose: 10 mg 3 times a day by mouth or intramuscularly.

H_3C O N Cl N

FLURAZEPAM HYDROCHLORIDE (Dalmane)
Dose: 15 to 30 mg, hypnotic.

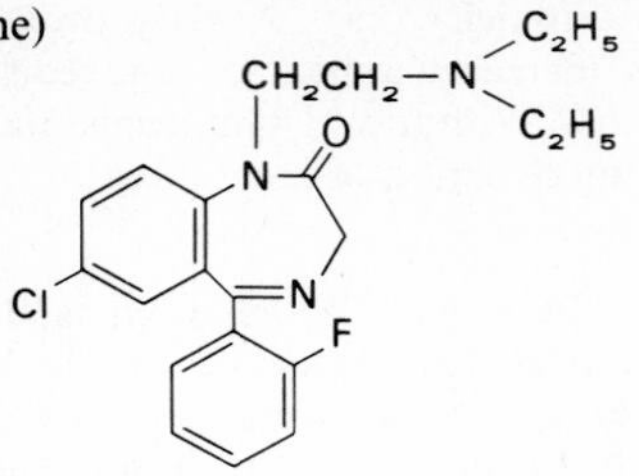

LORAZEPAM (Ativan)
Dose: 2 to 6 mg a day by mouth.

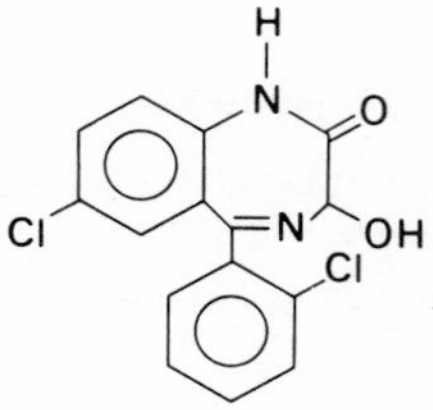

PRAZEPAM (Verstran)
Dose: 10 mg 3 times a day by mouth.

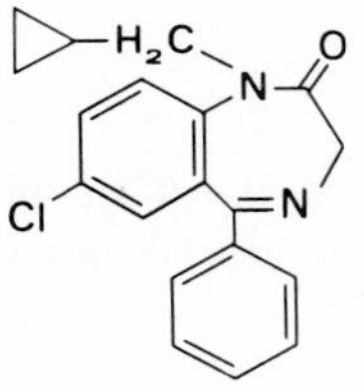

OTHERS

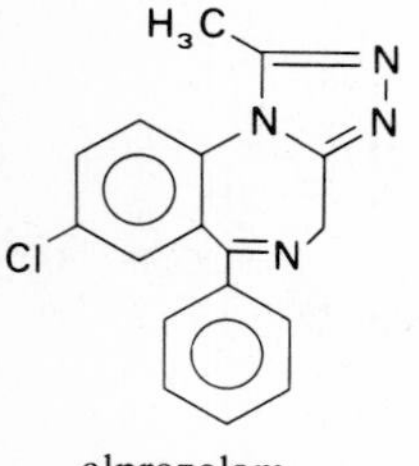

alprazolam

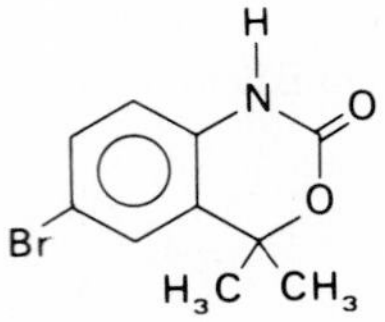

brofoxine

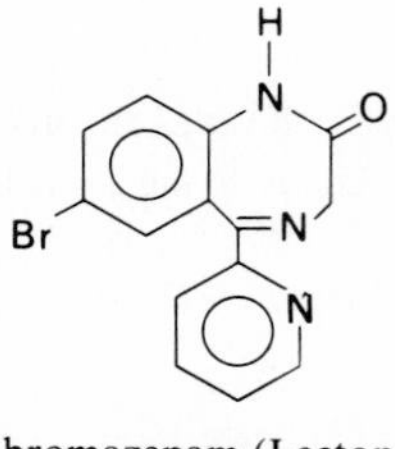

bromazepam (Lectopam)

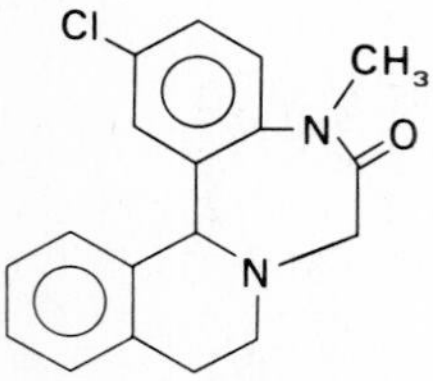

clazolam

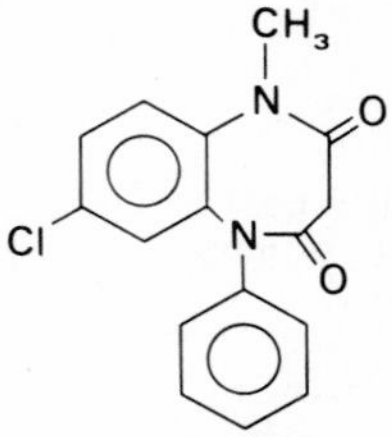

clobazam

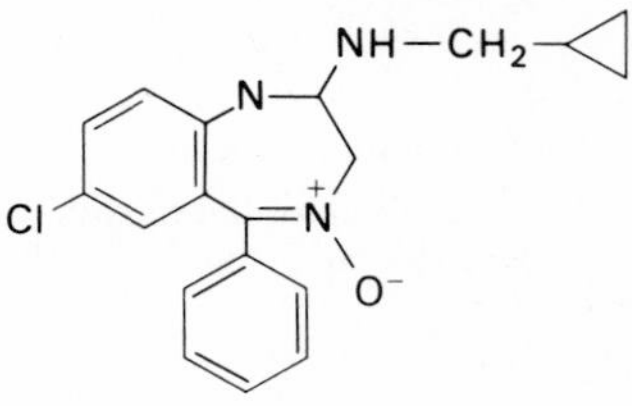

cyprazepam

fletazepam (See under Muscle Relaxants)

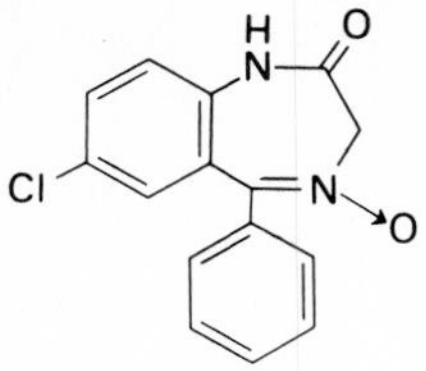

demoxepam

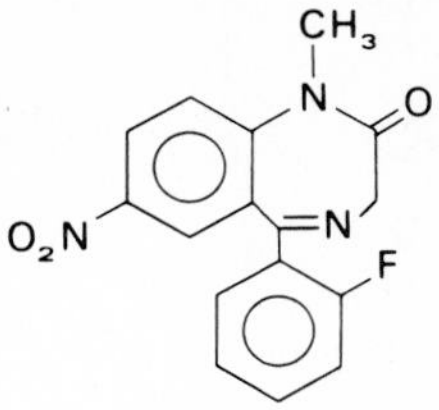

flunitrazepam (Rohypnol)

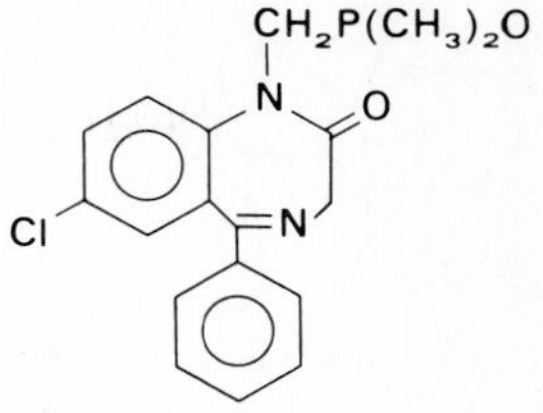

fosazepam

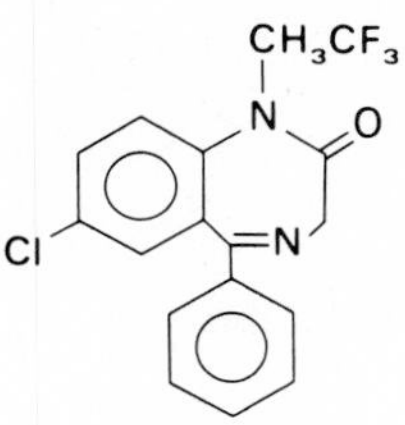

halazepam

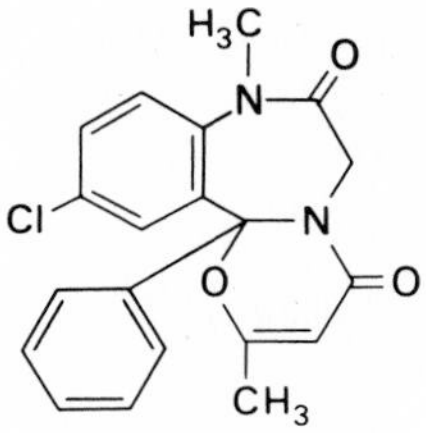

ketazolam

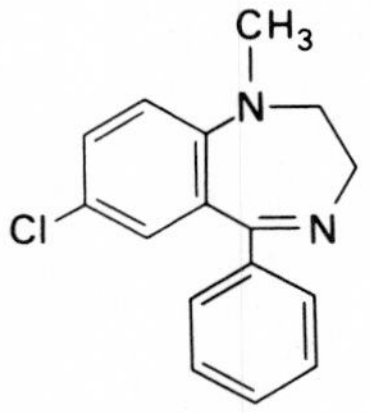

medazepam HCl (Nobrium)

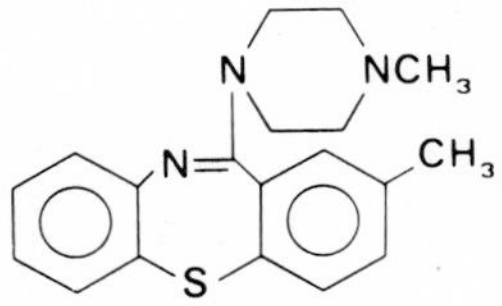

metiapine

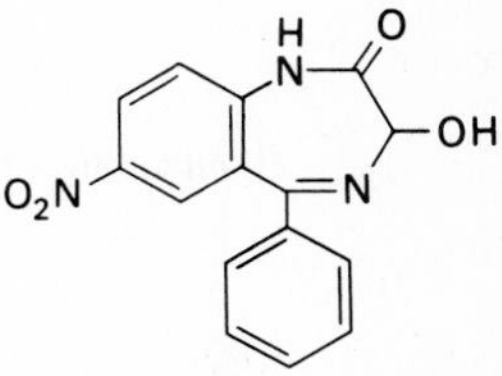

nitrazepam (Mogadon)

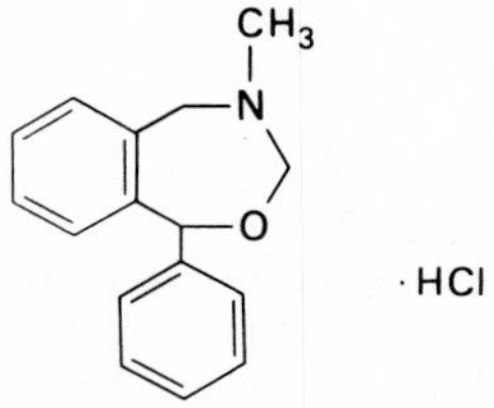

nefopam HCl (Acupan)

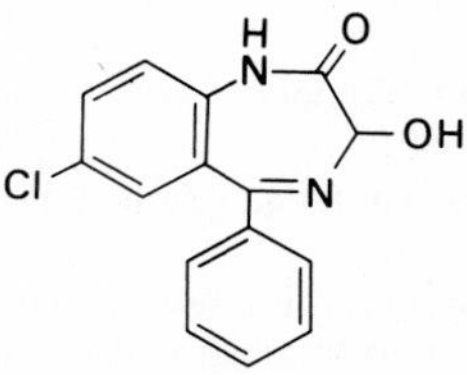

oxazepam (Serax)

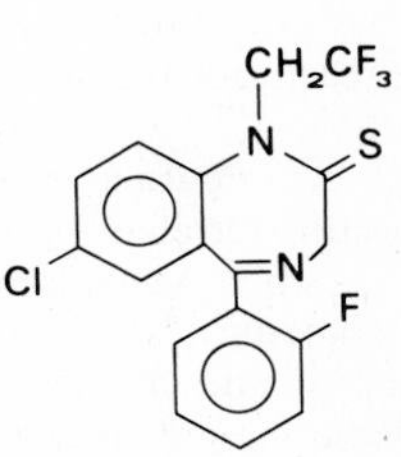

quazepam

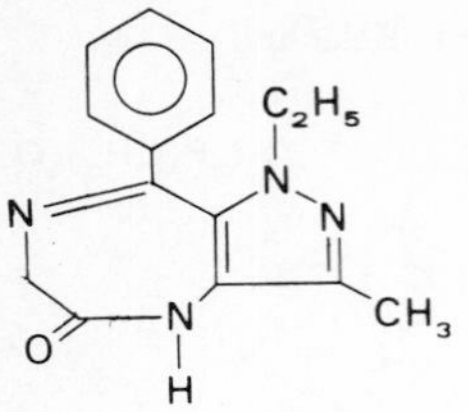

ripazepam

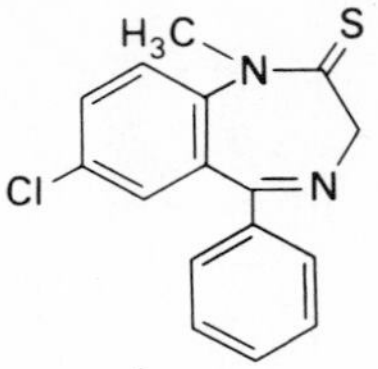

sulazepam

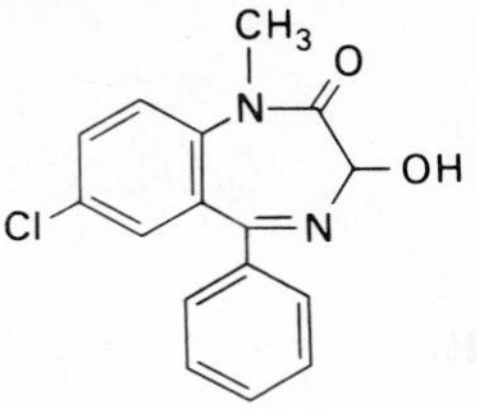

temazepam

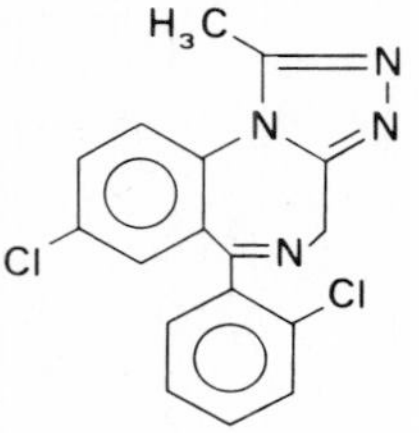

triazolam (Halcion)

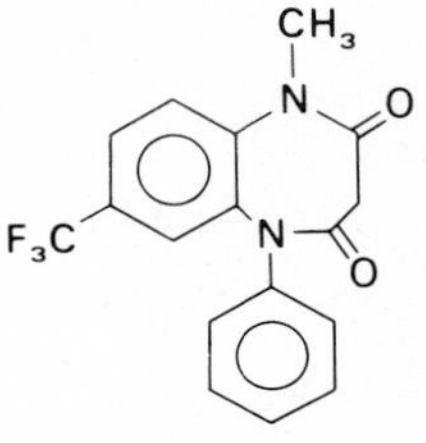

triflubazam

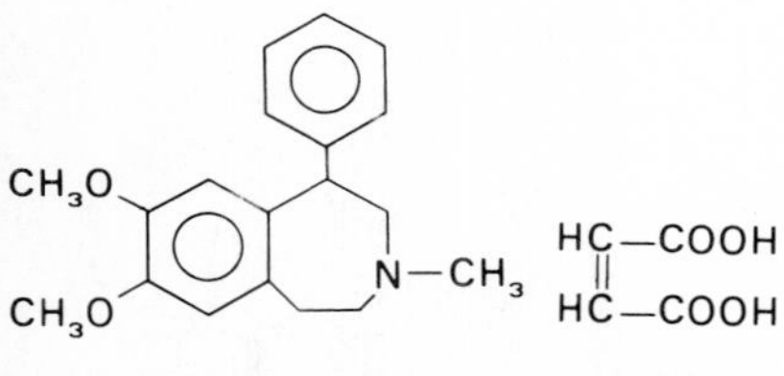

trimopam maleate

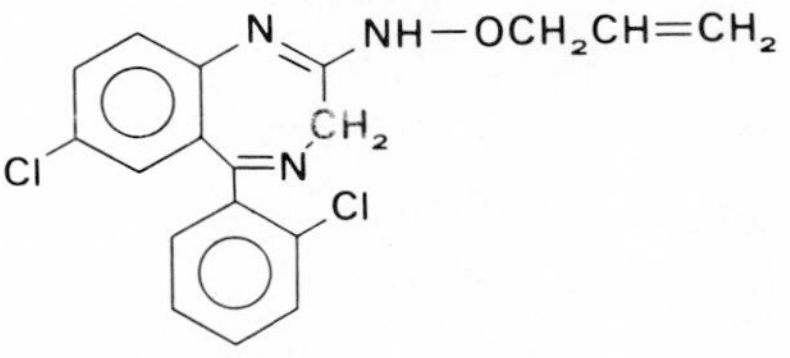

uldazepam

G. Lithium Salts

1. Action and Mechanism. a. Produce tranquility in manic states and possibly in depressions.

b. Suggested mechanisms include decreased availability of norepinephrine at receptors and shift in electrolyte balance.

2. Pharmacodynamics and Toxicity. a. Easily absorbed by mouth and rapidly excreted.

b. Nausea, polyuria, and diarrhea reached at a level only slightly above the therapeutic; severe toxicity follows excessive dosage, including tremor, nausea, slurred speech, confusion, lethargy, and death. This severe toxicity led to the abandonment of lithium salts as sodium substitutes in low-salt therapy for heart failure.

3. Uses. Used particularly in manic-depressive psychoses.

4. Preparation

LITHIUM CARBONATE (Escalith; Lithane): Li_2CO_3
Dose: 300 to 600 mg 3 times a day by mouth, reduced as required.

H. Other Tranquilizers

A number of other drugs have been described as having some of the characteristics of tranquilizers, but for the most part the resemblance is greater to the sedatives and hypnotics. As with meprobamate or chlordiazepoxide the effect appears not to be specifically on the mood but to be a part of minimal sedation and drowsiness; they are unsuited to the treatment of psychoses. However, they are useful in the treatment of emotional disorders in the general population, most desirably in augmentation of appropriate psychotherapy. Phenobarbital is usually as satisfactory as any of the newer drugs and cheaper.

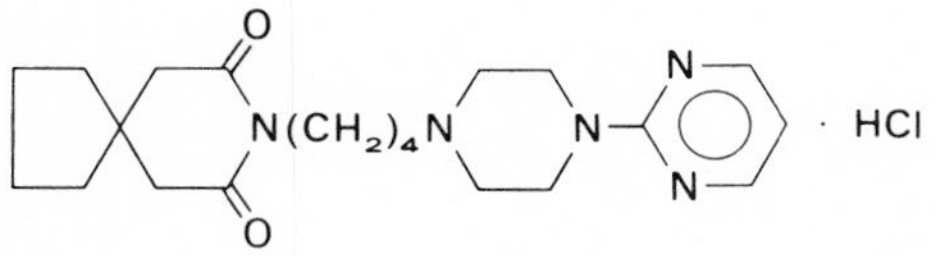

N(CH$_2$)$_4$N · HCl

buspirone hydrochloride

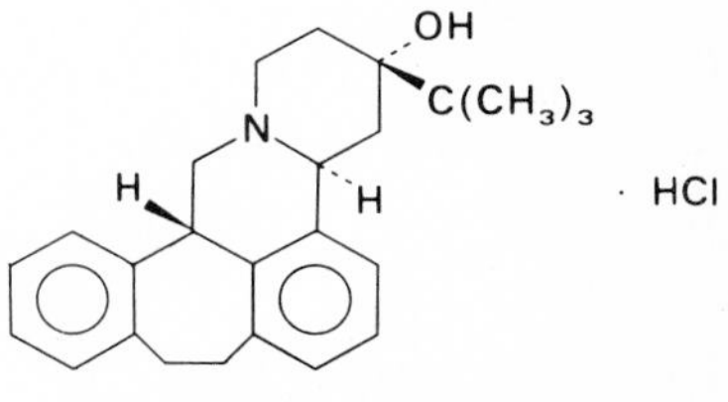

OH C(CH$_3$)$_3$ N H H · HCl

butaclomol hydrochloride

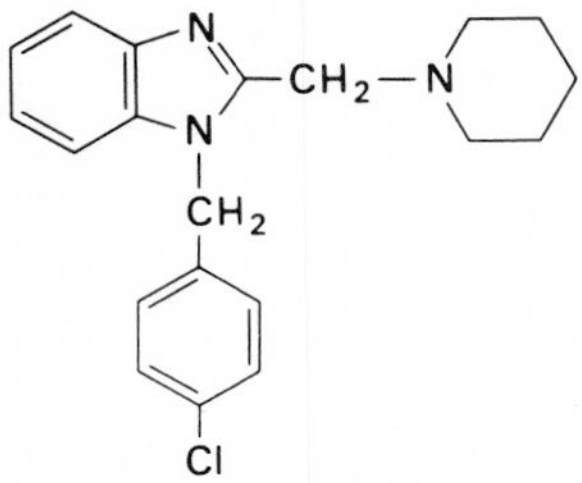

N CH$_2$—N N CH$_2$ Cl

clemizole (Allercur)

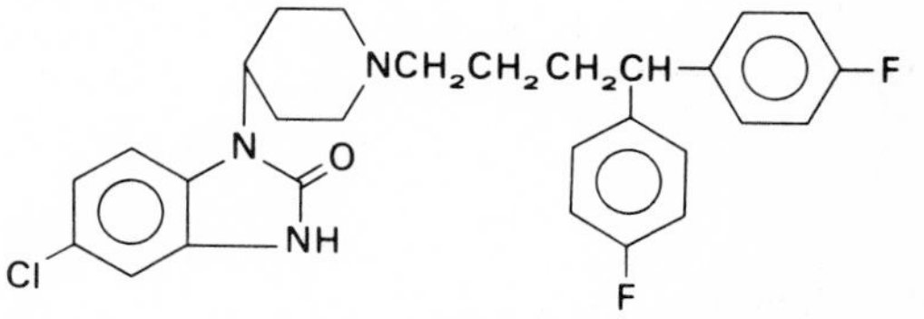

NCH$_2$CH$_2$CH$_2$CH F N O NH Cl F

clopimozide

C$_2$H$_5$ N N N · HCl C$_2$H$_5$OC O NH—N=C(CH$_3$)$_2$

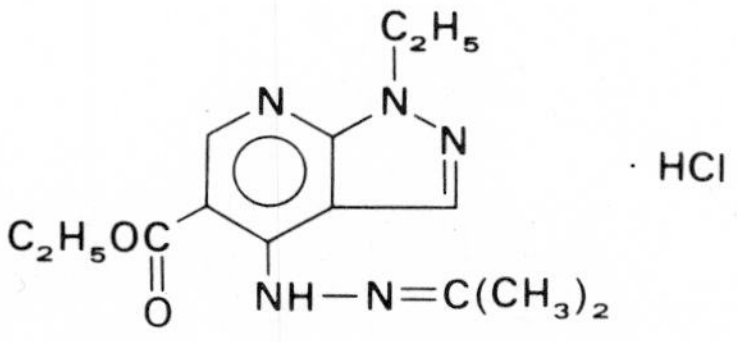

etazolate hydrochloride

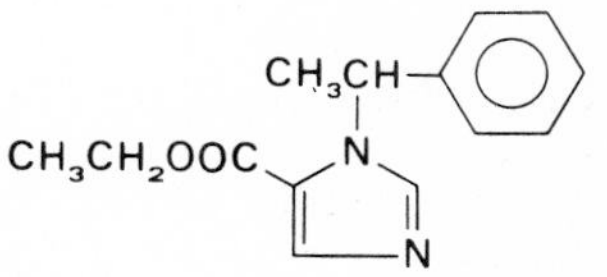

CH$_3$CH CH$_3$CH$_2$OOC N N

etomidate

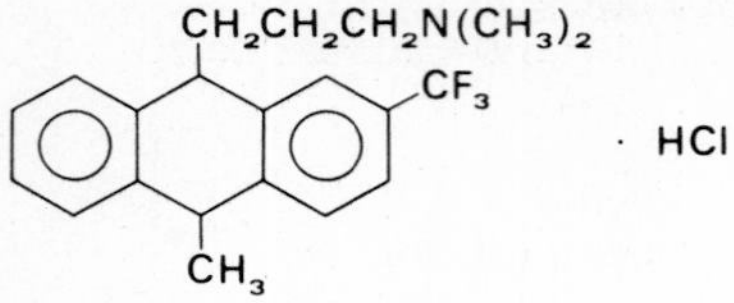

$CH_2CH_2CH_2N(CH_3)_2$ CF_3 CH_3 · HCl

fluotracen hydrochloride

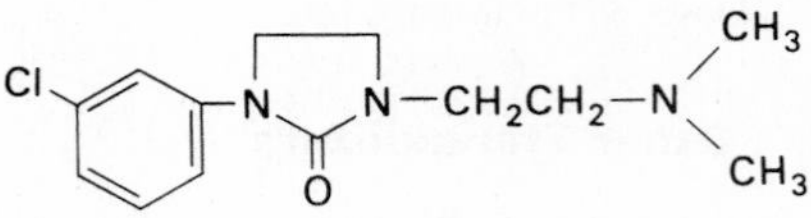

Cl N N—CH_2CH_2—N CH_3 CH_3 O

imidoline HCl

Cl $N(CH_3)_2$ · HCl OCH_3

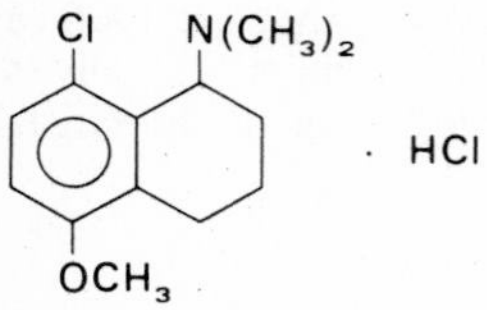

lometraline hydrochloride

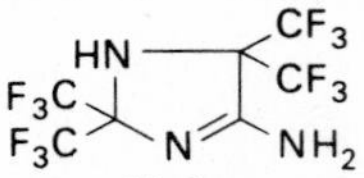

HN CF_3 CF_3 F_3C F_3C N NH_2

midaflur

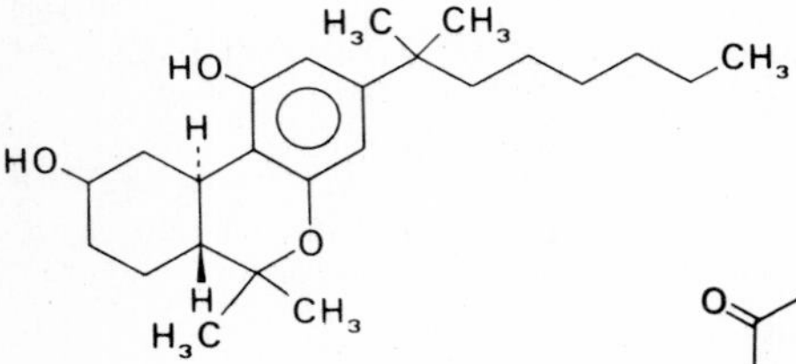

H_3C CH_3 HO CH_3 H HO O H CH_3 H_3C

nabidrox

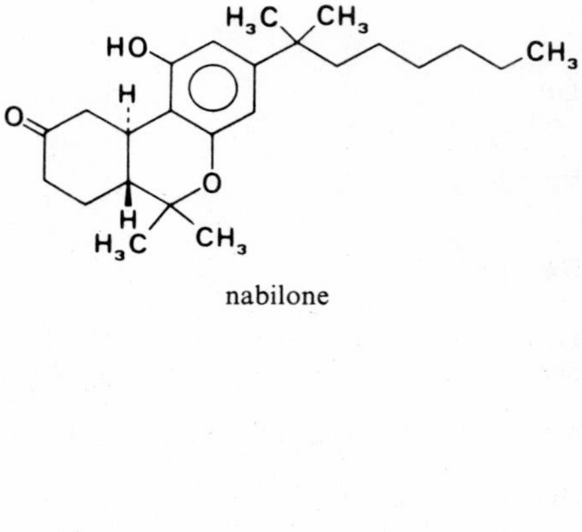

H_3C CH_3 HO CH_3 H O O H H_3C CH_3

nabilone

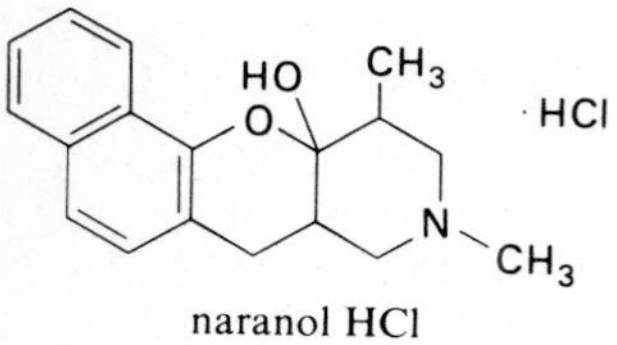

HO CH_3 O · HCl N CH_3

naranol HCl

N · HCl

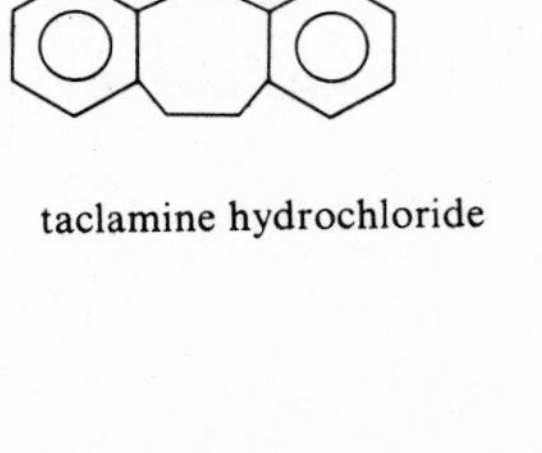

taclamine hydrochloride

SUMMARY: TRANQUILIZERS

TYPE	*ACTION AND MECHANISM*	*TOXICITY*	*USE*	*EXAMPLES*
Phenothiazines	Produce mental calm, probably by blocking access of nor-epinephrine to receptor and reentry into axon	Sympatholytic effects, extra-pyramidal syndromes, hepatitis, agranulocytosis	Excited psychoses, antiemetic	Chlorpromazine HCl
Rauwolfia derivatives	Produce mental calm, primarily by release of stored catechol-amines, which are then destroyed	Sympatholytic effects, bleed-ing in peptic ulcer	Excited psychoses, hypertension	Reserpine
Diphenyl-methanes	Induce calm Mechanism unclear	Sedation	Psychoneuroses	Benactyzine
Butyrophenones	Same	Sedation, extra-pyramidal syndromes	Excited psychoses	Haloperidol
Benzodiazepines	Sedation and muscle relaxation Mechanism unclear	Sedation, ataxia, dermatitis	Psychoneuroses, alcoholism	Chlordiazepoxide
Lithium salts	Induce calm Mechanism unclear	Nausea, tremor, confusion, lethargy	Manic depressive psychoses	Lithium carbonate

Reviews

Domino, E. Human pharmacology of tranquilizers. Clin. Pharmacol. Ther., 3:599, 1962.

Shore, P. Release of serotonin and catechol amines by drugs. Pharmacol. Rev., 14:531, 1962.

Moertel, C., Reitemeier, R., and Gage, R. Controlled clinical evaluation of antiemetic drugs. J.A.M.A., 186:116, 1963.

Hollister, L., Overall, J., and others. Triperidol in schizophrenia: Further evidence for specific patterns of action of antipsychotic drugs. J. New Drugs, 5:34, 1965.

Hollister, L. Human pharmacology of antipsychotropic and antidepressant drugs. Ann. Rev. Pharmacol., 8:491, 1968.

Gershon, S. Lithium in mania. Clin. Pharmacol. Ther., 11:168, 1970.

55. Stimulants

Stimulants of the central nervous system may be classified, somewhat arbitrarily, into two groups. The first, general stimulants, comprise medullary, reflex, and spinal cord stimulants, according to principal site of action. They have been much studied by pharmacologists, but in clinical use are relatively ineffective and some are dangerous. The second, cerebral or psychic stimulants, by contrast enjoy wide use.

I. GENERAL STIMULANTS

A. Medullary Stimulants

As a group, the medullary stimulants are convulsants, producing clonic seizures by stimulating higher levels in the CNS. However, in doses below the convulsant, they stimulate the brain stem and especially the depressed respiratory center. This has led to their use in respiratory and circulatory depression, primarily when caused by overdosage with other drugs.

NIKETHAMIDE GROUP

1. Chemistry. Derivatives, or phenyl analogues, of niacinamide; nikethamide possesses vitamin activity.

2. Action and Mechanism. a. Produce general medullary stimulation, respiratory and circulatory.

b. Mechanism unknown. Ethamivan may act by lowering a previously elevated threshold to CO_2 in the respiratory center (Rockwell, Clin. Pharmacol. Ther., 4:728, 1963).

3. Pharmacodynamics and Toxicity. a. Well absorbed by mouth, but may be given intravenously. Longer acting than picrotoxin or pentylenetetrazol.

b. Toxicity minor. Not convulsant in therapeutic dosage.

4. Uses. a. Nikethamide formerly used in anesthetic and morphine poisoning and in shock, but largely ineffective.

b. Ethamivan used as a respiratory stimulant to hasten the return of consciousness after anesthesia, for CO_2 accumulation, for CNS depression from sedatives; clinical value limited.

5. Preparations

NIKETHAMIDE (Coramine)

Dose: 1.5 to 3 ml of 25% solution by mouth or intravenously.

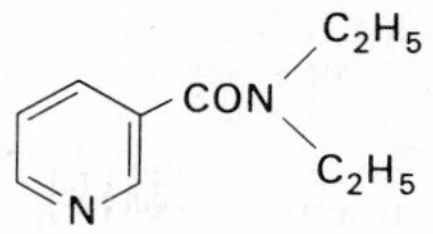

ETHAMIVAN (Emivan, Vandid)

Dose: 20 mg by mouth; up to 100 mg intravenously.

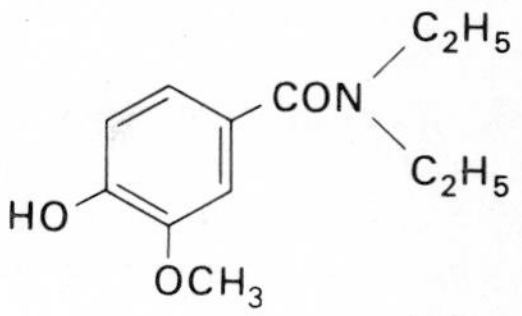

COTININE FUMARATE (Scotine)

Said to be a metabolite of nicotine; psychic stimulant.

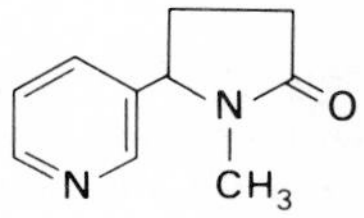

PENTYLENETETRAZOL

1. Chemistry. Unusual condensed structure.

2. Action and Mechanism. a. Primarily a cortical and brain stem stimulant with secondary cord stimulation.

b. In adequate dosage, produces a convulsive seizure about 10 seconds after intravenous administration.

c. Mechanism unknown.

3. Pharmacodynamics and Toxicity. a. Absorbable by mouth, but ordinarily given by vein; detoxified in the liver.

b. Dangers consist of unintended convulsions; bone fractures during convulsive therapy.

4. Uses. a. Limited use in anesthetic and barbiturate poisoning.

b. Formerly used to produce convulsive shock in depressive psychoses; displaced by electroshock therapy; activates EEG in suspected epilepsy.

5. Preparations

PENTYLENETETRAZOL (Metrazol)

Dose: 1 to 5 ml of 10% solution intravenously.

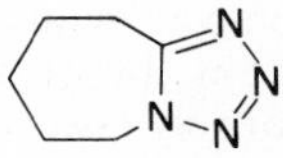

PICROTOXIN

1. Chemistry. a. A combination of picrotoxinin and picrotin (inert); former may be derived from a steroid.

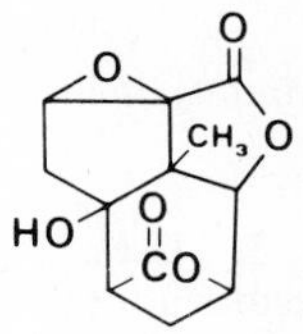

b. Obtained from *Anamirta cocculus*, fish berry; used as a fish poison in the East Indies.

2. Action and Mechanism. The most powerful of the classical medullary convulsants and respiratory stimulants; latter effect is not prominent except in the presence of respiratory depression.

3. Pharmacodynamics and Toxicity. a. Effects delayed; appear 10 to 15 minutes after intravenous injection.

b. Rapidly destroyed in an hour or two with minimal cumulation.

c. Great danger of inducing convulsions by overdosage; counteract with intravenous barbiturates.

4. Uses. a. Controversial use in barbiturate poisoning. Division of opinion as to whether potent respiratory stimulation valuable, or whether supportive treatment may not be as satisfactory and safer.

b. Supportive treatment: warmth, evacuation of stomach, oxygen, maintenance of ventilation (artificial respiration if needed), circulation, and kidney function.

5. Preparation

PICROTOXIN

Dose: 3 mg intravenously, repeated at intervals of 3 minutes; caution!

BEMEGRIDE

1. History. Shaw (1954) introduced as a specific barbiturate antagonist.

2. Chemistry. A glutarimide derivative, resembling glutethimide slightly, barbiturates less.

3. Action and Mechanism. a. General analeptic with about the potency of pentylenetetrazol; respirations increased in one minute; effect lasts 15 minutes.

b. Originally considered to be a barbiturate competitor on a chemical (competitive interference) basis; now competition believed to be pharmacological, that is, by competition at different receptors. Chemical competition, however, probably exists between the barbiturates and the experimental antagonist 5,5-ethyl-alpha-8-dimethylbutylbarbital.

4. Pharmacodynamics and Toxicity. a. Administered by vein.

b. Overdosage produces vomiting, twitching, convulsions (inject barbiturates), delirium; safer than picrotoxin.

5. Uses. Has been used in barbiturate poisoning, and to lessen thiopental anesthesia; of doubtful future.

6. Preparation

BEMEGRIDE (Megimide)

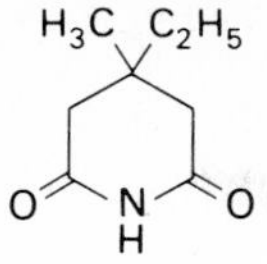

Dose: 50 mg every 3 to 5 minutes intravenously until improvement.

OTHERS

AMIPHENAZOLE (Daptazole)

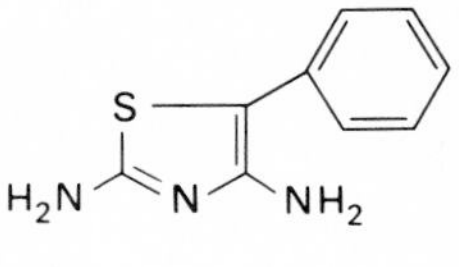

Moderately potent stimulant; no apparent therapeutic advantages.

Dose: 20 to 50 mg intramuscularly or 30 to 100 mg by mouth.

AZABON

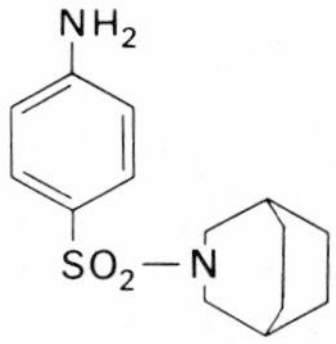

CNS stimulant; sulfonamide derivative.

DIMEFLINE HYDROCHLORIDE (Remeflin)

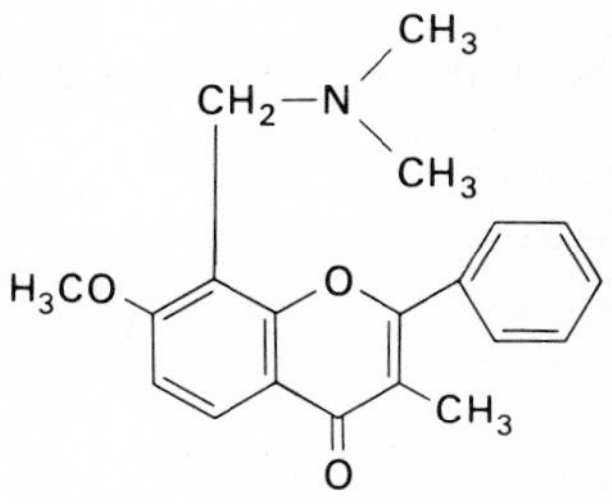

Respiratory stimulant.
Under investigation.

DOXAPRAM HYDROCHLORIDE (Stimulexin)

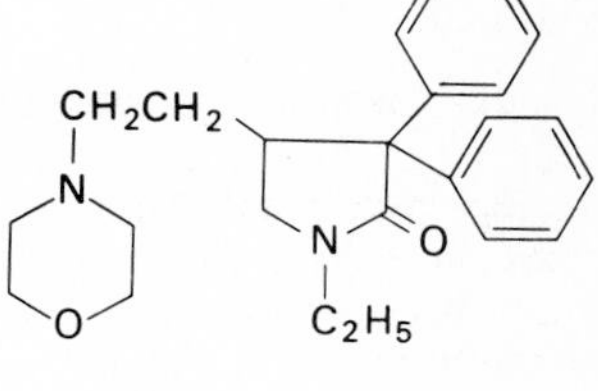

Stimulates all levels of the CNS; used as a respiratory stimulant in anesthesia (Stephen, Anesth. Analg., 43:628, 1964).

Dose: 1 to 1.5 mg per kg body weight intravenously.

FLUROTHYL (Indoklon)

See General Anesthetics.

METHASTYRIDONE

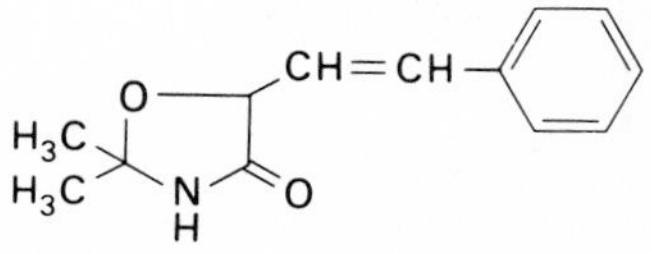

Analeptic.
Under investigation.

CARBON DIOXIDE

The natural stimulant of the respiratory center, and, to a lesser extent, of the carotid sinus; however, ineffective when center depressed. Used to cause deep inspirations and prevent postoperative atelectasis; ineffective in barbiturate or other drug poisoning (see Therapeutic Gases).

B. Reflex Stimulants

The medullary centers may be stimulated reflexly, as well as directly (as by the drugs in the previous section). The impulses may arise from various peripheral sites, including the carotid sinus.

1. Preparations

AROMATIC SPIRIT OF AMMONIA

Reflex arises from irritation of the nose and throat.
Dose: 2 ml diluted in water.

AMMONIUM CARBONATE (smelling salts)

Similar stimulation by ammonia.
Dose: by inhalation.

LOBELINE

An unreliable and obsolete carotid body stimulant.

CYANIDE

Also a strong stimulant of the carotid body, but excessively dangerous.

C. Spinal Cord Stimulants

STRYCHNINE

1. Chemistry. Alkaloid from seeds of *Strychnos nux-vomica.*

2. Action and Mechanism. a. Produces tonic convulsions without clonic phase, in contrast to medullary stimulants.

b. Removes synaptic resistance in cord. Blocks action of acetylcholine on inhibitory cells.

c. Shows anticholinesterase action in vitro, but this is probably not the basis of the in vivo effect.

3. Pharmacodynamics and Toxicity. a. Well absorbed by mouth.

b. May produce convulsions; control by barbiturates and mephenesin.

4. Uses. a. Old-time bitter and "muscular tonic," but no modern indication in medicine.

b. Rodenticide.

5. Preparations

TINCTURE OF NUX VOMICA
Obsolete bitter tonic.

STRYCHNINE SULFATE
Dose: 2 mg by mouth or subcutaneously.
Obsolete.

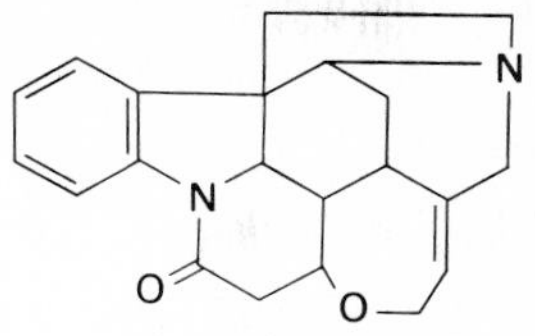

strychnine

II. CEREBRAL OR PSYCHIC STIMULANTS

Cerebral or psychic stimulants are stimulants used largely for psychic effects; that is, to heighten or improve the mood. Psychic stimulants are also called psychic energizers, a term coined by Freud long before the appearance of such drugs, antidepressants, and thymoleptics. The recognition that the mind could be influenced by drugs, somewhat apart from the CNS in general, was not widely appreciated until the advent of tranquilizers and renewed interest in psychotomimetic agents.

A. Xanthine Group

METHYLATED PURINES

Drinks containing methylated purines, especially caffeine, are almost worldwide in use. It is said that every known plant source was first discovered by primitive society. The drinks are mildly euphoriant and produce a sense of well being.

Moderate tolerance may develop. There is no physical dependence; only mild psychic symptoms appear upon withdrawal.

COFFEE

From *Coffea arabica*, an Arabian bush; beans contain 1% to 2% caffeine.

TEA

From *Camelia theca*, an Asian bush; leaves contain 2% to 3% caffeine, and theobromine and theophylline.

CACAO

From *Theobroma cacao*, Aztec chocolate; beans contain about 2% theobromine and traces of caffeine and theophylline.

MATÉ

From *Ilex paraguayensis*, a South American bush; leaves contain 2% caffeine.

GUARANA

From *Panela supana*, an Amazonian vine; contains 5% caffeine.

KOLA

From *Cola nitida*, an African nut; contains 3% caffeine.

CAFFEINE

1. Chemistry. Caffeine is the most stimulating of the methylxanthines.

2. Action. a. Stimulates all parts of the CNS, especially the cerebral cortex and medullary centers.

b. Small doses produce alertness, wakefulness, talkativeness (and diuresis).

c. Larger doses stimulate the respiratory center if it is depressed but still responsive. (See also Smooth Muscle Relaxants.)

3. Mechanism. Fundamental mechanism not understood; inhibition of phosphodiesterase, with consequent increase in tissue 3′5′-AMP, may be important (Butcher, J. Biol. Chem., 237:1244, 1962).

4. Pharmacodynamics and Toxicity. a. Rapidly absorbed by mouth or injection.

b. Widely distributed; excreted as various breakdown products.

c. Excessive dosage produces insomnia and restlessness, probably as a result of keener appreciation of sensory stimuli.

5. Uses. a. To induce wakefulness, but more often as beverage coffee than medicinal.

b. Contained in over-the-counter tablets for keeping awake.

c. Often injected as a harmless, final administration to the dying.

6. Preparations

CAFFEINE and SODIUM BENZOATE

Dose: 0.5 to 1.0 gm subcutaneously or by mouth.

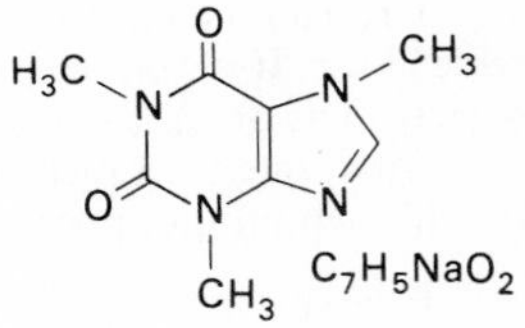

$C_7H_5NaO_2$

DIMETHAZAN

Tried in the depressed aged.

Dose: 200 mg 4 times a day by mouth.

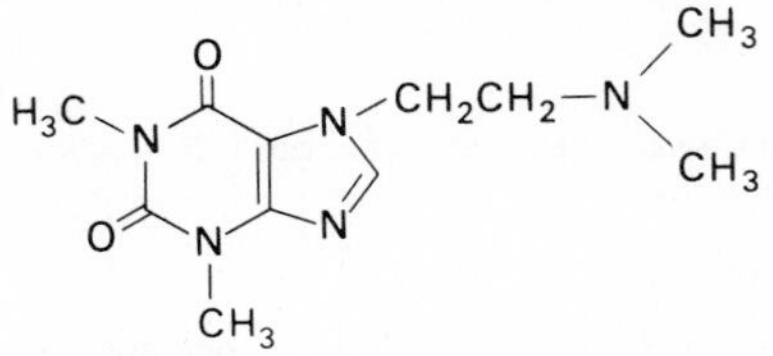

RIBAMOL (2-hydroxytriethylammonium ribonucleate)

Claimed to enhance memory and learning.

Under investigation.

B. Sympathomimetic Group

AMPHETAMINES

1. Chemistry. Sympathomimetic amines (see Sympathetic Stimulants for general consideration).

2. Action. a. Potent cerebral stimulants producing alertness, wakefulness, talkativeness, random motor activity, and a stimulation or heightening of the mood.

b. Larger doses stimulate the respiratory center if it is depressed.

c. Also produce general sympathomimetic effects to which tolerance develops rapidly.

3. Mechanism. Not clarified, but presumably related to mechanism of the sympathomimetic effects.

4. Pharmacodynamics and Toxicity. a. Well absorbed by mouth, effects prompt; excessive dosage may cause insomnia, mania, hallucinations, hyperpyrexia, convulsions, and death.

b. May be habituating.

5. Uses. a. To induce wakefulness.

b. To improve mood and brighten the outlook in mild depressions and behavioral problems.

c. As a respiratory stimulant in barbiturate poisoning.

d. In narcolepsy, often in large dosage; as an anorexic.

6. Preparations

AMPHETAMINE SULFATE (Benzedrine)

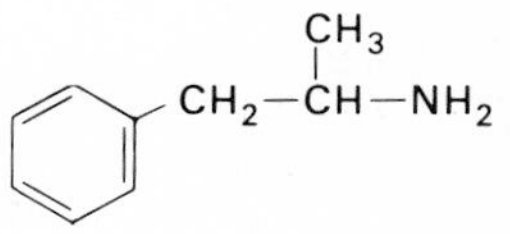

Dose: 5 to 10 mg or more by mouth or subcutaneously.

Dextroamphetamine sulfate (Dexedrine and others)
Dose: 2.5 to 5 mg or more by mouth.

$C_6H_5-CH_2-CH(CH_3)-NH_2$

METHAMPHETAMINE HYDROCHLORIDE (Desoxyn; and others)

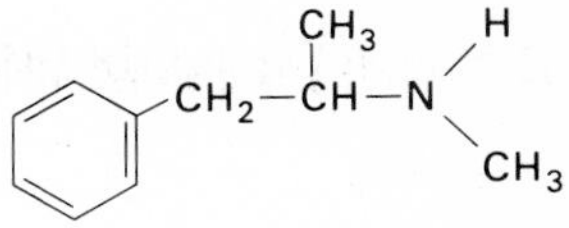

Dose: 2.5 to 5 mg or more by mouth.

$C_6H_5-CH_2-CH(CH_3)-N(H)(CH_3)$

PEMOLINE (Cylert)

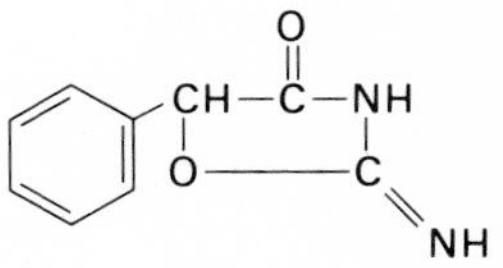

Central stimulant; psychoanaleptic. Helps some mildly depressed patients (Rückels, Clin. Pharmacol. Ther., 11:698, 1970).

Magnesium pemoline
Dose: 100 mg by mouth.

CH—C(=O)—NH, O——C=NH (with phenyl on CH)

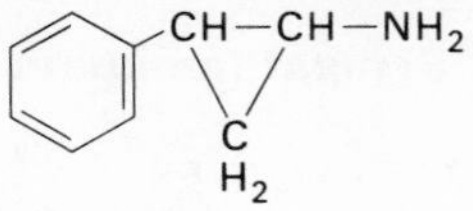

TRANYLCYPROMINE (PARNATE)

Potent MAO inhibitor; structurally resembles amphetamine. Side effects may include postural hypotension, insomnia, restlessness, photophobia. More seriously, hypertensive crises may appear with palpitation, headaches, vomiting, stiff neck, hypertension, and even death. The latter attacks are thought to be the result of tyramine poisoning by the following mechanism; tyrosine from food (cheese) is broken down by bacteria in the bowel to tyramine, which is absorbed; if there is inadequate MAO to destroy it, the tyramine rises to dangerous levels. Antidote: phentolamine mesylate, 5 mg intramuscularly.

Dose: 10 mg 2 times a day for 2 to 3 weeks; then increase to 3 times a day if necessary. Withdrawn from market; then returned for limited use.

OTHER SYMPATHOMIMETICS

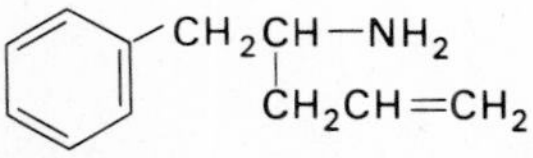

aletamine

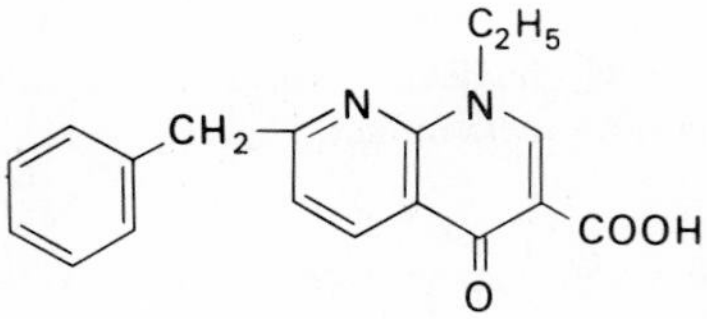

amfonelic acid

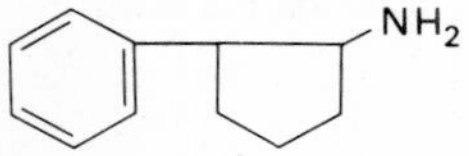

cypenamine

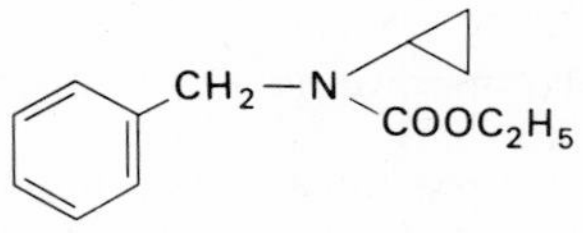

encyprate

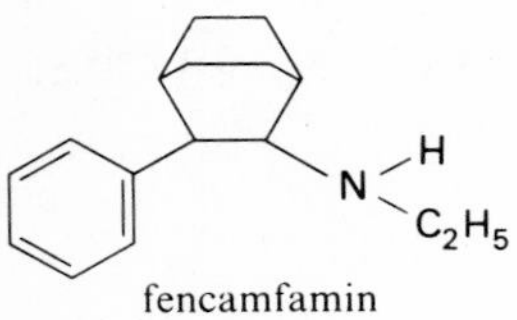

fencamfamin

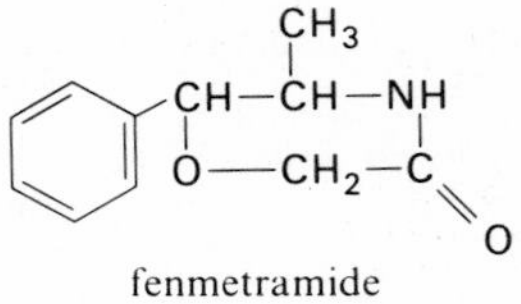

fenmetramide

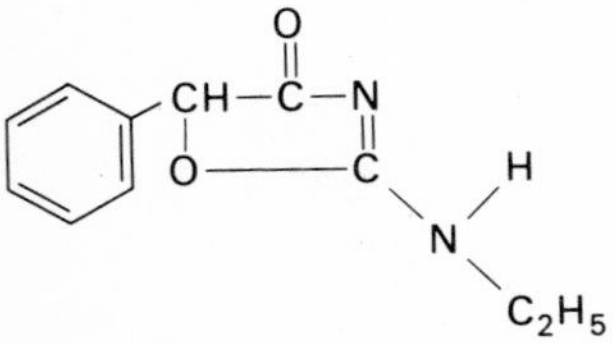

fenozolone

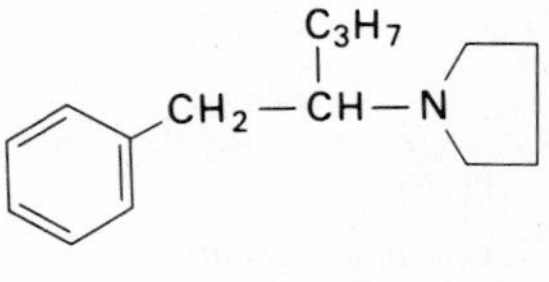

prolintane HCl

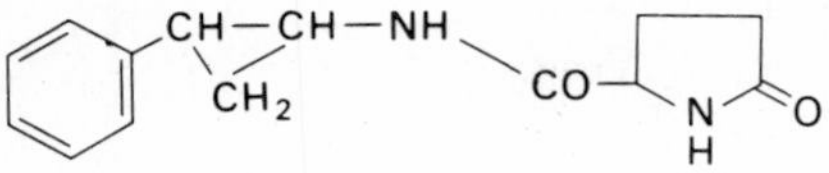

rolicyprine (Cypromin)

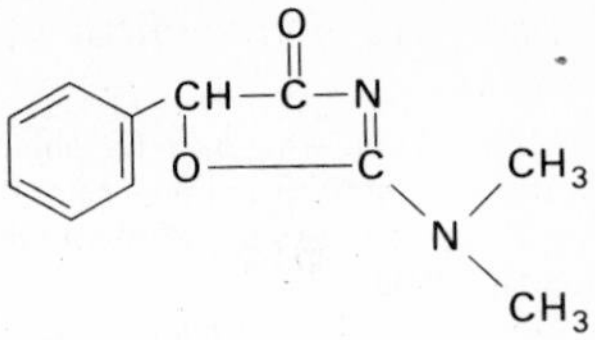

thozalinone

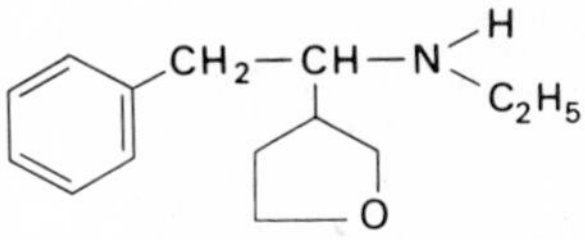

zylofuramine

C. Diphenylmethane Derivatives and Related Compounds

This group contains the stimulant counterparts of the diphenylmethane tranquilizers (see Tranquilizers), and like them may show spasmolytic and antihistaminic effects.

1. Chemistry. Diphenylmethanes, benzilic acid esters, and related compounds.

2. Action and Mechanism. Mild stimulants of mood; little effect on sleep.

3. Pharmacodynamics and Toxicity. a. Adequately absorbed by mouth. b. Toxicity minor; hyperexcitability, irritability, insomnia.

4. Uses. As mild psychic stimulants.

5. Preparations

DEANOL ACETAMIDOBENZOATE (Deaner)

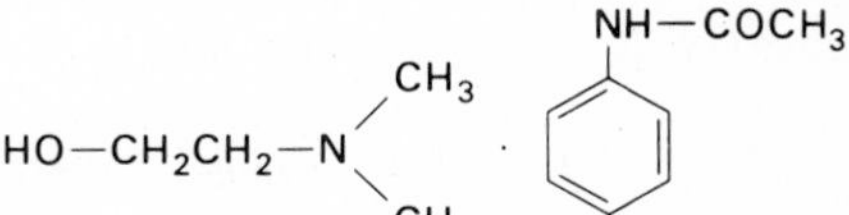

Mechanism suggested: to act as a precursor of acetylcholine which penetrates the blood-brain barrier better than choline. Slowly, over several weeks, stated to produce a mild, pleasant stimulation with improvement in mental concentration, muscle tone, sleep, energy, especially in children. Therapeutic claims controversial.

Dose: 10 to 50 mg once daily by mouth.

METHYLPHENIDATE HYDROCHLORIDE (Ritalin)

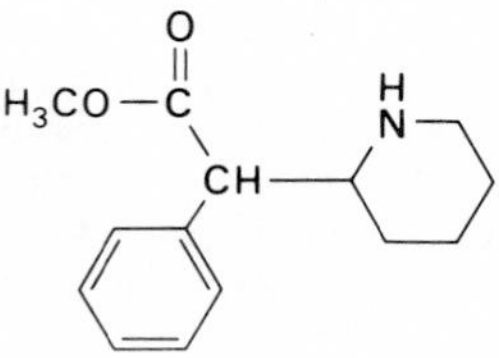

Also may be considered a phenylethylamine relative. Effects develop slowly over several days.

Dose: 10 mg 3 times a day by mouth.

PIPRADROL HYDROCHLORIDE (Meratran)

May also be considered a phenylethylamine (amphetamine relative). Promptly stimulates the mood and may reduce appetite.

Dose: 1 to 2 mg 3 times a day by mouth.

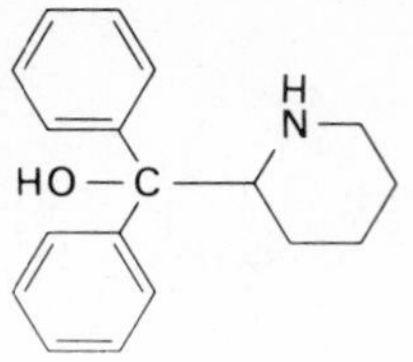

OTHERS

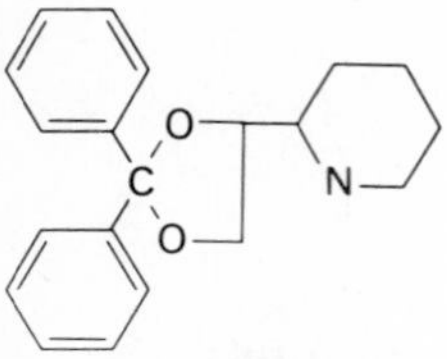

dexoxadrol (Relane) (also levoxadrol)

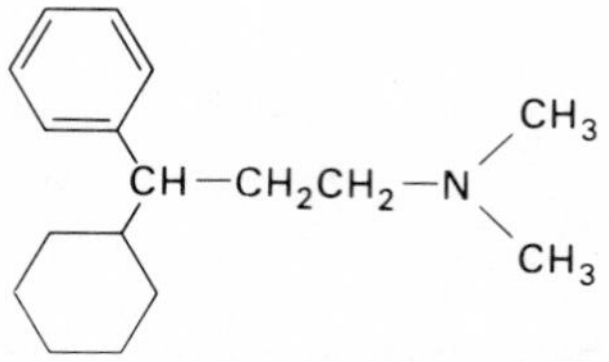

gamfexine

D. Amine Oxidase Inhibitors

HYDRAZINES

1. History. a. Bernheim (1928) showed that liver homogenates contained an enzyme, amine oxidase, which oxidized tyramine; later it was found in other tissues. Blaschko (1937) found that epinephrine was also oxidized; later that norepinephrine, serotonin, histamine, tryptamine, and other monoamines and diamines were oxidized; hence, mono- and di-amine oxidases.

b. Fox (1951) noted that iproniazid raised the mood in tuberculosis patients; Zeller (1952) found that it was a potent monoamine oxidase (MAO) inhibitor; Kline (1957) and others used it for psychiatric depression.

2. Chemistry. Hydrazines ($-NHNH_2$) and hydrazides ($-CONHNH_2$).

3. Action. a. Slowly (one to two weeks) exert a stimulant action on mood.

b. Appetite stimulated; blood pressure lowered; convulsive threshold raised.

4. Mechanism. a. Amine oxidase inhibition (theory): Inhibitors penetrate to the site of MAO in the brain, and there inactivate it by serving as irreversible substrate. Substances normally oxidized by it, especially serotonin and norepinephrine, therefore accumulate, and in some way produce stimulation of the mood (see Psychotomimetic Agents). The action appears to be related to the increase of norepinephrine, rather than serotonin (Spector, J. Pharmacol. Exp. Ther., 128:15, 1960).

b. Alternative theories:

a′. Action may be to inhibit release of norepinephrine from storage sites (Axelrod, J. Pharmacol. Exp. Ther., 134:325, 1961).

b′. The agents may stimulate CNS receptors directly (Quastel) as they are analogues of the pressor amines.

c′. They may interfere with penetration of pressor amines to intracellular sites, thus prolonging their stay at receptors (Koelle).

d′. DOPA decarboxylase is inhibited.

5. Pharmacodynamics. a. Well absorbed by mouth, but the onset of action is slow, over many days; presumably waits on gradual inactivation of all MAO.

b. Effect on MAO outlasts the apparent tenure of the drugs by many days.

6. Toxicity. a. Iproniazid may produce a number of toxic manifestations; dry mouth, constipation, impotence, visual disturbances, hypotension, rash, hyperreflexia, edema, and jaundice.

b. Other members less toxic.

c. May prolong and intensify actions of other drugs by interfering with their metabolism (CNS depressants; narcotic analgesics; anticholinergics; dibenzazepine antidepressants).

7. Uses. Tried widely in psychotic and nonpsychotic depressions, and may be highly effective agents: "produce extroversion." Now largely replaced by dibenzazepines.

8. Preparations

IPRONIAZID PHOSPHATE (Marsilid)

Excessively toxic; obsolete.
Dose: 50 mg daily by mouth.

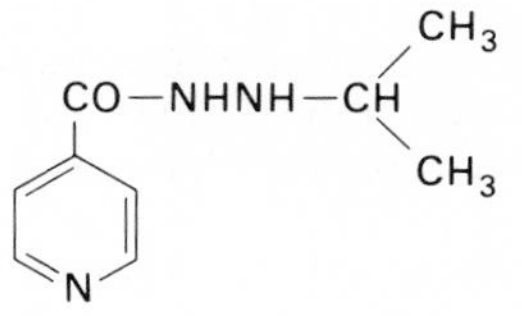

CH_3
CO—NHNH—CH
CH_3
N

ISOCARBOXAZID (Marplan)

Relatively nontoxic; satisfactory agent.

Dose: 10 mg 3 times a day by mouth.

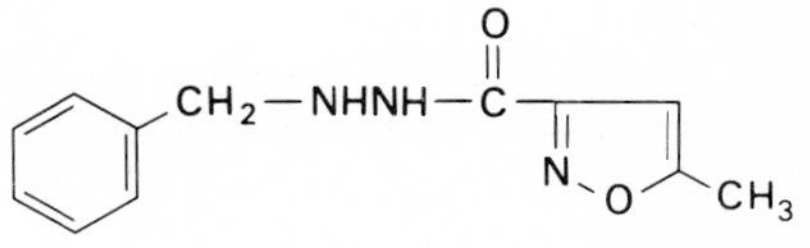

O
CH_2—NHNH—C
N O CH_3

NIALAMIDE (Niamid)

Less toxic than iproniazid, but less effective.

Dose: 25 mg 3 times a day by mouth.

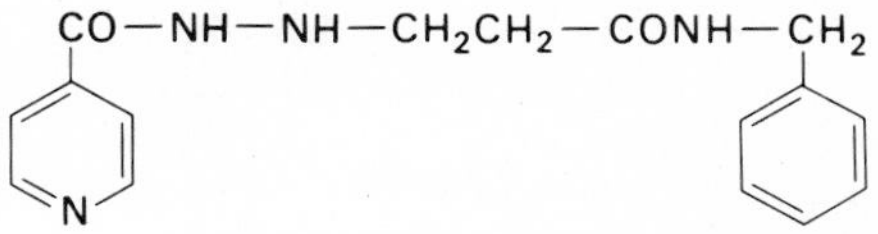

CO—NH—NH—CH_2CH_2—CONH—CH_2
N

PHENELZINE SULFATE (Nardil)

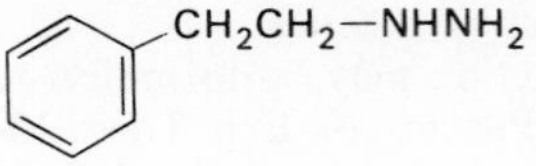

$C_6H_5CH_2CH_2—NHNH_2$

May cause toxic effects resembling tetanus, meningitis, or epilepsy, but a useful stimulant.

Dose: 15 mg 3 times a day by mouth.

PHENIPRAZINE (Catron)

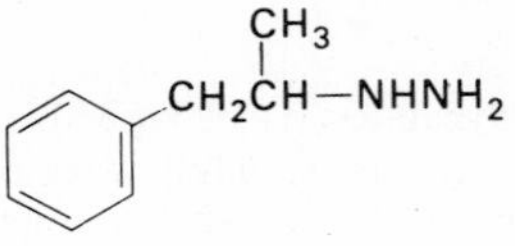

$C_6H_5CH_2CH(CH_3)—NHNH_2$

Severe toxicity, including transient red-green color blindness from retrobulbar neuritis. Obsolete and no longer marketed.

Dose: 3 mg 3 times a day.

E. Dibenzazepine Group (Imipramine)

1. History. Kuhn (1958) introduced imipramine.

2. Chemistry. Dibenzazepine derivatives and related compounds; analogues of the phenothiazine tranquilizers (promazine).

3. Action. a. Produce tranquilizing effects in animals and normal man, but antidepressant effects in endogenous and involutional depression.

b. Like the related phenothiazine tranquilizers, block pain arousal, produce the EEG of sleep, and large doses may be sedative.

4. Mechanism. a. Block uptake of norepinephrine by nerve cell, thus increasing the amine in the synaptic cleft and hence the effect on the receptors. This assumes a catecholamine deficit in affective disorders, but the evidence is complicated and often contrary.

b. Also block accumulation of serotonin in nerve cell.

5. Pharmacodynamics. a. Presumably well absorbed, but, as with MAO inhibitors, the onset of effectiveness is delayed for days to weeks.

b. Desipramine metabolized to desmethylimipramine in the liver; acts after a delay of only 24 to 72 hours.

6. Toxicity. a. Produce a number of atropinelike side effects: dry mouth, blurred vision, tachycardia, constipation.

b. Also may sensitize, producing eosinophilia, urticaria, angioneurotic edema, pruritis.

c. May produce hypotension; cholestatic jaundice and agranulocytosis rare.

d. CNS symptoms include parkinsonism, agitation, tremor, insomnia, excitement, manic swings, drowsiness, dizziness, anxiety, anorexia.

e. Should be avoided in glaucoma because of the atropine effect.

f. Severe toxicity may be seen when given during exhibition of MAO inhibitors: circulatory collapse, hyperpyrexia, death. May cause accumulation of a substance normally destroyed by MAO.

7. Uses. a. Beneficial in endogenous depressions: depressed phase in manic depressives, involutional melancholia; patients become more cheerful and animated.

b. Little influence in absence of depression.

8. Preparations

AMITRIPTYLINE HYDROCHLORIDE (Elavil)

Dose: 25 to 50 mg 3 times a day by mouth.

$\cdot HCl$

$CHCH_2CH_2-N(CH_3)_2$

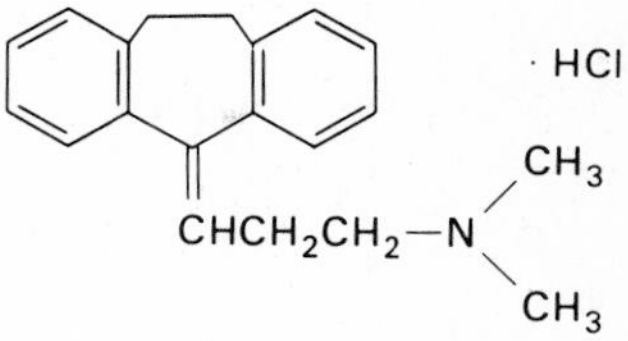

CYCLOBENZAPRINE HYDROCHLORIDE (Flexeril)

Muscle relaxant.

Dose: 30 mg 3 times a day by mouth.

DESIPRAMINE HYDROCHLORIDE (Pertofrane)

Dose: 25 to 50 mg 3 times a day by mouth.

$\cdot HCl$

N

$CH_2CH_2CH_2-N(H)(CH_3)$

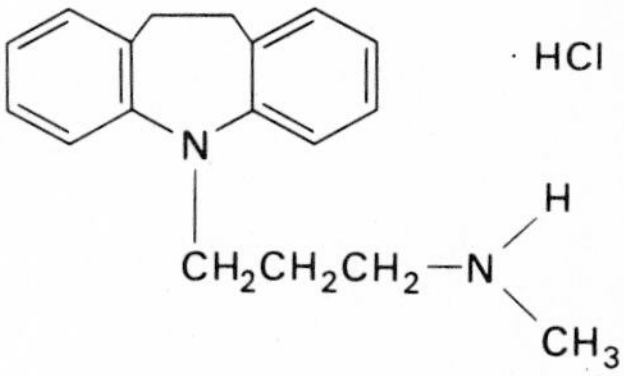

IMIPRAMINE HYDROCHLORIDE (Tofranil)

Dose: 25 mg 4 times a day by mouth, gradually doubled if required.

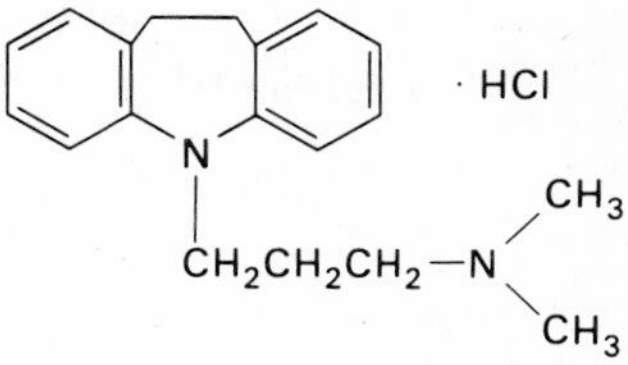

$\cdot HCl$

N

$CH_2CH_2CH_2-N(CH_3)_2$

NORTRIPTYLINE (Aventyl)

Dose: 10 to 20 mg 3 times a day by mouth.

$CHCH_2CH_2-N(H)(CH_3)$

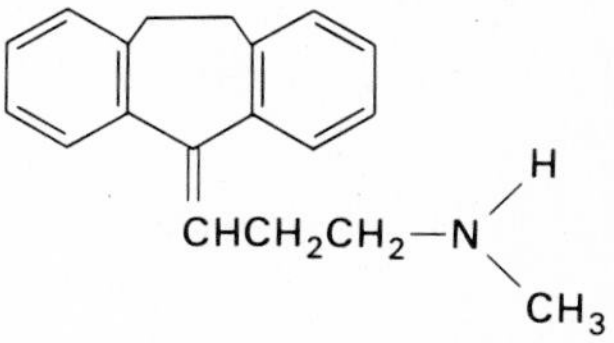

OPIPRAMOL HYDROCHLORIDE (Ensidon)

Dose: 100 mg by mouth.

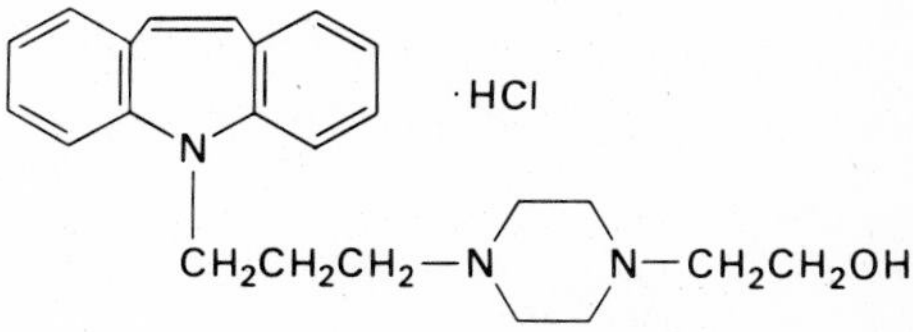

$\cdot HCl$

N

$CH_2CH_2CH_2-N \quad N-CH_2CH_2OH$

PROTRIPTYLINE (Vivactil)
Dose: 5 to 10 mg 3 to 4 times a day by mouth.

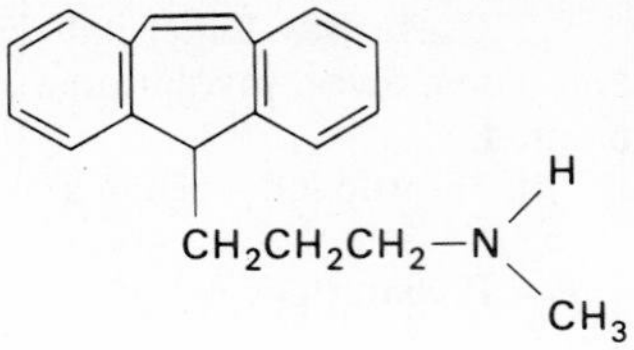
H
CH₂CH₂CH₂—N
CH₃

OTHERS

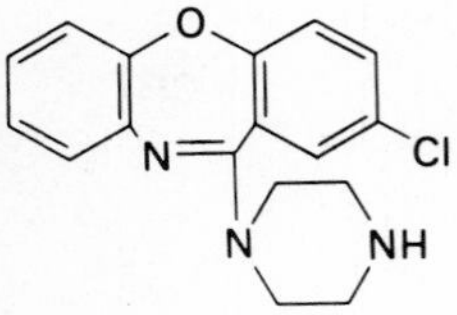
O
N
Cl
N
NH

amoxapine

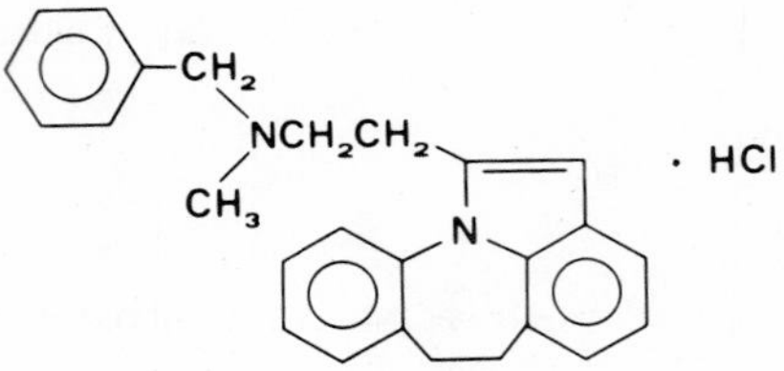
CH₂
NCH₂CH₂
CH₃
N
· HCl

azipramine hydrochloride

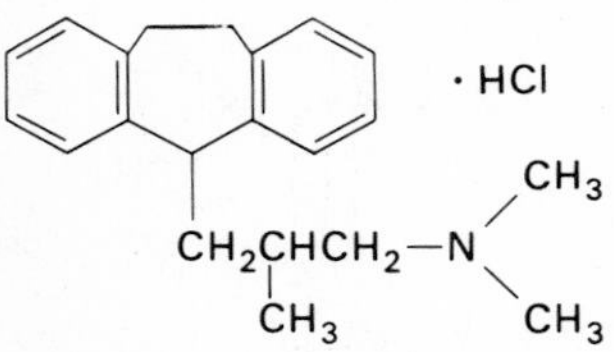
· HCl
CH₃
CH₂CHCH₂—N
CH₃
CH₃

butriptyline HCl

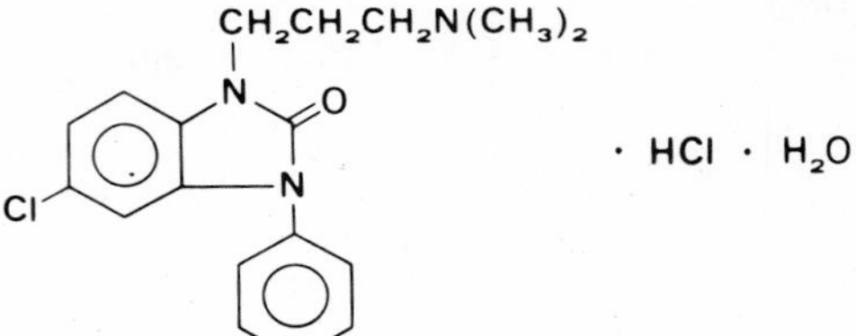
CH₂CH₂CH₂N(CH₃)₂
N
O
N
Cl
· HCl · H₂O

clodazon hydrochloride

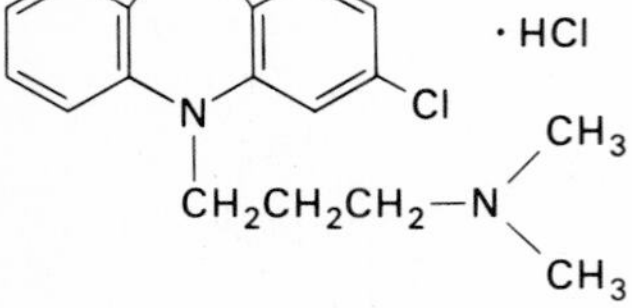
· HCl
N
Cl
CH₃
CH₂CH₂CH₂—N
CH₃

clomipramine HCl (Anafranil)

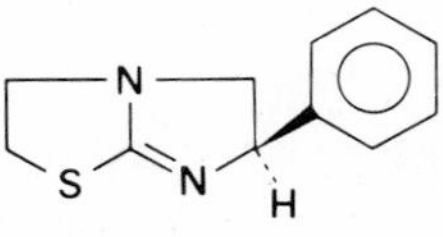
N
S
N
H

dexamisole

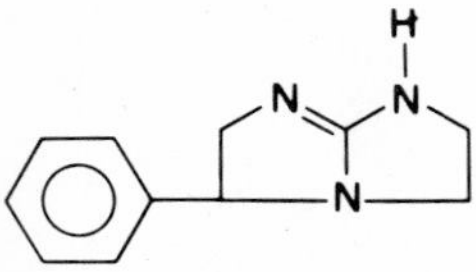
H
N
N
N

deximafen

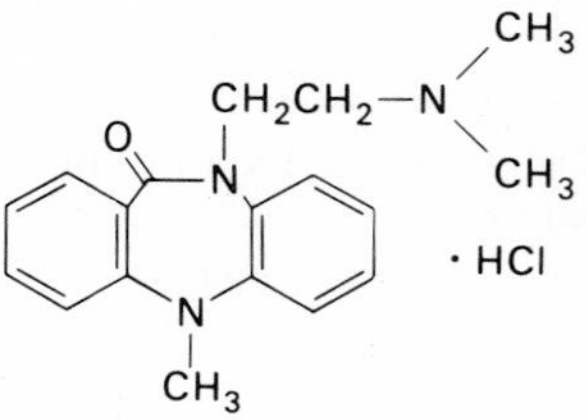
CH₃
CH₂CH₂—N
CH₃
O
N
· HCl
N
CH₃

dibenzepin HCl

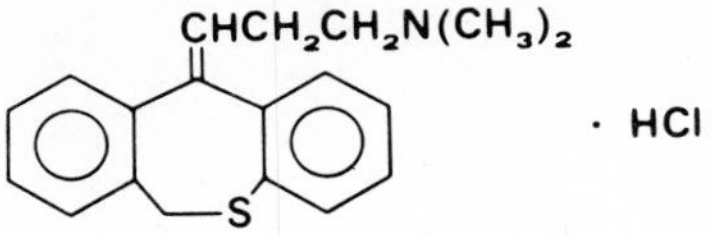

$CHCH_2CH_2N(CH_3)_2$ · HCl

dothiepin hydrochloride (Prothiaden)

fluotracen hydrochloride
(See Tranquilizers)

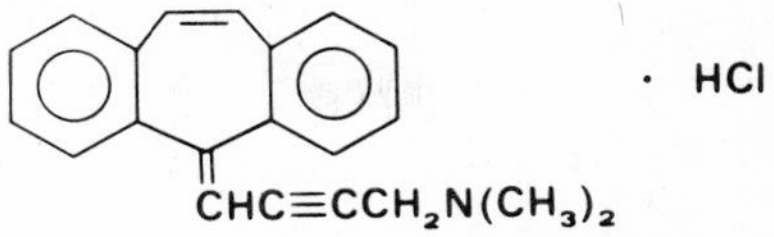

· HCl

$CHC{\equiv}CCH_2N(CH_3)_2$

intriptyline hydrochloride

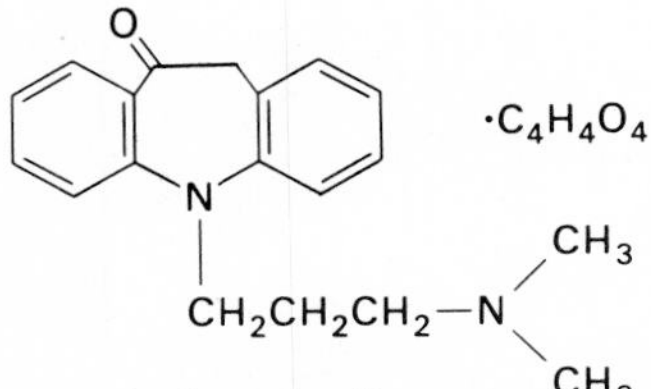

O

$\cdot C_4H_4O_4$

N

CH_3

$CH_2CH_2CH_2{-}N$

CH_3

ketipramine fumarate

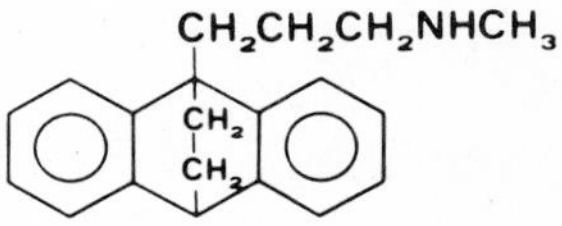

$CH_2CH_2CH_2NHCH_3$

CH_2

CH_2

maprotiline

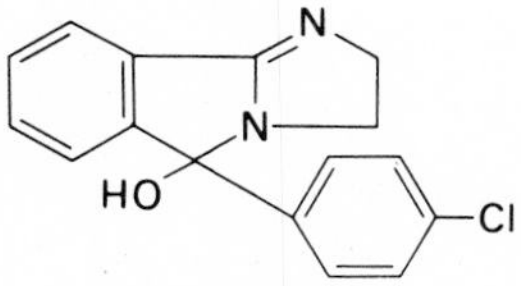

N

N

HO

Cl

mazindol (Sanorex)

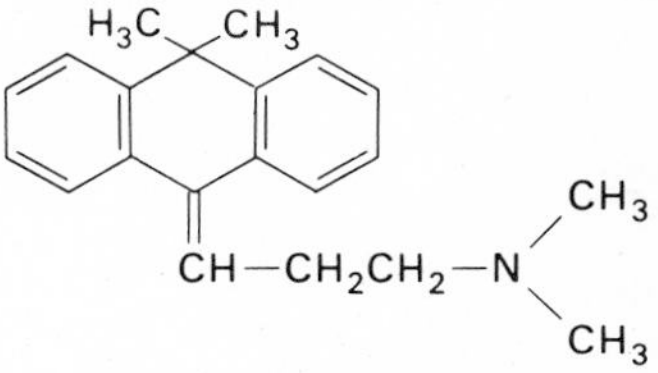

H_3C CH_3

CH_3

$CH{-}CH_2CH_2{-}N$

CH_3

melitracen HCl

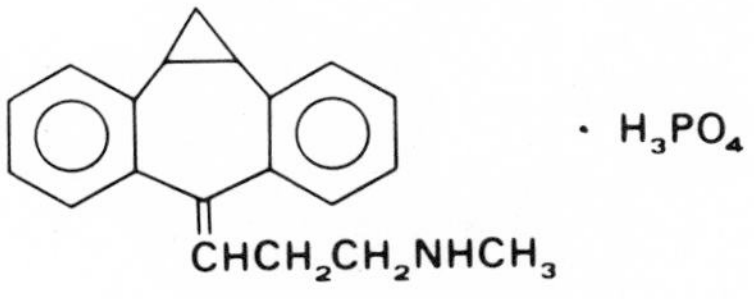

· H_3PO_4

$CHCH_2CH_2NHCH_3$

octriptyline phosphate

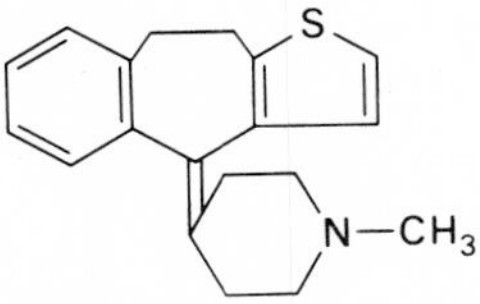

S

$N{-}CH_3$

pizotyline (pizotifin)

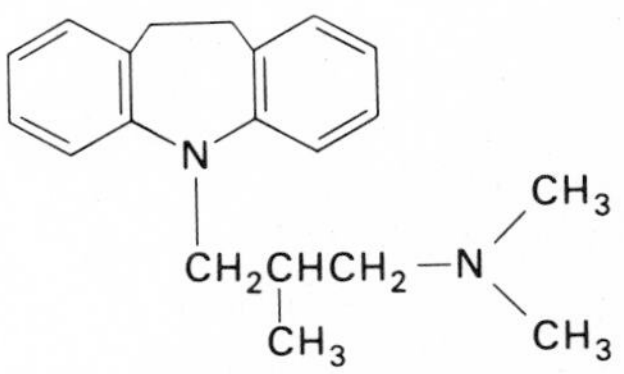

N

CH_3

$CH_2CHCH_2{-}N$

CH_3 CH_3

trimipramine (Surmontil)

F. Other Cerebral Stimulants

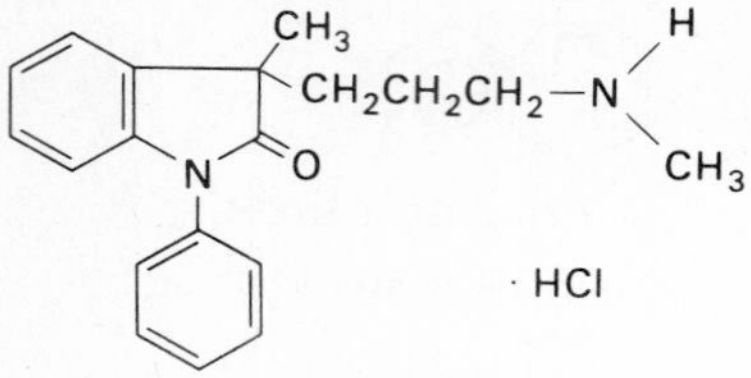

amedalin HCl

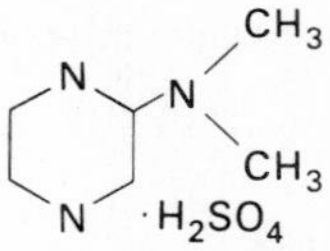

ampyzine sulfate

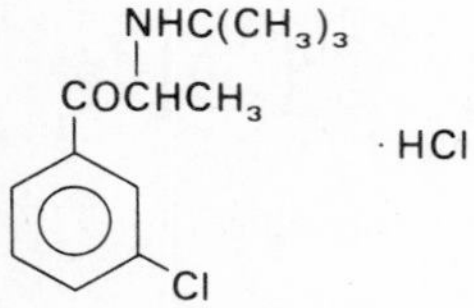

bupropion hydrochloride (Wellbatrin)

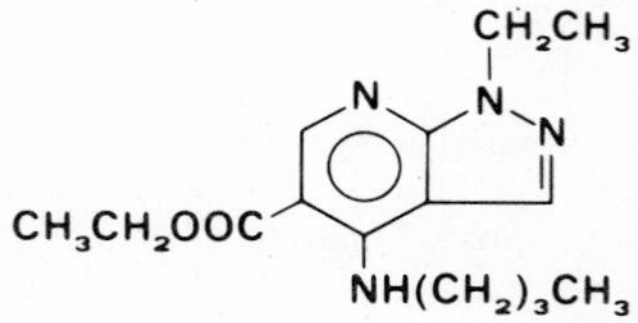

cartazolate

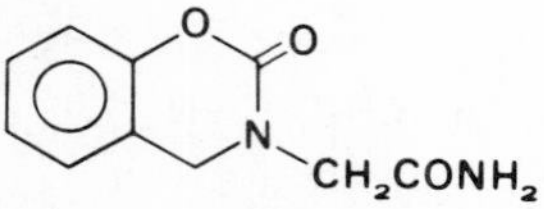

caroxazone

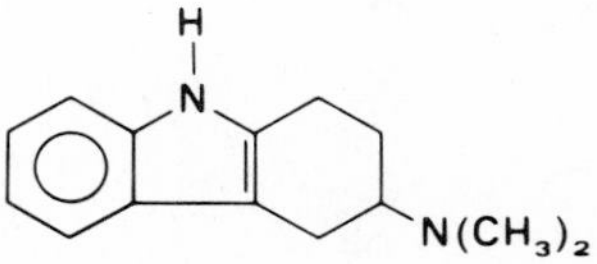

cyclindole

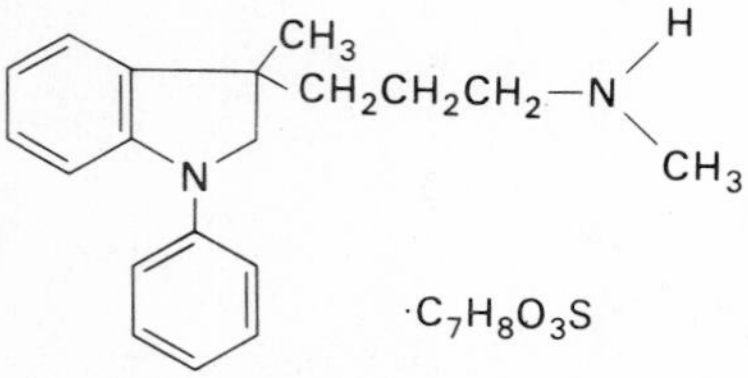

daledalin tosylate

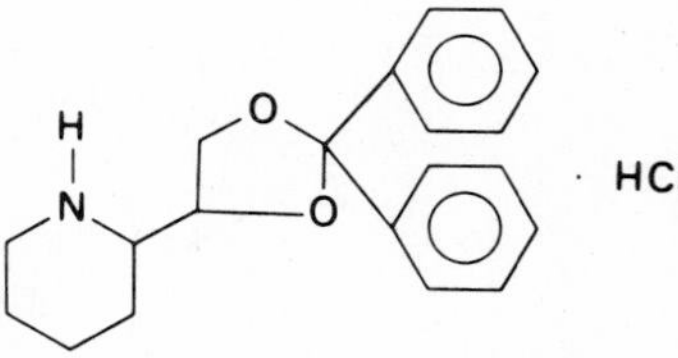

dioxadrol hydrochloride (Rydar)

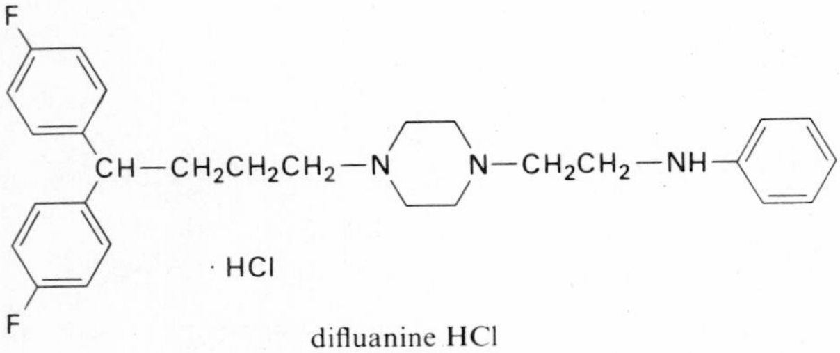

difluanine HCl

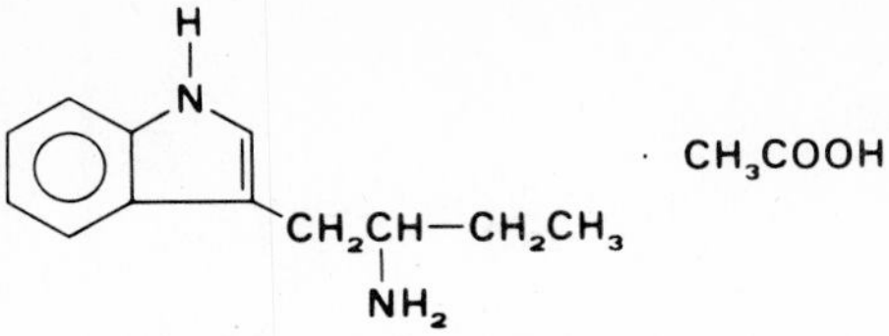

$\cdot CH_3COOH$

$CH_2CH-CH_2CH_3$

NH_2

etryptamine acetate (Monase)

$\cdot HCl$

CH_3

$CH_2CH_2CH_2-N$ $\cdot HCl$

CH_3

fenmetozole hydrochloride
(See Morphine Antagonists)

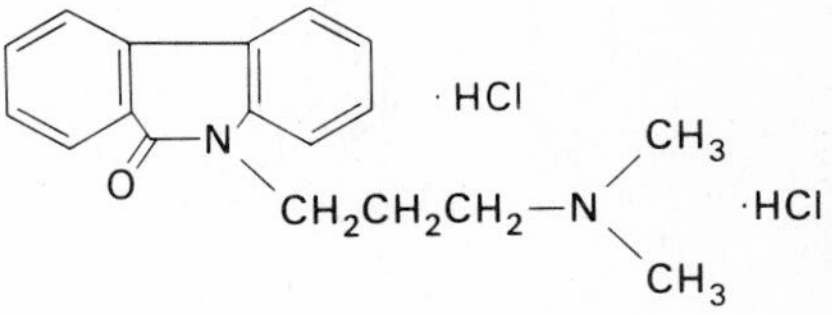

fantridone

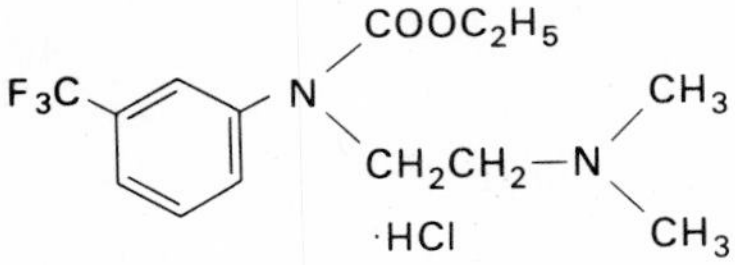

$COOC_2H_5$

F_3C N CH_3

CH_2CH_2-N

$\cdot HCl$ CH_3

flubanilate HCl

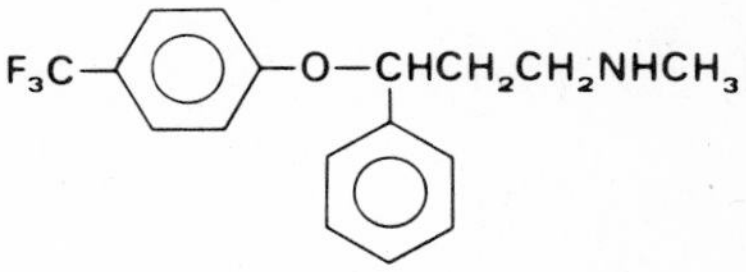

F_3C–O–$CHCH_2CH_2NHCH_3$

fluoxetine

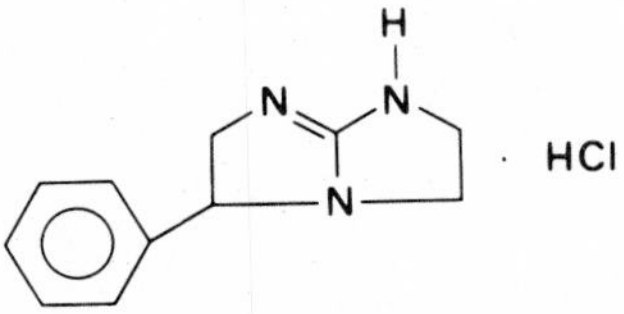

$\cdot HCl$

imafen hydrochloride

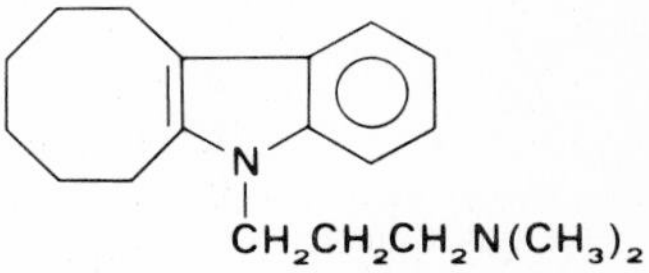

$CH_2CH_2CH_2N(CH_3)_2$

iprindole (Tertran)

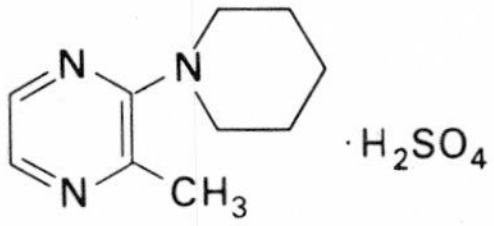

$\cdot H_2SO_4$

CH_3

modaline sulfate

OCH_3

–O–$CHCH_2CH_2NHCH_3$

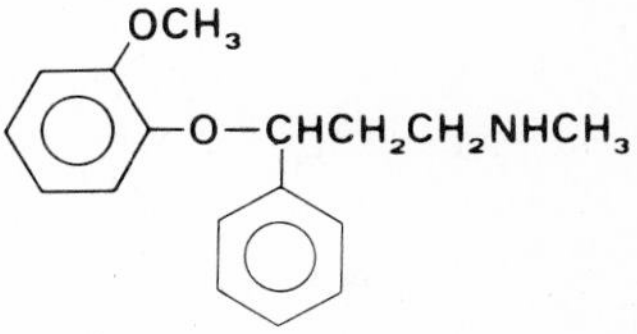

nisoxetine

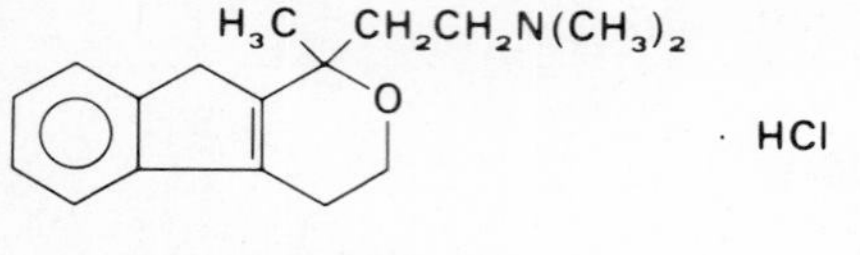

H₃C CH₂CH₂N(CH₃)₂ O · HCl

pirandamine hydrochloride

O CH₃CH₂CH₂CH—C—CH₃ N · HCl

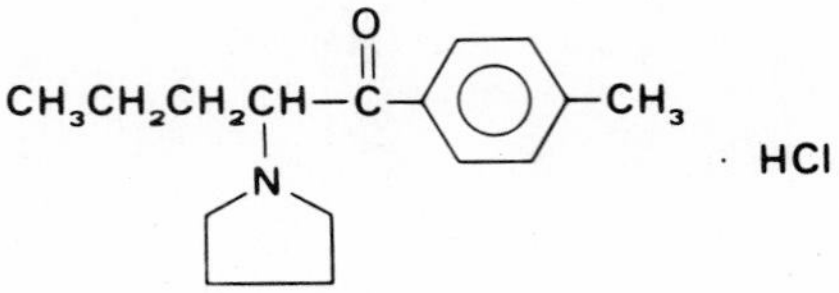

pyrovalerone hydrochloride

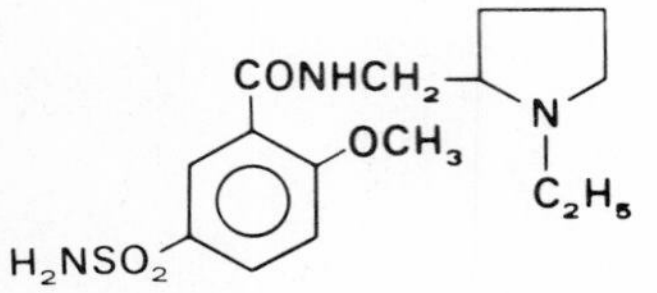

CONHCH₂ N OCH₃ C₂H₅ H₂NSO₂

sulpiride

CH₂CH₃ CH₃ CH₂CH₂N(CH₃)₂ N S ·HCl

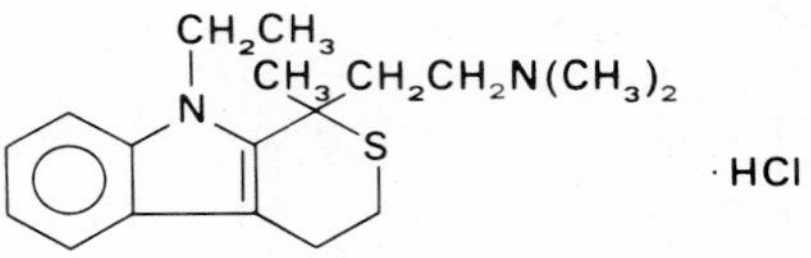

tandamine hydrochloride

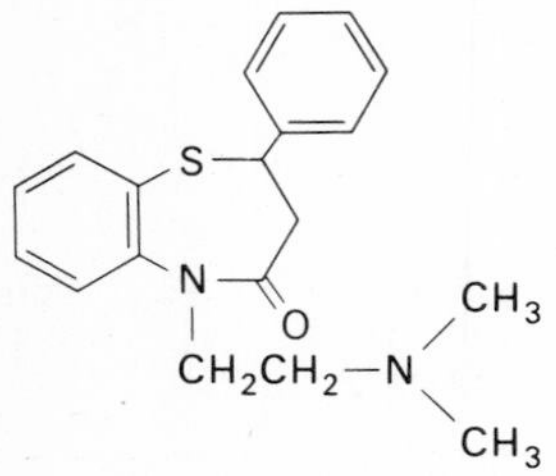

S N O CH₂CH₂—N CH₃ CH₃

thiazesim

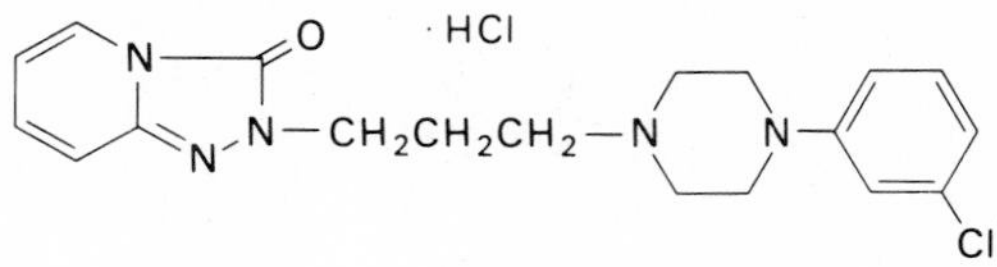

N O ·HCl N—CH₂CH₂CH₂—N N Cl

trazodone HCl

O CH₃ N(CH₃)₂ · HCl

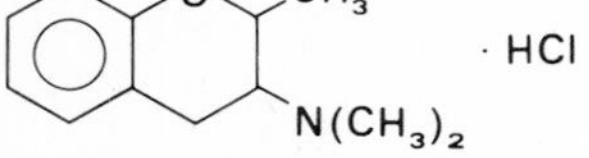

trebenzomine hydrochloride

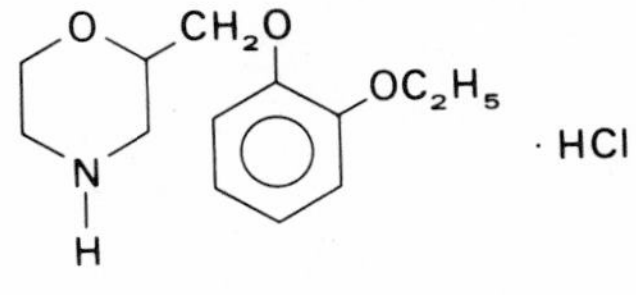

O CH₂O OC₂H₅ N H · HCl

viloxazine hydrochloride

SUMMARY: STIMULANTS

TYPE	*ACTION AND MECHANISM*	*TOXICITY*	*USE*	*EXAMPLES*
Medullary stimulants	Stimulate respiratory, circulatory, other centers in brain Mechanism unknown	Convulsions	Respiratory stimulants in drug poisoning	Nikethamide
Reflex stimulants	Stimulate respiratory center reflexly	Minor	Fainting	Aromatic spirit of ammonia
Xanthines	Stimulate all parts of brain, including cortex Mechanism unknown	Insomnia	To induce wakefulness, alertness	Caffeine
Amphetamines	Sympathomimetic	Insomnia, convulsions	Same, plus narcolepsy	Methamphetamine
Diphenylmethanes	Central stimulation Mechanism unknown	Insomnia	As mild psychic stimulants	Methylphenidate
Amine oxidase inhibitors	Inhibit MAO, allowing excessive norepinephrine action	Hypotension, cholestatic jaundice	Psychotic depressions	Iproniazid
Dibenzazepines	Elevate mood in depressions Mechanism probably similar to that of phenothiazine tranquilizers	Allergic sensitivity, cholestatic jaundice, agranulocytosis, parkinsonism	Psychotic depressions	Imipramine

Reviews

Cole, J. Therapeutic efficacy of antidepressant drugs. J.A.M.A., 190:448, 1964.

Goldberg, L. Monoamine oxidase inhibitors. J.A.M.A., 190:456, 1964.

Hordern, A. Antidepressant drugs. New Eng. J. Med., 272:1159, 1965.

Kimbell, I., Overall, J., and Hollister, L. Antidepressant drugs: Myth or reality. J. New Drugs, 5:9, 1965.

Garattini, S., and Dukes, M. Antidepressant Drugs. Excerpta Medical Foundation, Amsterdam, 1967.

56.
Addicting and Hallucinogenic Drugs

I. DRUG ADDICTION

Drug addiction may be described as a chronic or periodic intoxication with a drug in which the patient loses self control and becomes a liability to self and society (Isbell and Fraser, Pharmacol. Rev., 2:355, 1950). To cause addiction, drugs must produce pleasurable or unusual effects: euphoria, escape, fantasy, hallucinations, or relief from withdrawal symptoms. Addicting agents are of two types, stimulating and depressing. The depressing drugs, like opiates, barbiturates, and alcohol, may produce dependence, with physical and mental withdrawal symptoms; the stimulants, like cocaine and amphetamine, produce dependence, but with only mental symptoms upon withdrawal.

A number of factors may contribute to drug addiction: predisposition by personality defect, desire to escape, contact with drug from curiosity, associates, or medical use, approach by peddlers. In the United States addiction is most common in large cities. In our society, multiple drug use is common; addicts may combine drugs, or use whatever is available.

The several degrees of drug use or response are specified as follows:

a. Habituation: Frequent, often regular, indulgence but with psychic dependence only.

b. Addiction: Habituation with physical dependence.

c. Psychic dependence: Drug desired, but no serious physical effects if it is not obtained. Characteristic of stimulating drugs; may lead to antisocial acts.

d. Physical dependence: Serious physical effects, as well as mental effects, appear when the drug is withdrawn. Characteristic of depressive drugs; also may lead to antisocial acts.

e. Tolerance: An increase in the dose required to produce the desired effects; occurs only with sedative, depressing drugs.

Narcotic regulations:

a. The Federal Harrison Narcotic Act (1915) regulates the sale and use of opiates, cocaine, and cannabis.

b. State acts variously regulate the sale and use of alcohol, tobacco, barbiturates, and amphetamines.

II. ADDICTING DRUGS: DEPRESSANT

A. Opium and Derivatives

1. Action and Use. a. Use worldwide; heroin preferred. "Flash" followed by dreamy sedation is effect usually sought; often used as antifatigue measure in Orient.

b. Symptoms: Addicts may carry on activities normally if withdrawal not threatened, but show pinpoint pupils and constipation, for tolerance does not develop to these effects. If withdrawal threatened, they are consumed with the desire to prevent abstinence symptoms, and may show fantasies and confabulation. EEG may show increased alpha, decreased delta, waves.

c. Diagnosis: confinement and observation, or nalorphine test, with caution, to indicate continuous use by producing withdrawal syndrome.

2. Tolerance. a. Increasing doses required to produce pleasurable effects; eventually a stabilizing dose is reached, which is without "kick," and only serves to prevent withdrawal effects; doses may be as high as 5 gm of morphine daily.

b. Mechanism: Probably a biochemical alteration of cells in the CNS; related to a "permanent" attachment of the morphine molecule to intracellular receptors. Does not appear to be the result of increased degradation, of conjugation, or of adaptation or "learning" by the CNS.

3. Dependence.

a. All phenanthrene opiates addicting, with physical withdrawal symptoms.

a′. Early withdrawal: In 10 to 12 hours, exaggerated autonomic responses, possibly from the release of enhanced autonomic stabilizing mechanisms: dilated pupils, diaphoresis, rhinitis, yawning, gooseflesh, tremor, elevation of temperature; also crying, loss of appetite, insomnia, and weakness followed by restlessness.

b′. Late withdrawal: In 24 hours, vomiting, diarrhea, constant agitated movements, frantic and maniacal state of mind, severe abdominal pain, weight loss, high fever, death or recovery in 3 or 4 days.

c′. Pathology: No characteristic findings.

b. Relative addicting power: heroin (greatest), morphine, crude opiates, codeine (weakly addicting but may be used because of availability in over-the-counter prescriptions). Oxycodone about as addicting as morphine.

4. Treatment. a. Institutional withdrawal of morphine over a week, with substitution of methadone, which may then be withdrawn rapidly.

b. Rehabilitation: Difficult; success about 25%.

c. "Methadone Clinics" for replacement of opiate with cheaper and non-clandestine synthetic. Methadone orally once daily, by long action, prevents flash or "kick" from subsequent narcotic injections. Start with 10 to 20 mg orally every 4 to 8 hours to keep patient comfortable, and then adjust to a single dose of about 100 mg daily.

5. Antagonists. Nalorphine. Will unmask addiction at any time, probably by successfully competing with the morphine for receptors, "stripping off" the morphine, and leaving the receptors in "withdrawal." Will usually detect intermittent use by causing mydriasis if given within 6 hours of last narcotic injection.

B. Other Narcotic Analgesics

METHADONE AND DERIVATIVES

Severely addictive; similar to morphine.

MEPERIDINE AND DERIVATIVES

Also addictive, but usually less severe than morphine or methadone, possibly because it is less euphoric and shorter acting. Addiction not uncommon among physicians.

C. Barbiturates

1. Action and Uses. a. Common addicting agents. Morphine addicts may switch to barbiturates when opiates are difficult to obtain.

b. Short-acting barbiturates most addictive, probably because they produce the most sudden, forceful "kick."

c. Symptoms: Exaggerated mental depression, ataxia, slovenly habits, impaired judgment, somnolence, anorexia.

2. Tolerance. a. Differs from opiate tolerance in that a given dose gradually produces less effect, but the fatal dose does not increase. Hence, overdosage is easy and death not uncommon; confusion often contributes to acute overdosage.

b. In severe addiction, especially in late stages, there may be "sensitization" to barbiturates, in which a smaller dose may give symptoms, and even death.

3. Dependence. Physical withdrawal symptoms may be produced, but of a different nature from the "classical" withdrawal from morphine.

a. After about 16 hours (during which there appears to be improvement) symptoms appear: profound weakness, rise in BP (10 to 15 mm systolic and diastolic), dehydration, weight loss, tremor, anxiety; later, psychosis resembling delirium tremens may occur. At any time up to about the fifth day convulsions may appear, and may be violent and fatal.

b. Pathology: Liver damage and mucinoid deposits throughout the CNS have been observed in experimental animals.

4. Treatment. a. Gradual, institutional withdrawal over 2 to 3 weeks, with increase of dosage if symptoms regain severity.

b. Rehabilitation: difficult; salvage rate about 25%.

D. Tobacco

Indulgence widespread; habituation probably in part drug (nicotine) and in part conditioned reflex. Tolerance to ganglionic stimulatory effects marked, but disappears in a few hours. Dependence is purely psychic.

E. Common Sedatives

All of the sedatives and hypnotics may cause true, physical dependence with withdrawal symptoms after large doses long continued. In addition to the barbiturates, addiction may therefore be observed from chloral, paraldehyde, meprobamate, chlordiazepoxide, and others.

F. Ethyl Alcohol

1. **History.** Indulgence universal among all peoples, primitives and sophisticates, except in the Muslim world.

2. **Chemistry.** Alcoholic beverages contain the following amounts of ethyl alcohol:

BEVERAGE	*SOURCE*	*% ALCOHOL*
beer	cereals	3.5 to 6
ale	cereals	6 to 8
hard cider	apples	8 to 12
wine	grapes	10 to 22
whiskey	cereals	40 to 55
brandy	wine	40 to 55
rum	molasses	40 to 55
gin	alcohol	40 to 55
vodka	alcohol	40 to 55

3. **Action.** a. Exclusively depressant on the CNS; first on consciousness and performance, then on respiration and circulation.

b. The apparent stimulation is due to release of inhibitions: the "stripping of 1,000 years of repressions and civilization."

c. Local actions: astringent 50%, antiseptic 70%, coagulant (nerve block) 80% to 95%.

d. Diuresis from inhibition of release of antidiuretic hormone.

4. **Mechanism.** Probably similar to that of the general anesthetics, not biochemically defined.

5. **Pharmacodynamics.** a. Absorption good from stomach and intestine; distribution, with water, rapid to all tissues, including brain (later and longer in spinal fluid).

b. Metabolized, mostly in the liver, to acetaldehyde and acetate at a constant rate of 10 to 20 ml per hour (thus maximum whiskey which can be metabolized in 24 hours is about one liter). Furnishes 7 calories per gram (net about 6 after deducting for excretion; thus beer yields about 300 calories per liter).

c. Excretion: 5% in breath, 5% in urine, unless dose excessive (90% metabolized).

d. Chemical diagnosis of drunkenness: Blood and urine tests reliable; breath unreliable.

BLOOD MG %	*SYMPTOMS*	*APPROXIMATE INTAKE ML SPIRITS*
50	Relaxed	30 to 60
100	Impairment of some faculties	60 to 120
150	Legally drunk	120 to 180
300	Very drunk	180 to 240
500	Approaching fatal level	400 to 480

6. Toxicity

a. Acute: Drunkenness; treat by protection and sedation.

b. Chronic:

a′. Addiction common; tolerance only superficial; dependence may become physical, with appearance of delirium tremens and psychosis on withdrawal.

b′. A psychiatric problem, usually complicated by dietary and vitamin deficiency; characterized by excessive drinking, antisocial acts.

c′. Treatment by abstention from drinking, psychiatric guidance, possibly aided by disulfiram or related measure.

c. Additive with other depressants; patients on sedatives and tranquilizers should be warned.

7. Uses. a. Moderate social drinking comforting to most persons. However, social drinking may become compulsive drinking in certain people and lead to chronic alcoholism.

b. Medicinal use as a tranquilizer may be advantageous.

G. Special Agents in Ethanol Intoxication (Disulfiram)

Periodically agents have been proposed to hasten the metabolism or excretion of alcohol. None has so far proved to be of more than minor effectiveness, but agents are available to make alcohol unpleasant.

1. Action. a. Disulfiram arrests the oxidation of alcohol at acetaldehyde.

b. The acetaldehyde causes flushing, pounding of the heart and head, dyspnea, nausea; this discourages further drinking. The reaction may be fatal.

c. Calcium carbimide acts similarly but less severely.

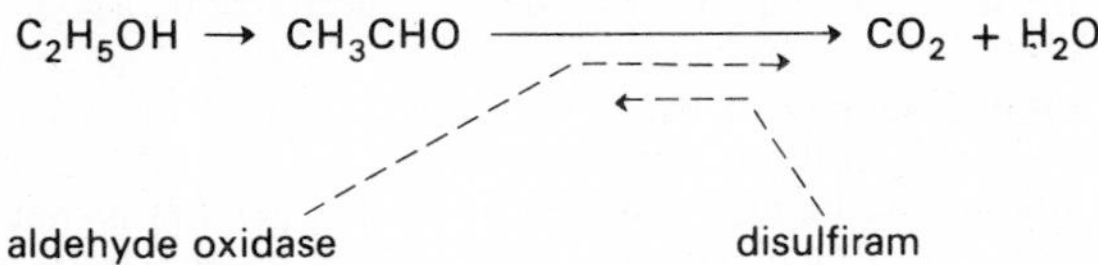

2. Mechanism. Inhibit aldehyde oxidase in the liver, which normally oxidizes acetaldehyde to acetic acid and eventually to CO_2 and water.

3. Pharmacodynamics. a. Disulfiram is slowly absorbed, and then slowly destroyed; effective concentrations may persist as long as a week.

b. Calcium carbimide is absorbed and metabolized more rapidly, so that administration twice a day is desirable.

4. Toxicity. a. Disulfiram may cause distressing side effects: nausea, vomiting, impaired taste, bad breath, drowsiness, and impotence; the reaction when alcohol is also taken may be severe, with collapse and psychosis.

b. Calcium carbimide produces less intense side effects, but has been reported to cause leukocytosis and retention of sulfbromphthalein; also asthma.

5. Uses. a. As adjuvants to psychotherapy in the reeducation of chronic alcoholics.

b. Therapy is difficult and may not be rewarding unless the mental security of the patient is also enhanced by a better interpretation of his problems.

c. Calcium carbimide is stated to be the drug of choice if drinking is likely to continue during medication.

6. Preparations

CALCIUM CARBIMIDE CITRATED (Temposil, Abstem) $Ca{=}N{-}C{\equiv}N$

Dose: 50 to 100 mg daily by mouth.

DISULFIRAM (Antabuse)

Dose: 500 mg daily by mouth for 2 to 3 weeks, then 125 to 500 mg daily.

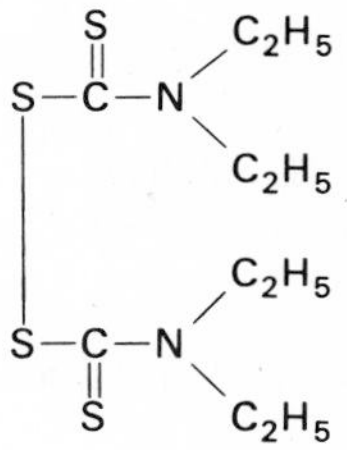

$(C_2H_5)_2N{-}C({=}S){-}S{-}S{-}C({=}S){-}N(C_2H_5)_2$

CONDITIONED RESPONSE TREATMENT

Another form of adjuvant treatment in chronic alcoholism is by association of the drinking of alcohol with nausea as produced by simultaneous administration of emetine. Every other day for 10 days, in the hospital, alcohol is given, and then followed by an injection of 60 mg of emetine (accompanied by ephedrine and pilocarpine). Booster treatments are then given subsequently for a year.

H. Methyl Alcohol (CH_3OH)

May be ingested in industrial poisoning or in bootleg whiskey.

1. Action. a. Causes an intoxication similar to that of ethyl alcohol, followed by acidosis (formic acid), pain, convulsions; blindness (also formic acid?) in hours to days, precedes death.

b. Metabolism: slowly transformed into formaldehyde and formic acid, and excreted.

2. Treatment. With alkali, or ethyl alcohol, which inhibits the metabolism of methyl alcohol by competing for liver alcohol dehydrogenase.

I. Isopropyl Alcohol [$(CH_3)_2CHOH$]

1. Action. a. Similar to ethyl alcohol as an antiinfective (50%); does not destroy insulin.

b. Ordinarily considered nonpotable; converted to acetone if drunk.

III. ADDICTING DRUGS: STIMULANTS

A. Cocaine and Coca Leaves

1. Action and Use. a. Use episodic in the United States and Europe, to produce occasional sessions of sensual delight; by contrast, is more or less continuous among native populations in Bolivia and certain other parts of South America, where the leaves are chewed to produce a sense of detachment and inurement to discomfort.

b. Symptoms (intermittent use): abolition of fatigue and hunger, increased physical activity, vivid hallucinations, tremors, tachycardia, sweating, toxic psychosis with compulsive, potentially antisocial acts.

2. Tolerance. None, increasing excitement conducive to sequential use of morphine, barbiturates, or alcohol to terminate the excitement.

3. Dependence. No physical dependence, but recollection of the excited release of the episode conducive to repetition.

4. Treatment. Acute intoxication: Neutralize excited symptoms with barbiturates, intravenously if convulsions are present.

B. Cannabinols

1. History. Use recognized in Chinese herbals about 2700 B.C.; assassin cult dates from A.D. 1100.

2. Chemistry. a. From *Cannabis sativa* (*indica* or *americana*); known as hemp, hashish, marihuana, marijuana.

b. The resinous exudate from the growing parts of the female plant contains a series of cannabinols. Oriental hemp is more potent than American marijuana.

3. Action and Mechanism. a. Euphoriant. May produce giggling, laughing, mild intoxication, exaggerated interpretation of objects and sensations, feeling of relief and escape, staggering, brightly colored illusions, loss of corneal reflex.

b. Ordinarily does not produce antisocial acts, but sometimes there may be aggressive behavior. Use is characteristically an occasional indulgence, but users are candidates for other drugs.

c. Chronic use may be accompanied by indolence and impaired mental functioning; chromosomal damage reported.

d. Does not produce tolerance or physical dependence, and little psychic dependence. Illegal.

e. Mechanism unknown.

4. Preparations

CANNABINOL

Basis of series, but inactive psychically.

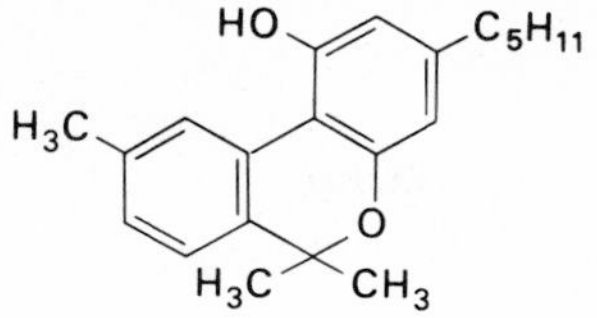

Δ′ TETRAHYDROCANNABINOL

Major psychotomimetic principle.

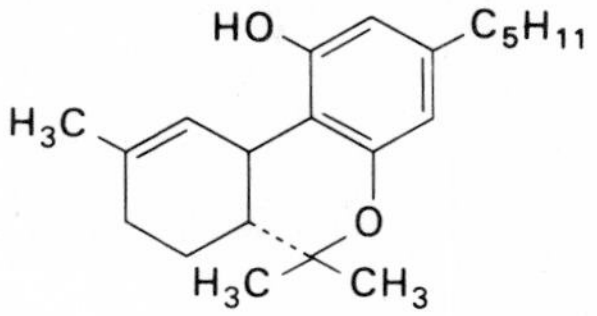

C. Amphetamine and Related Compounds

1. Action and Uses. a. May produce violent, excited, and even psychotic episodes.

b. Use increasingly common; represent a hazard that can be more serious than that from depressant drugs because of the more immediate violence involved.

2. Tolerance. Great tolerance may be produced, up to 1,000 to 2,000 mg per day, taken in "jolts" every half hour.

3. Dependence. a. Psychological dependence may be strong and produce effective addiction, even though physical dependence is slight.

b. A terminal, irreversible state may be produced in monkeys with ceaseless activity, anorexia, weight loss, and death.

4. Preparations

a. Amphetamine and related synthetics

AMPHETAMINE SULFATE

Strong psychic stimulant; habituating; psychoses reported after poisoning or excessive use (Beamish, J. Ment. Sci., 106:337, 1960).

Methamphetamine is favored by drug addicts because of availability in ampules.

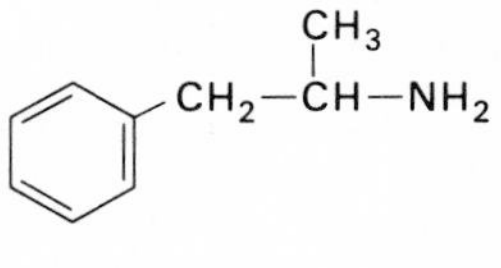

METHYLENEDIOXYPHENYLETHYLAMINE

Produces tremor, mild visual and space illusions (Alles).

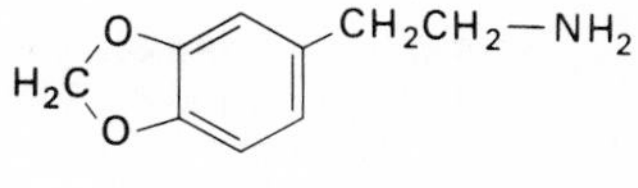

METHYLENEDIOXYAMPHETAMINE (MDA)

More active than mescaline; produces auditory hallucinations (Alles).

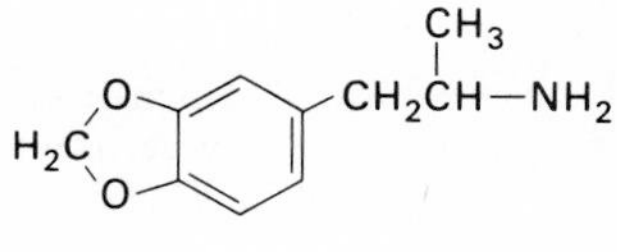

2,5-DIMETHOXY-4-METHYLAMPHETAMINE (DOM; STP)

Used as a psychedelic drug.

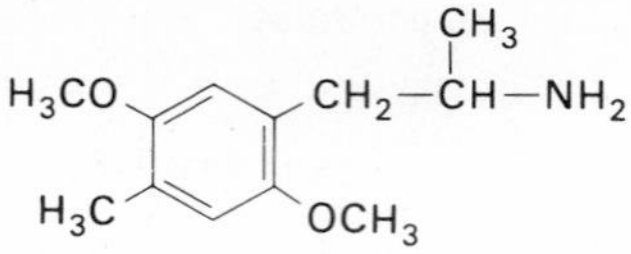

TRIMETHOXYAMPHETAMINE (MDA)

Less stimulating than amphetamine but more hallucinogenic than mescaline (Alles).

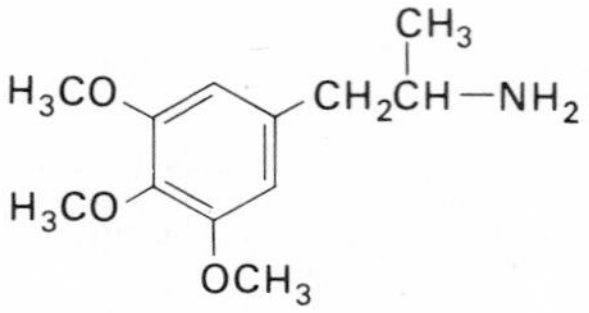

b. Natural alkaloids related to amphetamine

KAT

Catha edulis, or kat, is grown in Ethiopia and used by Arabs; it contains cathine (*d*-nor-isoephedrine). It is said to produce excitation and joy and to dull hunger; also "sweet exotic forgetfulness" and "delightful excitation and release from need to sleep."

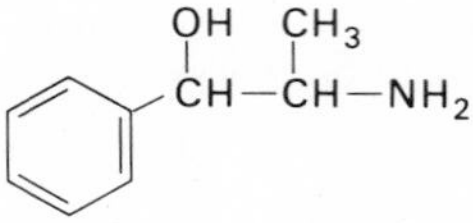

MESCALINE

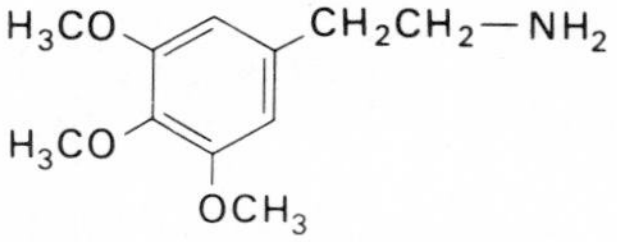

Present in "buttons" from peyote, a cactus of the Southwest; used in Indian religious services. Mescaline probably derives from phenylethylamine via trimethoxyindole (Zeller, J. Pharmacol. Exp. Ther., 124:282, 1958). It produces fullness in the head, photophobia, brilliantly colored visual hallucinations, and a sleepy trancelike state.

Tolerance probably can be produced, but little psychological dependence and no physical dependence.

D. Lysergic Acid and Indoleamine Derivatives

LYSERGIC ACID DIETHYLAMIDE

1. History. Hoffman (1943) accidentally discovered hallucinogenic effects.

2. Chemistry. Lysergic acid derivatives (see Smooth Muscle Stimulants) containing an indoleamine structure.

3. Action. a. Produces exaggerated imagination and visual illusions resembling those from mescaline. Ineffective in a state of sensory deprivation.

b. Most observers consider the effects not identical with symptoms of psychoses.

4. Mechanism. Deficient serotonin hypothesis: May block serotonin receptors and prevent access of serotonin. LSD produces a small but significant rise in serotonin in brain granules (Giarman, Pharmacol. Rev., 17:1, 1965).

5. Pharmacodynamics and Toxicity. LSD absorbed by various routes; little known of its metabolic course.

6. Implication in Psychoses. a. Hoffman's chance observation reawakened interest in biochemical explanations for psychoses. The latter had been relatively dormant for more than ten years during the ascendancy of the psychoanalytical school.

At present there are two principal theories to explain the origin of psychoses:

a. Emotional reflection of environmental history: In this thesis psychological factors are thought to cause schizophrenia and other psychoses; the possibility of secondary biochemical changes is not excluded.

b. Emotional reflection of biochemical predisposition: In this thesis biochemical abnormalities, inborn or acquired, are considered to underlie the psychoses. These abnormalities are presumed to cause cumulated metabolic deficiencies or excesses; there may or may not be responsible anatomical defects. In some variations of the thesis environmental factors are seen as precipitating causes.

Support for the second possibility comes in large part from the "psychotomimetic" agents which produce symptoms suggestive of the psychoses. Such agents may cause illusions, visual hallucinations, and less often, auditory hallucinations; others may produce a state of catalepsy. Although so far no sure association with natural psychoses has been demonstrable, and in fact most observers see considerable differences between natural and experimental states, the prospect of the discovery of chemicals responsible for natural psychoses does not seem inaccessibly remote.

7. Uses. Has limited use in psychiatry to give "LSD experience" as an aid to psychotherapy; it may be questioned seriously whether this use may not have been excessive, and associated with an element of the "thrill" of cocaine or marijuana, especially when not administered by physicians. Psychoses have been precipitated in some patients (Farnsworth, J.A.M.A., 185:878, 1963). Used by the laity as a psychedelic drug (Louria, New Eng. J. Med., 278:435, 1968).

8. Preparation

LYSERGIDE (Lysergic Acid Diethylamide (LSD-αS))

Dose: 100 to 1,000 μg, or more, by mouth; 50 to 500 μg intravenously.

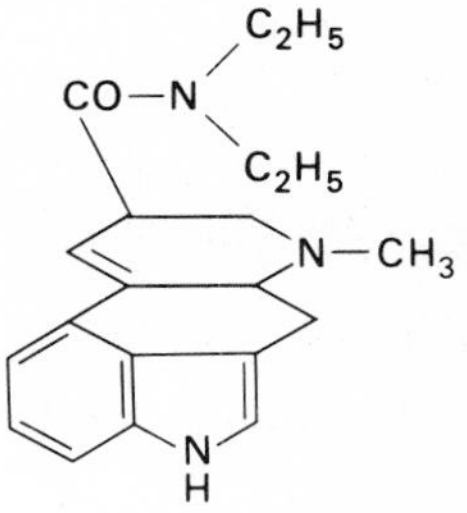

C_2H_5 CO—N C_2H_5 N—CH_3 N H

LSD-LIKE COMPOUNDS

BUFOTENIN

An indoleamine from a plant, *Piptadenia peregrina*, and a South American toad; actions like those of LSD.

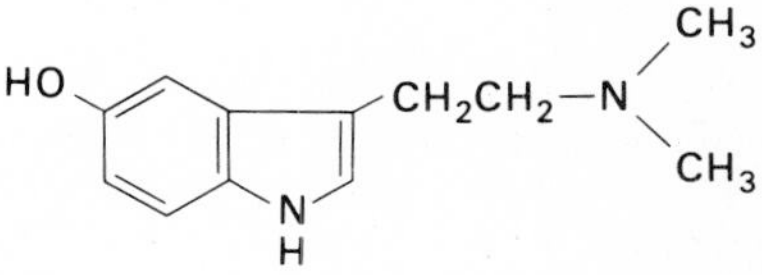

HO CH_2CH_2—N CH_3 CH_3 N H

CAAPI (aya huasca, wild rue)

From *Banistericopsis caapi*, a South American jungle vine; contains harmine. Produces frenzy, visions, psychoeroticism, and sleep.

COHOBA (niopo; parica)

From *Acacia niopo*, a Central American mimosa; contains bufotenin and other substances. Taken by natives as snuff or enema; produces burning mouth, purple face, vomiting; celebrants are drunk, then gay, and have colored visions.

HARMINE (banisterine; yageine; telepathine)

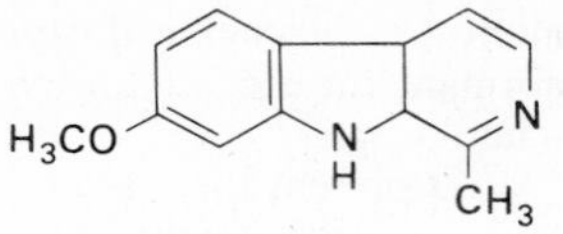

From *Peganum harmala* and other plants. Called a psychic sedative; isomer harmaline has been tried in parkinsonism. Potent MAO inhibitor.

H_3CO N H N CH_3

IBOGA

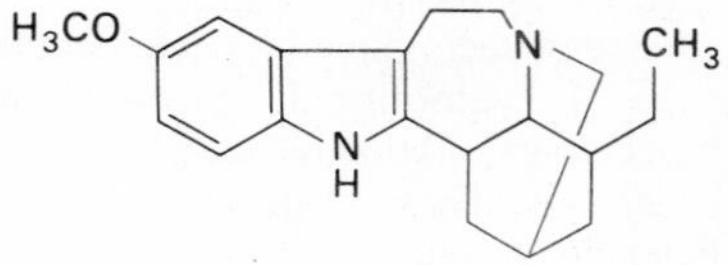

From *Tabermanthe iboga*, an African plant containing ibogaine and iboganine. Said to relieve fatigue.

H_3CO N CH_3 N H

METHYLTRYPTAMINE (indole amphetamine)

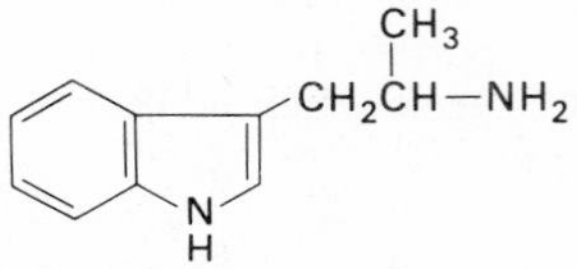

Produces visions; also sympatholytic effects including flushing, crying, aching, and gastrointestinal activity. Produces rise in serotonin in brain (Himwich, J. Neuropsychiat., 2: (Suppl. 1) 136, 1961). Related to stimulant, etryptamine.

CH_3 CH_2CH-NH_2 N H

MYRISTICIN

From nutmeg; produces bizarre CNS symptoms (Payne, New Eng. Med. J., 269:36, 1963).

N,N-DIMETHYLTRYPTAMINE (also diethyl- analogue)

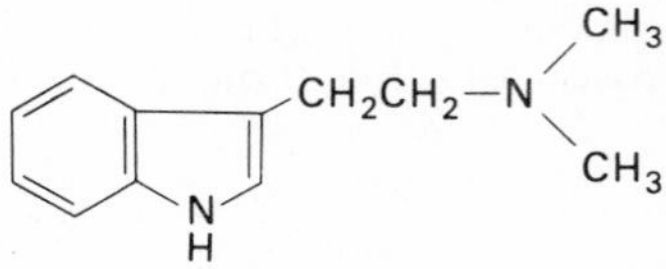

Powerful hallucinogen, 5 times as active as mescaline, but faster and briefer; effects appear in 3 to 5 minutes and disappear in 1 hour (Boszormenyi, J. Ment. Sci., 105:171, 1959). Noted to be strong MAO inhibitor (Grieg, J. Pharmacol. Exp. Ther., 127:110, 1959).

CH_3 CH_2CH_2-N CH_3 N H

OLOLIUQUI; MORNING GLORY

Lysergic acid monoethylamide or other amides from *Rivea Corymbosa*, the Mexican bindweed (flower of the Virgin), or domestic morning glory. Produce visual hallucinations and sleep; often taken alone, in quiet.

PSILOCYBIN (also teonanacath?)

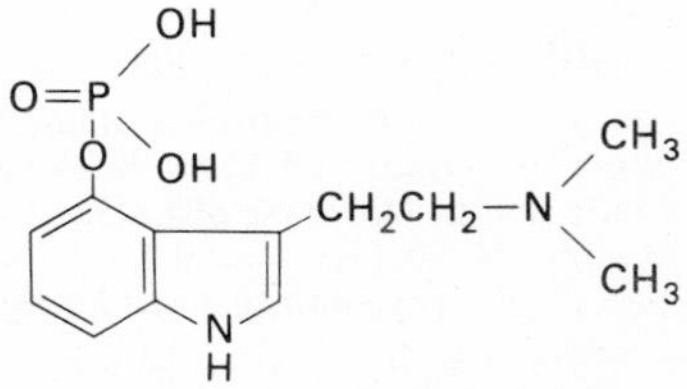

From *Psilocybe mexicana*, a Mexican mushroom; natural form phosphorylated, but easily hydrolyzed to 4-hydroxybufotenin. Used by Mexican Indians for the production of a narcotic state with colored visions, delusions, and hallucinations whose unreal nature is recognized by the partakers. About 1/100 as potent as LSD (Isbell, Psychopharm., 1:29, 1959).

OH $O=P$ O OH CH_3 CH_2CH_2-N CH_3 N H

YAGÉ

From *Haemadictyon amazonia*; contains harmine. Stimulates, then depresses with drowsy hallucinations.

E. Agents Related to Acetylcholine

ANTICHOLINERGIC AGENTS

ATROPINE SULFATE

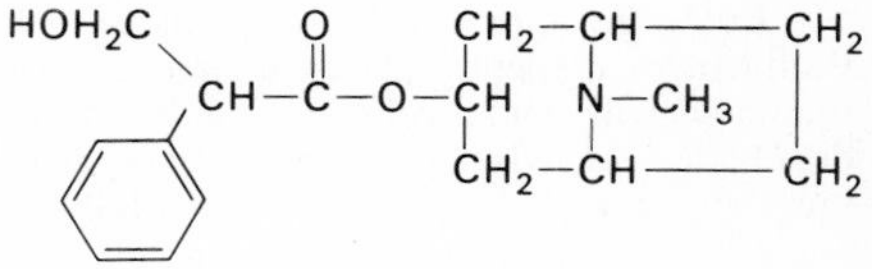

The atropine alkaloids, including atropine, l-hyoscyamine, and scopolamine, are found in *Atropa belladonna* (deadly nightshade) and other plants: henbane, mandrake, thornapple, and Jimson weed. They are among the oldest hallucinogens; taken in medieval Europe, and associated with mass hysteria, visions, and dances. The central effects are poorly understood, but euphoria and excitement or depression may follow administration. Atropine and related alkaloids have little modern use as psychotomimetic agents, but scopolamine has been used as a "truth serum." Also, atropine has been used in huge doses in a "coma treatment" of schizophrenia.

PIPERIDYL BENZILATES

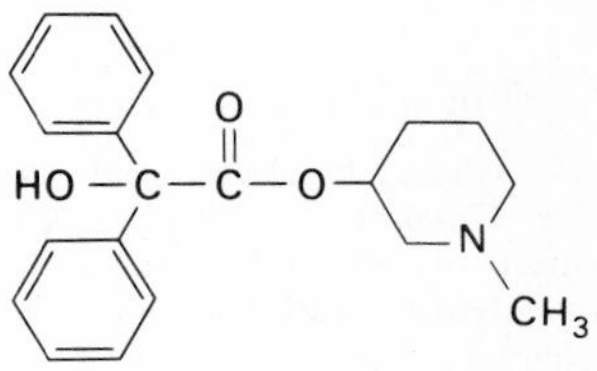

A series of anticholinergic drugs synthesized by Biehl (1958); N-methyl-3-piperidyl benzilate is the basic structure. They are strongly anticholinergic, and have central actions of various types. The central effects are said not to be antagonized by eserin; inhibition of electrical activity in the bulb has been observed in rabbits.

N-ETHYL-3-PIPERIDYLCYCLOPENTENYL-PHENYL GLYCOLATE (Ditran)

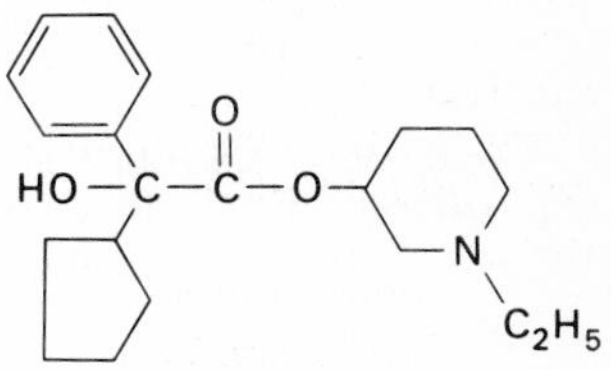

Psychotomimetic member of the piperidyl benzilate group. Produces olfactory, tactile, and visual hallucinations, delirium, disorientation, blocking of speech, hyperactivity, euphoria, and in general resembles scopolamine. Has been tried as an energizer in reactive, nonpsychotic depressions (5 to 10 mg by mouth; Meduna, J. Neuropsychiat., 1:20, 1959) but probably has no substantial use.

CHOLINERGIC AGENTS

ARECOLINE

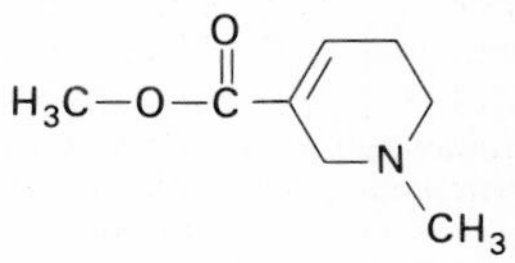

From areca or betel nut; ethylene bridge present in ring. Stimulates and produces a sense of well being; also produces red saliva and teeth when chewed with lime. Widely used as a mild euphoriant in Southeast Asia.

MUSCARINE

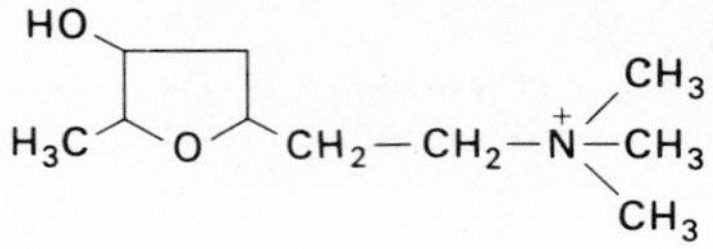

Alkaloid derived from *Amanita muscaria* (crimson fly agaric and Siberian mushrooms). Produces delirium, shouting; used in native orgies.

F. Other Psychotomimetics

BULBOCAPNINE

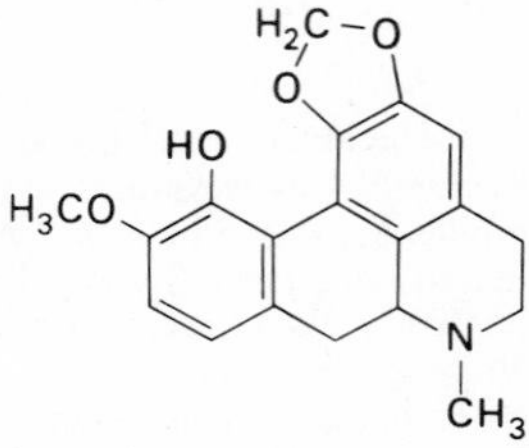

From *Corydalis cava*; possibly related to the indoles. Produces a cataleptic state; unique among psychotomimetics as most others produce excitement, or depression, and visual illusions. Isocorydine from the same source is similarly active. Sympatholytic.

KAVA (ken, kava-kava; ava)

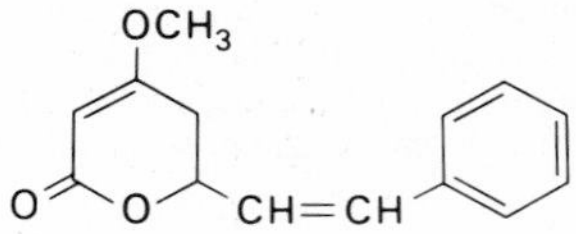

Drink prepared from the roots of *Piper methysticum* in the South Pacific; contains a resin, kawain. Produces gentle stimulation, then depression.

PHENCYCLIDINE (Sernyl)

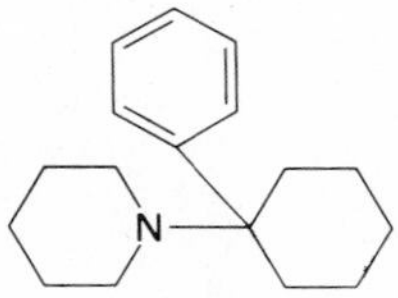

Sensory blocking agent developed as an anesthetic (see General Anesthetics). Reported to produce a variety of "schizoid" states, such as body image changes; to intensify schizophrenia; no visual hallucinations. Mechanism may be through a direct action on the cortex, or by a "defect in propioceptive feedback" (Luby, Arch. Neuropath., 81:363, 1959).

SOMA

Traditional Vedic ritual potion; thought to be the juice of the East Indian leafless vine *Sarcostemma acidum*; liquor personified and worshipped as a god; name adapted in Huxley's *Brave New World* for a panacea; more recently as a trade name for carisoprodol.

SUMMARY: ADDICTING AND HALLUCINOGENIC DRUGS

TYPE	*ACTION AND MECHANISM*	*TOXICITY*	*USE*	*EXAMPLES*
Addicting agents: depressant	CNS depression	Depression, addiction, convulsions psychosis	Analgesic, tranquilizing	Morphine, ethanol, seconal
Addicting agents: stimulant	CNS stimulation, psychic stimulation, hallucinations	Excessive agitation, convulsions	Mood elevation, psychedelic	Cocaine, amphetamine, marijuana

SUMMARY: ADDICTING AND HALLUCINOGENIC DRUGS (cont.)

TYPE	*ACTION AND MECHANISM*	*TOXICITY*	*USE*	*EXAMPLES*
Alcoholism control	Inhibit metabolism of alcohol at toxic acetaldehyde step	Nausea when alcohol taken, collapse	Alcoholism	Disulfiram
Lysergic acid derivatives	Psychic aberration from serotonin inhibition	Hallucinations	Investigative psychedelic	Lysergide (LSD)

Reviews

Shepherd, M., and Wing, L. Pharmacological aspects of psychiatry. Advances Pharmacol., 1:229, 1962.

Woolley, D. Biochemical Basis of Psychoses. New York, John Wiley & Sons, 1962.

Seevers, M. Medical perspectives on habituation and addiction. J. Amer. Med. Soc., 181:92, 1962.

New York Academy of Medicine Committee on Public Health. Report on drug addiction. Clin. Pharmacol. Ther., 4:425, 1963.

Cook, L., and Kelleher, R. Effects of drugs on behavior. Ann. Rev. Pharmacol., 3:205, 1963.

Hollister, L. Chemical Psychoses. Ann. Rev. Med., 15:203, 1964.

Cole, J., and Katz, M. The Psychotomimetic Drugs. J.A.M.A., 187:758, 1964.

Berger, H. Treatment of narcotic addicts in private practice. Arch. Int. Med., 114:59, 1964.

Ludwig, A., and Levine, J. Patterns of hallucinogenic drug abuse. J.A.M.A., 191:92, 1965.

Giarman, N., and Freedman, D. Biochemical aspects of the actions of psychotomimetic drugs. Pharmacol. Rev., 17:1, 1965.

Kety, S. Biochemistry and mental function. Nature, 208:1252, 1965.

——— Current biochemical approaches to schizophrenia. New Eng. J. Med., 276:325, 1967.

Cohen, S. Psychotomimetic agents. Ann. Rev. Pharmacol., 7:301, 1967.

Schildkraut, J., and Kety, S. Biogenic amines and emotion. Science, 156:21, 1967.

Weiss, B., and Laties, V. Behavioral pharmacology and toxicology. Ann. Rev. Pharmacol., 9:297, 1969.

INDEX

A

C

E

G

H

I

M

O

P

Q

R

S

T

U